F THO

KL SEP 2006

Outside The Ring

by

G. I. Thompson

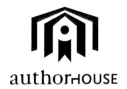

1663 LIBERTY DRIVE, SUITE 200
BLOOMINGTON, INDIANA 47403
(800) 839-8640
www.authorhouse.com

This book is a work of fiction. Places, events, and situations in this story are purely fictional and any resemblance to actual persons, living or dead, is coincidental.

© 2004 G. I. Thompson
All Rights Reserved.

No part of this book may be reproduced, stored in a retrieval system, or transmitted by any means without the written permission of the author.

First published by AuthorHouse 06/08/04

ISBN: 1-4184-6808-8 (e)
ISBN: 1-4184-3680-1 (sc)

Library of Congress Control Number: 2004092874

Printed in the United States of America
Bloomington, Indiana

This book is printed on acid-free paper.

Chapter 1

With the dawning of a new day, the fresh scent of the morning dew drifted in through the partially open living room window. Sabrina was still huddled on the couch as she was the night before. The nocturnal gloom had transcended so expeditiously; without observation.

I wonder if this is what true loneliness indeed is like; not being able to comprehend the passage of time. Then again, time was always like that; at least for me. Running headlong into eternity, always constant, never changing, that's how it was in my mundane existence. Forever watching, standing alone in the shadows, seeing, but not feeling or touching, that which went on around me; shackled to my life of shadows, yearning for a chance to be free of my bonds once and for all. To, if only for a little while, be a part of that life that I have only watched go by.

As she watched the sun leisurely announce its presence over the mountains, she repositioned her tall, voluptuous body into a more comfortable position. Incapable of sleeping for the past two days, she quickly gave in to the warmth and comfort that the sun was bringing to her this morning.

The burdens of the last week had taken their toll on her mind and her body. The anxiety that had ruled over every tedious day was finally being held at bay. As she drifted off, the early morning sounds of the neighborhood coming to life, bypassed her again, as they had for so many years. Her dreams and thoughts took her away from all this, taking her back, recounting the years that had brought her to this juncture in her life.

For all of her thirty-one years, Sabrina had never really been alone. Raised as an only child in a rural area of the Canadian west coast, she had only known her family for companionship, a child in a dominating adult world. No friends or playmates, only her parents and grandparents pervaded her world. Her life revolved around her family, and pleasing them. Needing more, their acceptance and approval for everything she did.

A strong, family connection was instilled in her at a very early age. Always abiding by the rule that you respected, and obeyed your parents; despite the perpetual inner turmoil this incited. Sabrina was always close to her parents, but it wasn't until the death of her father, that she began to realize the suppressing influence that her mother really had over her. Meticulously choking the life from her, taking her very quintessence, all her expectations and desires; leaving a barren canvas that cried out for paint and texture.

Sabrina's father was a compassionate man in every sense of the word. Never having to discipline her, for that was not his manner. With his calm demeanor they would discuss the events that had occurred; allowing Sabrina to ascertain for herself the true meaning of her actions. Then together they would workout a suitable punishment. Despite his tall stature and large build, he had never intimidated her; constantly agreeable to allowing his little girl to experience life and try new things. On his tragic death on her thirteenth birthday, Sabrina's world would irrevocably change.

Never again would she hear his words of encouragement or praise. This would be her first experience with death, standing at her father's bedside, watching his life come to termination. He had tried to prepare her for the inevitable outcome. She had been with him one afternoon when death crept into his hospital room and tried to take him. When he was brought back from that dreaded threshold he explained to Sabrina that she had watched him die and it was not to be feared. It was a peaceful journey that we would all eventually have to take. Despite their discussion it was still painful for her when death finally grasped his heart and took him from her forever.

There was no comforting arm for me that day, or any day after. All condolences were directed to my mother. I was left alone, to sit in my room, with only a picture of my father for company and solace and the longing to feel his embrace just one more time.

She stirred slightly on the couch. In her dreams she cuddled up to the father that she missed so much. Sinking deeper into the abyss, knowing that sleep could not prevent the memories from rushing back.

With her father now gone, Sabrina's mother began to keep her even closer than she had before; finding every possible reason for Sabrina to stay at home with her. Freedom was steadily being appropriated, and Sabrina didn't approve at all. Rebelling as any typical teenager would. Trying to take a stand against her mother; for she had found friends in high school and desired to be in their company. It seemed that her mother was always there, prepared to apply the guilt trips that she was so skilled at. Sabrina resided herself to the fact that this is how it would be.

Someday, somehow, I will be emancipated from this torment. I won't have to watch life from the shadows of hell.

As graduation day arrived, Sabrina thought that this would be her time, a chance for independence, but that faint flicker of desire was soon denied her. Mother had never approved of any of Sabrina's school friends, saying "that they were nothing but trouble and that she would be better off staying away from *those* kind of people." Sabrina could never figure that out. Who were *those* people? Her friends seemed normal enough. Graduation night was spent at home, alone in her room, the repulsion of her mother seething up to the surface.

Weeks passed like infinite years that summer, after graduation. Sabrina wanted to run away, but with no money of her own she was forced to remain at home. After weeks of searching the want ads, she found her first job. It wasn't the most desirable vocation around, but it was a way to distance herself from her mother; if only for a few precious hours. The new job took her into the city where she was immediately seduced by all the events.

The night life of the city was exhilarating; she couldn't get enough of it. Sheltered for so many years, she was beguiled. The clubs, the shows, the restaurants; they all beckoned to her; whispering to her. Every spare moment found her planning her evening with her new found friends. Where would they go tonight? Whom would she meet?

The feeling of freedom that she had lost with the death of her father five years before, began to surface. He would be happy for her, for the wonderful exhilarating experiences that she was encountering. Growing and learning; taking steps away from her shadows.

Sabrina's mother had vocally disapproved of what her daughter was doing, but Sabrina disregarded the remarks. She was legally an adult, nothing could stop her; until she found herself without a car. Her mother had taken the car away and without it Sabrina was forced to quit her job. Her mother had recaptured control once again. She regressed to being completely dependent on her mother for everything, from transportation to spending money.

Being so brusquely disconnected from this new life, Sabrina was more determined than ever to get away from home. Like an addict needing a fix, Sabrina was thoroughly ensnared by the night life, and would not give it up. It was in her blood now, guiding her. Good fortune found her a new job, this time closer to home, and surprisingly, with the approval of her mother.

Immersing herself in her work, she soon acquired new friends. She became accustom to her mother's daily visits, under the guise of shopping; but Sabrina knew better. With her new sense of independence, she purchased a car. There was no way that her mother could interfere now; the latch on the door to freedom had been opened.

Sabrina dated a few times, yet never managed to keep a relationship going. There was always a sense that there was something lacking. She knew that men were attracted to her for her looks, but sometimes that just wasn't enough.

Being self conscious and awkward about her height, she compensated by exercising, making her body the center of attention; instead of her height. The plan worked with great success, for she could not go anywhere that men did not stare at her. It was her creation and she loved to admire it; from her long natural golden blond hair, to her large firm breasts, curvaceous waist and long legs.

Men looked at Sabrina with desire, and she reveled in it. Being in the company of a man was thrilling. The mystery of sex was disclosed to her by a man, not her mother, like most girls. That was a subject never spoken about in their home and Sabrina's curiosity about the subject begged to be explored.

Somewhat promiscuous as a young adult, she was always prudent, but still there was always something missing in those relationships. No sense of belonging or commitment, that was what kept her searching. Her search led her to Will; he became her salvation in this life of torment.

Snuggling into the arm of the couch Sabrina pulled her blanket up close, sighing ever so softly. Her mind whispered out the name in her thoughts. "Will." A faint smile graced her lips as her dreams brought him back to her again.

Will was everything Sabrina's imagination could conjure. Tall, with light brown hair that had just a hint of gray at the temples. His lightly tanned skin, flawlessly fit over his firm body. The one thing that she could never forget was his eyes; they were a unique color of blue, almost gray. Looking into his eyes she could become lost within them. This had to be the man for her, the kind of man that every girl dreamed about.

Will taught her what it was really like to be a woman and with those lessons he showed her all the ways to please a man. The other lovers that she had before him, had not been able to captivate her senses the way he did. A gentle touch, a soft kiss, or being held close in his arms was euphoric. Every time that they were together they made love, and each time was as emotionally satisfying as the first. The true meaning of love was not overly clear to her, yet a small part of her kept insisting that this was what she wanted out of life.

Being away from him was like having a part of her own body missing. She yearned for him, longing to feel the passion. Daydreaming preoccupied her at work, thinking of him, and how he made her feel. Closing her eyes, she could feel his gentle touch on her skin, vividly recalling the sensation of his hand slowly stroking her breast. Making love with him was always pleasurable, leisurely discovering their bodies as is for the very first time. If this was what love was like then to her it was the most remarkable thing.

After being together for three months, they decided that it was time that Will met her mother. This was the man that she hoped someday she was going to marry. Things had become eerily tranquil between Sabrina and her mother, and she was convinced that her mother had finally accepted that her daughter was an adult, with a life of her own. Sabrina was now twenty-five and her mother couldn't control her forever; or could she? That was the one nagging uncertainty that lingered in her mind.

Will arrived at Sabrina's house with a bouquet of flowers for her mother and the encounter began without any incidents. They talked for a while and things appeared to be going quite well. Then, without warning, Sabrina's mother regressed to her old self. Yelling at both of them, voicing her disapproval of Will, because he was older than Sabrina, older by only 6 years.

So what did age have to do with love?

She had been following them, telling them that she knew about all the sordid things that they were doing together. Sabrina attempted to get dominion over the conversation, telling her mother that she was in love with Will, that they were going to be together; but it was no use. Her mother accused Will of hiding things. Saying that if he was an honest man, he would not need to take her daughter to a motel. It horrified Sabrina, to think that her mother could be so intrusive. She knew, in explicit detail, everyplace they had been together; every bar, every restaurant, and every intimate rendezvous.

The accusations continued until Will could not take any more of it. He rushed from the house; promising to call Sabrina in a few days, to try and work things out, but the call never came. In desperation she endeavored to contact him at his work, but he would not come to the phone, nor would he return her messages. She sent him letters, but they too went unanswered. Sabrina went to his home, to their favorite pubs, but couldn't find him. Finally one of his coworkers told her that he had taken a leave of absence and gone away. For how long, and where, they didn't know.

Sabrina was devastated; her mother had gotten her own way, again. She had succeeded in destroying her daughter's dreams of the future and along with that the meager remainders of self confidence. Distraught and depressed, Sabrina reverted back to being the devoted daughter that her mother wanted; but it couldn't stop her thoughts.

When depression began to affect her work and with the threat of losing her job, Sabrina convinced herself that it was time to put the past behind her and move on with her life. With great difficulty, she pushed all thoughts of Will out of her mind but the pain of lost love was still inside her.

It wasn't long before she was back to her old self, on the outside. On the inside she was hollow, an empty void that yearned for love again. She started to go out with her friends from work again; only with the anticipation that she might see Will again, but any man would have been a welcomed distraction from her loneliness. Her mother continued to express disapproval of Sabrina's socializing, but Sabrina had begun to ignore her. She tired of the same lecture day after day; a lecture that she could recite by heart, and did when her mother wasn't looking.

Before too long Sabrina found herself in the constant company of a coworker named Steve. He was nothing like Will. Steve was a little shorter than Sabrina and had short trimmed dark brown hair. Sabrina's mother had known Steve for as long as Sabrina had worked there, and for some strange reason she could not find anything to criticize him about.

It didn't take long for Steve to propose, and after a brief four month engagement they were married. A full, formal wedding, with family and friends that were only heard from at holidays. It was every young girl's dream; Sabrina's dream; to be loved and taken care of. Yet, even though, a small corner of her heart told her that this was all wrong, she pursued it anyway. Her fear of being alone spoke louder than her conscience.

Steve and Sabrina moved in with her mother, until they acquired a place of their own. Settling into the routine of being married was easy, this was what she so desperately wanted from life; but still she couldn't break the ties with her mother; she was constantly in the picture. Whether she phoned, or came to the apartment, she was always there; offering her daily dose of unwanted advice, on how to cook his meals or how to wash his clothes. How to butt out, and leave them alone, that conversation never came about.

They stopped going out with their friends from work, because Steve said that they no longer had anything in common with them. Everything that they needed was at home, according to Steve. Reality came as a hard blow to Sabrina's conscience; she was not in love with him. She had married him on the rebound from Will; and to get away from her mother. All she had succeeded in doing was to change the face of her dominator. After eighteen months of marriage, and perpetual fights, they were divorced.

Incapable of living on her own, Sabrina moved back home with her mother and settled into the belief that this is where she belonged. This was where she would grow old; alone. Her mother wanted to control her life, and Sabrina let her have it.

Four more years she lived at home, allowing her mother to make all the decisions and choose what she thought was right for Sabrina. They were inseparable; where Sabrina went, her mother went too. She never acquired any new friends and lost touch with all of the old friends she once had. Her mother had won; she had Sabrina all to herself, until a few days ago.

Awakening from her sleep, feeling more lethargic and fatigued than before; rising from the couch, Sabrina stretched, removing the kinks in her back and neck. Making her way into the kitchen, she began preparing breakfast. Filling the kettle to make tea, and retrieving the toaster from the cupboard the way she had done for so many years.

Patches, the cat, upon hearing someone moving about the kitchen made his presence known; lazily walking into the kitchen and meowing his good morning to Sabrina. She halted her routine to pick him up, giving him a big hug and a kiss. "Well, I suppose that you want your breakfast too?"

she asked. He purred and snuggled up against her. "You know, I think that you are about the best friend a girl could have. You don't interrupt when I'm talking, and you never tell me what to do. You are a good old friend, Patches." She carried him over to his dish on the floor and fed him his breakfast, then returned to the task she had begun before he had disturbed her.

She was about to make the toast when she stopped. A surge of reality washed over her; it had finally hit her. "You don't have to do this anymore. We can do what ever we want now, right Patches? She's dead; the old bitch is really dead."

Death had come swiftly to claim her mother just three days ago. "This is a new beginning, a chance to reclaim some of the years that have been lost." She smiled slightly as a tear rolled down her cheek. "I'm free, but I'm alone, and I'm scared." All of her emotions came rushing up inside her; she crumpled to the floor crying; crying for the loss of her mother or the trepidation of being alone?

The independence that I have dreamed about for so long is now within reach. Can I handle this freedom? I no longer have to account for my every movement, inside or outside this house. The fear that she was feeling was deep. *Have I regressed so far that I won't be able to move on? Will I become a prisoner in this house? Will my fears keep me locked away for the rest of my life?*

When the phone rang, she was able to pull herself back to the real world; away from all the questions her mind clung to. Hesitant to pick it up, not really wanting to talk to anyone, especially today, she took a deep breath and reached for the receiver. The voice on the other end was calm and very monotone.

"Mrs. Scott, this is Mr. Turner from the Glen View Funeral Home. I apologize for disturbing you this morning, but I just wanted to know if you had any last minute changes for your mother's service today."

Spending so much time lost in the past, Sabrina had forgotten that the funeral was today. After a brief pause the voice on the phone spoke again. "Mrs. Scott? Are you there?" "Yes, thank you for calling Mr. Turner. The arrangements that we made will be just fine. There won't be any changes." "Thank you; Mrs. Scott; and my deepest sympathies go out to you for your loss. Good-by Mrs. Scott." "Good-by Mr. Turner."

As she hung up the phone, Sabrina thought out loud. "Sympathy for my loss; you poor man, you have no idea just how much of a relief this is to me." A relief that her torment was over. The disdain that she had kept locked away for all those years had surfaced. Heading off to the bedroom to get dressed, she picked up Patches along the way, cuddling him. He never tired of her affections; willingly accepting her love anytime she wanted to give it.

Choosing an outfit for the funeral was effortless, as her wardrobe was primarily black anyway. She had never been one to buy bright colorful clothes. Never having felt the need to be bright and cheerful; the way colors made you feel. Black fit in with her beliefs as easily as it fit into her personality. While she dressed, she started thinking about what she should do.

Now that I'm on my own, with no one to hold me back, I don't know where, or how to start my new life. Mother's estate has left me quite well off. The house is paid for, and she had the good sense to transfer everything into my name before her death. Everything regarding the estate has already been taken care of; I now have the capability to do what ever I want. No more nagging about the clothes I wore. No more listening to mother tell me how to live my life, no more conversations, no more anything.

A single tear ran slowly down the side of her face, pausing for but a second at her jaw before it dripped off.

In my own way I do mourn for my mother, for so many years she has been my only source of adult company. It's time to make some changes in my life, now, before I became swallowed up by my loneliness.

She turned around to look at Patches, who was sitting on the bed cleaning his fur, the way he did just before having a nap. "Hey, Patches, how about we pack the car and go on a trip? Would you like that? We can start to see all those wonderful places that we've only read about. Well? What do you say Patches? Does that sound like fun to you?"

Patches, who had been watching Sabrina intently, let out a loud meow as if to signify his approval. He came trotting over to her, rubbing against her arm, purring loudly. "Well, I guess I have my answer; as soon as I get home today, we'll figure out where to go first." She gave Patches a big hug and headed out the door.

The journey to the funeral home was tedious. In her mind she rehearsed what she would say to people, but what she really wished was that it was all over.

If it wasn't for my mother's family, and friends, I would not have bothered with a funeral service. I'm only going because it's the appropriate thing to do.

When she arrived at the funeral home there was only fifteen minutes before the service was to begin. The parking lot was nearly full; some of the cars she recognized, but most she didn't.

This place has two chapels; some of these cars must belong to another funeral. The sound of gravel crunching under the wheels of the car, momentarily deafened her to the morose thoughts that crept through her mind.

In the silence and the privacy of the car she swallowed hard and took a deep breath; convincing herself that she would be just fine. She embarked on her journey along the path that directed her to the chapel. An old chapel, built of stones from the near by river bed, had served the community for over one hundred years. Sabrina hadn't been here since her father's funeral; but it all was as she remembered.

How many people have walked this same path before me, seeking closure with each laborious step, but how many of them felt as I do? Did they feel the relief? Were they delivered of their burden? There's no one standing outside the entrance; good.

She continued on through the doors, pausing in the entrance hall. *These places always give me a chill, and a headache.* She massaged her temple to alleviate the throbbing pressure.

The chapel was filled to capacity. As if queued by someone inside, the congregation turned to look at her, carefully scrutinizing her appearance and demeanor. She felt very self conscious. An usher appeared at her side and with a gentle grip on her elbow they began the slow walk up the aisle to the front seats.

It was difficult to maintain control of her emotions, especially when she made eye contact with someone who was already crying. Taking her seat in front, along side her mother's family; her body was in turmoil, wanting to cry, but more importantly not wanting anyone to see her cry.

After her father's death she had learned to lock away her emotions. She never cried in front of her mother as that would have brought on a tongue lashing about being weak and not in control. Besides, crying always made her blue eyes so much more intense when they were framed by those bright veins and puffy eyelids.

Another deep, cleansing breath; the minister approached the pulpit. As he spoke, Sabrina's headache intensified until she no longer heard what he was saying.

The contents of the service she couldn't ascertain as the rhythmic pulsing in her ears blocked everything out. Fortunately, it wasn't too long; she managed to keep her emotions in control all through the service, and through the multitude of hugs and well wishes from family and friends. A tea had been arranged for after the service in one of the chapel's halls.

Time just seems to drag on. I want to leave, to be away from this place, but I know that the proper thing to do is to make sure that I briefly visit with those who attended. This is truly the hardest thing I've ever had to do. My father's funeral was entirely different. I was just a kid then and no one paid any attention to me.

When no one was looking, she took a few minutes to sit in the garden, next to her father's memorial marker. She didn't speak aloud, but she did talk to him. There was a need to justify her actions of the past few years and to tell him of her intentions for the future. It gave her some comfort and reaffirmed her conviction to make a better future for herself. He would be happy for her, and she knew that he would understand her need to move on.

Having said her good-byes to the family, Sabrina was making her way to the car when she felt a hand grasp her shoulder. With a gasp she turned quickly, surprised by the unexpected touch. Her mothers best friend, Marion Pierce was standing there.

Marion was the same age as Sabrina's mother, but now, today, she appeared to be so much older than she did last week. The lines in her face were deeper, her dyed red hair, showing traces of gray, but her expression was still loving.

Sabrina had know Marion for all of her life, and many times had secretly wished that Marion had been her mother; she was so much more affectionate. As she quietly stood looking at Marion her emotional guard began to crumble away. The tears that she didn't want to shed came rushing forward. Marion reached out and took Sabrina in her arms; holding her tight, not saying anything.

After what seemed an eternity, Marion released her grip on Sabrina, and as she gently wiped the tears from her face she spoke. "I know how your life has been dear; I have watched you for many years. I know how frustrated, and tormented you have been. Despite all that, you still need to grieve for your mother."

Sabrina's tears began again. She knew that Marion understood, about what it was like to grow up in that house. Several times Marion had tried to get Sabrina to move away, to start over; but her mother's grip would never release her. "I know that you won't grieve for long. You are a strong woman, and you will get on with your life. Do you have any plans yet?" Marion asked.

"Yes, Marion I do, I plan to take a trip," Sabrina replied, trying to control her sobs. "I don't know to where yet, or for how long I will be gone; I just know that I have to get away from here right now, the sooner the better."

Marion smiled at Sabrina, pulling her close again. The two women hugged each other tight and Marion whispered to Sabrina. "You go, and enjoy yourself dear. This is finally your time, and don't you waste one minute of it. Keep it touch with me will you?" "Yes, Marion, I could never forget you. You've always been in my corner, and always so supportive. Thank you, for everything." They hugged again, and without saying anything, exchanged their good-byes. Sabrina got into her car and headed for home.

The tears had finally subsided. With the exception of scattered, uncontrollable sobs, Sabrina drove home in silence. The car radio played, but she wasn't listening; her mind was working on what she should do first. As she turned onto the street that led to her house, she recognized the sign for the local travel agent. Remembering what Marion had said; she promptly steered the car into the parking lot.

After an hour of collecting brochures, magazines and asking questions, Sabrina emerged from the travel agency with enough information to fill a shopping bag. With a renewed zest, she hurriedly made her way home.

Patches was sitting by the door, where he always was when she came home. She could never understand how he knew that it was her coming home, and not some stranger. He greeted her with many meows, and rubbed around and around her feet, nearly causing her to trip.

He's always happy to see me; a far cry from the way it used to be. If I ever had managed to go out without mother, the worry of coming home was worse. To be given the third degree every time; about where I went, whom I talked to, implanted the most degrading feelings. There was no trust, and never the slightest indication of love.

Scooping up Patches, she nuzzled her face against his. "Wait until you see what I brought home; you're gonna love it." She headed off to the bedroom; put the bag of travel brochures on the bed, and quickly changed her clothes.

Patches, being naturally curious, made his way inside the bag. "Well, aren't you impatient. You just can't wait to see where we are going; can you?" Making herself comfortable on the bed, beside the wiggling bag; she picked up the bottom corners of the bag and emptied it. Patches, and the brochures, landed on the bed with a thud. Disgusted with having his hiding place disrupted, he wandered down to the foot of the bed; watching intently as she began looking through all the information.

"What do you think of this one Patches?" She held up a brochure for Mexico. Patches, who had now curled up and gone to sleep, offered no acknowledgment. Sabrina continued looking through brochures until her eyes began to flutter. Unable to fight the feeling, she put down the brochure. Before long she was fast asleep, dreaming of the exotic places in the pamphlets.

Sabrina stretched and yawned; turning over to check the time, amazed to find that she had slept through to the next morning. With everything that had happened over the past few days, sleep had evaded her; but last night, her mind, and body relaxed enough for her to sleep undisturbed. Stretching again, she noticed Patches sitting at the foot of the bed, motionless as a statue; his eyes fixated on her, in his own way saying, it's about time you got up.

Shuffling her way to the bathroom, she started the shower. Patches trotted in behind her, taking his place on the counter beside the sink. As she stood in the shower, the warm water brought her back to full consciousness. Her mind began to go over all the brochures that she had looked at the night before.

Suddenly she was very alert. Pulling back the shower curtain, she looked at Patches. "You know; I just had a great idea. Why do we have to go to one of those tourist places? Why don't we just go wherever the road takes us? What do you think Patches? Sound like a good idea to you?" Patches stood up and meowed several times, expressing his approval of her idea. "Well then, that settles it; we go wherever. I like that idea." She finished her shower quickly, for she had many things to do today to prepare for her trip.

While seated at the kitchen table, she made a list of things that would have to be done. She had always been a person that liked things organized, bordering dangerously close to obsessive. People teased her about her lists, but in the end it was Sabrina who had completed her work for the day, not the others. As she drank her tea, she reviewed what had been put on the list so far.

Take Patches to the vet for a check up. Go to the mall for luggage and new outfit. Travel agency for road maps. Get a hair cut. Have the car serviced. Cancel newspaper and have the mail put on hold. Go to power company and make an advance payment for six months. Buy medical insurance. Have an alarm installed in the house.

"Well, Patches, I sure have a lot to do today. I probably won't get all of it done, but that's okay. We can leave tomorrow instead. We're not in a hurry are we?" Sabrina suddenly realized that she had been talking to herself; Patches was nowhere to be seen. After a brief search of the house, she stopped, running her hand through her hair as she scolded herself for saying things out loud.

"I swear that cat knows exactly what I am saying and thinking. Just the mention of the vet and he disappears." Taking a deep breath, she continued to search; finally catching up to him in the bedroom. Much to his disapproval, she put him into the pet carrier, giving him a stern lecture about hiding on her.

With the morning's misadventures behind her, she stopped for a bite of lunch at the cafe in the mall; pulling out her list she marked off what she had accomplished. It was past noon and she had only been able to complete two things on her list. She reminded herself that there was no need to get upset; time was on her side now.

She felt good. Her mood was up and it showed, in how she walked and how she greeted people along the way. Nothing was going to get her down; these changes were long overdue. By the time she picked up Patches from the vet, she only had two things remaining on her list. When she returned home there would still be time to take care of one of them and the other would be completed before noon tomorrow.

I am so pleased with myself. Everything is coming together nicely. The entire evening is mine to pack; but before I do that, I had better phone Marion and let her know what my plans are.

Patches was glad to be home again, he disliked being in the pet carrier, and he definitely did not like going to the vet. As soon as Sabrina released him from his portable prison he began a methodical inspection of the house; just to make sure that nothing had changed while he was gone.

Sabrina began unloading the car; she had so many packages that it took her several trips. By the time she had made her last trip in from the car, Patches had already begun to investigate the bags in the foyer; she scolded him for tipping over the shopping bags. Taking her new set of luggage into the bedroom, she prepared them for packing. They needed to be aired out. She liked the smell of leather, but she didn't want it on her clothes.

Before she did anything else, she reminded herself to phone Marion. Marion was very pleased to hear Sabrina's news. "I am so proud of you dear. You deserve this now; and don't even give a second thought to what people are going to say." "Say about what?" Sabrina asked. "You know that they will gossip about you leaving town, so soon after your mother's death. Their opinions don't matter. The only thing that matters is your happiness right now. If taking a trip is what you need to do, then do it. Besides, from the sounds of it you will be long gone before they even realize that you have left town," Marion softly chuckled. "That's right." They talked for a few minutes more, then ended their conversation with the traditional 'I will miss you' phrases and hung up.

Feeling hungry, and thinking that her packing could wait for just a little while, Sabrina picked up the phone again and ordered a pizza. Grabbing a can of pop from the fridge, she went out to the porch to await the delivery man. While she sat on the porch, a typical autumn wind began to blow gently through the yard. The branches of the old cedar trees swayed slowly like lovers caught up in the mood of this romantic wind song that only they could hear.

This is my most favorite part of the day, and of the year. The sun still lingered on into the evening, and the days were still comfortably warm. The neighborhood is beginning to come to life. Dinner is long over for most of the homes along the street and the contented people begin their evening ritual of walking off their meal. I can hear children's voices in the distance. The laughter that is so often associated with play time.

I envy those children, even now, wishing that that could have been me out there, playing, having fun. All those long lonely years, with only my imagination for a playmate, no one ever came to play with me. I had a cupboard full of all the popular games, but playing them by myself held no challenge, no fun. Neither of my parents liked to play games of any kind, which always made me wonder why they bothered to buy them for me.

People moved past the house, each in turn casually acknowledging her presence. None of them stopped this time; not like they did when there was no one outside. It was as if they didn't want to be caught looking at the gardens, that were to Sabrina, completely perfect. She had dedicated a lot of time to her gardens. What else was there for her to do anyway?

The flowers were still in bloom, turning the front yard into a vibrant artist's palette. There was very little lawn in the large front yard, for Sabrina always felt that the front of a house was for showing off, and the backyard was where you had a lawn; for relaxing.

It will be hard to leave this place. This home has been in my family for four generations. It's truly a heritage house, in every sense of the meaning. From the moment you stepped through the wrought iron front gate, it is as if you had stepped back in time. The house has a lot of history to it, along with it's well-kept secrets.

The meandering brick pathway guided visitor's slowly through the bright colorful gardens, the unique twists and turns giving them a complete view of each bed. The original path had been straight; but over the course of several months, Sabrina had changed the path; giving visitors more time amongst the gardens. The flower beds embraced both sides of the walk, to the base of the large stone staircase, that led up onto the porch. They also embraced the perimeter of the house. One was given the impression of being presented to the house, like royalty.

The gardens, near the gate, were delicate, with low growing primroses and bright faced pansies. The farther you went, the more dramatic the gardens became. Gradually transforming into denser and more vibrant beds, with collections of ruffled iris and spicy carnations. On the final turn you were led past the herb garden and onto Sabrina's true masterpiece; the rose garden; with its abundance of vivid colors, bright against the gray concrete foundation of the house. The multitudes of colors changed with the seasons. There was always life there, until the blanket of winter snow covered the gardens; allowing the earth to sleep and revitalize itself in preparation for the forthcoming spring.

Upon reaching the porch you were again embraced by flowers. A clematis climbed its way up the side of the house, while an old wisteria rambled along the full length of the porch. The heavy clusters of purple flowers creating a fragrant lacy veil. There were always hummingbirds and butterflies hovering about, fortifying themselves on the sweet nectar.

The porch alone, was very commanding; extending the full length of the house and nearly ten feet wide. Its rim was guarded by heavy white spindles, and supported by large square posts. Reminders of sentries on duty, carefully guarding and protecting all who entered. The large lead glass windows watched over all, taking care not to let too much light in, so as not to give up the secrets inside this magnificent fortress.

Sabrina's favorite place was the porch swing at the north end; she could sit there for hours, looking at her gardens; her creations. This was her place to dream. A place where she could become lost in fantasies. Even as a child she would curl up on the porch swing; one foot just barely touching the deck, giving the swing a gentle push now and again. The swaying motion had a hypnotic effect. This was a place for good memories, of her father, her grandparents, of times long ago.

She shook herself back to the present; there was packing to do and the evening was passing by rapidly. Collecting the remains of the pizza, she headed back inside; through the heavy front door with its ornate stained glass window. Hesitating just inside the entrance, she gazed about.

This is a family home, it needs the sounds of children playing; not the hollow emptiness that stands before me.

With a loud sigh, she started back to the bedroom. The inlaid hardwood floors squeaked under her step, letting her know that there was still life sounds in this old house. Sabrina had kept her room on the main floor; it was her only way of putting some distance between her and her mother, whose room was upstairs.

Sabrina didn't like the staircase that led up to the second floor; her mother used to make her clean the spindles once a week; and the staircase squeaked horribly. There was no easy way of going up or down that her mother didn't hear. Yet even being downstairs offered her little privacy. Her mother always knew what time she came in or how late she stayed up.

I remember that I always had one of those big ugly purses, big enough to carry all my junk plus a change of clothes. I didn't dare leave the house wearing anything that may have aroused mother's suspicions. Such a routine I had back then. I'd stop at a gas station and change my clothes and put on some makeup before going to any club. Just like Cinderella, by midnight I was back into my respectable clothes and headed home. My life was such a miserable joke.

Sabrina liked having the downstairs bedroom, even though she had installed a key lock on the door, to keep her mother from going through her things when she was at work. That move caused no end of arguments. Her mother was so quick to accuse her of having something to hide, if she had to have a lock on the door, but that was over now and the secrets that were contained in that room were no longer in threat of discovery.

When her great grandfather had built this house the room that Sabrina had for a bedroom was originally a parlor. When the house was passed down to her grandparents they had the parlor remodeled into a bedroom with an ensuite when they could no longer manage the stairs up to the second floor.

As she passed through the bedroom door, she stopped. "Well, you're sure not going to make this easy, are you?" she announced with her hands on her hips. Her gaze was fixed on the suitcase that lay on the bed, filled to the edges with cat. He returned her stare, knowing by her tone that he was being scolded, but made no attempt to move from his new found bed. She picked up the sleepy cat. "You crazy fur ball, you won't fit in there with all of my stuff. Too bad you don't think as highly of your pet carrier. Now you behave while I finish packing." She gave him a kiss, and placed him on the bed beside her pillow.

Sabrina was surprised at just how little time it took her to pack the suitcases and load them into the car. She didn't take a great deal. If there was something that she needed, or wanted, she could just go out and buy it. It would be easier that way, since she didn't know where she was going, or what the weather would be like.

After making one more check of the house, just to make sure it was all locked up tight, Sabrina returned to her bedroom and fell onto the bed. Patches was immediately by her side. She rolled over onto her back, lifting him up onto her stomach. As she lay there quietly stroking his head, she could only think of tomorrow.

Where do I go first? Which road should I take? It had been a long time since she had felt this excited over anything. It was late when she finally succumbed to sleep, but it wasn't a restful sleep. She tossed and turned most of the night, so much so, that even Patches gave up and went into the living room to sleep.

Sabrina's mind wouldn't let her relax. Too many dreams invaded her subconscious that night; but one kept returning, again and again; as it had for years. The shadowy image returned to taunt her, but gave her no clear view; yet it left her with such strong sensations that it made her moan softly in her sleep; a pillow clutched tightly in her arms.

The next morning brought with it the feeling as if she hadn't been to bed for a week. She slowly groped her way into the bathroom, hoping that a long hot shower would wash away this sluggish feeling. As she stood there, the water washing over her body, she began to come back to consciousness. Lathering the soap over her body, she lingered a moment, enjoying the slippery coating that now covered her breasts. She caressed them for a few moments more. "I need a man." It had been a long time since she had made love and she missed it. The very thought sent tingles down her spine.

Maybe I'll meet someone on my trip. A soft smile of anticipation came over her face. *Maybe. No. It's just a dream borne of frustration. He's not real.*

Dressed in a comfortable outfit, she went off toward the kitchen; as she passed the living room she yelled at Patches. "Come on lazy bones, its time for breakfast. This is our big day; so get a move on."

With breakfast done, the dishes washed and put away; there was nothing left to do but wait for the alarm installer to arrive. She was about to pick up the phone and call the company to remind them, when the doorbell rang, there before her stood the installer; strange coincidence.

She briefly went over the type of system that she wanted installed, and then left him to his work. She didn't interfere with the man, as she found him to be quite revolting. He gave off an aroma of someone who had not taken a shower, or changed his clothes for quite some time. The typical workman's outfit, of poorly fitting gray pants and matching shirt, that somehow couldn't come together at his waist, only added to her repulsion. *Why do all these guys look like beer drinking slobs?*

Using her extra time she did a little bit of dusting around the house, but gave up when she caught herself looking at her watch for the fourth time in twenty minutes. *Just be patient. He'll be finished soon.* Finally, after an hour and a half, the installer announced that his task was completed.

Touring her through the house, he showed her where he had put the motion sensors and the alarm panel. Sabrina really didn't care much. Following along behind him, but she committed none of it to her memory. The system would be monitored, and Marion would look in once in a while. She paid him for his services and handed him a note with Marion's name and phone number on it, making him promise her that he would show her how the system operated. As an added incentive, Sabrina gave him a nice cash tip, if he would do what she asked later in the day, or the first thing tomorrow. The incentive worked. As she closed the front door, she heard him on the cell phone with Marion.

Standing at the living room window, she watched until the man had driven away and was no longer in sight. Picking up Patches, and her purse, she headed out the door. As she turned the key to lock the door, she couldn't help feeling somewhat melancholy.

It will be awhile before I see home again, but if I don't get away now I never will.

She placed her hand on the panel of the heavy door, sighed and turned to leave the porch. Passing the porch swing, she gave it a push and went on down the stairs, through the gardens and along the driveway to the garage. She placed Patches on the seat beside her. He didn't need to be in his carrier now, for he was quite used to traveling in the car with her; but she kept the carrier in the back seat, just in case. As she backed the car down the driveway, she took a last long look at the house as she slowly drove up the street. Thoughts of misgivings entered her mind as she drove.

Is this truly the right thing to do? Am I making the right decision, leaving like this; telling no one, except Marion what my intentions are?

She mulled these thoughts over and over in her mind until she came to the line up for the border crossing. The urge to turn around and go home was strong, but she kept telling herself that it was now or never.

I have to be the master of my destiny. It was her turn to speak to the border guard. *There is no turning around now.*

The guard tried to give her a hard time, about having a cat loose in the car, and for not knowing how long she would be in the United States; he finally let her through and wished her a good trip. As she drove away, she thought to herself, what a jerk he was. Her attitude had changed.

No more will I be subservient. No more do I have to account for my every move. For the first time I'm following my heart; and chasing a dream.

Driving through Washington State, she found nothing that impressed her enough to stop. *Distance; that's what I'm doing, putting space between the memories and myself.* When her mother was alive they had traveled a little in Washington, and there was nothing new to see. Before she realized it she was in Oregon; she had to stop for the night. Even though she had got a late start, Sabrina was surprised at just how far she had driven. She took a motel room in Portland. Settled in for the night, it wasn't long before they were both fast asleep.

With the dawn of a new morning came a new enthusiasm, a feeling she hadn't had for a very long time. The decision was easy; she would go out to see the Oregon coast. She had seen the ocean before, but not this part. People that she knew always used to speak of it as the most sensational place on earth. They made it sound so intriguing.

Before too long she had reached a town called Astoria; she remembered that this was the beginning of the coast. Stopping the car at the far end of town, she was astounded at the width of the Columbia River, and of the bridge that spanned its mouth. Never before had she seen anything so spectacular as this. Its curving on-ramp reached high above, and then climbed higher to the bridge deck. She craned her neck to see all of it. It came down to a road that was built on the water; the far end was but a fine dot in the distance.

Continuing on, she began to catch glimpses of the ocean, but she was still too far inland, and there were no roads that indicated that they went out towards the ocean. She drove on, contented knowing that her opportunity to stop would come soon; and it did. Spotting a sign for a park with beach access, she pulled the car in and parked; mesmerized by the sight before her. The beach area was so immense. She headed down the trail. The tide was coming in and the sound of the waves hypnotized her.

Incredible. I can see for miles in both directions. This is definitely a place I have to get to know.

With an urgency in her step, she went back to the car and drove on until she found a motel that was on the ocean side of the highway. Taking the last available room, she got Patches settled and headed back out to the beach. Walking in the surf, digging in the sand, and thoroughly enjoying the wind blowing through her hair, she felt like a child again, reveling in her new experience. Hunger finally forced her back to the motel.

Upon returning to her room, with dinner from the local drive-in, she found Patches sitting in the window that looked out over the beach. His tail twitching back and forth, and he was smacking his lips; his attention was focused on some little birds that were hopping about; unaware that she had returned and was standing behind him. "Well, this isn't as good as a fresh bird but it will have to do," she said crumbling the plain hamburger into his dish. It wasn't the best meal she had either, but it was all right. There was no time for a proper meal tonight, she wanted to get back to the beach, to watch the sunset.

Pulling on a pair of sweat pants, she grabbed a sweater from the suitcase; patted Patches on the head and went back to the beach. Finding a driftwood log to sit on, she made herself as comfortable as she could. Quietly watching the ocean slowly devouring the glowing orange ball on the horizon; her mind became void of all thought. The only thing that echoed through her brain was the sound of the waves; she was so relaxed, so content. As the last sliver of the sun disappeared from view she sighed. Her eyes began to scan the beach around her, stopping momentarily to look at the couples that sat huddled together; their silhouettes just barely visible in the growing darkness; she hadn't noticed their arrival.

Sunsets are for lovers. A tear slid down her cheek as she stood to return to her motel room. *This night would have been perfect, if only I had someone to share it with.*

Sabrina carefully chose her way back; as to not disturb the other couples. Her room was cold, but the bed was inviting and within minutes sleep had taken her back into her memories, back into her dreams. She stirred once, only to pull the pillow, that lay beside her, even closer, unconsciously caressing the imaginary shape.

Chapter 2

Sabrina spent the next three weeks exploring the Oregon coast, with its many fascinating little towns to stop and visit, and the intriguing little shops that beckoned to travelers, come in and see what wonders we have to peruse. Oregon had so much to offer her; from its sea lion caves, to its wild animal parks, and rock hounding expeditions. She reveled in all the wonders she encountered.

If this one small strip of land held so many marvels, what does the rest of the country have in store for me? Even my imagination could not have conjured up the spectacular sights that I've encountered, how could it begin to comprehend what lay ahead.

She made sure that she picked up postcards to send back to Marion. She didn't write very much on the cards for her excitement did not allow for enough quiet time.

A letter is something that requires a good deal of time; something I just don't have. Marion will understand; and the brief notes will at least help her to stop worrying.

At the end of the three weeks she decided that it was time for her to move on; to see what else lay in waiting in this marvelous country. *If I don't like the inland area I can always come back out to the coast.*

After reviewing the travel brochures again, she decided that Reno appeared to be an interesting place to go next. The terrain gradually began to transform from the dense evergreen forests of Oregon, to the barren desolate plains of Nevada. Driving for what seemed hours, passing no signs for upcoming towns, only sage brush, and the odd lonely pine tree.

I wonder if I'm traveling on the right road? I haven't passed a car for miles. Feelings of desperation began to set in; the fuel tank registered just above a quarter tank. *What if I was to run out of gas, here in the middle of nowhere? Who would find me, and when?* "Stop it. Nothing is going to happen."

As hard as she tried, the feelings of worry kept returning, with an ever increasing urgency. Off in the distance something caught her eye, still too far away to recognize what it was, she pushed her foot down hard on the gas pedal. The object became larger and more distinctive. *A sign!* She brought the car to a full stop just in front of the sign post; it read, RENO 40 Miles.

Slumped forward against the steering wheel, she took a deep breath and instantly could feel her tension ease away. The muscles in her neck relaxed first, triggering the muscles in her arms and hands to do the same; her grip on the steering wheel lessened. Bringing her palms up, she wiped the perspiration off of her face, onto her shorts. "That's a relief, huh Patches. Only 40 more miles until we get into Reno. It's a good thing to, considering our current gas situation."

Taking a long drink of water from the bottle that rested between the seats, she did a quick calculation as to what the odometer should read when she entered Reno.

It was a curious habit that she had; taking the mileage off of a sign and adding it to the odometer. It was her way of knowing just how close she was to her destination. It was also a way of keeping her mind alert; always checking the reading, and counting down the miles. This quirky habit had come about when her mother had traveled with her, it let her know that the torturous trip was coming to an end.

Her mother used to continually nag her about how fast she was going. Not keeping her eyes on the road and always playing the radio too loud. Once, on a long trip, the nagging had become so excessive that Sabrina entertained, for a fleeting moment, the concept of running the car into a pole, but being unable to guarantee her own survival, she dismissed it.

With her calculations made, and her thirst quenched, she pulled her car back onto the highway and headed toward Reno. The scenery along the way didn't offer any changes, but that did not matter; she drove on eagerly; passing a dry lake bed, that was now being used as a race track.

Indications of human existence began to emerge along the highway. Retirement condos and industrial areas seemed to spring forth from nowhere. Sabrina glanced at the odometer. *Reno is only five miles away.*

At the crest of a hill she pulled the car onto the shoulder of the road; staring out at what lay ahead of her. "Oh my Patches, this is wonderful." The cat, who was trying to reclaim his bed, after being bounced onto the floor, when the car had stopped so abruptly, completely ignored her.

It was just starting to get dark, and at the bottom of the hill, spreading out as far as she could see was Reno; its twinkling lights awakening weary travelers. "It looks sort of like a carnival midway; but much bigger." Leaning her head out the window she tried to hear the sounds that should accompany the lights.

Bubbling with overwhelming anticipation, she continued on down the hill. The city opened up and she entered willingly. The sights and sounds of the main street were indescribable. The bright flashing hotel signs made it difficult for her to concentrate on the road; traffic lights blended in with the decor.

I want to stop the car and run into every building. "Not yet, first, we have to find a place to stay, then it will be time for fun." Locating a motel wasn't as easy as it looked. There were so many of them, but they didn't like having pets staying with their guests. The clerks were very quick to suggest a local boarding kennel, but Sabrina didn't like that idea at all. They were no different from a prison; and she would not tolerate her best friend being locked in a cage and away from her.

When she found a motel that would accept them both, checking in seemed to take forever. The clerk was slow, but quick to blame the delays on his computer than on himself; she began to feel that he was doing it on purpose. *He must sense my excitement.* He presented her with a room key; she thanked him and hurried off to get Patches settled. He had been cooped up in the car just as long as she had.

Over the years she had trained him well. He was well adjusted to wearing a harness, and not unlike a dog, very excited when she put it on him. He had learned what walks were for, and even though Sabrina had a litter box for him, he very seldom used it. Within minutes she was settled into her room, had changed her clothes, and fed Patches. She picked him up and cuddled him. "Sorry baby, I'm going out for a while. You be a good boy now." Placing him on the bed she gave him a pat on the head. Then, as if hearing a shot from a starting pistol, she was off, exploring this enchanting new world.

Fortunately, the motel was only a block away from the main street; if it had not been, she was sure that her anxiety would have gotten the better of her. Hurrying down the block, she soon slowed herself, thinking that people may notice that this was her first time here. "Stop being so eager; you have plenty of time." Her gait was finally back too normal when she reached the corner. Standing motionless, she took in the dazzling signs. *They look like electric fireworks.*

Not wanting to miss anything, and being the methodical person that she was, her plan was to start with the side of the street that she was on, and work her way down to the end of the strip and then back up the other side.

As she approached the first casino, there was a uniformed person standing out front handing out flyers for the casino, calling to people as they passed by, not that much different from a carnival barker. It was enough to entice her in.

Once inside, she moved leisurely about the slot machines and the gaming tables, captivated by all the sights and the sounds. Music played, but not loud enough to drown out the distinctive sound of coins dropping into tin trays. Even though the excitement was tremendous she wasn't quite ready to start gambling. Having never indulged in gambling before, she did not want to appear to be ignorant.

There was so much to see. She visited every gift shop, and every casino along the main street, and when she arrived back at her original starting point she was amazed to find that five hours had passed. Feeling a little bit tired, and quite hungry; she entered the restaurant across the street from her motel. Making her way past the line of slot machines, she stood at the cashier's station at the front of the restaurant. The waitress told her that she would have quite a wait for a table; but if she didn't mind the bar area, they would be happy to serve her there. That sounded all right; the thought of a nice cold beer had helped to make up her mind.

The bar was relatively quiet; considering that it served a dual purpose. The back wall had room enough for four booths that took the overflow from the main restaurant. A lone man sat at the end of the bar, watching a wrestling program on the TV, and seated at the booth in the corner, was a group of four men. She noticed that they were all dressed in the same color uniform; not recognizing it at first, but finally noted that they were bus drivers. She settled into a seat near the middle of the bar.

I'm not to close to the man at the end and just far enough away from the bus drivers, a nice safe distance.

The bartender caught her attention. "Good evening Miss, my name is Jim. What can I get for you?" he asked. Without hesitation she ordered a beer, and the special of the evening. She quietly watched first the TV in the corner and then the video poker machine that was installed in the bar top. Both were equally intriguing.

The TV with it's tanned, hard bodied wrestlers provoking her fantasies, and the poker machine, with its opportunities to make money. She settled on the poker machine. Feeling that watching the wrestlers would only cause her more sexual frustration; the poker machine offered her something new and exciting. She called to Jim the bartender. "Could you please tell me how these machines work?" she asked. His mouth opened to speak, but before he could answer her another voice from behind her said, "I can."

Startled by the unexpected voice so close to her, she jumped. Turning around she saw one of the bus drivers standing behind her. A tremor ran up her spine. "I'm sorry if I frightened you. My name is Larry." He was holding out his hand to her. Regaining her composure, she spoke. "Hi, I'm Sabrina." Accepting the handshake, Larry sat down beside her. "So you have never played poker before?" "I've never had the opportunity." "First, you will have to get Jim here to get you some silver dollars and then I'll show you what to do." Sabrina handed Jim a twenty dollar bill and he quickly returned with twenty silver dollars.

Larry explained the workings of the game. She could put in as little as one coin, or as many as five coins, and then push the deal button. Being conservative, she deposited two coins into the machine and pushed deal; the machine turned over five cards. Larry explained to her which cards she should keep, and which ones to throw away. He also explained the meanings of the poker hands. None of it really registered at first, for she was to busy discretely studying the man that sat beside her.

He is definitely attractive; or is it just that it's been so long since I had any male company?

They played and talked through two more beers; Sabrina won a few games and lost a few games, but it was of no significance, she was having fun; something that she had not done in a very long time. Swallowing the last mouthful of beer, she turned to look at Larry. "It's getting late and I should go," she said. "Would you allow me to walk you back to your motel? You shouldn't be out on the street alone at this time of night." "That would be nice; but it won't be much of a walk."

A look of puzzlement came over Larry's face. Sabrina smiled. "My motel is just across the street," she said. Larry started to laugh. "So is mine! Isn't that a strange coincidence?" As they stood up to leave, Sabrina had to steady herself; she could feel the effects of the beer. Larry was at her side, as if knowing how she felt. Putting his arm around her waist, he grasped her elbow; she felt the tremor again; Larry's touch stimulated her.

The cool night air aided in clearing her head. "What room are you in?" he asked. "I'm in two twenty-two," Sabrina answered. Larry smiled and chuckled. "I don't believe this! My room is right next door to yours.

It must be fate." They walked on, laughing at the odds of something like this happening. Stopping outside the doors to the rooms, Larry turned to Sabrina. "Would you like to come in for a drink; or a cup of coffee?" he asked. She hesitated.

He is wearing a wedding ring but damn he is definitely good looking. Her feelings were in turmoil. A man in his middle forties, Larry was tall and very well built. Sitting behind the wheel of a bus day after day had not altered his youthful physique. His uniform gave the appearance of being specifically tailored just for him; it outlined the shape of his body so very well. The thick mass of black hair had a scattering of gray at the temples; Sabrina found that to be attractive as well. He wore his hair in a similar fashion to an air force pilot, close cut at the neck and gradually lengthening on the top; just long enough to show off the natural waves that it grew in. The haircut finished off the whole look. Men in uniform were always pleasing to look at.

"Well, are you going to give me an answer or are we going to stand here all night?" Accepting his offer, unsure if it was the beer that had made her decision, or the anticipation of a romantic rendezvous; either way it didn't matter much, she longed for some kind of companionship.

Sabrina entered his room; it was completely different from hers; much larger, and with better furniture. The queen size bed was the most pronounced item in the room. Across from the bed was a large armoire, with two heavy doors on the top, and several drawers below that. It was quite unlike the typical motel dresser in her room. Across the room was a small round table with two chairs. On one of the chairs set a tote bag, its contents protruding through the open zipper.

To the left of the table she noticed two steps that led up to a landing; she could not see what was at the top. "Make yourself comfortable," Larry said as he slipped passed her. With him occupied in the bathroom, she could satisfy her curiosity; she headed toward the two steps.

What she was unable to ascertained from her previous vantage point, was that the landing was framed on three sides with mirrors, and off in the far left corner, sunk into the floor, was a Jacuzzi tub. The bubbling effervescence left a glistening coating on the tile floor. She scanned every detail until she noticed in the mirror that Larry had returned.

"This is unbelievable. Do all the drivers get rooms like this?" "No, we take turns with this one. I won't get to use this room again for a month now. It has more comforts than home; even a big screen TV." He walked back over to the armoire and pulled open the doors on the top, exposing the black faced monitor that was concealed inside. "They even have all those fancy pay channels hooked up in here just for the drivers. All the other rooms you have to pay for each channel. That's the one really nice thing about being a driver; the motels treat you better than their paying customers. What can I get for you?" "Beer, please."

Larry handed her the remote control for the TV and retreated to the fridge that stood beside the table. Positioning herself in front of the TV, Sabrina began scanning through the channels. Larry was at her side; leaning up against her shoulder, he whispered in her ear. "They even have the adult movie channel. Would you like to see?"

Unsure of just how to answer him, all she could do was look into his deep blue eyes. Handing her a can of beer, he took the remote from her. Without moving his eyes off of her, he programmed the TV to the adult channel. "They aren't the best movies ever made, but some of them do have a story to them."

He seems to be giving me an explanation for his action. Sabrina could not answer him. Wild thoughts raced through her mind as she looked at him. The tremors that had been teasing her spine now ran together repeatedly.

The picture on the TV tuned in on a couple at the peak of fevered love making; curiosity compelled her to watch. After a few seconds she walked over to the table; she placed her beer down and released a soft sigh. *I must gain control.* Larry was behind her; she could feel him; his voice broke the silence.

"It's warm in here; can I take your jacket?" he asked. Sabrina turned to face him; his drivers jacket no longer covered him and his shirt was half unbuttoned. Her heart skipped a beat. "All right," she answered in a breathless voice.

She started to remove her jacket when Larry spoke. "No, let me." Placing his drink on the table, he moved his hands up to cradle the sides of her neck. Her mind and body cried out for him to kiss her, but he did not. His hands slid down her neck and onto her shoulders, pushing the jacket as he went. Never moving his eyes from hers, he continued down her arms until the jacket slipped off to the floor. He wanted her. Moving his hands back to caress her shoulders; he stepped in closer and pulled her to him. He kissed her. Sabrina pulled away.

"Larry, this isn't right; you're a married man." "That shouldn't make a difference right now. I'm leaving tomorrow and I'll never see you again. I don't normally do this; I have been happily married for fifteen years. I have never had an affair before, or even thought about having one, until now. You are so beautiful and all I know is I want you. I want to make love to you."

The line he's feeding me is a classic; I've heard it all before. Yet she still fell for it. Leaning in he kissed her neck. "You want me too; I can feel it in the way you move." *What he says is true. This is something that I want.* That they both wanted and listening to the sounds of the people on the TV had only served to intensify the feelings that were rushing through her body.

She placed her hands on his chest and when he kissed her again she allowed him to explore her body. As they kissed, his hand found its way down to her breast; he gently caressed it unable to completely grasp its size with his palm. Unbuttoning her blouse, slowly at first, then with more urgency; he slipped it off her shoulders. His hands slid around her back to unhook her bra; she stopped him.

This isn't right; but it has been so long since I have felt the need. A primal, instinctive need that overrides all my doubts of why I'm doing this; with him. Yet there is a foreboding feeling, one of betrayal, but to whom, I have no one.

She pushed the feelings away. Undoing the remaining buttons on his shirt, she pulled it off to the floor, exposing the firm chest that had been taunting her. Kissing his chest, she ran her tongue up over his skin, until she had reached his mouth again. Holding each other close, she was unaware that he had slowly been moving her across the room, until she noticed the Jacuzzi behind him. Reaching for the light switch on the wall, he dimmed the lights. She allowed him to remove the remainder of her clothes. Sabrina reached down and undid the belt on his pants, eager to release his body from its confinement. They stepped into the Jacuzzi and amid the warm bubbling water began to explore the desire. She began to feel alive again.

It has been such a long time, but I don't want to appear to be too eager either. The anticipation was overwhelming for her; she wanted him; she was tired of foreplay.

The desire was building. Her mind locked onto a sound. "What did you say?" she asked, leaning back. "Nothing. Come here." Larry attempted to bring her to him, but she resisted. The overwhelming feeling of betrayal washed over her. The sound whispered in her head. Closing her eyes she focused intently on this annoying distraction. It was a voice, so faint, so distant, yet so clear; beseeching her to discontinue this shameful act.

This is not right, it said, *I'm the one who loves you. Follow your heart; let your soul be your council; let it guide you to me.*

The voice vanished as Larry grasped her shoulders. "What's with you?" Larry asked. Sabrina's eyes snapped open and she stared blindly at his face. "I can't do this," she said pushing herself away from him. "I'm sorry Larry but I have to go." Grabbing a towel, she wrapped it around herself and began collecting her clothes. Larry followed closely behind her, taking her into his arms. "Sabrina I don't understand, I thought you wanted to." "I did Larry, but I can't go through with it. Please don't ask for an explanation, because I don't have one."

Emotions that were foreign to her caused her to tremble and stammer. "Please Larry, I, I have to leave now." Larry relinquished to her request, more convinced that he had nearly made love to a certifiable psychopath. In his eyes she was no longer a beautiful, desirable woman, she was just a freak; and he wanted no involvement with anyone like that.

With her clothes bundled under her arm and still clad in the towel, Sabrina retreated from his room; frantically searching for the key that would open the door to her sanctuary. Patches was waiting on the bed. Scooping him up, she cuddled him tight.

What is happening to me? Am I losing my mind? Only insane people hear voices. Am I going insane? That question brought tears to her eyes; she could not begin to comprehend the full meaning of what had occurred. The slightest attempt to reason out what had happened gave her an intense headache. She lay back on the bed, hoping that sleep would cleanse her mind of these thoughts. Patches curled up against the curve of her stomach, understanding her need to be comforted.

A hundred miles away, tears dripped undetected onto a pillow. The lonely, abandoned soul within this body had called out to its eternal mate. They had been kept apart far too long in this life; they needed to be together. As separate entities they were inadequate, without direction or purpose. They needed to be together. They were strong when they were united, resilient against all forms of oppression. Their love was perpetual, transcending centuries of change, to reunite in each new life where they could once again partake in the physical pleasures of their undying bond. This physical body was just now beginning to understand what was happening to it. The heart, beat with a purpose that was coming clearer with each dream. The mate was advancing closer. The dreams would come more frequently now, with more intensity.

Morning came too soon for Sabrina. Her seemingly brief repose was shattered by noisy motel guests coming and going from their rooms. Car engines revved and backfired; heavy trucks rambled down the street and a train activated the crossing signal up the block. Covering her head with a pillow could not block out the annoying sounds. She exchanged them for the sound of the shower.

With Patches fed, and herself dressed, she peered out the window. Her stomach begged to be fed but she was fearful of going over to the restaurant, in case she ran into Larry. She waited until nine o'clock, until she was sure that all the tour buses had left for the day.

After breakfast, she continued to meander around Reno; visiting a couple more casinos along the way. Gambling was fun, but she could find better things to do with her money. Directing her attentions to the clothing stores; she found these especially appealing. They had styles that she had not seen before. She found that spandex was very pleasing to her figure it hugged her curves and defined her body. She treated herself; why not?

There is no longer any reason to be the conservative dowdy looking woman that my mother expected me to be. Now I can do what ever I want, and if spandex pants, high heels and a revealing top is what makes me feel good, then that's just how I'm going to dress. Sexy; I want to feel sexy. More importantly, I just need to feel good. To do something that will exonerate my unexplainable behavior of last night. I refuse to let myself get caught up in the what if game.

With so much to see, it was easy to rid her mind of those nagging feelings. Having seen enough of Reno, she headed the car south, to Carson City; making sure to stop at all the tourist sights along the way. Carson City was not all that appealing; merely a down scaled version of Reno; crowded and bustling with traffic; typical of a state capital. She quickly found a park to pull into, to get away from the traffic for a while.

Sitting in the car, she shared a snack with Patches, and reviewed some of the brochures she had picked up. She came across one for Virginia

City. An old west mining town; the pictures and write up made this place appear very interesting. Packing up the remains of their snack, she drove out of the park. The traffic was getting worse and Sabrina was having difficulty watching for signs, as well as watching for other drivers. Finally she spotted the turn for Virginia City. She headed off up the mountain leaving the noise and commotion behind.

As she climbed higher up the mountain she began to daydream. *Was this one of the original routes up to the town? If it was, it must have taken a very long time with just a horse and wagon.*

Pulling into a view point, she got out to take a few pictures. The panoramic view was breathtaking. Far below her lay the town of Carson City, relatively small compared to the size of the valley that it rested in. The road clung to the cliffs, periodically turning inward between two hills, only to reemerge along another precipice; switch backs and hills that seemed to go on forever.

The constant upward climb was taking its toll on the car; the temperature gauge went up, as did her anxiety. She breathed a sigh of relief when she saw the town before her. Slowly cruising through its main street, she looked for a place to park. A sign on her right indicated a parking lot. Turning in, she paid the attendant and cautiously maneuvered her car through the tourists and the buses. "Tour buses? No. There is no chance in hell that one of those buses is Larry's." *The last thing I need is to confront him.*

Despite the altitude, Virginia City was hotter than she expected, and finding a parking spot away from the sun was not easy, it took her two turns around the lot before she located a suitable place. She felt bad at having to leave Patches in the car; it was in partial shade and there was a breeze blowing; but just to be sure though, she covered the windows with a reflective screen and placed a bowl of water on the floor of the front seat; patted him on the head and went to explore this wonderful looking town.

Virginia City was even more intriguing than the brochures let on. It was living, breathing history. Yet, for her it had a homey feeling. *Strange, it's like I've been here before. I must have seen something about it on TV and not really paid any attention.*

The history that the town represented was phenomenal; from the board sidewalks, to the saloons with their strange sounding names. The architecture and the craftsmanship, so lavish for the time period.

Some of the buildings had been restored, but it in no way disguised their original elegance. Yet amongst all this history, the presence of modern times had encroached onto this oasis. Souvenir peddlers were everywhere trying to get rich off of this town; but not like the original founders, who dug their fortunes from the earth, these modern day miners were very astute at digging into the wallets of tourists.

By far the most engrossing place was that of the cemetery, erected at the far end of town on a gentle slope. The headstones related a story of a very hard life. The men that had died in mining accidents, the women that had died in childbirth, and entire families lost to epidemics. The stones were not just markers for those who had passed on, but of testimonials to a way of life that these people had chosen.

Sabrina wandered amongst the graves for a long time; stopping to read the names of as many as she could. Sadness engulfed her as she passed plots that contained entire families, that were lost within a few days or months of each other.

The wind whispered to her, with sad, mournful gusts. The voices of long ago were caught in the wind, reaching out to anyone who could, or would hear them.

What had driven these people to be in such a desolate place, other than the chance of getting rich? No amount of money seemed to be worth it when so many lives were lost looking for it. Why would they crawl deep into the earth, searching for that one vein of ore that would make them rich? Why? When at any time a simple mistake, or act of nature would seal them inside forever.

As she stood atop the hill of the cemetery, she perceived herself riding over the rolling hills. She had always thought that she belonged to a time other than this.

If reincarnation is a reality, then my past life is somehow connected to the old west; to this place. Her mind began to drift.

She believed that she had walked this earth before. There were the feelings of déjà vu. Pictures flashed into her mind, of events, places, things she had not experienced before, yet they were so familiar, so fresh. There were two images that appeared quite frequently, a frontier scene and the other of a town torn apart during the witch trials.

Pushing these images aside, she felt that they were just segments of her lonely imagination. There was one other image that used to visit her. *I* had almost forgotten it. The image of a man, but his face was never visible. The image was only clear from the neck to the waist; but the sensations of touch, and smell were very strong. She could feel the skin of this man as her hand caressed his chest, his powerfully strong chest.

It's not an image of someone that I recognize, unfamiliar, yet exhilarating; but what does it mean?

"Stop it. This is not real. Get a grip on yourself," she said stomping her foot on the ground and turned back to town. So engrossed in reading the headstones, she had not noticed that the sun was beginning to set; she hurried back into town. The last thing she wanted was to have to drive down the mountain in the dark. Driving in a strange place was stressful on its own, but driving in a strange place in the dark frightened her.

I have to come back to this place again; I need to find out the rest of its secrets.

Patches had survived the afternoon; the sun had not penetrated the window screens. The car was warm but not unbearable, but she still turned on the air conditioning anyway; more for him, than for her. Darkness was setting in fast. Her heart raced as she drove down the mountain. By the time she had reached the bottom, darkness had enveloped the valley floor. She felt a bit more at ease once she was back on the highway with the other cars to help break the darkness.

Her attention was drawn to the big motorcycle parked at the side of the road; the man seated on it gave her a cold chill. She couldn't see his face, but he unnerved her anyway. The ominous dark figure was hard to push from her mind.

She pressed on until she reached Lake Tahoe. Taking the first available motel, she went straight to bed. The day of touring, and the drive, had taken its toll, she was more tired than she realized, but sleep was far from restful, her mind drew forth the vision that had taunted her for so many years, but this time it became intermixed with the vision of the man on the bike. Weaving the two together until they were no longer separated. The haunting whisper of last night returned to narrate her vision.

The show was finally over for the night. It had been a long grueling evening that had put the Warlock in a handicap match, against two opponents in the wrestling ring. His body was tired and bruised from the evening's ordeal of being thrust into ring posts and hit with metal chairs, sometimes caught off guard by his opponent, only to be unprepared for the move, or the impact. Yet he had prevailed, as he was supposed to.

Wandering slowly back into his dressing room, the sound of the spa perked him up. *I need a good soak tonight.* Peeling off his spandex costume, that was stuck to his body by sweat, he stepped into the awaiting spa, relaxing against a bank of water jets. The warm water swirled furiously about his body, stinging now and then when it contacted a bruise. His mind wandered; far away from the wrestling ring, to a special place; a place in his heart where a tiny light of hope still flickered.

If only I had a special lady to share this with, I would not feel the pain that surges through my body tonight. Love is what I want to feel, soft passionate love. The love of a woman who loves me, and not what I am.

There were plenty of opportunities for him to take a lover in this business; fans congregated around the entrances, and the cars, with the hopes of being selected by one the wrestlers for a night of unbridled passion. This was not to be for Warlock; he could not bring himself to take any of these women; no matter how much they begged or pleaded for his company.

Settling for a life of solitude; a recluse, keeping his distance from even the other wrestlers, his mind had become fixated on a persistent fantasy. A fantasy of the ideal woman; the woman who had disturbed his dreams for so many nights, so many years. Never able to clearly see her face, but he knew her body, strong and supple. She loved him, the man, not the wrestling celebrity that he had become.

If only she were real, how complete my life would be. He laid his head back; the warmth of the water took him back into his dreams, back to her. His mind envisioned her making love to him; her sensuous, shapely body straddled over his, loving him. He could feel her, taking all of his love with soft sighs of pleasure. The gentle touch of her hands caressing his body; her sweet, luscious lips pressed against his. His eyes snapped open; he sat up straight as a cold chill ran over his spine.

Damn, that was intense. Vividly recalling the sensations he licked his lips, he thought he could almost taste her. *That's impossible; she isn't real. Yet I can't shake the feeling that there is something different about this dream tonight, it's more intense than I've ever experienced. Is it a sign? Is this fantasy a premonition? Could this woman be somewhere near by?*

Dressing quickly, he packed his gear onto the truck and took off on his motorcycle; scouring the streets of Reno.

She must be here, but where? My senses are so strong this time.

He drove into the night, through Reno and into Carson City, the sensation of her presence forcing him onward, without direction or regard. Searching the cars that passed him, hoping for some other sign that he wasn't losing his mind. The big bike came to a stop near the turn to Virginia City.

I can feel her slipping away from me again. She had been so close, but I couldn't find her. How can I find her?

He lifted his eyes up to the dark night sky. "Oh God, if there is truly a woman out there for me, then please guide me to her. Let me find her someday soon I'm tired of being alone. I need, I want to love someone, and I want to know what it's like to be loved. Please help me." Wiping the mist from his eyes, he turned the bike around; he had to get back to Reno before the tour moved on without him.

I will never abandon my search for you, this elusive woman who toys with my mind, and makes my heart beat with life. She is out there, waiting for me to find her.

Patches woke Sabrina when he jumped onto the bed from the night stand. Having slept away most of the morning, she took her time at getting up. Traveling, although a pleasurable diversion, was tiring; she needed a couple of days to recuperate before moving on. When she finally had herself organized for the day, the first thing she did was to book her motel room for another night. "Now to see where I am."

She drove around the lake; so blue and clear, the air so fresh. She treated herself to a swim in its gorgeous waters. It was cold at first, but so refreshing. She attracted the attention of the men on the beach, for how could they not look at this tall, shapely blonde, clad only in a bikini. It didn't leave much for their imaginations. A couple of them tried to pick her up, but she showed them no interest.

While she laid on the beach, she thought of the ocean. It was calling to her; she pictured the waves in her mind, and could almost hear the surf call her name.

I want to go back to the ocean, but not to Oregon. This time I want to experience the beaches of California; if I don't like it then I'll go back to Oregon. Deep inside she felt some primal need to go to California; as if some other force was directing her. *It couldn't be merely curiosity. What if? Oh enough of this nonsense.*

She spent the remainder of the afternoon on the beach of Lake Tahoe, periodically going in for a swim when she felt the need; her mind wandering from one thing to another not content with just one single thought, almost a dream state but not asleep. Then the image of that man again; so intense this time, that she found herself looking about the beach for an answer.

This is crazy, but what does it mean? It's just your imagination for crying out loud. She waded back out into the lake. *The cold water will wash my mind clear, and free myself of this cursed apparition.*

Staying the extra night in Tahoe had been good; she was rejuvenated and prepared to continue her adventure. Patches, however, didn't care one way or the other; as long as he had something to eat and a place to sleep he was cooperative. Sabrina had used this time to sit down and write a proper letter to Marion, recounting most of her trip, but not everything.

Liking her new found independence, especially not having to report to someone about where she was, or what she was doing. She kept her letter to Marion short, but filled with more information than was truly necessary. She took one more drive around the lake, making sure that she had some good pictures of it before she made the turn that took her back to the highway.

Driving into California she noticed how quickly the evergreen trees gave way to the towering palm trees and to the heat. As she drove farther into southern California, she noticed that the clear blue skies of Lake Tahoe were now being replaced by the dull gray smog that hovered over the urban communities. "It will be better when we reach the coast," she said aloud, rolling the car window up and turning on the air conditioner.

Air conditioning was something she didn't much care for. Preferring to drive with the windows open, the wind blowing on her arms and into her hair, but the smell of the exhaust fumes made her nauseous, and the dry heat was giving her a headache. With the exception of filling the car with gas or getting something cold to drink, there was no need to stop. To see the ocean again, that thought kept her moving on through town after town.

It had taken her most of the day to reach her goal, and with the ocean now in view she stopped at the first available pullout. Leaning against the car, taking deep breaths of the salty air; the wind blew her hair wildly about until she restrained it in a ponytail. Even then, the wind fought to release it from its captivity. "This is were I want to be. Tomorrow I'm going to try to find just the right spot and stay awhile."

California feels right; I don't understand the feelings that I'm having, but I know that I have to be here; now.

She sat on the hood of the car for a few minutes more, before forcing herself back into the car and back on the road. She didn't much care that she could not find a motel with an ocean view, she was tired, but she was where she wanted to be. The drive had been lengthy and the sticky heat and the smog had drained away her excess energy. Sleep was difficult this night; the air conditioner didn't work, nor did the windows open. Twice she got up and took a cool shower, hoping that it would help her to sleep. It wasn't until around four AM that the necessity to sleep overcame the tenacious heat; but it only lasted until seven.

Still hung over from the lack of sleep, she dragged herself into the shower, optimistic that this time it would wash away this awful feeling. The cool water relieved some of the grogginess, enough anyway, for her to pack and move on.

The morning drive was tedious. Despite the ocean breeze blowing in through the car windows, she had to stop frequently to recharge herself. The excursion took her along the California coast, oblivious to the towns that cropped up along the way. Still tired from the night before, she knew that she would have to stop soon or run the risk of falling asleep behind the wheel. By late afternoon she had reached the extreme outskirts of Los Angeles, and that was as far as she could go. She pulled into the first motel that had a vacancy sign. Exhausted, she didn't care if they had an ocean view, or even an air conditioner; all she wanted to do was to sleep, and that she did without interruption.

Before heading out, she made sure that she left a very nice tip for the maid, who was kind enough to leave the room alone for two days, contrary to the rules of the management. People like that were hard to find nowadays, and Sabrina had greatly appreciated the woman's kind gestures. She tucked forty dollars into an envelope and sealed it; placing it on top of the TV along with the room key. The time off from driving had done her considerable good; she was now physically and emotionally prepared to resume her journey.

Continuing along the coast highway, she stopped every once in a while to admire the beauty of the ocean, or to bask in the cool breeze that it offered to her. She spotted a sign for a local real estate agency. Upon entering the office she was immediately approached by the secretary. "Can I help you?" The prim little red head asked. "Yes, you can; I would like to speak to one of your agents about renting a beach house." "If you would like to have a seat I'll check and see who is available."

The secretary disappeared into a hallway behind her desk. Sabrina thought her to be a little odd; she had been scanning Sabrina as if trying to figure out what *she* would want with a beach house. Dismissing the woman's odd looks, Sabrina took a seat near the desk. The office was very lavishly decorated with fine plush carpeting; intricately embossed wallpaper and very expensive oak furniture.

I wonder if I've chosen wisely? Maybe this agency will be too expensive? Oh well, it will be fun to look anyway.

Sabrina had hardly got comfortable when another woman came out of the hallway. She was an older woman, who showed her age by the conservative way that she was dressed; in a powder blue linen suit and white blouse, buttoned all the way to the collar, her black hair pulled back tight into a bun. *She looks more like a school teacher than a real estate agent.* Her dress was very business like, but it didn't fit with Sabrina's ideas of southern California living. "Good morning, I'm Mrs. Walters and I understand that you would like to rent a house." "Yes, I am, a beach house."

The two women exchanged cordial greetings and handshakes as Mrs. Walters directed them into her office. The office was not as lavish as the waiting room, very ordinary in fact. There was no wallpaper on the walls, no plush carpeting just cold tile and a standard metal frame desk with two arm chairs waiting in front.

This room suits Mrs. Walters very well, plain, and unimaginative. "Please have a seat; it will take me just a minute to pull out some information for you to look at. Is there a certain price range that you have in mind?" "No, cost is not really the issue here. I am looking for a beach house, that's not overly large, to rent for a few months. Nothing fancy; just a comfortable place, for my cat and me."

Upon hearing Sabrina say that price was not important Mrs. Walters began pulling sheets of paper from a different file folder in the cabinet. "Here are a few of the houses that are currently available for a long term lease. If any of them piques your interest, we could go and look at them today."

Sabrina scanned through the information before her. The easiest way was for her to sort them into categories; definite no; possible and last resort. When she was done Sabrina handed the pile of possibilities to Mrs. Walters. "I would like to take a look at these please." "Not a problem we can go right now if you like." "That will be just fine."

Leaving the office, Sabrina quickly checked on Patches, who was asleep on the floor of the front seat, and then settled into the passenger seat of the white Cadillac convertible.

Such a flashy car for such a conservative person, it must be a company car. She probably has a beat up old station wagon parked around back.

Sabrina had picked out six houses to look at, and fortunately they were not all that far apart. Mrs. Walters told her not to make a decision until she had a chance to look at all of them; but that was something that Sabrina had already made up her mind about. She was not about to make a hasty decision concerning a house.

If there is nothing here that I like there would always be another agency to go to. I'm in no hurry.

Mrs. Walters led and Sabrina followed, through all of the six homes. By the time they had reached the last one Sabrina was getting a little tired of hearing about all the features. That was not her concern; she was looking for a place that gave her a good feeling; a place that felt like a home not a show piece. Fortunately, all the homes were fully furnished, some a little more than others.

When they left the last house Mrs. Walters took Sabrina to a little cafe for a glass of iced tea, where she began the conversation. "Did you like any of the houses that we looked at?" "Yes, they are all very lovely homes, but I think that the third one is the one that I like the best. It's not too big, which is good; but it has a real homey feeling to it. When do you think I could move in?" "Today, if you like."

Sabrina could see that the woman's expression had definitely changed from when she first met her just a couple of hours ago. Somehow she almost looked younger. "We'll finish our tea, then head back to the office to get the paper work completed." Mrs. Walters tried not to appear to be anxious, but Sabrina could sense it.

They engaged in some light conversation; Sabrina didn't offer up too many details; this woman was a stranger, and as such not privileged to her life history. They chatted on for a while longer, but Sabrina's thoughts were of the house and a couple of times she found herself completely tuned out to what Mrs. Walters was saying. As they drove back to the office, Mrs. Walters made a point of driving past the house one more time; Sabrina was pleased with her choice.

Once back inside the office Mrs. Walters began to fill out the rental agreement; they read over the standard agreement and Sabrina gave her a check for six months rent. "I will have to contact your bank to verify this check, but it won't take long. Can I get you something to drink while you are waiting?" "No, thank you." Mrs. Walters left the office; Sabrina could hear her talking to the secretary out front. After fifteen minutes, Mrs. Walters returned; she congratulated Sabrina as she handed her the keys to the beach house.

"If you have any questions, or if there is anything that you need, please do not hesitate to give me a call. Here is my card; it has all my phone numbers on it." "Thank you, but I'll be just fine. I will let you know if I am going to stay longer than the six months." Sabrina turned and left the office; the secretary congratulated her as she passed by on her way to the door. She was relieved to be away from Mrs. Walters; despite her prim look, she had found her to be a bit arrogant and pushy, and that did not sit well with her. Fortunately for Sabrina she would not have to deal with her very often.

The opening of the car door startled Patches from his nap and he was quickly onto the seat to get a better look at what was going on. Sabrina reached over and scooped him up into her arms; she gave him a big hug and a kiss. Patches didn't understand her joy but the attention he was getting was not going unnoticed; he nuzzled around her face and purred.

"Oh Patches I have found the most wonderful house for us to live in. It's right on the beach, just like I wanted. We'll be there soon and you can run around all you want. I imagine that you're getting a little sick of this car." Giving him a kiss she placed him back on the seat beside her. "I have to make one more stop first; there is a market not to far from the house, and I had better pick up a few things before we get there."

Slowly browsing through the market, she picked up the necessities as well as some treats. Sabrina enjoyed shopping in American grocery stores, for her they were like department stores; everything you could think of was in there, including a liquor section. She selected a couple bottles of wine and set out toward the check-out, stopping briefly to pick up a couple of treats for Patches as well. The excitement was overwhelming; she couldn't wait to get to the house; catching herself tapping her foot as she waited in the check out line.

The day had gone so quickly and she didn't want to miss the sunset from her new home. The customer in front of her was visiting with the cashier, and that only added to Sabrina's anxiety. Generally, easy going and patient by nature, she did have one pet peeve, and that was having to wait in a line up. The cashier glanced at her, and noticing the annoyed look on her face, quickly finished with the other customer. She greeted Sabrina politely and began scanning through her purchases. Sabrina could only nod her head in acknowledgment; she was pissed off; and the cashier knew it too.

With her packages stored in the trunk; she was all set to start the car when she noticed the motorcycle parked two stalls over.

How beautiful it is, so well taken care of. The paint job is unblemished, and the chrome, blindingly beautiful.

The entire bike sparkled in the sunlight, showing off every feature. It had always been a secret desire of hers to have a motorcycle; but like so many of her dreams it had never come to fruition. Admiring the bike, she fantasized about the man who owned it.

Would he be dressed in a tight black leather outfit, or just plain old jeans and a muscle shirt? Her fantasy didn't last for long, as a man approached the bike; Sabrina gasped slightly, as she looked at the man. He was average height, wearing a pair of tight black denim jeans and a T-shirt, which had the sleeves torn out to expose the tattoos on his arms. His black hair was pulled into a pony tail that hung just below his collar. *Please turn around so I can see your face.*

As if he had heard her silent thought, he turned to look at her. His face was badly scarred on the left side; Sabrina felt a cold spike rush up her spine. Quickly looking away, she started the car, embarrassed that she had been caught staring. She left the parking lot rather quickly; driven by the inner fear that this guy may belong to a gang. She had heard many stories about the bike gangs here, and the last thing she wanted was trouble from one of these guys. She drove on towards her house, but frequently caught herself checking the rear view mirror; just to make sure that he wasn't following her.

Every time she looked, she would reassure herself that she had done nothing to provoke him. *There's no reason for him to follow me. I was only admiring his bike.* Her mind recalled the biker she had seen on the side of the highway after she had left Virginia City; even though she had not clearly seen him, her mind still clung to that image. His large, dark frame, silhouetted by the street lights; just sitting there, staring up at the night sky.

What would make me think of him? He had done nothing special to make his image stand out in my mind so vividly. Was it simply that he aroused my curiosity? He was only a shape in the darkness. She tried to reason it out, with no explainable answers. *He was just a man, resting, fatigued from his journey; nothing more.*

She arrived at her new home with plenty of time to get everything into the house before the sunset. The first thing into the house was Patches. "I'm not going to take a chance on losing you. Sorry old man; this is only for a few minutes." She quickly closed the bathroom door. Sabrina went back to the car and began bringing in the groceries, and the suitcases that filled her trunk.

Within minutes, everything was relocated to the entry hall; she closed and locked the heavy oak door, picked up a bag of groceries and headed for the kitchen. As she made her way down the hall she paused briefly to let Patches out of the bathroom. He wasted no time in making his escape but soon stopped in his tracks, realizing that this wasn't his familiar home. "Come on now, are you going to be my first statue, instead of my pet?" Patches didn't budge, observing his new surroundings.

Sabrina hurried with her tasks, sunset was approaching fast and she wouldn't tolerate missing it. It was nice to be able to rent a house that was fully furnished. Grabbing a blanket from the closet she wandered out to the sun deck; remembering how cold it had been along the Oregon coast, and shivering wasn't going to be part of her plans tonight. She opened the sliding door to the deck, then closed the screen door so that Patches wouldn't get out. The house hadn't been occupied for some time, and it required a good airing to remove the stale scents that still lingered.

What a perfect sun deck, everything you could possibly want and more. Californian's sure know how to live. A large gas barbecue stood against the left hand railing, complimented by a white wrought iron table and chair set. On the right side of the deck was a gate and stairs leading down to the beach. Across the front of the deck was a lounger, and beside the patio door stood another lounger, and two regular white deck chairs. Laying her blanket down on the lounger nearest to the patio door; she strolled over to the white iron railing that embraced the magnificent deck.

Gazing out at the ocean, watching a sea bird gracefully riding the waves; her eyes scanned the beach, both left and right; there was no one.

Maybe these people have grown so accustom to the ocean that they don't bother with it anymore. Her eyes wandered towards the houses. *There are no lights on in any of these houses, how strange? These beautiful homes can't be merely summer homes? Maybe they are out for the evening; but all of them; there is no point in puzzling over it.*

She imagined the people who lived in these houses. *Maybe they're movie actors; or singers, and they're just away on a tour.*

Sabrina felt a shiver go up her spine; it made her entire body shudder. She wasn't cold; it was a feeling of uneasiness, thinking that she may be all alone out here. Her thoughts raced wildly from one chilling thought to another.

What if someone broke in? What if? "Stop it; you have nothing to worry about." She was trying hard to reassure herself. *There are first-rate locks on the doors and windows, as well as an alarm system. As long as I remember to keep things locked up at night, and while I'm out, there is nothing to worry about. This is where I need to be, I don't understand why, but there is something about this place; I felt it from the first moment I saw the house.*

The house was nothing spectacular; considerably smaller than the others along the street; but there was a feeling that she couldn't shake. Hugging herself tightly, she returned her attentions to the gentle rolling surf; standing motionless for a few more minutes, before returning to the house to get herself a glass of wine, and to give Patches his dinner.

On her way back outside, she stopped and put a CD into the stereo. *A little mood music couldn't hurt.* The music started off very loud, it surprised her; she quickly turned the volume down. "Don't want to disturb the neighbors," she said looking out at the houses on either side. *Still no lights.* She turned the music up a bit louder and went outside.

Placing her glass of wine on a little table that stood beside the lounger, she picked up the blanket, and was about to sit down when she noticed a light in the sixth house down from hers. "Well, I'm not completely alone." She stared at the windows until she saw movement inside.

With a more relaxed feeling, she stretched out on the lounger and covered herself with the blanket. The sun was going down, and the warm orange glow gave her a feeling of contentment; she sipped her wine, and became absorbed in the music that played in the background.

The sunset was as spectacular as she had hoped for. She felt so privileged to be viewing such a wondrous event; the ocean slowly teasing the sun into its depths. It was hypnotic, like a drug to her; she was calm and relaxed; she began drifting off to sleep. The combination of the wine, the blanket and the intoxicating breeze coming off the water had succeeded in bringing her body, and mind into this peaceful state. Drifting in and out, she was startled into alertness; she sat upright, listening.

What was it that startled me? She looked at the door for Patches, but he was nowhere to be seen. Then she heard it again; a mans voice called to her from the direction of the beach. The cold chill returned to her spine as she stood up. Wrapping the blanket around her; she cautiously moved toward the railing, hesitating with every step. The voice called again. "Hello?"

Her eyes strained to see through the darkness, searching for the voice. She could see nothing. The lights from the deck formed an abyss of blackness beyond the railing. The voice called to her again, and this time she established its location. Straining her eyes, trying to pierce the darkness; finally something moved below her on the beach.

She could barely make out the shape of the man that stood calling to her. Her heart was pounding hard; she pulled the blanket tighter across her chest. The voice spoke again. "Hey, how are you?" It was a deep gravely voice. "You must be new in town?" Sabrina was frozen in place, still trying to see some details of this person; this man. The chills were creeping faster and faster up her spine; thoughts raced through her mind.

Is this the biker from earlier? Had he followed me? How fast could I run to the safety of the house, before he overtook me?

The voice broke through the darkness again. "Do you talk? I'm sorry if I scared you, but I just thought I would be neighborly and stop and say hi. I live in that house down there." "That big house over there, the one with all the lights on is that yours?" "Oh, so you can talk; and yes that's my house. So would you mind if I came up for a visit?" Without any hesitation she blurted out her answer. "Not right now."

She hurried toward the patio door. Before she shut the patio door she called back to the man on the beach. "Maybe another time would be good but not now." Not waiting for a reply, she shut the door and locked it; pulling the curtains shut as well. Her heart still pounding, she ran to the alarm box and set the system for the doors and windows.

Dropping her blanket on the floor, she went to the dining room to shut the curtains on that window. She hesitated a moment. The figure of the man walking along the beach had caught her attention. She continued to watch, still trying to see some features, but couldn't make out anything. Suddenly he stopped, and it appeared to Sabrina that he had turned around. She couldn't make out his face, but she knew that he was staring at her. He took a step and she closed the curtains. Running frantically from room to room, she closed all the curtains and made sure that the windows were all securely locked.

With her task complete, she returned to the living room and fell onto the couch. Laying back, trying to regain her composure she heard a noise from behind her. Spontaneous reaction made her leap to her feet; fully expecting to see someone standing there. A loud sigh passed through her lips when she realized that the noise was only Patches playing with his new toy around a table leg. "You're a silly fool."

Knowing that the house was secure, she went to bed. Sleep didn't come easily tonight; she turned the light out, but soon turned it back on again. Every sound made her nervous; every creak of the house made her stomach jump. She finally succumbed to sleep just before dawn.

Chapter 3

Sabrina finally came to consciousness after being repeatedly nudged by Patches. Rolling onto her back, she stretched; lifting the sheet up for him to crawl under. He curled up tight beside her purring. Stretching again she rubbed her hands across her eyes and looked at the alarm clock 11:45 was what stared back at her.

How could I have slept so late? So what, I can stay up late, and sleep late, whenever I want too now, no more being pestered about how I'm wasting the best part of the day.

Patting Patches, who was still pretending to sleep, she went to take a shower. The European style shower had been the first thing that had caught her attention when she viewed the house earlier, she couldn't wait to try it out. Stepping into the shower, her body was instantly aroused by the way the water sprayed onto different parts of her body. *How delightful this would be if only there was someone to share it with.*

The warm water had swept away all of her tension from the night before; she felt invigorated. Pulling her hair back into a ponytail she set off to begin her day. Feeling a little silly about her behavior last night, she resolved to put it behind her. *This isn't going to turn into a prison.*

Retracing her steps of last night, she opened the curtains, and admired the view. The house had an appealing view from every window; but the layout of this house, and the ones on either side, in no way compromised each other. None of the windows allowed you to look into the other homes. They had been built very close together, and privacy was obviously a very important factor.

On her way through the kitchen, she had stopped to pick up an apple; having only taken a couple of bites by the time she reached the patio door. She gripped it in her teeth while she pulled open the curtains. The sight before her took her by surprise. Sometime during the course of the night, the tide had gone out and had left behind it a vast expanse of beach.

She could barely make out the tiny waves that slowly pushed their way back towards the house. A flock of little birds was scurrying back and forth across the sand, stopping only seconds as they pecked for food.

This is about as close to heaven as I'm gonna get. She was about to return to the kitchen when she spotted something resting beside her wine glass from last night; it brought the chill back to her spine. On the table was a single white rose tied with a tiny red bow. Beneath the rose she could see an envelope. Satisfied that no one was out there, she carefully opened the patio door and stepped outside. Still scrutinizing the area, she cautiously picked up the rose and inhaled its sweet scent. Putting it down, along with her apple, she picked up the envelope.

Maybe it's from Mrs. Walters? That must be it. She must have dropped by this morning and since the curtains were still shut assumed that I wasn't up yet. That's it. Smiling to herself, she opened the envelope and removed the note from inside.

The smile disappeared; it wasn't from Mrs. Walters. Sabrina read the note aloud. "I hope that you will forgive me for last night. It wasn't my intention to upset you; all I was trying to do was be friendly; and to welcome you to the beach. I realized after I got home that you must not have been able to see me because of the lights from your house. I am very sorry if I frightened you. I won't try to visit you again; but please feel free to come down to my place, strictly on your own terms. I will be here for the next three weeks and then I have to go away on business. Please, don't be afraid of me; I promise that I will keep my distance. Again my deepest apologies for what happened. Sincerely, Sean."

Sabrina's mind momentarily went blank her body numb. *I can't believe it. For this guy to do something like this, he must really be sincere, but words can hide lies, and I'm not about to rush over to his house and possibly find myself in a compromising situation. I can afford to take it slow, test this man, to see if he truly means what he has written. Sean. What is the meaning of his name? Oh I remember it means God's grace. We'll see.*

Folding the note, she placed it into her pocket. Picking up the rose, she turned and looked down the beach towards his house, not at all surprised to see him standing on the deck. He waved at her, but she didn't respond. She went back into the house to make herself something to eat. Taking her snack into the bedroom with her, nibbling at it while she unpacked her suitcases.

Her clothes hardly took up any space in the enormous walk-in closet; which also had a dressing area across from the drawers and racks; a multi-directional, full length mirror and a small settee. The bedroom itself was massive, with the large king size four-poster bed as the center piece. There was a gas fireplace along one wall, a love seat, and a recliner across the corner.

Back home people were fortunate to get an apartment this size, let alone just one room. I really like this house, it makes me feel like Cinderella, only without a Prince. This clean, white California home, with its bright red tile roof, here I can be anyone I want to be; imagined or real. This will be a good place to dream.

Finished with her snack and all of her unpacking, she decided to go for a walk on the beach. Looking towards Sean's house, she decided to go the other way. Having only taken a few steps, she stopped to slip off her shoes. The sand was warm on her feet and she wiggled her toes until they were buried in the warmth. The wind coming in off the water tossed her hair over her shoulder. She walked out to where the water was coming in over the sand; it lapped at her feet. Every once in a while a clam would squirt at her through the sand, annoyed that she had disturbed its resting place.

When she finally stopped to take her bearings, she noticed that she was quite a long way from her house; she could tell which one was hers, by the windsock that oscillated on the deck. *Better head back.* As she made her way back along the beach, she took careful notice of the homes along the way. Every one of them had their curtains drawn shut; some of them had driftwood littered up to, and under their decks. *It appears as if these homes have not been occupied for some time now.*

Getting nearer to her own house, she looked down the beach towards Sean's again; making sure that he wasn't outside. Her eyes roamed over the houses between them. They too were giving the appearance of being empty of occupants. One of them even had heavy shutters covering its many windows.

How strange, that no one is around. How could people have homes like this on the ocean, and not want to live in them all year around? Standing by the railing, a mischievous smile came across her face. *If I have this much privacy then I could really get a good tan by sunbathing in the nude.* Her gaze again relocated to Sean's house. *If he had meant what he said, then he wouldn't be a bother, besides, he said he was leaving in three weeks anyway. Better not to tempt fate, a bathing suit will do just fine; at least until he's gone.* She went back inside the house to change; entirely unaware that she was being observed from close by; and it wasn't Sean.

Concealed amongst the shrubs of the house next door, was a man in his mid twenties; his heart pounding loudly, as he sat crouched, watching her. *I'm gonna have that bitch.* He almost gave himself away, when she returned to the deck, wearing a bathing suit. He was so turned on by her that he momentarily lost his balance, catching himself before he fell over into the pathway. Sweat began to bead on his forehead. His palms were wet too; he rubbed them down over the front of his jeans slowly, paying great attention to the tightness of his pants. He squeezed his crotch. *This is for you bitch.*

He had followed her home from the market the day before; he had caught her staring at him, while he readied his bike. She had not noticed him before that moment, but he had been watching her in the market; fantasizing over her; careful to keep his distance as he followed her. *Soon this bitch will know me and she'll never forget me.* While watching her, he decided that he would wait until he was absolutely sure that she was alone, that there was no one else around.

Then I will have her; with no one to hear her, I could do what ever I wanted to her; without interruption. She could cry and scream but it would be no use. Thoughts raged through his mind; thoughts of having that body solely for his deranged pleasure. His eyes rolled back; he rubbed the front of his jeans harder and faster.

Having treated herself to a new bikini, Sabrina felt that this was most definitely the perfect place to wear it; a place where she wouldn't be hit on by every guy that passed by; like at Lake Tahoe. Reclining the lounger back, she spread a blanket over it; lying down, she closed her eyes. The warmth from the sun, and the wind off the water soon lulled her into a peaceful sleep. She stirred once; only to turn over onto her stomach, and was soon asleep again.

She was awakened by a dog barking. Rising up, she turned towards the sound, and saw a golden retriever chasing after a ball; she also saw a man running along behind the dog. He stopped and looked up at her; never speaking, he only waved to her, then continued on his way. She watched, but did not acknowledge his gesture.

It's him, Sean, from last night. In the daylight he doesn't look so intimidating. His long bleach blonde hair, tied back into a ponytail; his tall, darkly tanned, well-muscled body, covered only by a pair of tight fitting black shorts. The sun sparkled off of his body. *He must have been out for a swim*. When he returned to his house, he waved to her again, from the deck, but still she didn't respond.

He looks perfectly harmless, then why is the little voice inside my head telling me that I should be wary. Dismissing her annoying voices, she went back into the house to change.

The man, obscured in the shrubs, hadn't taken any notice of Sean or his dog; his mind was solidly consumed by his fantasies of Sabrina, and what he was going to do to her.

The end of the first week was approaching rapidly. Sabrina had not left her home for anything. She spent languid mornings writing a letter to Marion and afternoons basking in the sun, and nights contemplating the sunsets. Every afternoon Sean would go by on his customary run; he would wave at her as he passed by. She had finally begun waving back to him only two days ago. She had acquired a sense of comfort, feeling that he had genuinely meant what he had written. He would not encroach on her space unless she invited him. Sitting at the dining room table, she finished her letter, and began working on a grocery list. Patches was running low on food and so was she.

"A quick trip into town and I'll still have the afternoon to work on my tan," she said to Patches as he strolled along the table top. She lifted him off onto the floor and went around the house making sure that everything was secured. As she drove past the other homes, she checked to see if there were any cars around; seeing none, she resigned herself to the fact that she would probably be alone until sometime in the spring.

With the market in view she remembered the biker; how he had scared her, yet secretly thrilled her at the same time. She remembered his tight jeans, his large arms.

How exciting it must be to ride a motorcycle. Her mind wandered the open roads, as she sauntered through the grocery store. Pausing at the wine section of the store, an idea formed in her head.

Today I will make the first move; I will invite Sean up for a drink. If I am going to meet any one, I guess it's going to be my decision as to when and how. As she cruised through the aisles, she purposefully selected some specialty items. *These should come in handy just in case I have to make dinner for two.* Sabrina was just about to the cashier when she remembered that she hadn't picked up food for Patches; so preoccupied with her daydream, that she had forgotten about her best friend, and that would never do.

Guiding her cart back to the pet aisle; she stopped at the magazines and books; selecting a new novel for her evening reading. As she leaned over to put it into the cart a magazine attracted her attention. It wasn't really the magazine, but the picture on the front cover that actually made her look; she stared at it.

It looks so much like Sean; but it couldn't be. She had only seen him from a distance, and this picture showed a man with blonde wavy hair framing his face. Placing the magazine back on the rack, she didn't give it another thought. She picked up the cat chow for Patches, plus a couple of cans of tuna for a treat.

If I'm going to be entertaining then I had better include that fur ball, or he will become a complete nuisance. I'm used to him sitting on the table, but other people may not be so receptive or forgiving.

Patches was waiting just inside the door when she got home; his habitual place; even here. He had settled in quite nicely, but Sabrina was still a bit leery of letting him outside just yet. With her groceries unpacked, she tossed the empty paper bag onto the floor. Patches was there immediately, circling around and around the bag before crawling inside. Sabrina touched the bag with her foot and it promptly flipped over, writhing and wriggling. "That should keep you happy for a while." She went to change into her swimsuit.

There is still plenty of time before Sean goes by on his afternoon run. Putting a CD into the stereo she took up her place on the lounger; still completely unaware that her actions were closely supervised.

The man had returned unnoticed. Coming and going at deviating times all week, and she hadn't suspected anything. Concealing his bike down the street, so she would not hear him arrive or leave. He had her routine down perfectly; knowing every move she made all day, and all night. Even going so far as to check the houses next door to hers, just to make sure that there was no one around. He didn't want anything to disturb him, or his plans; he was going to have her, and he was going to relish every glorious minute of it.

I could remain here for days with her; until I've had enough of her. This is incredible luck, finding a woman alone, on a deserted beach, how perfect. He licked his lips and shuddered. Sweat was forming on his brow; he wiped it away with the back of his hand. *I've waited long enough; today I will have her.* His thoughts instantly aroused him. *She will make a mistake and I'll know it.*

Sabrina basked in the sun all that afternoon, trying to read the book that she had bought, but that was a futile endeavor; her mind had but one thought.

How should I start the conversation with Sean? Rehearsing the speech repeatedly in her mind, she got up a couple of times to scan the beach.

No sign of him but it's still early. Stop being so impatient. If it is meant to be, it will happen; stop worrying about it.

The time dragged on and on, and still no sign of Sean. *I had better go and put on a shirt; it just doesn't seem respectable to greet someone wearing only a bathing suit, even though we live at the beach.* Her self conscious nature had won over. Still role playing the conversation in her mind she neglected to lock the screen door.

Her every move had been under careful scrutiny, and when she went inside the house he immediately detected her oversight. Without hesitation he leapt from his hiding place, quickly climbing up the side of the deck; pausing briefly near the patio door, listening for any movement inside. Hearing nothing, he peered inside. The living room was empty; she was nowhere to be seen. Painstakingly slow, he slid open the screen door and entered the house; his heart pounding in his chest.

The rush of adrenaline precipitated his gait across the room, to her bedroom. He could hear her moving about in the room, quietly humming to herself. *I'll give you something to sing about, ya bitch.* He entered the room; he couldn't see her; frantically searching every corner. *Where are you?* He heard a noise coming from the closet; he pulled a knife out of his belt and waited.

Sabrina came out from behind the closet door, wearing a long white gauze shirt. Without a sound, he grabbed her from behind, covering her mouth with his free hand. She tried to fight him, but he had her at a disadvantage. Terror ripped through her body as she saw his other hand slide over her breasts; the icy cold knife blade against her skin. "I've been watching you for a very long time, and now you're gonna be mine. I'm gonna have you, and there's no one around who can stop me. If you scream, or make one single sound I'll kill you," he said holding the knife up before her.

Sabrina stared at the blade, so clean and shiny, reflecting the tiniest of light rays into glistening star bursts. Still holding his hand over her mouth, he turned her around to face him. "You won't scream, will you?" Sabrina shook her head no. He slowly removed his hand from her mouth; dragging his raspy palm over her cheek. His kiss was unyielding, forcing his tongue deep inside her mouth; it made her gag. His unshaven face burned against her skin.

Stopping to take a breath, he moved her towards the bed, and with immense force pushed her backwards, leaving the tattered remnants of her shirt still clutched in his hand. Sabrina scrambled away from him, seeking refuge at the head of the bed. The recognition flashed in her mind; the tattoos, the scar on his face. *He's the biker I saw at the market.*

Standing at the end of the bed; his knife still firmly clutched in his fist; he observed her movements. She was paralyzed with fear. Crawling onto the bed, he pulled her down under him, his legs straddling her body restricting her movement. Reaching behind her he grabbed a pillow, pulling off the cover. The distinct sound of cloth ripping sent tremors through her body. With his knife he slashed several long pieces of cloth.

Sabrina couldn't speak; the words were cemented deep in her throat. When he grabbed her arm she cringed. He tied the cloth to her wrist, then to the post of the bed. Repeating the motions until she was completely bound, immobile and prone, thoroughly helpless beneath him. Her body trembled uncontrollably; she tried to speak, but he was on top of her; his vile fetid breath made her sick to her stomach. "Have you forgotten what I said? Not a sound, remember?" Sabrina could only nod her head, but inside she was screaming.

He kissed her with intense cruelty, she tasted blood; he had bitten through her lip. Leaning back, he studied her; slowly running the blade of the knife down her throat, across her heaving chest; cutting the straps of her swimsuit. She felt the cold steel in between her breasts and with one brisk jerk the blade sliced through the center of her top.

Pulling the remnants of her suit off of her breasts he fondled them, kissed them. She felt his teeth biting at her nipples. Never speaking, he only uttered bestial sounds as his stubbly unshaven face moved across her stomach. Unable to look at him; Sabrina alienated herself, staring at the ceiling, thinking of anything but the harsh reality of the moment.

The frigid steel was against her skin again; he was cutting off her bikini bottoms. In her mind she cried out for him to stop, for this to be over, to awaken from this distressing dream. When she felt his tongue touch her skin, she jumped. He slapped her leg cruelly. The sharp sting made her cry. "Lie still, bitch!" he snarled. She complied as best she could, but fear had her shaking uncontrollably. He lay beside her; she heard the zipper on his jeans and felt his hard erect cock pressing against her thigh as he licked at her breast, while forcefully fondling the warmth between her legs.

The soul inside this body screamed out to the mate. It didn't want this to be happening. It sought forgiveness from the other; the comforting embrace of their timeless love.

His fingers were inside her. Sabrina tensed as he prodded deeper. In a swift move he was on top of her, squeezing her breasts as he spoke. "You're never gonna forget this ya bitch." When he forced her legs apart, her fears intensified all at once and with all the power that she could muster up, she screamed. He slapped her hard across the face, making her lip bleed again. Once she had released that first scream she couldn't stop. He hit her again and again, even after she slipped into unconsciousness.

Sean was out for his afternoon run, with his dog Rex. As he passed Sabrina's place, he thought it strange that she was not out on the deck. Not giving it another thought he continued on his way. On his way back home, he threw a ball; Rex would run after it, bringing it back to his master to throw again.

Sean threw the ball again, but this time Rex didn't go after it; this time he ran towards Sabrina's and climbed the stairs to the deck. Sean called him, but Rex did not respond to his master's voice. He went after him; at the top of the stairs he found Rex pawing and whining at the gate. "What's the matter with you boy?" The dog continued his frantic pawing. Sean grabbed Rex by the collar and was attempting to pull him away when he heard Sabrina's screams. Without thinking Sean leapt over the gate and was inside the house.

The screams had abruptly stopped, but there were noises coming from the direction of the bedroom. Racing across the room, he entered the bedroom just in time to see the man raise his knife high above Sabrina's body. Sean took a running leap and tackled the man off onto the floor. Caught by surprise, the attacker had no time to respond. The strength of Sean's blow rendered the man unconscious. Working quickly Sean untied Sabrina's legs and used the cloth to bind the man on the floor before he came around again.

Working at a frantic pace, Sean dialed 911, requesting an ambulance and the police to her address. *I have to do something for her.* Finding a sheet in the closet, he covered her body. As he pulled the sheet up, he noticed the bleeding bite marks on her breasts, and the bruises that were beginning to form around them, and on her face. He laid the sheet on her, and untied her wrists. She was still unconscious, as was her attacker.

Holding her limp hand in his, he waited impatiently for the police to arrive, partly blaming himself for this horrible scene.

If only I hadn't scared her so bad last week, maybe this would not have happened. Maybe we would have become friends. Maybe this, maybe that; it was still too late to have prevented this. Sean gently squeezed her hand. "I promise you; you won't have to be alone; I'll make sure of that." The sound of the sirens was getting closer, the wailing echoing off of the cliffs across the road.

The police entered first, wasting no time in securing Sabrina's attacker and taking him away. The man, still groggy from the blow delivered by Sean, staggered as the two policemen dragged him from the room. Sean overheard one of the officer's speak to the half naked man.

"You've really done it this time Frank. You're going away for a very long time, you sorry son of a bitch." As the officers passed Sean, Frank looked up at him. "Hey man, that guy broke my jaw." "For Christ's sake Frank shut up! You're damn lucky that's all he did to you," the officer said giving Frank a shove toward the door.

Sean paid little attention to the man with the officers, his thoughts were trained on Sabrina, and the paramedics that were tending to her. His mind raced like a train out of control. *Was I too late? Did that bastard rape her? Someone so beautiful didn't deserve this.*

Staring at her limp form; the sheet that he had placed on her was now dotted with blood. A lump came up in his throat; he didn't know whether to weep for her, or to go and throw up. He swallowed hard; at the same moment a deep voice from behind him broke the tension.

"Excuse me sir; I'm Sergeant Doyle. I understand that you are the person responsible for catching the guy who did this?" "Yes," Sean answered. "I know that it may seem cut and dried to you, but I'm still going to need a formal statement from you. Let's go into the living room, and let the paramedics do their job."

Sean didn't want to leave, his gut kept telling him to stay with her, but the Sergeant had placed his hand on Sean's shoulder and was directing him out of the room. The paramedics performed their examination of Sabrina very methodically. With the guidance of a Doctor, via a radio, they began to awaken her.

In the living room Sean paced back and forth in front of the patio door, recounting the incident to the Sergeant. "What's going to happen to her now?" Sean asked. "Well, they'll try to bring her around before they take her to the hospital. She's going to need to have a Doctor's exam to find out if she was raped; and we're gonna need photos for the Judge." "Is she going to have to go to court?" "Heaven's no, thanks to you, she'll never have to go through that ordeal. This guy has a record so long that nothing will keep him out of jail this time. Besides, he's violated his parole, and that gives him an automatic ticket back to jail. You're a real hero, Mr. Malloy. You risked your life to save her. God only knows what that piece of trash would have done if you hadn't happened by when you did."

Sean was about to speak when the air was cut by Sabrina's piercing cry. He ran to the bedroom, stopping in the doorway. She was awake, and fighting the paramedics. The Sergeant was right behind him, with his hand on Sean's shoulder holding him back. He shrugged off the officer's hold and moved to Sabrina; she was hysterical. Her hands lashed out at the paramedics every time they came close to her. She had pushed herself up to the head of the bed, and in doing so had lost the protection of the sheet. She sat, bare to the waist, her knees drawn up towards her chest; crying hard.

Sean managed to grab her flailing hands, but that just made her struggle harder. Sitting beside her, he spoke softly. "It's okay; you're safe now. No one is going to harm you," he said. Through the tears, and the fear, Sabrina heard Sean's soft comforting words, she cautiously looked up at him. She knew his face and in his blue eyes she could see kindness, and concern.

Feeling her arms relax under his grip, he let go, bringing her close to him, cradling her like a child. Pulling the sheet up over her, he wrapped his arms around her quaking body. Her tears slowly subsided, but her sobs sent shudders throughout her body. She was in shock; he held her tight.

The paramedics, who had stepped back to talk to the Sergeant, returned. "Miss, we have to take you to the hospital now." Sabrina concealed her face against Sean. "No, no, no!" she pleaded loudly. Sean felt her tears against his skin; he hugged her tighter. Looking at the paramedics, then at the Sergeant; he knew what he had to do. Reaching his hand around he found her face; lightly brushing away the tears from her cheek he spoke calmly to her. "You have to go with them; you need to see a Doctor. You'll be all right; I'll make sure of that because I'm going with you."

The Sergeant could see the determination on Sean's face; he nodded his approval to the paramedics and left the room. The paramedic touched her arm and she tensed. "Miss, you're gonna have to get onto the stretcher, so we can take you out to the ambulance." Sabrina pressed her face against Sean's chest; he motioned the paramedics to back off. Repositioning his hold on her, he rose up, lifting Sabrina up off the bed, carrying her out of the house to the waiting ambulance.

With her resting on the stretcher, he sat down opposite her. Brushing the hair from her face, he pulled the blanket up close to her neck and picked up her hand. The ride to the hospital seemed to take forever, the wail of the siren adding to Sabrina's pounding headache; her emotions were running wild. Sean squeezed her hand wiping away the tears as best he could. *I want to hold her, to ease her fears.*

At the hospital, Sean stayed with her in the examination room, holding her hand. The Doctor loudly announced that Sean would have to leave the room. Sabrina tightened her hand around Sean's and tried to speak. "No, I want him to stay; please let him stay," she whispered hoarsely. Her mouth was dry, permeated by a horrid taste of that man in her mouth.

The Doctor repeated his command more sternly; Sean looked at him and made his own announcement. "I'm staying. I promised her that I wouldn't leave and I am not going to break my promise." With that said, he pulled a stool over with his foot, and sat down next to her; his back to the medical staff.

The Doctor proceeded with his examination; annoyed at the tone Sean had taken with him. Sabrina's feet were put into a set of stirrups. When her knees were spread apart she began to shake. Sean saw the fear on her face. "Look at me. I want you to focus only on me. No one is going to harm you. Just look at me, and listen to my voice," he said calmly. Sabrina stared at this man who was comforting her. She knew by his hair that it was Sean. She was still very aware of what the Doctor was doing but concentrating on Sean's face made her feel more at ease. *How kind he looks, how concerned. I need to trust someone.*

When the examination was completed, the Doctor came up behind Sean, looking at Sabrina. "Ms. Scott." Sabrina was preparing herself for the worst; she tightened her grip on Sean's hand. "Ms. Scott, you have some minor cuts and bruises and you're going to be quite sore for a few days. I'll give you a prescription for some pain medication and a few days of sleeping pills. I suggest that you use ice on your bruises, it will help them to disappear faster." Before he left, Sean turned to speak to him. "Was she?" "No, Ms. Scott, there is no evidence of rape. You were lucky. You can go home anytime you're ready; I see no reason for you to stay."

A nurse stayed in the room, quietly cleaning up the work area. Without warning Sabrina's tears began again. Sean helped her to sit up. He put his arms around her and held her tightly until he felt her relax. "Are you ready to get out of here?" Sean asked. Sabrina nodded, but then looked down at the sheet that covered her. Sean rolled his eyes back and smiled at her. "I guess you need some clothes to wear? Let me make a phone call," he said going to the phone on the far wall of the exam room.

"Hey Charles, it's me. I need you to bring the car down to the hospital emergency ward. No, I'm fine. Oh, and bring that blue track suit from the closet. See you soon, bye." He turned back to Sabrina. "Charles will be here soon and I'll take you home. Is there anything that you want while we're waiting?" "I'm thirsty," she answered her voice still hoarse. "Okay, I'll see what I can find. I won't be gone long. You just lay back and rest." He lightly brushed her forehead with the back of his hand before leaving to go find a vending machine.

She was startled when Sean came back into the room; he had a can of soda in one hand, and a blue track suit in the other. "Charles is here with the car and you can wear this to go home," he said. Taking it from him, she laid it down beside her, what she really desired was the can of pop he had in his other hand; she reached for it. "I'm sorry," he said handing her the can.

Opening it, she drank nonstop until it was nearly empty. She was so thirsty. Her throat was dry, even breathing made it burn. "Thank you," she said. He smiled at her. "Get yourself dressed and we can get out of this place. I'll wait outside for you." "Stay with me." "Okay." Turning around, Sean gave her what little privacy he could.

"I'm ready," she announced, sliding off the side of the table to stand. Her knees buckled and he caught her before she fell. Lifting her into his arms, he carried her out of the room and down the hall to the exit. People in the hallway stopped and pointed; whispering amongst themselves. *This must look strange; being carried out of the hospital instead of in.* Little did she know that this was the farthest thing from these people's minds; they recognized Sean.

As they reached the exit door Sabrina spoke. "I think I can walk to the car from here. Where is it?" Sean turned her around. "It's right there, and I'm not going to take a chance on you falling." She looked in the direction that Sean had pointed her, but all she could see was a small black limo. Pulling forward, it stopped in front of them; a man stepped out from behind the wheel and trotted around to the passenger side; he opened the door and waited. Sean stepped toward the open door; Sabrina looked at him with surprise. He smiled at her, as he placed her inside on the back seat. Intrigued, she stared at him out the corner of her eye.

Who is this man, this angel that has liberated me from this horrible ordeal? Her head still ached horribly. She ran her hands through her hair, trying to soothe the intense throbbing. Sleep was beckoning to her, the sedative was working quickly; her head rolled to one side.

"Tired?" Sean asked. A nod was her only response; even opening her eyes was a painful struggle. Sean reached across to a compartment opposite him, removing a small pillow and a blanket. Nuzzling her head into the pillow, she pulled the blanket up close to her face. Giving into the effects of the sedative, she was no longer aware of the movement of the limo, or of Sean's voice. "Sleep my pretty lady, sleep," he whispered. Feelings of rage seethed in his gut.

How could that bastard do this to her? I wish that he would have fought back, given me an excuse to beat the hell out of him. In all the fights that I've been in over the years, never, until now, have I had such feelings of anger toward anyone. Breathing deeply, he forced himself to relax.

When Charles opened the door of the limo Sean was much calmer. "Will you be needing my assistance sir?" "No, Charles, I can manage." Sean leaned into the limo and picked up Sabrina's limp, sleeping body. He carried her into the house, up the stairs to his bedroom. Repositioning the blanket over her, he left to go and find Charles.

Charles was waiting for Sean in the living room. "Sir, is that the young lady who lives in the small house up the beach?" "Yes, Charles it is." "May I ask what happened sir?" "An animal, Charles, a pure, unadulterated, vicious, bastard of an animal is what happened to her. I really don't want to get into the details right now, all I want is for you to go down to her house and make sure that it is all locked up. Oh, I noticed that she had a cat, could you find it, and bring it and Rex home. When you've completed that I would appreciate it if you would take a few days off, right now the fewer people that are around her the better." Sean handed Charles a set of keys that he had found in Sabrina's purse.

Feeling at loose ends, Sean fell back onto the couch. He was weary, it wasn't late, but tonight he felt emotionally drained; it had been a very intense day. He looked at the purse that lay on the coffee table; the wallet peaked out from inside. His curiosity being what it was, he picked it up and opened it, taking out the drivers license he read aloud. "Sabrina Scott, six feet tall, blonde hair, blue eyes." He put the license back inside the wallet, but not before he had another long look at the picture. Pushing everything back inside the purse, he took it up to the bedroom.

Standing at the foot of the bed, he watched her sleep. *All curled up like a child. She'll probably sleep for the rest of the night.* He made himself comfortable in the big chair in the corner of the room. It wasn't long before his own exhaustion claimed him, and his fantasies became his reality.

In the darkness of his bedroom, Warlock listened intently for what it was that had awakened him. Something had brought him out of a sound sleep so suddenly that he was wide awake.

The cries of the other had disturbed the soul with such an urgency. It had felt the pain, suffering along with it. This body has to know; the pain must stop, and it will once they were reunited.

Reaching over to the bedside lamp, he felt a sharp pain in his right chest. Running his hand over the area only intensified the feeling; he went into the bathroom to investigate. It took his eyes a few seconds to adjust to the light. "What the hell is this?" What he saw when he looked in the mirror confused him. There was blood on his lip and a large red mark on the right side of his chest; encompassing the nipple and a wide area toward the sternum.

I haven't been in the ring for over a week. Is this some sort of delayed reaction? He tried to think back, but he couldn't remember being injured there. The blood on his lip was easier to understand. *I must have bitten it in my sleep.* He wiped it clean.

Dismissing the entire episode, he crawled back into bed. Laying on his back, he soon began to drift into that void, still partially conscious, but traveling closer to the threshold of sleep.

The wind blew gently outside, until it found the open window of his bedroom. A strong gust rushed into the room, like an unwanted intruder; the curtains flapped frantically. Warlock was brought back to consciousness, as the wind swirled over him, teasing at the sheet that covered him. He listened as the gusts continued to invade his room, but there was something more; there was a sound being carried by the wind, the sound of a woman crying. It was faint, distant, but it was unmistakable, the woeful lamentation of a woman in pain, crying out to him in the darkness. His fist pounded the mattress.

Damn this! It's just the wind, nothing more. Turning on his side, he pulled the spare pillow over. Covering his ear; it hushed the sound of the wind enough for him to get to sleep; only to have it return to haunt his dreams. He dreamed of her again, but the love was not there this time; he felt the physical pain and the deep sadness. It kept him moving all night, tossing and turning, trying to get to her, to comfort her; but she was just beyond his reach.

Hours had passed; the sun had begun its trek across the sky. The sedative had begun to wear off, and Sabrina's mind was vividly recounting the events of her attack. She cried out, not completely asleep, but yet not fully awake either. Sean was at her side in seconds. "Sabrina, you're okay. There's no one here to hurt you. Can you hear me Sabrina?"

Her mind remembered that voice; she opened her eyes. "Where am I?" she asked. "You're at my place. I thought it best, considering your situation. My name is Sean Malloy. You know I've never had the opportunity to properly introduce myself. How are you feeling this morning?" "Stiff and sore," she replied, sitting herself up. "Can I get you anything?" "No, thank you, not right now. I would like to take a shower though." "Sure, the bathroom is right through there," he said pointing across the room. "There's a clean robe behind the door, and fresh towels on the counter."

Helping her to her feet, she wobbled momentarily; he secured his arm around her. "Are you sure you're okay?" Sean asked. Sabrina could hear the concern in his voice. "Yeah; I guess it's still some of the effects of that shot; I'll be fine." She was reassuring herself more than Sean.

Sean departed only when he heard the shower start. She paid little attention to the elaborate room. The warm water washed over her head and down her back; the warmth soon vanquished the tension that burned in her shoulders. Picking up the bar of soap, she turned to wet down the front of her body; the water stung hard as it splashed against her breasts. Looking down, for the first time she saw the cuts and bruises that were causing her such pain.

Frantically she took stock of the rest of her body. Dark red marks encompassed her ankles and wrists, covering her face with her hands her fingers felt the thick scab that had formed on her lip and the swelling on her cheek. The memories of last night were rushing into her mind like a film in fast forward. She slid down the shower wall. Crouched in the corner, she tried to force these images from her mind.

Sean was on his way to the bedroom when he heard her cries from out in the hallway. Running into the bathroom, he grabbed the robe from the door and shut off the shower. Pulling the robe tightly around her, he held her close to him. She pulled away from him in a jerk. "I remember! I remember what happened, all of it." A single tear rolled down her cheek. "It's okay. Do you remember what the Doctor said?" Sean asked. She looked at him with a blank expression. "You weren't raped. Did you hear me? You were not raped." Sabrina melted into his arms, accepting his embrace and his comforting manner. There was a sense of security, even in the arms of this stranger.

He has a kind face, but who is he really? Who is this Guardian Angel that was sent to me? She closed her eyes in a silent prayer of thanks.

The days passed slowly; Sabrina spent a considerable amount of time sleeping. There had been little or no conversation between herself and Sean; she wasn't ready to talk, and he didn't press. The physical reminders of the ordeal were healing well, the swelling around her jaw had gone down, and the cut on her lip was now barely visible.

Standing in front of the bathroom mirror, she took a deep breath and gave herself a lecture. "It's time to go home, you're all right now, and there's no need to burden Sean any further. You weren't raped; and what's a few bruises anyway." The reflection in the mirror agreed with her. "That's settled; I'm going home. Besides I need some clothes of my own to wear." She headed down stairs to tell Sean her decision.

She located him out on the sun deck; he was on the phone and locked in a deep conversation. When he spotted her, he abruptly ended the conversation. "Good morning Sabrina," he greeted her with a smile. "Good morning, I'm sorry that I interrupted your phone call." "No, you didn't, it was just business, and I can take care of that anytime. So how are you feeling this morning?" "Really quite good," she answered taking the seat beside him.

"Sean, I need to talk to you. It's time that I went home, soon, like today maybe." "Are you sure you want to do that? You know I've told you that you're welcome to stay here as long as you like." "I know, and I am grateful for everything that you've done for me; but I need to go home. Please understand; I have to go back if I am ever to get completely over this ordeal and put it behind me."

Sean took her hand in his. "Okay, but I'm going with you." She opened her mouth to speak, but he quickly cut her off. "I won't hear any arguments from you. I will not let you go back there alone; not yet anyway. So when did you want to go?" "Now Sean. Right now, right this very minute," she said pulling him up with her.

Her pace was quick as they walked the beach toward her house; but she began to slow as they neared the stairs to the deck. Her feet were like lead weights as she ascended the stairs, each step a laborious effort. Once on the deck she became stock-still, standing at the patio door. Without thought to her action she slipped her hand into Sean's, he squeezed it gently. "Are you sure?" Sean asked. "Uh huh." Unlocking the door, she stepped inside; a flurry of butterflies came alive in her stomach; she swallowed hard, repeating one phrase over and over in her mind.

You can do this. You can do this. She nearly jumped out of her skin when Patches bounced onto the back of the couch. She picked him up, hugging him and scratching his chin. "Oh you poor baby, you've been here all alone; you must be hungry." "No, he's not. I had Charles bring him to the house, but he didn't like Rex, so I brought him back here. I've been feeding him for you. I also had Charles clean up in the, you know." "Thank you."

Keeping a tight hold on Patches for a sense of security, she proceeded to the bedroom, hesitating at the doorway before going inside. The bed was made. The room is tidy. *No one would have ever known what went on in here. Except me.* Charles had taken all the bedding, replacing it with fresh linens from the closet. The police had taken the strips of cloth for evidence. *The room is perfect; just like when I first viewed it.*

"Charles has done an excellent job. By the way, where is he now?" Sabrina asked. "Oh I gave him some time off." "I would like to thank him for all he's done, when he gets back. Well, I think I had better get myself dressed; I've borrowed this robe long enough." "I'll wait for you out in the living room." "No! Please stay; I'll only be a minute," she said peeking around the closet door. "Stay and talk to me." "Okay, what would you like to talk about." "Oh I don't know; tell me about the work that you do."

Sean was speechless for a moment. *I guess she really doesn't know who I am.* "Sean?" "Yeah, I'm still here. What do I do? Well, I'm in sports." "Sports eh, let me guess, baseball. No, football, am I right?" "Well, not exactly. You didn't let me finish my sentence. What I was about to say was that I'm in sports entertainment." "Sports entertainment; what is that, exactly?" "Well, in simple terms it's called wrestling."

Sabrina appeared from the closet wearing a floral short set; she looked at Sean with a strange expression. "What?" He asked, confused by her look. "Now I know where I've seen you before; your picture was on a magazine cover at the market. A wrestler, huh, I never would have guessed that."

That would explain his incredible physique. I've seen some of the wrestling shows on TV; all of those guys are always so well built. That's about the only reason that I had to have ever watched such a program. All those perfect bodies helped to bring out my fantasies; and now, here before me, stands one of the most perfect bodies that I've ever seen.

In her mind she began to take inventory of this young Adonis. *He's at least six foot two, and all muscle; even through his T-shirt I can see the fine definition of his chest and abdomen. The sleeves of his shirt had to be cut away to expose his powerful arms; no wonder he had been able to carry me. I can't begin to estimate the size of his biceps, but I would guess that both of my hands together wouldn't be able to enclose them. How handsome he looks.*

"Is everything all right?" Sean's voice disturbed her concentration. "Huh? Oh I'm fine," she said bringing herself back to reality. "I'm hungry; how about you?" Not waiting for an answer, she was already off to the kitchen. "It's my turn to cook for you; and no arguments."

Sean shook his head at hearing his very own words being thrown back at him. He picked up Patches. "You know cat, that is one special lady; and maybe with time and a little luck, she'll think of me the way that I think of her." Patches rolled about in his arms, he liked him, but then again he liked everyone who scratched his chin and paid him some attention.

Sabrina called to him from the kitchen. "Brunch is ready." Sean was already there by the time she had finished her sentence. "Where were you?" "Oh we were just having a nice conversation," he said continuing to stroke Patches on the head. Sabrina gazed at him with a whimsical look.

They ate in silence, neither of them sure how to begin another conversation. Finally finding her courage, she took a long drink of lemonade and began. "So tell me all about your work." "There's not much to tell. I'm a wrestler; that's basically all there is to it." "Oh come on there has to be more. I've seen those programs on TV. Do you use your real name or do you have a stage name?" "No, I have a character, called the Guardian." "You're kidding! This is so strange." "What is?" "It's nothing."

Sabrina shook her head in disbelief at this sudden revelation. "I don't know if you remember, but I told you that I would be going away soon on business." "Yes, I do remember." "Well, soon is the day after tomorrow, and I would really like it if you would come with me. I don't think it's a good idea for you to stay here at the beach house alone."

How do I respond to that? Picking up their plates Sabrina retreated into the kitchen, grasping the sink for support. Following her, Sean could see her tension; placing his hand on her shoulder, he turned her around to face him. "I'm sorry if I upset you. I'm just worried about you, being here alone." "I'm not upset; you've done so much for me already. I just don't know how I'll ever be able to repay you for your kindness." "It's not necessary; just let me be your friend."

Putting her arms around him, she hugged him. Somehow she felt safe surrounded by his strength. Releasing her, he brushed the hair away from her face, looking into her eyes. "Will you? Will you come with me?" "Yes, I'd like that very much," she answered. He leaned into her, and kissed her cheek.

In my heart I wish that he had really kissed me. Despite what has happened, I still long to be loved.

Sean could see her eyes scanning his face; he could feel her hands, gentle against his back. His mind was in turmoil. *I want to kiss her, I feel that it's what she wants too. The look on her face tells me everything.*

Placing his hand on the side of her face, he stroked her cheek with his thumb. Her eyes closed; she tilted her head slightly. He drew nearer and kissed her mouth ever so softly; her arms tightened around him. Their kiss deepened.

Our bodies feel good together. I want to take her up into my arms, to carry her to the bedroom, to make love to her; slow, passionate love. From the first time I saw her, I wanted her in my life, and definitely in my bed.

Sean pulled away; his action surprised her. "What's wrong?" Sabrina asked. "Nothing's wrong; this just isn't the right time; you need time to recover from this." "Shhh, I don't want to talk about that anymore; it's in the past already. If I am to recover, then I have to carry on with my life; I refuse to be a prisoner of the past any longer." "I'm not going to rush you; if we are supposed to make love, then it will happen when the time is right."

Sabrina hugged him tight. "You are an incredible man." "Now; how about we pack up your things, and move you into the guest room at my place?" "That sounds nice; but what about this place?" "Don't worry Charles can check on it throughout the day. Besides we're only going to be away for a couple of weeks. The only thing he'll have on his schedule is feeding the dog."

"What about the cat, what will I do with Patches?" "Move him too; he'll be fine. It will take some getting used to, but he should get along just fine with Rex." Sabrina smiled at him. "There it is! I've been waiting for you to do that. You have such a beautiful smile," Sean said. She blushed. Sean kissed her again; holding her tight for a few more moments.

By mutual agreement they conceded that they couldn't stand there all day; there were things to be done. As soon as she had a bag packed he took it to the car. She took a final look around the house. Everything was packed up; the closet was empty, the fridge and cupboards bare. Standing at the front door, she took one last look at her dream house. She had fallen in love with this house; but she wasn't regretting that she wasn't spending another night here.

This is the end of one adventure, and the beginning of a new one. She turned to look at Sean, who was waiting by the car. When she was settled into the passenger seat he took her hand and leaned over to kiss her cheek. He could barely contain his excitement; it hadn't been that long since he had the companionship of a woman, but not one as especially beautiful as her.

Sabrina took immense interest in Sean's house as they approached it. The monumental house dwarfed the one's on either side of it. The ten foot iron gate, and red brick perimeter walls made it look like a fortress. *A castle built for a Prince.* From the road, all that was readily visible was a portion of the top floor and the red tile roof. Large stately palm trees grew just behind the red wall, giving the house both privacy and mystery.

The car passed through the gate into a courtyard; she was impressed by what she saw. The driveway was done in similar bricks to those of the wall. There was no lawn, but clusters of flowers cascaded from large cement urns set throughout the yard. A fountain was the main centerpiece, with its stone cherub gracefully pouring water from a jug. Spellbound by the vision of the house; its clean, bright white plastered walls towered high above her, high enough that she had to tip her head back to see the roof top. The windows that faced the yard, were protected by heavy iron rails, like those of the gate.

Is this a fortress or a prison? Sean called to her but she was lost in her thoughts. *Either way it's still the most magnificent home I've ever seen.*

He touched her arm. "Coming?" he asked. "Oh yeah." She picked up a bag and followed him. "The rent on this place must be outrageous," she said. Sean laughed heartily. "Not really, I don't rent it; I own it." *How could anyone afford a house like this?* "It didn't look like this when I bought it. I've had to do some major renovations. It was badly neglected for many years; but I liked the location and I thought it was a good investment at the time. When I bought it, the place was only worth a hundred thousand; but now I've had offers for as much as three million for it; but I won't sell."

He guided her towards the front door, which was obscured in an alcove. She admired the heavy oak door in front of her with its curved upper edge and stained glass inset depicting a sunrise. No detail had been overlooked. During her brief stay, she had not really taken any notice of the interior of the house; now, without the veil of pain killers and sedatives she could see the house clearly for the first time.

The door opened onto a large entrance hall; the floor, laid with black and white marble tiles. There was nothing in the entrance way except for a bank of four BI-fold doors along one wall. The hallway led into a large living room; she couldn't begin to estimate it's size, but in the center was a conversation pit, consisting of four large, off white leather sofas with a square coffee table in the middle. The windows, beyond the sofas, had to be at least nine feet high, and extended the full length of the room; they looked out over part of the sun deck, and beyond to the ocean.

Following Sean, they walked through the living room, into what she could only describe to herself as a family room. She had seen this room before and thought that it was the living room. This room was far more informal, and had another set of patio doors that led to the sun deck. It was decorated in a south west theme. Navajo blankets lay across the back of a couch, and a large cactus stood in the corner of the room.

They continued through the dining room, the kitchen and up the stairs to the hallway that led to the bedrooms. To her left was Sean's room, with its own private sun deck. "There's four guest rooms up here, they all have an ensuite; but this one," he said opening the last door on the right side of the hallway. "This one is a bit bigger, and it has a small deck that overlooks the ocean." She followed him into the room; it took her breathe away. "This is beautiful."

The room was decorated in soft pinks and warm maroons; it had a skylight above the bed, a gas fireplace along the outside wall and a walk-in closet that led through to the ensuite. "I thought you might like this one," Sean remarked, as he placed her suitcase inside the closet. "I do; I love it. It's so beautiful; thank you." "You're welcome. You start unpacking and I'll bring in the rest of your things."

Sabrina opened the French doors to the deck, allowing the ocean breeze to blow in. She began putting her clothes away when Sean returned with the rest. "Where is Patches?" she asked. "Oh he's exploring downstairs. Don't worry; the doors are all shut, so he can't get out. Can I help you unpack?" "No, thank you anyway; I can manage just fine." "All right then, how about I make you a cup of tea?" "That sounds good; I don't have a whole lot left to do and then I'll be down." He left her to her tasks; bounding down the stairs like a teenager.

I've had other women in my life, quite a few in fact, but none of them ever made me feel like this. Make my heart skip a beat every time I see her. He stopped and put on some music before going into the kitchen; his body began to move to the beat, unaware that he was now being observed from the doorway.

She watched intently, and quietly, as his body shook and gyrated to the music. *Could something come of this new found friendship? He is definitely one hot stud, and he has made it very obvious that he wants me as more than a friend, but I'm not about to rush into anything, at least not right now.* Her curiosity about his career intrigued her more. *I want to know more, and going with him will hopefully give me the answers that I want.*

Clearing her throat; trying not to startle him; she let him know that she was there. He turned around quickly and she saw the blush on his face. "Tea is just about ready why don't you go out to the sun deck and I'll bring it out in a minute." She quietly complied with his request; knowing that she had embarrassed him and he required a few moments to regain his manly composure.

The surf was beating against the shore. It was never the same, and that was one of the things that she liked about the ocean.

Every moment of every day it's changing, washing away the memories, then running full in, depositing something new. That's how I will deal with my attack; I'll envision this horrid event trapped inside a bottle, and with each movement of the tide it will drift farther and farther out to sea; eventually disappearing forever.

"A penny for your thoughts?" Sean asked, distracting her concentration. "Not this time; my thoughts are between the ocean and me right now." He was puzzled by her comment, but didn't pursue the issue any further. "Come and sit down; tea's ready." He touched her shoulder, gently caressing the curve of it and fantasizing about the moment when he would be able to really touch her.

They spent the remainder of the afternoon on the sun deck; sometimes conversing but mostly just watching the ocean. During their times of conversation Sabrina was able to ascertain that Sean was born in a small town in southern Texas; he was 30 years old, had no brothers or sisters, and he had been an active wrestler for more than ten years. She tried to find out more about his wrestling career, but all he would tell her was that she would have to wait and see. Her curiosity was eating away at her; but she respected his wish, and didn't pry any further.

Sean made dinner for them and then excused himself from her presence; he told her that he had to get started on his packing. Sabrina returned to the sun deck to await the sunset. Sean had been gone nearly an hour when he returned with a blanket in his hand. The sun was starting to go down, and the evening breeze had turned cool. "Here, you're gonna need this," he said unfolding the blanket. He put it over her and sat down. "What about you?" She looked at his bare legs stretched out beside her. "I'm fine." "I don't think so." She lifted the blanket and placed half of it over Sean.

It didn't quite cover them both due to the gap between them; she slid herself closer. Taking his arm, lifting it up and behind her, she wiggled closer to his side. Sean rested his arm along the back of the bench, unsure if he should put it around her or not; he decided to take the chance, and cautiously embraced her shoulder.

They sat through the sunset, and on into the darkness; Sean soon realized that she was asleep. Trying not to wake her, he carefully picked her up in his arms and carried her up to bed. He kissed her softly on the forehead and left the room. Standing outside the door he prayed silently, for the day that she would accept him into her bed.

Chapter 4

On the day that they were to leave for the trip, Sabrina watched Sean's disposition, and mannerism change. He went from a placid, conservative person, to that of a hyper, over excited child; bounding up and down the stairs, checking and then rechecking the luggage; muttering to himself constantly.

He bounced over to her at the couch, stopped, kissed her and was about to bound away but she had a firm hold of his shirt; the unexpected restraint snapped him back in front of her. He kissed her again, but this time she was prepared, responding to his touch; putting her arms around his neck, he slipped his around her waist.

She tried to get him to kiss her longer, but all she received were short frequent kisses on her face and neck. "Wait a minute, how much coffee have you had today?" she asked. "None. Why?" "Why? You're bouncing around here like someone on a caffeine overdose that's why." Sean laughed as he picked her up, twirling her around and around, until she thought she would be sick. "I'm excited, that's all. I always get like this before a tour, but this time it's even more exciting, more special than ever before because you're going with me." He twirled her again, this time giving in to the passionate kiss that she desired.

Charles cleared his throat, as he entered the room. "Excuse me sir; but it's time to leave for the airport." Sean lowered Sabrina down, her feet were touching the floor but her head was still spinning. "Are you ready?" he asked. *What a loaded question you ask.* "Yeah I'm ready; I just have one more thing to do." Picking up Patches from the couch, she cuddled him. "Now you be a good boy, and I'll be back soon." She nuzzled him again before returning him to the couch. Sabrina took Sean's outstretched hand, and walked with him out to the limo.

On the way to the airport he went over the itinerary with her. "Tonight we'll be in Seattle. Tomorrow night Portland, Wednesday Reno, Thursday Las Vegas, Friday San Diego and Saturday Sacramento; and the next week will be worked out later." "Wow, when you work you really work! At least it's all in the same time zone." "Yeah, sometimes it's really hard to stay on track, when one night you're here in California, and the next night you're somewhere in New York; it plays havoc with your internal clock. That's why they rotate us around, so we can get at least a few days off between tours; it's the only way to stay sane."

Can I keep up with this outrageous schedule that he has? But like he said, it is only for two weeks, and then home for a week to recover.

As they neared the airport, Sean pulled his hair back into a ponytail and put on a baseball cap and a pair of sunglasses. "What are you doing?" she asked, perplexed by his conduct. "Hopefully you won't have to find out." Sabrina was even more baffled, and it was evident in her expression. "It's a way of dodging photographers and fans," he said. *I still don't understand why he would have to do such a thing, but it's none of my business.*

The luggage was loaded onto a cart by the time they stepped out of the car. "Have a good trip sir. You will be returning Saturday morning is that correct?" "Yes, Charles, that's right; unless something comes up in which case I will call you. You know the routine for Saturday night?" " Yes sir; everything will be ready when you get back." Sean nodded to Charles, and crooked his elbow for Sabrina; she willing took his arm and he wasted no time in crossing through the terminal to the departure gate.

Looking about the relatively quiet terminal, she saw nothing that resembled a photographer, or a mob of anxious fans. She thought Sean was being a bit pretentious, taking such precautions to disguise himself; but who was she to say any different.

Once they were seated on the plane, their bags stored above, she had to ask him about what he and Charles had been talking about outside. "What did you mean when you said to Charles you know the routine for Saturday night?" "Oh that, well it's kind of become a tradition that when we have a west coast tour, I always host a party at the end."

"What do you mean a party?" "A party, I don't know what else to call it. The guys that are on the tour come to my place; we have a barbecue, drink a few beers and just generally unwind from the time on the road. Does that explain it for you?" "Yes, it does. Thank you."

Turning away from Sean, she looked out the window; they were already in the air and she hadn't noticed the plane take off. She took a deep breath; her nerves were trying to get the better of her; she was apprehensive at just going with Sean, but now to find out that she would be socializing with these people he worked with was a bit overwhelming for her. She took another deep breath and listened to bits and pieces from the monotone voice on the intercom. When it fell silent, she didn't notice, her thoughts were wrapped up in envisioning this party at Sean's; even the firm squeeze of his hand on hers had no effect at that moment, she was lost, adrift in the clouds that wafted past the window.

    As rapidly as they had maneuvered through the Los Angeles airport, Sean advanced them just as quickly through the Seattle terminal; not at a run, but at a fast enough walk that it was hard for her to keep up with him. Outside they were greeted by another chauffeur and another black limo; Sean hustled Sabrina into the back. "That was close," he said slumping back against the seat. "What do you mean?"

    No sooner had the words spilled from her lips when hands began knocking on the limo, and vague faces appeared through the darkened windows. The commotion outside startled her. "What's going on?" "Fans. I spotted them and they spotted me. That's why I was rushing you so."

    Sabrina looked out into the crowd that had formed around the limo. Fans, comprised mostly young girls, were carrying signs, with Sean's name and picture on them, some of them even crying. Sean pressed a button on the console beside him. "Hey Syd, how about getting us out of here and away from this zoo?" "You got it sir," was the response on the intercom.

    Slowly the big limo began to move away from the curb; Sabrina observed a few of the girls chasing after it, waiving their arms and their signs. "Looks like you're quite popular, at least with the female fans," she said. Detecting the hint of sarcasm in her voice, Sean put his arms around her, whispering into her ear. "I guess; but they're just fans; they're not as important as you are."

    When he nuzzled at her neck, she tried to bring him closer. Resisting the temptation he sat back. "At least we won't have to go through this at the hotel; that place has a private underground parkade. The valet will meet us down there and then take us up to our room via a service elevator. It's the same at the arena; the limo drives right inside. No one knows who's arriving, or who's leaving."

    Sabrina was very much overwhelmed by all of this. *For someone so common as myself to be enjoying all the privileges of celebrity status just doesn't seem possible.*

    "What do you do about meals?" she asked. "That's easy; room service." "So this is how you live when you're on tour." She saw the confused look on his face. "Airport, hotel, arena, hotel, airport." "Yeah that's it all right; really glamorous, isn't it? Oh and every once in a while they throw in a public interview, or autograph signing; but that's only to encourage ticket sales." "Do you ever get the chance to really see the cities that you're in?" "Sometimes I do, but not very often."

In a way, he's like a slave to this job; to be able to travel to all of these cities, and only be able to see them from the hotel room, or from the airplane, such a waste.

The limo came to a stop. The engine went quiet. It was just as Sean had described it; underground parking, and a valet, with a room key in one hand, and a luggage cart in the other. They were escorted to the elevator where the young valet pushed the last button on the elevator panel before turning to face Sean. "The manager was able to make the changes to your room as you requested. I hope you will find them satisfactory." Sean did not respond to the young man, as the valet had already turned away, not expecting a reply.

The hotel room was much more than she had imagined; she had been in hotels before, but never had she been in a room like this one. A small sofa and two arm chairs were the main attraction, as well as the entertainment center, the bar, and the dining table. *Where are the beds?* She scanned the room again. The valet spoke again. "This was the only two-bedroom suite left available sir; we hope it meets your needs." "Yes, it's fine," Sean replied; handing the young man a tip and showing him to the door.

The valet went off to tend to his next client, but couldn't help wondering, why a man, traveling with a woman like that, would want a two-bedroom suite. With a sudden look of discovery he thought to himself that she must be his sister; satisfied with his answer, he dismissed the issue from his mind.

Sean obtained Sabrina's attention when he spoke. "So which one do you want? They're really pretty much identical," he said opening the two doors behind the sofa. "It doesn't matter to me." She tried not to let her disappointment show through. *I was sure that he would make his move now.*

"Okay then I'll take this one," he said throwing his bags onto the bed in the first room. "Hungry?" "Just a little," Sabrina answered." "Well, let's see what room service has to offer." He began to peruse the menu on the table. "Sean, what time do you have to be at the arena?" "Well, the show is scheduled to start at seven and I'd like to be there by at least five. It takes me a while to get ready; and the show schedule never runs exactly. I could be on early or late; depending on if there has been any changes to the roster, or if something else is going on."

I'm not sure if I'm ready for this. "What would you like?" he asked handing her the menu. "I don't know; surprise me. I'm gonna have a rest; if that's okay." "Sure, go right ahead; room service will take at least an hour; I'll call you when it arrives."

Needing some personal space, the plane ride, and the conversation, all these had agitated her; she began to question her motives for making this trip. Laying on the bed she stared up at the ceiling, thoughts raced through her mind.

Am I doing the right thing? Maybe it's too soon. He is younger than me. Is he the one? The one that has been invading my dreams for so long. Her mind became stuck on that question. She tried to remember, but her vision never had a face; at least not that she could recall. *Maybe if I went to sleep it will return; hopefully with more detail this time.* She turned on her side to get comfortable.

It was going onto three, when Sean knocked lightly on Sabrina's door; she didn't respond; she was in a deep, dreamless sleep. Sean knocked again, louder, and called to her once more. This time she awoke and answered him. "Yeah, I'll be out in a minute." Sitting on the edge of the bed, she tried to clear the fog from her mind. The vision had not come to her this time and it saddened her.

For the first time I wanted this dream to materialize, I need to make some connection, to get some answers. It's disheartening to realize that I can't summon it at will; it comes to me when I least expected it; trifling with me. If only I could see his face, then, perhaps, I could put this perplexing apparition to rest. There has to be a logical reason behind this, or is it my sanity that is slipping away?

Rubbing the kink from her neck Sabrina couldn't help thinking that since she had embarked on this odyssey she had become more ensnared in this vision than she ever had at home. *There has to be some significance to it; but what?*

Sean was seated at the table when she entered the sitting room. "What time is it?" she asked. "It's nearly three; room service was late and we're gonna have to leave here just after four." "I can't believe I slept this long." She stretched before sitting down at the table. He acknowledged her with a soft smile. They dined quietly, as Sabrina was still consumed by her thoughts; having slept for nearly two hours, with no vision, no dream; she vanquished all thoughts from her mind.

Things will happen if they are meant to. I'm not going to let that vision haunt me anymore. There is no point in holding on to something that may very well be a product of my vivid imagination.

Sean brought her back to reality when he touched her cheek. "We have to leave soon; you had better get yourself ready to go." His voice was soft when he spoke to her. He knew her mind had drifted off to some secret place; but to where, and about what he could only imagine.

"Should I change into something a little dressier?" Sabrina asked. "No, it's not necessary; what you're wearing is just fine." He looked over her denim shorts and tank top. Watching her walk away to the bathroom, his eyes were fixated on her form. *I can't remember when I've seen a pair of shorts fit a woman as good as those fit her.* He exhaled hard, rolled his eyes and shook his head. "Man what that woman does to me, and the things that I want to do to her, oh man. I just have to be patient."

Warlock's eyes snapped open. He sat bolt upright on the bed. He had been awakened by an extraordinary feeling, that sense of urgency. That same feeling that had consumed him back in Reno; that sense of presence.

I must have been dreaming again; dreaming of that woman that bedeviled my most private moment's time and again. It's only my imagination. There is no woman like that. Not for me anyway. Face it; I'm going to be alone for the rest of my life. His lecture did little to alleviate the sensation that coursed through his body.

It's so strong; much stronger than ever before, but how could that be? Am I losing my mind? Have I fixated on this dream for so long now, that it has thoroughly taken control of me; unable to distinguish between fantasy and reality. Get over it. I've got two weeks of shows to do; and then there's the party at Sean's. Yes, a party, that's what I need, anything to take my mind off of this damn feeling. He threw his bag over his shoulder and headed for the arena.

Through the dark lenses of his sunglasses, he scanned the faces of all the women he passed in the hallway and the elevator. *Nothing. Not one of those faces brought forth any of the feelings that I had when I dreamed.*

Tying his bag onto the back of his bike, he left the hotel. *Feeling the wind on my face will help to clear my mind.*

The soul had awakened this body; it had to become aware. The mate was near. The barriers had been weakened; the body will respond to the commands. It will hear us clearer and be more receptive to our voice. The other body is still resistant, the will is strong in that one; but our bond will break that barrier, we will be together once again.

They left the hotel the same way they had entered; the black limo waiting for them in the underground parking. A motorcycle sped past them at the entrance; Sabrina became engulfed by that same feeling.

Damn it it's just a guy on a motorcycle nothing to get upset about. She couldn't let go of the feelings this time. No matter how many times she told herself to forget it. *If only I could have seen him more clearly, but what's the point, he's real, my dream is not.*

There was a faint whispering in her head. *Hear me,* it said, *see me. We are close my beloved. Open your heart and let our love reunite.*

"I'm sorry Sean, what did you say?" "Nothing, why?" "Never mind." *What is wrong with me? Get out of my head!* At her command, the whisper was hushed, but did not terminate. It couldn't; she had to hear.

They arrived at the arena just before five; and as Sean said, the limo drove down a ramp and into the arena. He opened the door and stepped out. She hesitated, nervous. Sean leaned back in and took her hand. "Come on; it's okay." She acquiesced and took her stand at his side. Scanning the area, her eyes fell upon the motorcycle parked far away from the other cars. *Damn these feelings. It's just a bike, nothing more.*

Sean picked up his bag and led her down a corridor to a locker room that had his name taped across the door. They had passed other people in the hallway, but none of them even gave them a second look. Sean stopped a young man, who was tending some electrical cables. "Hey man, I want you to make sure that a TV monitor is put into my dressing room," Sean said pointing toward the door. "Yes sir, right away; I'll tell the video guys right now." His voice was shaky, but he managed to jog back down the corridor. It was the first time one of the shows stars had ever talked to him and his excitement made him nervous.

Sean opened the door and allowed Sabrina to enter first; the room was nothing special; a folding table with a couple of chairs, a bench, and a wall of open wooden lockers. Sean made a move to put his bag on the table, but he was held back; Sabrina still had a hold of his hand, she was not moving. Dropping his bag on the floor, he turned back to her.

"What's the matter?" he asked. Her voice cracked when she spoke. "Nerves, I guess." He brought her into his arms; her body trembled under his embrace. He held her tight; gently rubbing her back until he felt her relax. "Feel better now?" "Almost." She looked into his blue eyes, a look of longing, wanting.

I hope I'm reading her body language right. Leaning in he kissed her. She willingly accepted him, sliding her hands up his back, motivating him to kiss her more deeply. When she finally released him, he leaned back. A breathless 'wow' escaped his lips. "I would like nothing better than to hold you like this all night long; but I do have to go to work." He kissed her quickly, before she could distract him any further.

Not satisfied, her voice became soft and low. "Is there anything that I can do for you?" Sabrina asked. Sean swallowed hard. *There is a lot of things you could do for me, and to me.* He pushed those thoughts away. "Yeah, if you like you can unpack my costume for me while I take a shower." "Sure." "Hang it up on one of those hooks; I won't be long." He disappeared around a wall and soon she heard the sound of a shower running.

Picking up the bag, she unzipped it; carefully removing the contents. She could see the sequins glittering under the fluorescent light. With the first item removed and in her hand, she unfolded it for examination, a white sequined, waist length jacket. She turned it around; on the back, designed in gold sequins, was the image of wings. *How appropriate this is for someone called The Guardian.*

The next item from the bag was a pair of white and gold sequin leather pants, that had a gold buckle in front, and gold colored zippers down the outside of each leg. She hung these beside the jacket. Returning to the bag, she retrieved a pair of white spandex pants, followed by a pair of white boots; these she laid across the bench, then stored the bag on the shelf below the jacket. With her task done, she sat down at the table and listened to the sound of the shower. A part of her wanted to go in there, to surprise him. *No, the first move is up to him.*

Sean had his hands braced against the shower wall, the cool water washing over his body. He was trying to wash away the feelings of arousal he had. As his body calmed, he turned up the warm water, fighting off the thoughts of her.

With a towel wrapped around his waist, and without thinking clearly, he headed back into the locker room. Sabrina watched him cross the room; his body glistening with moisture. Every muscle in his chest, and abdomen perfectly sculpted. The hair on his chest, wet from the water, laid flat against his tanned skin. It formed a dark line down the center of his abdomen, that she followed with her eyes until it disappeared beneath the towel. Sean grabbed at the towel to remove it. "Excuse me," she said reminding him that she was still there. "Oh I'm sorry; I'm so used to my routine that I just plain forgot myself."

His apology was not as sincere as she expected. Turning away from him while he dressed she focused her attentions on the sounds coming from the hallway. Sean dried himself quickly and began to put on his pants; but his skin was still moist, and the spandex stuck repeatedly. He pulled and tugged until success was finally achieved. "You can turn around now," he said. She stood up to move her chair a bit closer to him when there was a knock at the door. "Do you want me to get that?" she asked. "I would appreciate it."

Standing in the hall was the young man that Sean had spoken to earlier. He was laden with a TV monitor, and numerous loops of electrical cable. She held the door open for him to enter, and he was immediately apologizing to Sean for being delayed. Sabrina took a quick look down the hallway, noticing all the people milling about. Some in costume, and some in regular clothes, while others had what appeared to be a type of uniform T-shirt that had EVENT STAFF written across it.

The whispers returned, making her stop, and take another look down the hall. At the far end of the hallway stood a man, a very tall man, a man who towered above those who were close to him; he was dressed in black attire, whether it was street clothes or a costume she couldn't determine. She couldn't see his face clearly, but she knew that he was looking at her. Her blood ran cold. An icy cold, that sent rocketing shivers up her spine. She shut the door to the locker room quickly, her heart pounding, about to break out of her chest. *Why? Why is this happening to me?*

Warlock had abandoned the sanctuary of his private dressing room, being drawn to the backstage area by that strange sense. Scanning the mass of faces, that milled about; searching. *For what? For whom? For her!* Through the mass of faces he saw her. To far away to really see the details of her face, but he knew she was looking at him. For a moment, everything moved in slow motion; he felt his heart stop. He was captivated, compelled to look at her. He blinked his eyes, and she was gone. *Damn it, it's only your imagination; she's not real.*

The young man, who had been setting up the TV, bumped into Sabrina as he was backing up to the door, unrolling cable as he walked. She ignored his apology, needing to be away from the opening door, just in case. Sean beckoned her to him, and she took refuge at his side. "Now you can watch the whole show from here, with nothing to bother you." "That sounds fine," she said, endeavoring to hold her nerves in check.

"I'm gonna have to leave you now. I have to do a couple of interviews and they want some publicity shots; if you're nervous about being here alone then just lock the door behind me." She nodded her answer, while unconsciously stroking the softness of his chest. He had already put on his leather pants, and he reached for his jacket, pulling it on as he walked to the door.

His hand had only touched the knob when she called to him. "Sean, wait a minute." With a touch of despair in her voice she ran to him, and kissed him full on the lips. "What was that for?" Sean asked. "Luck." That was the only answer she could come up with. She locked the door, and leaned against it, giving herself a moment to calm down. The monitor was already turned on; she fiddled with the knobs. "Oh great, a picture and no sound," she grumbled quietly to herself. She shrugged it off and pulled her chair closer to the table.

As scheduled, the show began right at seven. She watched the monitor periodically, waiting to see Sean, or worked on a crossword puzzle, when the show didn't hold her interest. She could hear the clamor of the fans in the arena, but it didn't make up for the fact that there was no sound coming from the TV. Sean appeared on the screen, she watched intently as he moved about the ring, graceful, yet very acrobatic, defeating his opponent in what seemed like only seconds.

She was about to turn the monitor off, when the camera panned the entrance way to the ring; she again saw the man dressed in dark attire. Goose bumps crawled in waves over her skin as she watched this mysterious man descend the ramp to the ring.

Who is he? Why is he causing these creepy feelings? The camera fixed on him again. She felt as if he were looking right at her, through her, into her very essence. Unable to watch any longer, she turned the monitor off.

When the door knob rattled, she jumped; hearing Sean's voice, she unlocked it. She waited quietly while he changed his clothes; she wanted to ask about that man she had seen, but then thought better not. They headed for the limo; Sabrina walked with her head lowered slightly, fearful that she might see him again.

The time progressed quicker than she expected, and the rigorous schedule kept Sean exceedingly occupied; Sabrina was beginning to feel a bit neglected. Before the tour they had spent so much time together, and she liked it, but now, with his time taken up with the shows, photo sessions, and interviews, when they did have some time together he was even too tired to talk. She questioned herself, about going home; but then there was Reno. She had been looking forward to that; a little shopping and maybe some gambling. She didn't need Sean around for that; but even that dream was not to be.

Sean's schedule for that day was overbearing. He had asked Sabrina to remain at the hotel. She respected his request and waited, until she was too tired and went to bed. She was sound asleep when he returned; he peaked at her through the crack of the door, then leaned against the frame.

I had promised her that I would come back and get her, but the way the day went, I was kept isolated from her. Suddenly his eyes widened as an idea formed in his mind. *Tomorrow we will be in Las Vegas. The show is scheduled for five, and when it's over, I will make it all up to her. I will make tomorrow a special day for her.* Falling onto his own bed he called the front desk and requested an early wake up call.

The six o'clock call came, but Sean was already awake; he had showered, packed and ordered breakfast, before going to knock on Sabrina's door. "Sabrina it's time to get up." Not waiting for an answer, he opened the door and went in, calling her name again. Her body jumped, from being awakened so abruptly. Sitting up, she rubbed at her eyes trying to get them to focus. "What's the matter?" she asked through a yawn. "Nothing's wrong, it's time to get up. Breakfast will be here soon and we have a plane to catch; so get a move on."

She sat on the edge of the bed, trying to shake off the sleepiness. Pulling on her robe, she looked at her watch. "Sean for God's sake it's six thirty; the plane doesn't leave until eleven." "No, it doesn't," he said as he peeked his head back in the doorway. "I have booked us on a private jet that will be leaving at nine; so I suggest that you get a shower and get your things packed." "Why do we have to leave so early?" "Ah, it's a surprise; and that's all I'm going to tell you." He disappeared from the doorway. She shuffled towards the bathroom. *Maybe a shower will help me to think more clearly.*

The smell of fresh coffee greeted her at the door; Sean was standing at the window, staring off into space. "Good morning," she announced her presence. "Good morning; and don't you look lovely this fine morning," he replied, holding out a chair for her at the table. She couldn't figure out what had brought on this strange mood that he was in; she scanned his face.

He's, what can I call it, beaming. That's it he's beaming, but why? What is he up to? "We should leave right after breakfast, that is, if you're ready," he said sitting down across from her at the table. "Sure, what ever; but what's the big rush?" "Ah, no more questions; you're gonna have to wait and see. Don't try to guess and don't try to make me tell you, because I won't." Shaking her head, she picked up her coffee and toast and went back into the bedroom to finish packing.

Before she knew it, they were in Las Vegas. Sean whisked her through the airport and into another waiting limo. They had barely spoken during the flight, just some casual comments about the shows, or a brief touch, nothing very exciting, but now in the limo she could detect Sean's anxiety. He fidgeted on the seat; looked out the windows, and checked his watch repeatedly. "Are you okay?" she asked, concerned over his behavior. "I'm great, just great," he answered. Yet she detected a hint of nervousness in his voice.

The limo came to a stop, in front of a huge hotel casino; through the darkened windows she could see the twinkling lights of the entrance. "You wait here; I'll only be a minute," he said. She felt the trunk lid shut, and saw Sean talking to a man in a dark colored uniform; he handed something to Sean and then took the luggage cart into the hotel. Sean disappeared from her view momentarily, but then she spotted him talking to the driver. They spoke briefly and in seconds he was back inside the limo.

In one unexpected move, he had her in his arms. "You are so beautiful. Beautiful women deserve beautiful things; and they deserve to be treated special." He kissed her. She was even more perplexed. "What exactly is going on?" "What is going on pretty lady, is that I am taking you shopping." "Sean, you don't have to do that." "Yes I do. I feel so bad about the way things have gone this week and I'm going to make it up to you; and don't try and tell me any different; my mind is made up and you are gonna have the most special day ever."

A smile came across her face. *If he's going to treat me to a special day, then I'm gonna treat him to a special night. Tonight Sean. Tonight I will have you in my bed. I will make love to you.* She kissed him tenderly and then withdrew. *If he can keep secrets, then so can I.*

The limo stopped in front of a clothing store. The front windows displayed an assortment of evening gowns. *This looks expensive.* Sean guided her towards the door. "Sean the sign says that they're closed." "No, they're not." He had no sooner said the words, when a dark haired woman opened the door. "Mr. Malloy?" "Yes ma'am." "We've been expecting you. Please come in," she said holding the door open for them. Sabrina stared at Sean intently. Catching her gaze, he offered up an explanation. "I arranged for a private shopping spree."

The dark haired woman was beside them; she was dressed in a lavender silk suit. "Is there anything special you'd like to see first Miss?" Sabrina was lost for words. *I've never shopped in a place like this before.* She looked to Sean for help. "Well, let's see. We need two evening dresses, a couple of casual outfits and the rest we'll figure out as we go," he said. "Very well sir," the woman replied, stepping off to speak to her staff. "Sean, what is going on?" "Remember I said no arguments; you deserve this. Now go pick out some things to try on." He patted her ass, as a way of getting her to move.

She had taken a couple of steps when the dark haired woman called to her. "Miss, if you would come with me, we can begin." She escorted Sabrina into the fitting room area and began to show her some of the items that they had selected. Sean called after her. "Everything that you try on I want to see."

After a few minutes Sabrina emerged from the dressing room, wearing an ankle length, black satin dress with thin straps. Sean looked at her, the vision took his breath away; the satin hugged her body, showing off her womanly curves. She turned around to reveal a slit that ran from the hem almost to the top of her thighs. The back of the dress was cut deep, exposing her back almost to the waist. Without any hesitation Sean spoke. "We'll take it!"

Sabrina returned to the dressing room, to continue her fashion show. The performance continued for almost an hour, until she had amassed a large collection of clothes. It seemed that everything she tried on, Sean approved of. "Enough," she said taking up his hands. "It's getting late; you have to get ready for the show tonight and I'm a bit hungry."

"Yeah; I know I'm gonna have to leave pretty soon, but you're not finished yet." "Yes, I am. I don't need anything else. Just let me go and change and we can go." She went to pull away but Sean held her hand. "Well, you see it's not that simple; I've also arranged for these ladies to do your hair, and make-up too. The limo will return for you about three thirty, and he's been instructed to bring you straight to the arena." "Why?" "I told you I have something really special planned for you tonight, so wear that pretty black dress; you know the first one that you tried on. I have to go, but I'll see you later." She had no time to respond; he was already out the door.

Sabrina was escorted to the back of the shop. She had never been so pampered. While one person worked on her hair, two others worked on her nails. They finished up just as the limo pulled up out front. The driver collected her packages, having to make three trips to get all of them. With his chore completed, he positioned himself at the limo door, waiting for Sabrina. She thanked each of the ladies for all of their help.

I feel like a Princess. Getting into the limo was done with great care. Long dresses were something that she was not accustom to wearing, and she had to watch that she didn't step on the hem. On the back seat lay a bouquet of white roses held together with a red velvet bow. Attached to the ribbon was a card; she picked it up and read. "These are for the most beautiful woman in the world. Sean." Sabrina held the card to her breast, trying to imagine just what he had planned next.

The limo arrived at the arena just passed four. Her nerves kept her on the edge of the seat. The backstage area was busy with people. The previous nights they had always managed to arrive long before any of the others, and had left before them as well. The show was due to start soon, and she felt very uneasy about having to walk through this mass of wrestlers and staff. Sean had never introduced her to any of them.

The door opened, and Sean's face appeared. Extending his hand to her, she took it, but was still wary about leaving the security of the limo. As they walked towards his dressing room, they passed many people; all of who stopped whatever they were doing, just to look at her. She felt uncomfortable and never returned any of the glances; focusing only on the approaching door.

Breathing a sigh of relief as she entered the room, away from the stares and whispers, she was half way across the room when she realized that Sean was not beside her. He was standing at the doorway just staring at her. "What?" Sabrina asked. "My God, you are so beautiful." A blush consumed her trembling body. He continued to stare at her. The gown fit her so perfectly; clinging tightly to her full round breasts, showing off her hard protruding nipples. Her hair was pulled up, with the exception of a few wisps that trailed around her neck.

Sabrina broke the silence. "So what's next on your agenda?" "Oh you'll find out soon enough," he said moving towards hers. "However, I will tell you, that when I'm done here, I'm taking you out to dinner and then for a night on the town. What ever you want to do, all you have to do is ask."

Now that, is a truly loaded question. Oh Sean if you only knew what I genuinely wanted to do tonight.

A knock came to the door, and a dull voice called, "Ten minutes Sean." He took her hand. "Come on let's go." "Go where?" "You'll see." Hooking her arm around his, he ushered her through the door and down the corridor. They walked past a collection of staff, and into a darkened alcove. Before them was a heavy black curtain, she could hear the tumultuous outcries from the fans inside the arena.

Sabrina suddenly had the horrible realization that he was planning to take her out there. She tried to release his arm but he held tight. "I'm not going out there!" "Yes, you are. You're going with me, not alone. It'll be all right, I promise." The music started; her stomach knotted. Her feet felt like they were cemented in place. Sean kissed her lips. "For luck, remember?"

Luck, like hell, I don't want to do this. He continued his coaxing until she was finally moving. They were at the top of the ramp. The black curtain was only an arm's length away. The noise from the crowd was getting louder; her stomach was slowly creeping up into her throat. "Damn it, Sean; I can't do this!" "Yes, you can." He reached out to part the curtain and they stepped through onto the platform.

The noise was deafening; Sean's hold on her was unyielding as he waved to the crowd. Walking her down the ramp, they headed towards the ring in the center of the arena; he talked calmly to her. She tried to stay focused on him, and not on the screaming masses that were leaning over the guard rails trying to touch him, and her. Reaching the ring, he led her up a set of stairs at the corner. He sat on the second rope that surrounded the ring, creating an opening for her to step through.

Once inside the ring, he paraded around the ring, almost dancing to the beat of the music. The spotlights were fixed on him, and the reflections off of his sequined outfit gave him an almost heavenly glow. When he had given his fans enough attention, he took Sabrina's hand and escorted her across the ring, where he again held open the ropes for her to step through. Helping her down the stairs, he guided her to an empty chair beside the time keeper. Her nerves were frayed. Removing his jacket, and leather pants, he handed them to her. Touching her cheek briefly, he gave her a wink and a smile before returning to the ring to await his opponent.

Flashes from a multitude of cameras were going off like fireworks. Sean flexed and posed for the fans, giving the fans what they wanted. His music faded off and another euphony began. The noise level increased, as the fans cheered the next competitor into the arena. From where she sat, Sabrina could not see clearly the man coming down the ramp to the ring; the announcer called him Lorenzo. Sean had moved off into a corner of the ring to allow this guy his moment with the fans.

Lorenzo entered the ring; he was about the same height as Sean, and Sabrina estimated at least thirty pounds heavier. He wore a pair of black trunks; his hair was jet black, wavy and shoulder length. A thick matting of black hair covered his chest and abdomen. His tanned well-muscled body shimmered under the spot lights as if covered with oil. A bell sounded, and

Sean and Lorenzo were locked in combat. Sabrina cringed as Lorenzo sent Sean over the top rope onto the floor.

The urge to go to him was strong, but she resisted. Sean climbed back into the ring, launching his offensive on Lorenzo. Supremacy of the match alternated several times, until Sean initiated a flying leap from the top rope; knocking Lorenzo to the mat. Laying across him Sean grabbed at Lorenzo's leg while the referee began to count. His hand slapped the mat three times and again the bell sounded. The referee raised Sean's hand, as the announcer proclaimed him the winner.

The fans cheered, and Sean's music started playing again. He climbed through the ropes and came to Sabrina. Taking her arm, he walked back up the ramp, stopping briefly on the platform to give his fans one last wave before they disappeared through the curtain. "That wasn't so bad was it?" Sean asked. "No, I guess not."

The fluttering of butterflies in her stomach were suddenly replaced by that cold, creepy feeling she had before. Standing at the end of another hallway was that same man as before. She still couldn't make out his face, but her instincts told her that his stare was fixated on her. She turned away, even though the whispers were telling her not to.

Again, Warlock was compelled to observe the crowd in the backstage area. Every night, since this tour began, he performed the same ritual. Telling himself that he was losing his mind, searching for a vision that wasn't real; his eyes widened as he caught sight of her.

How graceful, this vision in black, that glides through the crowd like a goddess. Still too far away to see her face clearly; he closed his eyes. *This can't be real; it's just an illusion.* He opened his eyes; she was gone. Bracing himself against the wall, he took a deep breath. *My God, I am losing my mind.*

Sabrina sought out the dressing room door as her place of refuge. When they were inside, she locked it. "What did you do that for?" Sean asked. "What? Oh that, habit I guess," she answered, masking her nerves. "I'm gonna take a quick shower and get ready for dinner." He was gone before she could blink. Taking a seat, she used her time alone to contemplate what had been occurring.

I can't deny that these sensations are getting stronger, but I have no concept as to why. Who is this man and why is he watching me all the time?

She was so engrossed in her thoughts that she never heard Sean walk up behind her. He touched her shoulder lightly, and she nearly jumped out of her skin. Standing quickly, she snapped at him angrily. "Christ Sean, don't ever do that to me again!" Her anger, and her words, trailed away as she looked at him. He stood before her dressed in a black tuxedo.

"Oh my," she uttered barely above a whisper. "Does that mean I pass the inspection? I'm sorry I frightened you." She was beyond words. He extended his hand to her. "Well, my pretty lady; your carriage awaits." "So where are we going for dinner?" "Now, no more questions." They made their way to the limo. Sabrina was watchful. Keeping her eyes alert for any sign of that man again.

Taking one of the roses from the bouquet, she placed it in the buttonhole of Sean's jacket. The limo was slow in maneuvering its way out of the arena. She watched out of the windows, as the lights of the arena gave way to the glittering lights of the Las Vegas strip.

This can't be happening. I'm gonna wake up, and find myself back at the beach house. Her concentration was broken as Sean spoke. "Champagne?" he asked holding a glass out to her. "A toast," he held his glass up. "A toast to the most extraordinary, beautiful woman I have ever had the pleasure to meet."

Tears welled up in her eyes; she tried to blink them away but couldn't. A single tear escaped and rolled down her cheek. Sean caught it with his finger, wiping away the moist trail that it had left behind. "There's no need for that; this is supposed to be a happy evening." "I am happy Sean; very happy. I'm just not used to all of this." He smiled at her and took another drink from his glass. *If she only knew the true meaning behind my actions.*

After a tour of the strip, the limo pulled into a large hotel/casino complex; the name was obscured. Sean walked her through the large casino. *I thought that the casinos in Reno were big, but this place is enormous.* They walked straight back to the bank of elevators at the far end of the casino; it took only seconds for them to reach their destination.

The doors opened up to a dimly lit restaurant. They were met by the host. Sean told him his name and a waiter was summoned. They followed him down a hallway, away from the main dining room; she didn't even venture to guess as to where they were going. The waiter stopped in front of a door. "Here we are sir. I will be your waiter for the entire evening; should you require my assistance then please just press the button at the side of the table."

Sean allowed Sabrina to enter first; she stopped in her tracks after only taking three steps into the room, gasping at the sight. The entire private dining room was illuminated solely by candles; a table for two sat against a picture window that overlooked the city. Two high-back, ornately carved chairs framed the table ends. The table was set with sparkling crystal stemware and bright silver cutlery. A bottle of champagne rested in a silver bucket beside the table.

"Do you like it?" Sean asked. "Like it! It's incredible!" That was the only word she could find; but even then, it didn't do justice to the room. She had only read in stories about places like this; never imagining that they really existed.

The mood was delicate. They talked a little, and dined on a wonderful meal. She felt very much relaxed and contented after her strenuous afternoon; her moment in the spotlight so to speak. "So, it's still early; what would you like to do now?" Sean asked. She shrugged a noncommittal answer. "Would you like to go dancing?" "No, I'm not in the mood to go dancing," she answered, scrunching up her nose. "I know what we can do," he announced, helping her to her feet. "We can go down to the casino for a while."

She wobbled for a brief moment; Sean put his arms around her. "No more champagne for you," he said with a slight chuckle. Feeling a bit light headed; she was grateful for his arm around her, as they went down to the casino. "What shall we play first?" "I'm not sure; all I've ever played is the slot machines." "I know; we'll try blackjack." Directing her to one of the tables, she took the seat beside him. There were no other players, so she didn't feel bad about taking a seat away from someone else.

Taking a roll of cash out of his pocket, he turned some of it in for chips. Before the game even started, he turned to her and kissed her. "For luck," he whispered. He placed his bet on the table and the dealer dealt out the cards; Sean got a blackjack right off the bat. "I knew you were my good luck charm," he said.

He continued to play, winning nearly every game. Sabrina finally persuaded him to quit when she realized that he had amassed quite a large stack of chips. With no second thoughts he cashed in. "So what would you like to try? The slot machines maybe?" "Actually, I would just like to go back to the hotel if you don't mind." "Your wish is my command."

The drive back to their hotel only took a matter of minutes. Sean began searching his pockets while they waited for the elevator. "What's the matter?" Sabrina asked. "I can't find the room key. Damn it; I must have left them in my other pants. No problem, I'll be right back." He crossed over to the hotel desk and engaged the clerk in a brief conversation; he soon returned tossing a key in the air as he walked.

I want to touch him; to really touch him and to make love to him. Soon, it has to be soon. She kept silent all the way to their room. Their room, the first one that she hadn't seen yet, they had been busy all day and this was the first time either of them had been in here.

Sean opened the door for her, and began turning on the lights. "Sean please don't. Not so many lights. My eyes have become accustomed to the low lighting." *Besides, dim lights just might make for a better mood.* Complying with her request, he turned out all the lights, with the exception of a small lamp on top of the entertainment center. "Is that better?" "Oh yes, much better; thank you," she answered walking over to the window. "Now you can see the lights of the city much better."

Sean took off his jacket, and went to her side. "Would you like a drink?" "No, thank you. I had a wonderful time today. Thank you so much for everything." She watched him intently as he unbuttoned the top of his shirt. "You don't need to thank me." "Yes, I do," she whispered.

He reached to undo the next button on his shirt; she put her hands on his, stopping him. Slipping her hands under his, she began to loosen the buttons. When she had five of them undone, she cautiously slid her hands inside, gently running her fingers over his chest. Parting the shirt wider, she kissed his chest. She felt him take a deep shuddering breath. She kissed his neck; then his cheek, hesitating briefly to moisten her lips before she kissed his lips.

"You don't have to do this," he struggled, even at a whisper. "I know; but I want to; I really want to." Her arms encircled his neck; he caressed her back. She pulled herself tightly against him, and took his tongue deep into her eager mouth. Sean picked her up and carried her into the bedroom; he kissed her softly as he put her down. "Are you sure?" he asked. "Yes, I'm very sure."

Helping him to remove his shirt, she was finally getting the chance to touch this magnificent body. He ran his hands over her shoulders pulling the straps of her dress down her arms. The dress fell away to the floor. She could feel the tightness of his pants against her. Working quickly, she freed him of his confinement.

Sean eased her back onto the bed and lay down beside her. He kissed her gently as his hand slowly drew up along the inside of her thigh, across her stomach and onto her breast. Her body tingled under his touch, as his hands caressed the fullness of her breasts. Her hands eagerly explored this body next to hers. Every muscle of his body was so firm, so finely honed for his craft.

His kisses progressed down her neck, until they reached her nipples. She moaned as his tongue tenderly teased at them. Moving his hand against her thigh, it traveled slowly upward until he found the moist warmth. Her hips rocked against his touch. She ran her hand through his hair; she could wait no longer. Lifting his face to hers, she kissed him, pulling him on top of her.

With her hands running down his back and over his hips she slowly wrapped her legs around his. With one upward push of her hips he entered her. Her body moved in time with his, and with each thrust she was closer to her climax. When it came, every muscle in her body went rigid, causing her to arch her back. Sean held her tight, feeling her body shudder under his. Exhausted, he rolled off beside her; Sabrina slid herself closer to him, resting her head on his shoulder. She couldn't see the smile that was on his face.

I got what I wanted, again. It took a little longer than usual, but I have achieved my objective. She has a great body to make love to. I think that I'll keep her around; at least until something else catches my attention.

The soul was distraught; this physical union was not with the true mate. It felt the physical need of this body, but it yearned for the tender, endearing passion of long ago. The other was so near; its essence was so strong. This body has to know, it has to see; the mate will know how to stop this pain of isolation.

Sabrina was awakened by Sean's kiss, the touch of his hand against her skin. She stretched her body, still in his embrace, rolling onto her back, resting her arms above her head. Sean supported himself up on one elbow beside her; looking down at her he smiled. "Good morning beautiful." "Good morning." Stretching again, she brought her arms down around his neck, pulling him onto her, eagerly awaiting his kiss.

Their bodies were aroused by the closeness, and the sensations of touch. As his body lowered onto hers they made love again. Only this time Sean was more forceful; taking her harder and faster than the night before. Sabrina noticed the change in intensity, but the physical loneliness within her let him have his way, this time.

Gratified, yet tired, she rolled on her side, nuzzling her head into the pillow. It had his scent on it; she breathed deep while drifting in and out of sleep. She felt Sean leave the bed and soon heard the faint sounds of water running as he turned on the shower. *Oh good; I can have a few more minutes of sleep.* She pulled the sheets up close around her neck, letting the warmth soothe her into slumber.

Sean came back into the bedroom and sat down beside her. "You should have been up already." "I don't want to." "You have to; we have another plane to catch." Lifting up the sheet, she exposed her nude body to him. "You come back to bed." "Well now, with an offer like that, who could refuse."

She eagerly awaited his body next to hers; but with a grasp of the sheet, and one tug, she lay fully exposed to him. He bent over her, slipped his arms under her body, and lifted her up against him. Startled by his actions she spoke abruptly. "What do you think you're doing?" "You're getting in that shower whether you want to or not."

The water splashed over her head and sprayed onto Sean's robe; she kissed him. "Close the door," she whispered. He was somewhat surprised by her comment, but the look on her face was hard to ignore. *She wants me again, and who am I to refuse such an opportunity.*

Her kisses were fast and frequent; she backed up against the shower wall for support. The cold tile was uncomfortable but the feeling of Sean's slick, wet body against hers, soon melted away the cold sensations. Their ecstasy could have lasted much longer if not for the persistent ringing of the telephone. He left the shower to put an end to the nuisance. Sabrina smiled to herself. *It has been a long time since a man has made me feel this good.*

Sean opened the shower door and turned off the water; he handed her a towel. "We really gotta hustle, that was the front desk; the limo is here already and our flight leaves in just over an hour." She put her daydreams aside and got ready to leave.

The flight to San Diego hardly took any time at all, but for Sabrina it seemed to take forever. Unable to get comfortable, she shifted frequently in her seat. Sean had noticed the perpetual fidgeting. "What's the matter?" he asked. She began to blush. "I. It's," she stammered nervously. She was unsure just how to answer him. "It's a little uncomfortable; sitting; here." "I'm sorry," he began, lines of compassion cutting deep into his forehead. "I knew that it was too soon for you. Will you forgive me?" He pulled her as close as he could. "No, Sean you don't understand. You know that I wasn't raped; it's just that it was too many times; last night and again this morning." She was embarrassed to even be talking about it with him.

"I'm still sorry; I never intended to hurt you." His voice was shaky, hoping that she believed him. He had a tendency to get carried away where sex was concerned, and it wasn't often that he was able to view the after effects of his actions. "Shhh, you have nothing to be sorry about; I was a willing participant in this to you know; and this minor discomfort is just a pleasant reminder of your passion." With her cuddled into his embrace; he breathed a sigh of relief.

They went straight to the hotel in San Diego. Sabrina tried to coax him into bed, but he refused her advances. "You should get some rest," he said. "I'm not tired!" "I didn't mean that you should take a nap; I just meant that maybe we should abstain for a little while, until you feel better," he tried to convince her. "Mind you a nap is not such a bad idea now that I think about it."

The look on her face told him that she didn't understand what he meant. "It's going to be quite late by the time we get back from the show tonight; and then there's the early flight tomorrow." He hoped his explanation would have some effect; it wasn't like he was trying to put her off, but he had always avoided sex just before a show; it tired him, and his show quality suffered for it.

Sean had moved over to the couch, and Sabrina followed, easing herself onto the seat beside him. She tucked one leg under her, trying to hide the discomfort from him. He saw her wince. A knot formed in his stomach.

I caused this. I have to get her out of this uncomfortable situation. "Hey why are you over there? Come here," he said patting his lap. "How can

I say no to an offer like that?" Turning around, she lay across his legs, resting her head against the arm of the couch. Her discomfort eased tremendously as she stretched out. "Now this is much better." Sabrina nodded her agreement, but her mind was overwhelmed with thoughts. She closed her eyes, and took in a deep breath, slowly releasing it, chasing away the whispers. Sean watched as her chest heaved upward, tightening against the fabric of her sun dress. He looked away, forcing himself to think of something else.

Her soft voice broke the tension between them. "So, tell me more about this party." "There's not a whole lot to tell; it's just a party." "Just a party; that's not a good enough answer. Who's coming? What time does it start? What do you do at these parties?" "Whoa. Slow down. As for who's coming, well that I won't know until they arrive. The guys all know that I do this; if they can come, great. If they can't make it, it's no big deal. When the party starts, that's hard to say. I've had some show up at noon and some not until midnight. Some of them may stay over if they've had too much to drink; so we'll have to move your things into my room; if that's all right?"

There was still an uneasiness about this whole thing; being with Sean, and this party. "Maybe I should just go back to my place," Sabrina said. Sean's face snapped around to look at her; she saw the distraught look upon it. "Or not. I'd like nothing better than to share your home; and your bed." She kissed him quickly before returning to her reclining position. "So continue on about the party," she prompted.

"As I was saying, some of the guys may need to stay over; and they may not be alone either." He hoped that she wouldn't explore that answer. "Generally, what we do is have a few beers, and sit around and talk. Sometimes a poker game gets going; but basically we just relax and unwind. Sometimes these tours can get pretty hectic and we just need a change of pace for a little while."

"Is there anything that I can do to help?" "Not a thing, Charles knows the routine and I can guarantee that he has everything ready even now. Oh, there is one thing that you can do." "So what would that be?" "This," he leaned down to her kiss her. "And often." "Oh I think I can handle that, no problem. I don't mean to spoil this moment, but what time do you have to be at the arena?" She knew full well what his reaction was going to be. He looked at his watch. "Oh shit; I'm gonna be late."

She moved out of his way so that he could collect his gear for tonight's show. With total disregard, he stuffed his costume into a tote bag.

"You are coming with me tonight?" "Of course, but only if you promise not to drag me out to that ring again." "I promise; cross my heart." "Good, then I'm not going to change my clothes. This dress is really comfortable," she answered, running her hands over the black and white checked garment.

His eyes followed her hands as they glided over her curves. Those feelings were coming back, but now was not the time. "If you're ready then let's blow this place," he interjected, taking his mind off of his thoughts.

Once we're back home, at the beach house, I won't have to keep my thoughts at bay, I will be able to make love to her as much as I want, whenever I want.

The San Diego arena was no different from the others they had been in during the past few days; the roadies were used to seeing Sabrina with Sean and they no longer paid her much attention. She had been granted permission to move about the back stage area whenever she wanted; but she always chose the security of the dressing room. They were never very comfortable, but they were safe.

Sean still had not bothered to introduce her to any of the other wrestlers; but then again the opportunity never really presented itself. They had kept pretty much to themselves at each event, never mixing with the others. That would change at the party. Sabrina found it difficult to occupy herself while he performed his pre-match rituals. Even with him there, the dressing room was becoming a lonely place.

So much has happened to me over the past few weeks. She began having thoughts, doubts even, if being with him was the right thing. *These haunting whispers keep telling me it's a mistake; yet I can't deny that he makes me feel good. Is it that I've been alone for too long, and am merely infatuated by his attention, his affection, or is he the man in my visions? If only I could remember more details, to find something that linked the two together.*

Unknowingly she was pacing the length of the dressing room when Sean returned from the shower. He could see that she was deep in thought, and it had caused deep lines to form across her forehead. "Hey, you okay?" he asked. "Hmm, yeah; I guess I'm just a little anxious." "Are you sure that's all there is to it?" "Yes, I am very sure," she answered hoping that her face had not given away her lie. The knock at the door gave her a chance to change the direction of their conversation.

"Time for you to go." "Walk me to the entrance?" "Sure, but you had better not have forgotten your promise to me." "I haven't forgotten. You can watch from the side of the entrance, near the edge of the curtain." Taking her hand, they walked down the corridor to the entrance way. Except for a few people wearing EVENT STAFF shirts the hall was nearly empty.

The noise coming from the arena made it impossible for them to talk, so they didn't. Sean guided her to the right hand side of the entrance; a small part in the curtain would allow her a view of the ring. Even with her, he had become ritualistic. As the entrance music began to play, Sean gave her a kiss on the cheek. "For luck," he said, whispering into her ear. A quick wink, and he made his entrance into the arena.

She observed as he performed for his fans. He truly enjoyed what he was doing and the fans liked him. The match began, she smiled when he was in control; and cringed when he wasn't. She didn't understand what all the wrestling moves were but some of them looked painful as well as dangerous. She continued to watch, but that feeling of unease began to crawl over her again. Looking around, she only saw a couple of guys working with some cable.

No one else is around, so why do I feel this way? Putting it out of her mind, she returned to watching the events in the ring; the feeling refused to go away gaining strength; she trembled, as a chill shot up her spine. She wrapped her arms around herself, holding tight. Feelings of paranoia ran through her mind as she again scanned the backstage area.

There's no one else here. She scolded herself for being so silly. She was about to refocus her attentions back onto Sean when, out of the corner of her eye, she spotted movement at the far side of the curtain; her eyes strained to see through the darkness. *There was definitely movement, not my imagination.* A wave of fear overtook her. She wanted to run, but couldn't. Her body refused to respond to her commands. The shadows moved forward, into the light. *Oh God, it's him; that man, again all dressed in black.*

Hear me, the soul whispered, see me. Know me for who I am.

He moved towards her; her heart was pounding; he moved closer, his eyes staring into hers. She could see him more clearly now; his long black robe moved silently with each step he took; his long dark hair shadowing his pale, ghostly face. She didn't know whether to faint or run; but it was impossible to tear herself away from his stare. There was recognition that went deeper than the physical facade. The chills in her spine had been replaced with searing spears of panic; beads of perspiration formed on her forehead.

If I don't make a move soon I'll be trapped. She commanded her body to move and slowly it responded. Taking small steps at first, brushing against the wall as she moved; every step put more space between them. His robe moved again; his hand appeared from beneath it; reaching out to her. A wave of panic rushed through her. Gaining the power that she needed, she turned and ran as fast as she could back to the dressing room; back to her realm of safety behind a locked door.

With his head slumped downward, Warlock turned away. *I've scared her terribly; the one thing that I never intended to do. All I wanted to do was to talk to her. My instincts tell me that I must; she has to know; but it's more than that. That urgency that I had felt before, had willed me to her. Why? There is more to this, more than just her needing to know about Sean.* Humbled by his own guilt, he returned to the shadows, to await his turn in the ring.

Sabrina's body shook violently as she leaned against the door; her stomach churned. She ran to the bathroom to be sick; she knelt on the floor until her body stopped heaving. Tears rolled down her face. *Who is this man? Why does he affect me so? My mind is so mixed up.*

When Sean returned from the ring, he was surprised to find that Sabrina wasn't waiting for him. Shrugging it off, he walked back to the dressing room. Finding the door locked, he knocked and called out her name; there was no response. He knocked again, louder, still calling to her; still no response from inside. His fist pounded against the door now. "Sabrina open the door!" His pounding and yelling drew the attention of some of the workers. Worry was over taking his mind. "Hey you!" he snapped at one of the workers. "Yeah you, go and get the damn key for this door. Now!"

The worker took off at a run, searching for the security guard. Sean continued to call to Sabrina. Now throwing himself against the door he tried to break the lock open. Lorenzo heard the commotion and came to see what was going on. Sean told him that Sabrina was locked inside, and not answering him. Lorenzo suggested that they try kicking the door in; Sean followed Lorenzo's lead but it was a useless effort; the steel plated door refused to budge.

Sean's thoughts ran wild. *Is she okay? Has something happened to her?* Driven by his own fears, he continued his attack on the door, until the head of security returned with his pass key in hand. Unlocking the door, Sean burst into the room, Lorenzo behind him.

Sean searched the room. Listening, he heard her sobs coming from the bathroom. She was huddled on the floor, rocking back and forth. His heart sank as he knelt beside her. Lorenzo backed away, ushering the inquisitive congregation of people out of the dressing room.

She looks so fragile, like she did that horrible night not so long ago. He spoke softly to her, reaching out to her with his hand. Recognizing his voice, she looked up at him; her face paled by the tears that poured over her cheeks. She couldn't speak, but limply raised her arms to him, seeking comfort. Sean held her tight; her tears spilled onto his chest as he rocked her. It took her a long time to calm down and when she was relaxed against him, he lifted her face up. Her eyes were so red and puffy, the tracks of her tears still boldly visible.

"I'm taking you out of here," he said helping her to stand up, but her balance was poor. He lifted her into his arms. She concealed her face against his neck when they went into the dressing room. Lorenzo was sitting on a bench near the door; he stood up as they entered. Sean passed close to him and stopped.

"Thanks man; I'm gonna take her to the hotel right now. Hey, could you do me a favor?" "You bet Sean, anything." "Would you mind collecting my stuff and then just bring it with you tomorrow?" "Hey, it's no problem." "Thanks again; it's just really important that I get her out of here." "Don't worry about it; I'll see you tomorrow." Sean left the dressing room, still carrying Sabrina; past the crowd of workers and wrestlers that had gathered in the hallway, and on to the limo that was waiting for them.

Reclining against the seat, her body came to rest partially atop his. He stroked her hair, and rubbed her back; soothing the tension in her muscles. "Do you want to tell me what happened?" he asked. She pulled back from him; rubbing her face, and running her hands through her hair.

He coaxed her again. "Can you? Will you tell me what happened?" She took in a deep, shaky breath, and let out a long sigh. "I got scared." "What do you mean you were scared?" Sean asked. She began to explain, but her anxiety showed through. "You left me at the curtain; it was dark. I heard something and I got scared." Her tears began again.

"I'm sorry Sabrina. I shouldn't have left you there alone. The memories of your attack are still relatively fresh. I just didn't think; I'm sorry." "No, Sean, it's not your fault. I've tried to put that night out of my mind; but I guess that the circumstances tonight just brought it all back to me. Please don't blame yourself." "In a way I do blame myself. We have never really talked about that night. The Doctor told me that I should encourage you to talk about it; he said that it would help you to deal with it and move on; but I never took the initiative. I never tried to get you to open up. I just didn't know how."

That was a bold faced lie; he just didn't care. Talk was the farthest thing from his mind, right from the first time he saw her. She could see the mock look of concern on his face but disregarded it anyway. "Sean I appreciate that you didn't force me into talking about it; all I wanted to do was to forget it; and I thought I had succeeded, until tonight." "I want you to tell me about tonight; the truth this time." "I did tell you." "I don't think so; I get the feeling that there is a lot more to it than you just being afraid of the dark or a noise." She lowered her head, away from his piercing eyes; his hand lifted it back up. "Tell me what happened?"

"I told you I heard something; but I also saw someone." "Go on." "On the far side of the entrance way, there was someone standing in the shadows. He moved towards me and I panicked. I felt trapped, so I ran, back to the dressing room, where it was safe. I was so scared." "Did you get a look at this man? I didn't see anyone when I came back." "Not really; all I know is he was wearing a black robe." "That sounds like the Warlock." "The Warlock?" "Yeah. His real name is Mark Cassidy, but around here he's known as the Warlock. You'll get to meet him at the party."

Sabrina pulled away from him in surprise, and fear. "It's okay; he's an all right kind of guy. His character does make him appear a bit creepy; but he's nothing like that, really," he said giving her a reassuring smile. She was having second thoughts about this party, but she didn't want to disappoint Sean.

It's important to him that I be there, no matter how awkward it makes me feel. Mark Cassidy; his name means a warrior and defender. From the little that I have seen of him he does look like a warrior. Maybe that's what it is about him that sets me on edge every time I see him. He's probably and Aries too, ruled by Mars, that's what gives him his warrior qualities.

Sabrina laid her head against Sean's shoulder and drove all of her thoughts away. Sean was still dressed in his ring costume. Her hand began to trace over the muscles in his chest. "I need you so much," she whispered. Sean responded to her gentle touch with great passion. Sliding her body over his, she repositioned herself so that her knees straddled his body. "Make love to me," she whispered, teasing his earlobe with her tongue.

Sean straightened her up in front of him; bracing her from kissing him again. "No, we're almost to the hotel." "I need you to love me, now, not later." "Soon, Sabrina, I promise." "Then touch me." She loosened the buttons that held the straps to her dress; it fell away exposing her breasts. His hold on her eased as his self control slipped away.

How can I resist such a creature? He kissed her deeply letting their bodies touch. Sean broke away from her, and pulled the dress back up over her. "What's wrong? Don't you want me?" "Oh God Sabrina; I want you so bad right now; but I want to wait. I don't want to make love to you in the back seat of a car like some sex starved teen-agers."

They cuddled together, each quietly anticipating their arrival, and the pleasures that awaited them both. He could have taken her right then; but he had no condoms; and he never had sex without them, just in case.

How she turns me on, never have I met another woman that has the same strong sex drive as I do. It will be a long time before I become bored with her.

Warlock sat alone in his dressing room, contemplating his actions of this evening. *What had possessed me to approach her the way I did; scaring her half to death? What is it about her that compelled me to go to her? She's with Sean, I know that; but she shouldn't be. It isn't my place to interfere with Sean's relationships; she will have to find out, on her own, what kind of a jerk she is involved with. But those feelings that flooded my mind; it couldn't be her; it just couldn't.*

Chapter 5

The next week of shows took them through Texas, New Mexico, Colorado and back to California. Sabrina was physically exhausted; from the perpetual traveling and from being Sean's love slave. He never overlooked an opportunity to take her to bed. The changes that had occurred in him were very noticeable. When they made love it wasn't the lingering, passion filled experience like the first time, but now much swifter and almost forceful. Long soaks in the tub, helped to ease her physical pain that his seemingly unsympathetic actions had caused her.

I long to go home, to my beach house, it would be good just to relax, and sleep. With Sean's voracious appetite for sex, I know that sleep will only come when he's exhausted. It doesn't seem to matter to him that I'm not in the mood all the time. He has to satisfy his compulsions, no matter what.

It distressed her slightly, but just to have the affections of such a handsome man dashed all of her misgivings. He never pressured her to go out to the ring with him again. The anxiety of seeing the Warlock caused her to conceal herself in the dressing room. The distant image of his face still sent goose bumps crawling over her flesh. Not that he repulsed her, but he was such an enigma. Swarthy and spectral, that was what had piqued her own dark side. Something about him had awakened a strange feeling inside her.

Yet with all the shows that they had been to, Sean still had not introduced her to any of the guys he worked with and that bothered her more than she really wanted to admit. He kept her segregated from the others. Even their flights were different. She recognized some of the faces at the airports but none of them were ever on the same flight as they were. She thought it strange but then again maybe that was how Sean was. Maybe he didn't need the social interaction of his coworkers, but why a party at the end of a tour?

The last show of the week, took them to Anaheim, California. They were supposed to drive home from there to the beach house; but that was not to be. The tour had been extended. In a way, Sabrina was relieved; the extension also deferred the party she was dreading. After touring through the Pacific Northwest and Canada, they finally ended up back in Los Angeles.

Sean had a car waiting to take them home. Sabrina managed to sleep for most of the way, since Sean never touched her while they were in the car.

It was good to be home. Patches made himself a perfect pest; he missed his master and was not about to let her out of his sight; she didn't like it much when Sean bounced the cat off of the bed their first night home. To lie down on a comfortable bed again was heaven; hotels were nice, but the beds were always so hard and uncomfortable.

Sean was excited about being home; he had told her that he couldn't wait to make love to her in his bed; and he did, repeatedly, until he succumbed to the exhaustion. Sabrina sneaked Patches back onto the bed and cuddled him for the night; away from Sean.

Sabrina was awake early; before dawn. Her stomach was upset. It burned in her throat. Turning on her side, she hoped that it would go away; but it didn't. She left the bed and hurried to the bathroom to be sick. Crawling quietly back into bed; she tried not to rouse Sean, but it was too late; he was awake. Her hasty departure had awakened him and he had heard her in the bathroom.

"Are you okay?" he asked. "I've been better. Maybe I've got a touch of the flu; or maybe it's just my nerves getting to me after three weeks of traveling, and now the party today." Sean touched her forehead. "You don't seem to have a fever; and I wouldn't worry about the party. Everything will be just fine. Now try and go back to sleep." His voice seemed so far away as she drifted; her dreams took her away to a tranquil place. Free from anxiety; lost amongst the clouds; and her visions.

They were awakened, when Charles knocked on the bedroom door. Sean acknowledged him, stretching himself beside Sabrina. He pulled the hair away from her face. "Feeling better?" "Much, thank you." "So, do you want the shower first or shall I?" "How about we take a shower together?" Sabrina suggested. "No, I don't think so. I'm having a hard enough time just getting out of bed; don't tempt me with that shower bit. There are still things that I have to do before our guests arrive." In his face she could see that he was trying to be firm with her, but his eyes told her that he was in conflict. "Fine then, you take the shower," she said pushing him toward the edge of the bed.

Slipping on a robe, she padded off down the hall, to her old room, and began searching for something to wear. Her closet was quite empty; she looked around for her luggage but didn't see it. *The bags must be in Sean's room.* There were no suitcases on the floor, or in the closet. "Where could it be? Maybe Charles knows." She called to him from the top of the stairs. "Charles?" "Yes ma'am." "Is our luggage down there anywhere?" "No ma'am; none came in with you last night." "Thank you, Charles." Sabrina was even more bewildered. *It couldn't have just vanished.* She returned to the bedroom and sat on the bed.

When Sean came into the bedroom, he caught immediately, the frowning look, that was directed at him. "Hey, what's with that look?" "Do you happen to know just where my luggage is?" "Yeah, there was a mix up at the airport. Tony ended up with it; he'll bring it along later. Why?" "First of all, who is Tony?" "Oh sorry, you know him as Lorenzo." "And secondly, what do you recommend I wear, since my clothes are somewhere in Los Angeles!"

"You didn't pack everything, did you?" "No, but all that's left is just some old shorts and tank tops." "What's wrong with that, at least for now anyway. When Tony arrives you can go and change if you want to; but it's not really necessary, this party is really casual." "Maybe to you it is; but I've never met any of these people and first impressions are very important." "Honestly, it really doesn't matter what you wear. Just pick out something that's comfortable for you." He kissed her on the forehead and began steering her towards the bathroom. "Your turn; and stop worrying." *Easy for you to say, you know these guys I don't.*

Stopping at the kitchen, Sabrina picked up a glass of juice, and a fruit salad; she took it out to the deck, and sat down at the table across from Sean. "You look terrific," he said. She had managed to find a pair of shorts, and a tight pink tank top to wear. "This is the best I could do; considering." "It's great; perfect for a beach party."

He stared at the low cut tank top that she wore. She handed him a napkin. "What's this for?" "You're drooling, just carry on reading your newspaper and let me have my breakfast in peace." She avoided his continued glance by gazing out at the ocean; it was breathtaking, hearing the waves and inhaling the salt air.

Being on tour with Sean has been an extraordinary diversion, but I much prefer the solitude of the beach, over the commotion of the cities. She took in a deep breath of the sweet salty air. *It's so placid, so mesmerizing.*

In reflection, she drifted back to her mother. *She would so disapprove of what I was doing, living with a man in sin, and the attack, well, I know exactly what mother's response would be to that. She would have told me that it was my own fault; that I had brought it on myself. Things like that don't happen to respectable girls. If I had only stayed home, like I was supposed to, then I wouldn't be in this predicament.* Sabrina rolled her eyes back. "Bitch," she muttered.

"Excuse me?" Sean was surprised by what he had just heard. "Nothing, I was just thinking." "What were you thinking about?" "It was nothing very important." He thought better than to ask again. *It must be something that really bothers her, for her to use a word like that with such anger attached to it.* "Any idea what time your friends will be arriving?" Sabrina asked.

"Maybe two or three, I'm not really sure. Why?" "I just thought that if I had some time I should write a letter to a friend back home; just to let them know that I haven't dropped off the face of the earth." "Sure, you have plenty of time for that. Charles has everything under control here; and I can disappear if you want some privacy." "You don't have to do that; I like having you around."

He smiled at her. Sabrina looked at his face; it seemed different somehow, softer, more relaxed. The lines of fatigue that only two days ago seemed to age him greatly were all gone now. His face had that youthful appearance that she saw when she first met him. *He's glad to be home too.*

"Would you like to go for a walk on the beach first?" he asked. "Now that sounds like a good idea." "Oh I have to do just one thing first." He leaned in through the open patio door, to tell Charles where they were going. "I wouldn't want him to worry you know."

The surf washed over their feet; Sabrina picked up a long piece of driftwood, using it as her walking stick. Poking it into the sand, annoying the clams, until one would squirt at her in retaliation. They stopped to rest upon a large log that had washed ashore. *Such power the ocean has, the ability to advance huge logs far onto the beach. From what distant shore had they traveled?*

Prodding blindly at the sand, she stared out into the horizon. "This is a dream," she said. "What do you mean?" "Being here, being with you; I can't help feeling that I'm gonna wake up and find myself back home." She felt his arm slide around her shoulders. "You're not dreaming," he said softly. "Could a dream do this?" His lips searched out hers. He kissed her, a long, slow, sensuous kiss.

They continued to cuddle together, contemplating the rhythmic movement of the water. Sean looked at his watch. "You know we've been gone for nearly two hours; we had better start for home." Standing in front of her, he took her hands, giving them a playful tug. Knowing what he was doing she played along. She let his tug pull her up and to him.

He steadied himself, as her body settled against his. Embracing her, his hands roved over her body; his eyes traveled around her face, down to her breasts and back up again. She took his face in her hands; leaning in close, close enough to kiss him, but she didn't. "Let's go home," she whispered. Pushing out of his embrace, she ran ahead of him; glancing back to see if he followed. Sean ran after her, getting almost to her, then deliberately backing off.

Catching her near the stairs to the sun deck, he took her up in his arms and spun her around, before bringing her down into the warm sand. He lay beside her, his leg constraining hers. They were both winded from the run, but laughing; both of which dissipated when he leaned down to kiss her. Their lips touched briefly, as a voice from above distracted them both. "Christ, get a room why don't ya." Sean looked up towards the voice. "Tony! Hey man how are ya?" "Obviously not as good as you." Sean helped Sabrina up, brushing the sand from her back. He ascended the stairs, with Sabrina slowly behind him.

The two men immediately exchanged hand shakes. "Sabrina." Sean summoned her to his side. "I'd like you to meet Tony Underhill. Tony this is Sabrina Scott." "I'm pleased to meet you Sabrina. I see that you're feeling much better than the last time I saw you." "Yes, I am," she responded, with some confusion. Sean saw the look.

"You should remember; I told you that Tony was in the dressing room that night that you were sick; and he's also the one that is bringing our luggage home." "Oh now I remember. That was some time ago. I'm sorry that I." "Hey don't worry about it; stuff happens." She smiled at his sincerity. "Where is the luggage?" "Charles said that he would take care of it." "Well then; if you gentlemen will excuse me." She left the sun deck, to go in search of her clothes; and to get rid of the rest of the sand that still clung to her legs.

Their bags were neatly stacked by the closet door; she tore through them, looking for one specific item. Finding it, she quickly stripped away her shorts and went into the bathroom to wash away the remains of the sand. Brushing her hair, sand fell about the counter top; she wiped it away and slipped into her new outfit.

She gazed at her image in the mirror, first one side, and then the other. A peacock blue dress, with thin straps, that had no practical purpose, but with the small amount of spandex in it, she had no fear of it falling down; straps or not, her breasts took care of that. It hugged every curve of her body, clinging to her thighs. She smiled, liking what she saw in the mirror; convinced that everything was in place, she made her way back to the sun deck.

Sean and Tony sat chatting. Sean took the opportunity while Sabrina was away, to enlighten Tony about how he had come to meet her. He also filled in some of the particulars of the past few weeks. Not to many components, but just enough that she wouldn't be agitated if it came up in a conversation some other time. The dialogue was abruptly averted when Sean heard Sabrina talking to Charles. There was a sudden silence as she stepped onto the deck. Tony leaned back in his chair, nearly tipping over. "Oh wow," was all he could manage to say.

Sean was speechless at the sight of her; he took a couple of steps forward; she met him halfway. "Do you like my dress?" she asked. "Like it! I think you know what I'd like to do with you in that dress; or out of it." He was playing with her ear as he spoke. His breath was hot with passion, his heart beat loudly against her. "Okay you two, knock it off before I get a bucket of water," Tony interrupted.

Sean escorted Sabrina to a chair, between Tony and himself. She felt awkward knowing that both of them were still staring at her. The silence was tedious; no one wanted to talk; she decided that she had better get things rolling. "Tony; thank you so much for bringing our luggage home." "Hey no problem, I'm happy to do it for you. Ya know in this business we're all kind of like a family; we take care of each other." "Speaking of taking care," Sean interrupted. "Can I get you a drink?" "Sure man; a beer would be good right now." "I'll have one too please," Sabrina added.

Sean disappeared into the house; Sabrina seized the moment. "Excuse my boldness, but Tony Underhill doesn't strike me as being a Latin name; or am I mistaken?" "No, you're not wrong; I am about as far away as you can get. I was born and raised in Florida, and so were my parents." "Why did you choose the name Lorenzo?" "Well, it has a lot to do with the guys that I work for; they thought that with my dark hair and dark skin I fit the Latin profile." "Well, I would have to agree with them. Anyway, how long have you been doing this; wrestling I mean?" "Let's see now; I started in school; I guess about twenty years; but I've only been in pro wrestling for the past twelve years." "Obviously you enjoy it." "Ya that I do; but it's not been easy, for me or any of us. I don't know of anyone who hasn't had something broken, or had to have surgery to fix a banged up knee or shoulder."

Sean had returned with their drinks, only to turn and leave when he heard the doorbell. "That should be the rest of the guys," Tony said. Sabrina fidgeted in her chair. Tony saw her nervousness. "That's right, you haven't met any one else; have you?" "No, I haven't." "Hey don't worry; they're an okay bunch of guys."

His reassuring tone did nothing to console her. She felt the butterflies in her stomach again. They fluttered wildly as the men's voices grew nearer to the patio door. Sean stepped through first, followed by three very tall men; she gasped at the sight. *So many good looking men in one place and all at one time, it's hard to believe.* All of them exchanged handshakes with Tony, but maintained their gaze on Sabrina.

Her body was trembling slightly as Sean put his arm around her waist. "Guys, I'd like you to meet Sabrina. Sabrina this is D'arcy Virtue, Brent Shea and Sam Ellis." They each, in turn, stepped forward to shake her hand. She searched her memory for the details of each man.

D'arcy Virtue, he's known as the Vulture. Brent Shea, the Master of Misery and Sam Ellis, Suicide Sam. She greeted them each politely.

Sean reinforced his hold on her, not for her reassurance, but as a declaration of possession. He was communicating to these guys that for now she belonged to him; and he wasn't about to share. "Sean, where ever did you find this lovely woman?" Sam asked, as he kissed her hand. "Well actually, she rented the beach house down there a while ago." "Why have you kept her a secret for this long?"

Sean only smiled, proud of his current appropriation. D'arcy, who had been leaning against the railing, glared at Sean. "Sean you know this is gonna be a real pain in the ass with." "That's not a topic for discussion!" Sean had rudely cut him off. Sabrina ignored the tone; she was engrossed in her own thoughts.

How different these guys look, away from the ring. Sam is the tallest, standing six foot nine at least; his curly light brown hair accentuates his dark brown tan and gently frames his bright blue eyes. How powerful he looks, yet under all that power he has a boyish charm that is hard to resist. His muscled body taught yet smooth; he must shave his chest, why I don't know. He sported a tank top with a pair of denim cutoffs, that had the side seams split to allow his massive thighs more comfort. *His body is exquisitely honed; every muscle visible, from his face to his toes. He would be the perfect subject for a sculptor.*

Her gaze slowly moved to D'arcy, still leaning on the railing. *How could he have come to be known as the Vulture? Sam is easy, because of his almost suicidal acrobatic exploits in the ring; but D'arcy.* She thought hard, trying to see the personality that was this man; envisioning a vulture, the similarities revealed themselves.

D'arcy is bald, so is a vulture, sort of. The eyes, they both have spooky dark eyes and he's always watching. I noticed that even at the arenas. He likes to stand back from the crowd and observe. I wonder what he's watching for; his next prey perhaps? He has a robust frame, but not very well defined. His strength is in his arms and his thighs. He's slightly taller than Sean, maybe six three or four; his tan, pale, compared to the others. I'm not too sure about him yet. He is a strange one that's for sure. His body was almost shiny in appearance under the black denim vest that he wore. It revealed to Sabrina, a man who enjoyed everything that life had to offer. His jeans cut deep into his waist.

Not wanting to be caught staring, she shifted her glance to Brent. *This one is even harder to figure out. He has an arrogance about him; the way he moves, the unchanging expression. It's like he's always locked in deep thought. His brow is always taught and that draws his eye brows together giving him an intensity I don't understand. I've never seen him smile. His dark brown, thick wavy hair, resting upon his shoulders, it doesn't look right; it should be shorter, much shorter.*

The T-shirt and loose fitting jeans, give up no clues as to his physical form. Even his ring costumes don't show off his body. The scars on his forehead tell a story all on their own. I suspect that he's a guy who likes to fight; with anyone, anytime and probably anywhere. Of the few matches that I have seen Brent in, he is intense in the ring like he constantly has something to prove to the world. He comes by his title honestly; he sure likes to inflict pain upon his opponents. I wonder if it truly is an act? I don't want to find out. I've never seen him without sunglasses. Is he hiding? From whom or what I wonder?

Her concentration was cut short when Sean touched her shoulder. Startled by it she shuddered. His hand drifted down her arm to her hand, and he gently tugged her up out of the chair. "This is a party; no wallflowers allowed. May I have this dance?" She was only now aware of the music that flowed from the speakers on the deck. Sean never waited for her answer, gliding her across the deck. It was a slow, romantic song that played; she pressed herself tight against him. Their bodies swayed together, long after the song had ended.

There's a sense of safety in his arms; yet there's still an uneasy feeling gnawing at me; a feeling that I can't quite grasp, yet alone shake.

Everything had gone quiet; no music playing, no voices talking. Their guests were all absorbed in watching them; she pulled back from Sean. "I think your friends need a little attention." "Yeah, but so do I," he winked at her and turned to his friends. "Ah, sorry guys; I got a little distracted." "Yeah right," was the echoing response from the group. "I hope that you're not gonna be selfish Sean," Sam proclaimed. "Well, that's up to Sabrina; if she wants to risk her feet with you guys; then it's all right with me." "Well Sabrina? Would you honor me with the next dance?" Sam asked. "Why most certainly sir, I would love to dance with you."

The music started up again and Sam seized his opportunity. They danced through two songs, and her tension eased. Finally she had begun to relax and was actually enjoying the afternoon. Within a couple of hours she felt very comfortable with these guys. They were just a regular bunch of guys, unwinding after work; having a few beers and a lot of laughs. Sabrina had become involved in a conversation with D'arcy when she overheard Brent speaking to Sean. "Hey Sean, where is Mark?" "Warlock? Oh he'll be along anytime now; he said he was coming." A cold spike shot up her spine. Her uneasiness returned in a multitude. *Sean had said he was coming but I had forgotten.*

Excusing herself from D'arcy, she went into the house; needing some space to regain her composure. Standing by the window, in the den, she took three long deep breaths, with each exhale she commanded her body to relax; it refused. The incessant whispering had returned to persecute her.

Going to the bar, she poured herself a glass of bourbon; knocking it back in one shot. She had poured another when Sean opened the door.

"What are you doing?" He spoke harshly to her. "What does it look like, I'm having a drink!" she snapped back at him. He took the glass from her hand and set it down. "What's the matter with you?" he asked. She rolled her eyes back. "What's the matter? I don't know if I can deal with this guy Mark." "He's just one of the guys for God's sake. A bit of a recluse but he's not someone you should fear. He's just like Sam and D'arcy once you get to know him."

"There's something about him that bothers me." "Like what?" "I don't know; just something!" "Come here. There's nothing to worry about you'll see." He held her close. "We should go back outside, or their gonna think that we're in here doing something that we shouldn't." He lifted her face up, a devilish grin across his lips. She smiled back and tried to laugh. "See you're feeling better already." She kept repeating to herself that she could handle this; driving the whispers in her head into a far away place.

They stepped back out onto the deck, amid a volley of cat calls and whistles. "Snuck off for a little afternoon delight," Tony smirked. "Now boys, if you think that we disappeared for some private play time you are absolutely wrong." "Why should we believe you?" Brent asked with a touch of sarcasm in his voice. "It's really simple gentlemen you would not have seen Sean again until sometime tomorrow." She blushed, caught off guard by her own words. The cat calls echoed again. "That is one sassy lady," Sam remarked, shaking his head.

Sean stepped in, changing the conversation, annoyed by their insinuations. Her body and her passion were for him only, at least for now. "Okay you've all had your fun; now let's get this barbecue going." Sabrina took a seat amongst the group of men and struck up a conversation with anyone who was willing to talk.

The afternoon had gone quite well; she had broken the ice, and was accepted into the fold. The guys relaxed around her, feeling that they could talk about any subject, now that she had relieved their own tensions about her. Sean kept himself busy; he had donned an apron and was preparing to put the steaks on the barbecue.

Sabrina felt that cold chill again. *It's just the breeze.* The doorbell rang; her body tensed as Sean went into the house. She waited, gripping her hands to the edge of the railing. Sean returned in moments, followed by a man. *It's him!* She braced herself against the railing as the two men moved towards her. Everything was in slow motion, each step bringing them closer.

This man towered above Sean. *He must be nearly seven feet tall.* His pale, colorless face, partially concealed by a pair of dark sunglasses; his hair was a dark auburn nearly black and it was pulled back into a long pony tail. Another step closer; she breathed deep, feeling it burn in her throat. Her eyes were riveted on this man. She scanned his body quickly.

He wore a black sleeveless shirt that was only partly buttoned; and with each step that he took, it parted slightly to reveal a smooth, yet very powerful chest. His arms were large, strong, and covered in many tattoos, most of them from the elbows up to his shoulders. The figure of a snake coiled around and around his right arm, stretching from his wrist to his shoulder. The head of the snake she couldn't see as it was hidden by his shirt. Another step closer; Sean had stopped in front of her.

"Sabrina," Sean called, snapping her back to reality. "Sabrina I'd like you to meet Mark Cassidy; the Warlock." Sabrina stood quietly; suspended in place and time. She stared as this leviathan as he removed his sunglasses, revealing his emerald green eyes. The hair on the back of her neck stood up as his hand reached out to her. She knew that her own hand was reaching back to him, but tearing herself away from those eyes was impossible. The sensation that he was looking deep inside her was so intense. Their hands locked, and she was overcome by a surge of energy. An electrical charge, that ran up her arm into her body. He spoke. "It's nice to meet you Sabrina."

His voice, it's so deep and commanding; yet oddly soothing; his expression never changing. I can't detect any emotion on his face. He presents all the outward qualities of a true warrior. She felt herself being drawn into the depths of his green eyes. As she looked deeper into his eyes she felt the sadness and the loneliness that was all too familiar to her. There was a feeling of recognition, a kinship of some kind that she had never before felt from any other living person.

The souls had touched once again. The dynamic convergence sent invigorating tremors through the physical bodies. They reveled in the enlightening pleasures of their immortal bond of pure love. The bodies will come to understand the need. We will not be separated my love; they will know.

Sean gave her a slight nudge that broke her concentration. Mark released her hand and the pulsating wave that had been pouring through her stopped abruptly. "Yes, it's n, nice to meet you too," she stammered nervously. Sean grabbed Mark by the arm. "Hey man, you're way behind; let's get you a beer and start these steaks cooking." He ushered Mark over to the cooler; fishing around in the ice, he found a beer and tossed it to Mark.

Sabrina exhaled, seeking a diversion from her tension, but it was pointless. The others began to gather around Sean, giving him instructions on how to cook the steaks. Her eyes followed Mark; even in street clothes there was still something about him that she couldn't quite grasp. *He doesn't look as intimidating as before; but what is it about him?*

Unable to shrug off the feeling, she told Sean that she was going in to see if Charles had any appetizers ready. She made a swift exit from the deck, and away from Mark. *Just a few minutes alone, that's what I need.* Busying herself in the kitchen, she arranged snacks on a tray, concentrating on the music that drifted in from the living room; but her mind drifted back to Mark and his incredible green eyes.

They are such a remarkable color, he must be wearing colored contacts, but that feeling that went through me, when we touched, that I can't explain away. She took another sip of her beer; a shudder went through her. *Damn, this beer is colder than I thought. No, it isn't the beer it's something else.* She turned quickly.

Mark was standing in the doorway, watching her. He was unable to tear himself away from her. *I should speak, but I can't. I felt the surge of power when we touched, but it was more. She is genuine, not part of my imagination. I have to be near her, yet she confuses me so.*

A chilling wave swept over Sabrina, and she became very defensive, feeling like a caged animal. "How long have you been standing there!" He offered up no response, and that infuriated her even more. "It's very rude to sneak up on someone like that!"

Picking up her tray, she moved toward him, to her only way out. "I have to take these out to Sean." Mark shifted his weight from the door frame and stood straight, blocking the doorway, and her escape. She felt so insignificant near him.

"This is not a good time for you to go out there," he said. "What do you mean by that?" "Please be quiet and listen." The music had stopped; Sabrina could hear loud voices coming from the sun deck. There was a man's voice; Sean's voice; and a woman's voice loud and angry. "Who's that? Sean never mentioned," she was confused. "She must be with one of the guys, right? Why is Sean so angry? I have to go out there." She made another attempt to get passed Mark but he stood fast. "Please; I ask that you remain in here; just for a little while longer." "Fine, if I am to stay in here, then I suggest that you explain to me just what in the hell is going on out there!"

Mark lowered his head. *I don't want to do this, but she has a right to know.* "Well, I'm waiting!" Her voice was becoming more agitated than before. "All right, that voice you hear is Robbie. She's been a part of this business for a couple of years now; and," he paused to think before he said anything else. "And what? Oh for Christ's sake would you just say it!" She was angry, yet afraid to hear what he was about to say.

"Sean and Robbie, well, they have a history together. They have a very personal and intimate history." He was trying to pad his response, to ease her into this. "So what you're saying is that they were lovers; right? Once upon a time they were lovers, so what?" "It's not quite like that. They have been close for a very long time and up until very recently." "How recently?" "They haven't seen each other for the past few weeks; that's when Robbie went away on a long promo tour."

"That can't be; I only met Sean a few weeks ago. There's no evidence that another woman has been in this house." "That's right, because when you went on tour with him that's when he had all of her things packed up and shipped back." "How do you know so damn much?" Her defenses were rising.

"I overheard him talking about it to one of the guys." "What!" "When he met you, that's when he decided to ditch Robbie, again." Sabrina stepped back, leaning against the counter for support. "I can't believe it. Sean has been carrying on a long time relationship and then just like that he decides to switch from her to me. I don't understand." She lowered her head, fighting back her tears.

Mark decided to take a bold chance. *I have to, even if she pushes me away, I have to do this.* He moved to her, putting his hands on her shoulders. "I'm sorry that you had to find out like this, but there's more that you need to know." "More?" She wasn't overly surprised. "What more could there possibly be?" Mark made sure she was looking at him. "This isn't the first time that he's done this; Robbie has been given the boot before. Sean has a real strong attraction to beautiful women."

Her heart was in her throat; she had been falling for Sean, and Mark's words cut her hard. She looked into his eyes; searching; but all she saw was sincerity and truth. "What are you going to do now?" Mark asked. "In the long term; I don't know yet; but right now I most certainly do not want to confront that bitch, and as for Sean; I guess I'll just wait and see what happens; see if he tells me or not." "I suggest that you find yourself another room in the house and wait this out; it could take a while."

Sabrina left for the seclusion of the den; Mark followed. Locking the door behind them, she went straight to the bar. "Damn it I need a drink." She poured herself a bourbon; downing it in one swallow then poured another. Mark attempted to speak, but she quickly cut him off. "Don't you dare tell me that I don't need this! You don't have to be here; and if you choose to stay I don't want to hear another word from you unless I ask for it." She poured another drink and slumped down onto the couch; her mind lost in their conversation. Mark took a seat near the window, where he could hear the argument outside.

Robbie had arrived only moments after Sabrina had gone into the house. She came onto the deck from the beach, and immediately commenced her verbal assault on Sean. "You son of a bitch!" Sean, and the others, had not noticed her arrival until the gates of hell opened up. Caught off guard Sean jumped when he heard her voice. "What are you doing here?" "You know damn well what I'm doing here you bastard!" Her shoulder length brown hair tousled wildly by her anger, and the wind.

"Here we go again," D'arcy said quietly to Brent. "You think he'd learn by now." The two men stepped aside, out of the line of fire; but ready to step back in should they be needed. Mark slipped unnoticed into the house. He had to prevent Sabrina from walking into this mess.

The argument continued very much one sided. "You spineless, gutless bastard, why can't you just tell me what you want? Why do you have to do things this way? If you don't want me, then just tell me to my face. Answer me damn it!" Sean silently looked at her; her beauty still captivated him.

Even when she was angry, she was still attractive. His eyes moved over her body, as if seeing her for the first time. Robbie was petite, only five foot four, but her curves made up for what she lacked in height. She stood before him, wearing a halter top and a pair of tight shorts; he watched her round breasts heave with her every breath.

God she is beautiful. I haven't made love to her for weeks, but I can vividly remember our last night together. A faint smile came to his face, but was chased away when Robbie spoke again.

"Well, you bastard; answer me. Damn it Sean; answer me!" "Robbie, there's no need to get so upset; you should know me by now. You were gone and I got lonely; that's all." "This is the last time Sean; you are not going to hurt me any more. If you want to be with this bitch so bad, then you can have her. I'm done with you, you bastard!"

Sean moved closer to her. "It's not like that; you know I still care about you." "Oh yeah; well this is what I think of you." She slapped him hard across the face. Satisfied, Robbie turned and ran back to the beach, around the side of the house to her car. Sean was in shock; his face hurt and he could feel the lumps that her fingers had left behind.

"Man when are you going to learn," D'arcy said, shaking his head. "Yeah Sean; and just what are you going to do about Sabrina? Whether you're aware of it or not, she's in love with you," Tony added. "No way!" Sean announced adamantly. "I've never told her that I loved her. Christ she's bright enough to know that this isn't a permanent thing." "I don't know Sean; I've seen the way she looks at you; and I've seen first hand how you treat her," Tony said.

"Ya know your screwing around is really starting to hurt people; people who obviously care about you," Sam interrupted. "Sometimes you can be a real sadistic creep," Brent added. "Enough! Knock it off; all of you! In a couple of weeks this will all be over and forgotten; and I for one plan to start right now. Sabrina doesn't need to know anything right now; let's just have dinner and forget that this ever happened." Sean returned to his barbecue.

The men shook their heads in disbelief at what Sean said. "By the way," Brent asked looking around. "Where is Sabrina; and for that matter where is Mark?" "They're both inside," D'arcy answered. "And hopefully, he was able to distract her from this bull shit." "She's gonna be devastated when Sean leaves her behind," Tony added, releasing a loud sigh.

It wasn't a thought that they really wanted to have, but all four were entertaining the idea of getting closer to Sabrina, once Sean dumped her. Brent dismissed this thought early on, settling for another beer. Yet in a dark corner of his heart the seed of lust was beginning to grow. He knew how Sean operated and he would bide his time and wait until Sean was done with Sabrina. Sean's cast off's were always worth the wait.

Mark continued his quiet vigil in the den; he could make out the words of the argument, and was quite sure that Sabrina could not hear them where she was seated. He watched her consume three more glasses of bourbon. *I wish that she wouldn't take another drink.* Something deep inside him kept trying to tell him that he should stop her; that she shouldn't do this. In some way, that he was not sure of, it was going to have a bad effect on her; but understanding why, or how was just beyond his comprehension.

My senses have always been so sharp, so in tune with others; but she confuses me. I'm intensely drawn to her, but I don't know why. There was silence at the window when he turned back; the argument had stopped, at least for now. Sean would probably be looking for them; he unlocked the door.

The bourbon had done just what Sabrina had wanted; she was numb and drunk. The glass slipped from her hand and fell to the floor unbroken; she never noticed it as a shock induced sleep controlled her body now. Mark picked up the glass and set it back on the bar; he watched her for a moment before returning to the sun deck to check out the damage.

"Hey Mark, where have you been?" Sean asked. "I was inside, waiting for the dust to settle." "Did you see Sabrina in there?" Mark paused, thinking through his answer. "Yeah I did; she's in the den." "Well, I better go and get her; steaks are just about ready." Sean moved towards the door. Mark stopped him. "She's asleep Sean." "What?" "She must need it man; so let her have a few more minutes." "I guess so; she was up really early this morning," Sean replied, returning to the grill. "It must be the flu." "What?" "Yeah that has to be it. She woke up this morning sick to her stomach; she said it was the flu."

Thoughts raced through Mark's mind; he tried to shake it off. *That can't be it. She couldn't, not now. They haven't been together long enough. Oh God, maybe they have.* His heart ached for her; having to learn about

Sean like this; and if his suspicions were right, she probably hadn't even realized what was happening to her yet. *I wish with all my heart that I'm wrong; but my senses keep telling me something completely different. I have a purpose here; I'm sure of it now.*

"Dinner's ready," Sean announced. "I'll go and get Sabrina and then we can eat." "I'll go," Mark offered. "You look after the dinner." "Thanks Mark." Mark went back to the den, thankful that Sean had accepted his request so readily. Sabrina needed to be prepared on how to face Sean without causing a scene.

Sabrina's sleep had not been a comfortable one; clouded with dreams and reruns of Mark's conversation. Off in the distance she heard her name being called; it got closer and closer, until she opened her eyes, to see Mark down on one knee in front of her. "Dinner's ready; do you think you're up to it?" "Oh my head hurts." "That's because you drank too much, too fast. Do you think you can stand?"

Still holding her head, she pulled herself up, with the aid of the arm of the couch. Her head pounded harder. She rubbed at her temple trying to make it stop. Her balance was poor, and Mark allowed her to lean against him. "Oh man, I don't feel very good," she said rubbing at her stomach.

Grabbing her by the shoulders he guided her down the hall to the bathroom. *As bad as she feels at this moment, this is the best thing for her. She has to get the alcohol out of her system.* When his vigil turned into a five minute wait, he knocked on the door. Hearing no response from her, he cautiously opened the door. "Sabrina; are you all right?" "Yeah I guess." He opened the door wider; she was standing at the sink; a wet face cloth draped across her neck; she looked so gaunt. "Is everything okay?" "Yes, thank you. I do feel a bit better now."

Opening the medicine cabinet, she found a bottle of aspirin and a bottle of Gravol. Removing tablets from each container she took them with a small sip of water. "You know you should try to eat something," Mark said. "You're right." Mark's expression turned serious and as much as he didn't want to he made eye contact with her. "I would like you to try and do something else too." "What?" Sabrina asked. "Please do no let on to Sean about what I've told you; not tonight anyway" "I'll try, but," she caught her words. "You're right; tonight is not the right time."

Still unsteady on her feet, part way into the living room she kicked off her shoes, and her balance improved a little. She padded her way back out to the sun deck; Sean grabbed her unexpectedly and gave her a hug. She wanted to recoil away from him, but Mark's words were still fresh in her mind. She reluctantly returned his hug. "I guess you really do have the flu," he said. Seeing her puzzled look he continued. "You're so pale; and sleeping through the best part of the day; well that could only mean that you have the flu." "I guess so; I know that I really don't feel well at all."

How can I feel good, knowing that our relationship is a fabrication, he has no feelings for me. I am so naive, to have willingly succumbed to this deceptive seduction. I have been beguiled, caught in his award winning performance.

She picked at her dinner, hungry but not really, forcing herself to eat something. D'arcy and Sam tried a couple of times to start up a conversation, but she politely declined. Her headache had eased up, and now the Gravol was making her sleepy. Excusing herself for the evening, she went upstairs to bed. At the top of the stairs, she internally debated over going back to her old room or going to Sean's. *I must keep up the charade.*

Slipping her dress off, leaving it in a crumpled heap upon the floor; she slowly crawled into bed. The Gravol allowed her to have an undisturbed and much needed sleep; she never even felt Sean slip into bed beside her.

Sabrina was awake early again; her stomach was still upset. She was quick to dismiss her nausea as a hangover. *That's exactly it; too much alcohol, and too much stress, that's what is making me sick.* Putting on her robe, she went back to the bedroom. Sean was still asleep, but very restless.

He's dreaming. His eyes are fluttering beneath their lids. Whom are you dreaming of, your other lover Robbie or me? He must know how I feel about him. I was so sure that he truly cared for me; or was this just a fling, like Mark had said; and I am just another of his many conquests. As hard as it will be, I will honor my promise to Mark, and not let Sean find out that I know about his masquerade; no matter how much it hurts.

Tears welled up in her eyes and she choked them back. Sean would probably sleep most of the morning and she needed some time alone. Tightening her robe, she crept quietly down the stairs, unsure if any of the others had stayed, and she wouldn't want to disturb them either.

She had the kitchen all to herself; Charles wasn't up yet either. Making herself some tea and toast she took it out to the sun deck, where she could enjoy the morning sun, and the solitude. Balancing her toast atop her mug, she opened the door and stepped outside; the fresh morning breeze made her feel a lot better. A voice behind her made her jump. She turned around quickly, and that made her stomach queasy.

Mark was stretched out on a lounger, still dressed in the same clothes as the day before, only this time his shirt was completely unbuttoned, laying agape against his chest. "Damn it; don't scare me like that!" she scolded. "Sorry."

She approached the lounger next to his, and as she bent over the top of her robe parted, permitting Mark an intimate look inside. Her full round breasts barely moved as she fussed about. *This is not right.* He looked away from her; waiting for her to settle down before he spoke. "How do you feel this morning?" "Ah, so, so, I guess I have a hangover. I was sick again this morning; but it could also be the flu. That's why the tea and toast."

Dear God I hope that's all it is; time will soon tell. "What are you doing up so early?" Sabrina asked. "I don't sleep much anymore." "Oh, too many lady friends keeping you up at night?" "No, it's nothing like that! I don't have a girlfriend!" "Why not? You are an attractive man; I would expect that women would be dripping off of you." "No, I, I have been celibate for over ten years now."

Why am I telling her this; my most personal secret? How is it I feel so comfortable talking to her? She thinks that I'm attractive. Stop this damn foolishness. She's only being kind.

Sabrina could detect a degree of sadness in his voice, and she felt bad for having made such comments. "I chose to make my career my only priority; and personal relationships just didn't fit into the schedule; and that's all I'm going to say about it." "I'm sorry I said what I did." Reluctantly she reached for his hand. "I didn't mean to upset you." "It's okay."

When her fingers slipped into his palm, a warm feeling washed over him. Tightening her hold on him she began to feel that same electric charge as she did yesterday. It coursed through her veins, giving her that pins and needle's effect. She removed her hand quickly as the feeling began to intensify.

What is happening to me? Why does he excite me so? She changed the subject abruptly. "So when did last night's festivities come to an end?"

"Somewhere around two, but I'm not really sure." "Who else has stayed over?" "Only me; the other guys have homes not too far away so there was no need for them to hang around." "So where do you call home then?" "I have a place a lot farther south, and inland."

Another taunting, yet evasive answer; if he wants me to know, then he would have told me. He is so mystifying, elusive, yet something about him is so intriguing.

They both went quiet for a long time, each of them unsure where, or how to continue the conversation. They were lost in their own private thoughts and intimate fantasies. Mark sighed deeply. "So what do you plan to do about Sean?" "Well, I've decided to play along with this charade of his; and from what you told me last night it shouldn't be very long before it's over," her voice cracked as she fought off her tears. "I am grateful that you had the guts to tell me; it somehow makes it easier; but damn it, it still hurts."

She lost her fight with her tears and they spilled down her face. Turning to the edge of the seat, she concealed her face in her hands, hiding her shame from Mark. He was in turmoil. *Should I or shouldn't I help her? The hell with it, she needs somebody right now.* Rising from his lounger he walked over to her and sat down beside her, placing his arm around her shoulders, comforting her as best as he could.

"Please don't," she sniffled. "Don't what?" "I don't want you to see me cry." "Why not?" "It's a sign of weakness that up until now I've managed to keep relatively controlled." "That's bull shit. You're hurting, not weak. You don't have to hide things, not from me." Sabrina leaned into him. He held her until her tears had stopped; not wanting to ever let her go.

Taking in a long breath, she straightened herself. "It just makes me so damn mad; he's so smooth; and I got sucked in; hook, line and sinker. How could I have been so stupid?" "Don't blame yourself. You met him at a very vulnerable time in your life; and he knew it." "Yes, I did; and I was so overwhelmed by his kind words and his total attention. It's been so long since anyone had made me feel like that." "Like I told you before, you are not the first, and you most definitely will not be the last."

"That's just a small part of what makes this charade so hard to deal with. I just don't know how long I can keep this up." "Do you think you can play along for two more days?" Mark asked. "Two days; what do you mean by that?" "I have a suggestion, if you're willing to listen." "Sure, I'll entertain anything at this point."

"Okay then. Sean got a phone call last night, and they've scheduled him to leave in two days for a twenty-one day east coast tour. What you have to do, is to convince him, that you're not well enough to go with him. Then, while he's away, you make the first move and get the hell out of here." "You don't think that I should wait for him to give me the brush off?" "No, I don't. If I know Sean, your time together is coming to an end; and fast; and the last thing that you need is to be stranded somewhere in the eastern United States."

Sabrina gave serious thought to what Mark had just said. *His plan sounds good enough.* "Where are you going to go?" Mark asked. "Oh that's really easy for me to answer." Raising her arm she pointed up the beach. "You see that house over there; the one with the windsock on the deck; that's my place." "Ah hell." "Yeah I leased it for six months." "Good thing you didn't give up your lease." "Sean tried to convince me that I didn't have any need for it, since I would be living here. I almost bought it too. Maybe deep down inside I knew that this wouldn't last so I renewed my lease on a month to month basis."

She tried to laugh, but her tears wiped it away. Mark gently squeezed her shoulder. "It's gonna be okay; you'll get through this." "Will you help me; or are you going away too?" Sabrina asked. Mark was completely stunned by her question, but also flattered that she would trust him so soon. "Sure I'll help you; I'm not going on tour for about another month. So if you need a friend I'll be here for you. I'll get a hotel in town, and after Sean is gone, I'll come back and help you move." "That's absolutely ridiculous." "Well, I sure can't stay here; it wouldn't look right." "I didn't mean that. Why don't you stay in my house? It's just sitting there empty."

Mark hesitated. *I'm not sure if that is such a good idea; but I do like the idea of being near her. I need to be near her. When her world falls apart, I want to be here for her.* When he didn't answer, Sabrina took the initiative. "It's settled. I'll get you the keys after Sean gets up." She shifted beside him, rubbing at her stomach. "You okay?" Mark asked. "I guess so; still a bit nauseous; that's all." Mark watched her walk to the railing and stretch; she rubbed her stomach again, and then her back. His thoughts and feelings were so mixed up.

If what I sense about her is true, then she is really going to need a friend. I want so desperately to be that person. I've been close to women in the past, but none ever inspired me the way she does. She makes my heart race, and I want; need to know her better. That's why I requested time off of work, before I had even met her.

The sun caught her hair, dazzling like strands of gold; even in an ordinary bathrobe he thought her to be extraordinarily beautiful. It wasn't her physical elegance that enchanted him, what he saw in her was much deeper, more significant. For well over ten years he had abstained from sex; renouncing all thoughts about it; until now. Now, at the age of thirty two, there were perceptions now of commitment; of his future. He truly wished that she would be the one, the one who would complete his dream.

Sabrina walked back to him and sat down; her hand lightly touched his and without any hesitation she kissed his cheek ever so softly. "Thank you; for everything," she said softly. Mark felt his heart skip a beat; he could not speak. Her hand was slow to slide off of his, and when it did, she left him to return to the house, taking with her a piece of his heart.

It has to be her; the one that has disrupted my dreams so frequently. The one I was compelled to seek out; the incentive that had brought me to this party.

Mark and Sabrina had spent the majority of the morning enjoying the sun, but engaging in little conversation. She had tried several times to get him to open up about himself, but her questions were met with short, noncommittal answers, or silence. Not that he didn't want to answer her, but he hadn't really heard her, lost in the feelings that she had awakened in him. He never questioned her about her history; but there was one question. He wanted to know if she was any where near Reno a little while back, but his pride stopped him from asking. She never volunteered anything, keeping her life as deep and secret as he did his own.

When Sean stepped onto the deck, he came straight to Sabrina; sitting beside her, he kissed her. She wanted to push him away, but reminded herself that she had to play along. "Are you feeling better today?" he asked. "Not really." "So what have you two been up to this morning?" Sean looked first at Sabrina and then at Mark.

"Nothing, it's just been a real quiet, lazy morning," she answered. "So why aren't you dressed yet?" "I didn't want to disturb you; but now that you're up, I'll go and put some clothes on." "So Mark, I thought you'd be long gone by now?" "Oh that's my fault, I persuaded him to stay for lunch," she said, giving Mark a pleading look from behind Sean's back. "Yeah that's right, she can be very persuasive," Mark answered. "That she can," Sean muttered, rubbing his hand over her ass. She made a hasty departure, putting some distance between her and Sean. *Keeping up this charade for two days isn't going to be easy.*

In the privacy of the bedroom, she dressed quickly, but paused at the foot of the bed. *How many women have shared this bed with him?* She remembered how caring he had been, when she was attacked; how he comforted her. *I can't believe that it was all an act; and I had given him, so freely, the prize he wanted all along, my body and my passion.* She wanted to cry, it would relieve her tension, but she refused to give in to it this time, she had to stay focused.

Finding the keys to her house, she stuffed them into her pocket. Somehow it gave her a sense of security, knowing that Mark would be so close. *It wasn't easy for him to tell me about Sean, but I am so grateful that he did. Better to end it now, like this, than to wait until he dumps me. The anger I feel will aid in overcoming the pain.*

Patches rubbed around her ankles until she picked him up, cuddling him tightly. "Soon, Patches, we'll get our life back in order, and we'll be back in our own place." She laid him on the bed, rubbing at his tummy until he began playing with her hand. With everything that had gone on, she felt a little guilty that she had been neglecting him so much, he was her one best friend. Rolling him up in the blanket, she left him to play in the wrinkles. She had to get back downstairs, to get Charles to prepare some lunch; and to wait for the opportunity to give Mark the keys.

"Lunch will be ready in about half an hour," she announced. "Good, that gives me time for a swim," Sean said. He came to her, putting his arms around her waist, pulling their bodies close together. "Wanna join me?" "Not right now Sean, maybe later." He kissed her, before trotting off down the stairs to the beach. Sabrina wiped the back of her hand across her lips, eliminating the revolting taste of him that still lingered.

She walked to the railing, watching Sean, as he ran out into the surf and dove in. Her hands tightened around the rail. "I don't think that I can do this. It's so hard; having to lie to him and all." She stared out at the ocean;

secretly wishing him to get caught in a rip tide. "Sabrina," Mark called. "Look at me, please."

Reluctantly, she turned around to face him, still using the rail as a support. In his expression she could see the indications of sympathy and compassion, but she avoided his eyes, they could see right through her. "You can do this. You have to, for your sake and for," he stopped himself. *I can't tell her my suspicions.* "For what?" she asked, wondering why he hadn't finished his sentence. "For your own satisfaction."

As he reached his hand out to her, she watched her own hand disappear into his. That same feeling began surging through her body, but she held on to it, feeling its power; drawing on the strength. "I know you're hurting, but you have to get past that. The time will go quickly; you'll see. Then you'll have the satisfaction of being the first woman to do to Sean what he has done to so many others."

Mark's words were calming to her, and empowering. The impulses ran stronger, engulfing her body. As much as his touch electrified her, something about it made her more relaxed and safe. She felt the sincerity; the overwhelming trust.

He isn't pretending; his words, his demeanor are all authentic. "You're right," she said unconsciously entwining her fingers with his. "I can do this, and I won't let it get me down; not now, not ever." Remembering the keys, she tugged her hand away, and pulled them from her pocket. "The house number is on the key tag." She folded his fingers in, over the small bundle; holding his hand in hers for a few more moments.

Her touch is so gentle. She's only holding my hand, but it feels like she is embracing my heart, warming it, making it really come alive for the first time in my life.

From the corner of her eye, Sabrina caught sight of Sean coming up the stairs; she let go of Mark. Sean reached the deck at the same moment Charles brought forth their lunch. The conversations during lunch focused primarily on Sean's tour itinerary. He never approached the subject of her going with him, so she only listened to bits and pieces. She was engrossed with her own itinerary of getting through the rest of today and tomorrow. Her freedom awaited her on Tuesday morning and that was all she needed to concentrate on.

"Sabrina?" Sean called to her. "Hmm, oh I'm sorry. What did you say?" "I asked you why you're not eating?" "I don't know. I thought I was hungry, but this isn't really what I wanted." "Then get Charles to make you something else." "Maybe; I'll go and see what there is in the fridge first," she said excusing herself from the table.

When he was sure that she was out of range of his voice, Mark spoke to Sean. "You know she's still not feeling very well. Are you planning on taking her with you on this tour?" "Of course I am!" "Do you think it's a wise move, when she's ill? You know how bizarre this tour is going to be; and she should be getting a lot of rest, or she's not going to get over this." "Oh come on; she'll snap out of it soon. So what makes you the expert all of a sudden?" Sean sounded annoyed. "Look man, I'm only stating the facts; you're asking her to follow you on a tour of eighteen cities in twenty-one days. You're used to it; she's not. Even if she wasn't sick, it's a hell of a tour to put her through."

Sean leaned back, contemplating what Mark had said. *Maybe he's right. Maybe I should let her stay behind. It would give me a chance to make peace with Robbie.* He made up his mind. *If Sabrina doesn't feel up to going, then I won't push her into it; but I'm not ready to give her up yet either. Being with her is different somehow; but I can't deny my feelings for Robbie.* "Mark, I think you're right," Sean patted the table affirmatively. "If she doesn't feel up to making the trip then at least she'll have Charles here to look after her until I get back."

In Mark's mind he breathed a sigh of relief. *For once Sean has taken someone's advice.* For a moment he thought that Charles would be a problem, until he remembered that he would be driving Sean to the airport, and that would give them about four hours to get her moved out. Mark knew that this was the ethical thing for her to do. *Sean would never make a commitment to her; even if my suspicions are right.*

There was a rumor a few years ago, that Sean had paid for one of his lady friends to have an abortion. *If he could do something like that back then, then he would be capable of persuading Sabrina to do the same thing now; if he had to.* Mark felt a knot tighten in his stomach. "I have to go," he announced; pushing back from the table. "Gee, that's too bad. Sure you can't stay longer?" Sean smirked sarcastically. "No, I really have to go. No need to get up; I can see myself out." "See you on the tour," Sean called after him as he entered the house. *See you in hell, you son of a bitch.*

Sabrina was just entering the living room as Mark entered the house. "I'm gonna take off," he said, nearing her. "Now!" Mark could only look at her and nod. "I'll walk you out." She was almost begging for his permission. Again, he could only nod his agreement. He could not decline the opportunity to have one good, last, look at her; to sustain him until the next time they would meet. Sabrina closed the heavy front door behind them and walked with him to his car.

As he opened the door to get in, she grabbed his arm. "Please wait," she said nervously. Mark waited, anticipating her next words; but all she could do was bite her lip. *I don't want him to go, not yet; but I don't fully understand why I want him to stay.*

Leaning down, he gave her a kiss on the forehead. He wanted to surrender to the uncontrollable urge to take her in his arms; he forced himself to resist. *I could never take advantage of her vulnerability. I'm not like Sean.* "You'll be just fine," he said looking into her blue eyes. "I'll see you Tuesday morning; call me when you're ready to go." She kept silent, watching his car pull out of the driveway. Somewhere, somehow a small part of her went with him.

The sound of the fountain bubbling in the front yard distracted her; she walked around it several times, occasionally dipping her hand into the water. Preparing herself to return to the house she repeated one phrase over and over in her mind. *You can get through this.*

Sean was waiting for her in the living room, startling her when he spoke. "Finally, we have the house all to ourselves again," he said motioning her to come to him, and she obliged. Putting his arms around her, he pulled her tight against him. "So what do you want to do for the rest of the day?" His hips were firmly against hers.

A simple 'I don't know' was the only response she had; but she knew precisely what he wanted to do. He kissed her lips, her cheek, her neck. "We could go upstairs," he whispered into her ear. "I really don't feel like it right now." "Still not feeling well?" "Not really; maybe I should take some more aspirins." "Well, if you're not feeling up to engaging in sex then how about we rent some movies and spend the rest of the day relaxing on the couch?" "That sounds good to me." She was grateful that she had diverted his mind off of sex, at least for a while.

Mark had not gone directly to Sabrina's house; presuming that there wouldn't be any groceries left behind, he went shopping. On his way back, he passed Sean heading into town; he was quite sure that he had not seen him, as he was driving a rental car. Mark parked the car inside the garage out of sight; he packed in the two bags of groceries he had with him; the rest was being delivered later on.

He paid little attention to the house itself; things like that never really impressed him anyway. He took his luggage to the guest room; it had a king size bed. He had been up so early because he had spent a sleepless night in Sean's guest room. It only had a double bed and because of his height he was incapable of getting comfortable. Tossing his bags into the corner, he stretched out across the bed; his mind invoked a vision of Sabrina, and her face stayed constant, all through his afternoon dreams.

Sean and Sabrina had spent the remainder of the afternoon, and part of the evening, on the couch watching videos; they even ate their supper there. Sabrina was content with a bowl of soup. Her stomach had settled down, but she was not going to take the chance on messing it up again. She allowed herself to be held by Sean; even though it disturbed her greatly. After dinner she became fidgety, shifting from one position to another. "What's wrong?" Sean asked. "I've got a backache," she answered. He leaned over to start rubbing it for her; she quickly stood up. "I think I'm gonna go up to bed; maybe lying down will help." "Sure, I'll be up in a bit."

She ploddingly ascended the staircase, each step only adding to her pain. She began peeling her clothes off just inside the door. By the time she reached the bed she was completely nude. *It must be muscle tension from being sick.* That sounded like a reasonable explanation.

Her movements were cautious as she got into bed. Laying flat on her back she commanded her body to relax, but it wasn't working. She turned from one side to the other, searching for relief. When Sean walked in she was to the point of tears; he sat down beside her. "Will you let me help you?" "Yes, anything, just make it go away." She clenched her fist on the pillow.

Sean went into the bathroom and returned with a bottle in his hand. "Lay on your stomach," he commanded. She cautiously obliged. He began to run his hand slowly down her back. "Tell me when I've reached the sore spot." "There," she said flinching away from his touch. Sean's hand had stopped in the small of her back. He poured some liniment into his hand and began a soft, gentle massage of the area. The liniment warmed as he rubbed; his hands caressed other parts of her back, not wanting to apply to much constant pressure to the one area. When he returned to the primary area she would flinch; he repeated his motions until her body no longer reacted to his touch. Thinking that he had massaged away her pain, but all he had done was to put her to sleep.

He carefully lay down beside; frustrated; he wanted to make love to her tonight. It was only yesterday that they were together that way but for him it seemed an eternity. *I understand that she doesn't feel well; but she looks all right. She couldn't be giving me the brush off. No. I have felt her intensity when we made love. I will give her tonight, let her rest; but I'm not going to go away without having her again. If she wants to stay home, then I require her passion to sustain me; but then again if she denies me, there's always Robbie, she never turned me down, even when she was mad.* He pulled the sheets up over her, and settled himself down for the night, on his side, away from her.

Sean awoke to find himself alone in the bed; the shadows under the bathroom door told him that Sabrina was in there. He stretched out on his back, awaiting her return. Sabrina emerged from the bathroom; her robe pulled tight around her; her face pale, her eyes red and puffy. She sat down on the edge of the bed; Sean reached over and gently rubbed his hand over her back. "You're shaking," he said. "I can't seem to get warm." "Come here; I'll warm you up."

He carefully laid her down beside him; pulled her close, his leg over hers, and the blankets pulled up over them both; yet Sabrina still shivered uncontrollably against him. "Still not feeling well?" "No, I'm not; but it will pass. It's always worse in the morning." "What do you mean?" "I guess it's because the aspirins have worn off during the night; that's why I feel so crummy in the morning." "Maybe you should see a Doctor?" "I don't think so. It's just the flu; and all a Doctor is gonna tell me is to take some aspirin and get lots of rest."

Sean didn't say any thing else for a while; he lay with Sabrina; holding her tight, pondering how he would ask her to go on tour with him.

She is visibly ill, and I don't want to jeopardize her health, or mine. This is going to be a very arduous tour, even for me, and there would be no way that she could rest properly. He rolled it over and over in his mind. *I desire her to go with me, but if she needs to stay behind, then I will have to be understanding; maybe in a few days she could join me.*

He released a sigh. "What?" Sabrina asked. "Huh." "Did you say something?" "No, I was just thinking. How do you feel now?" "Better, thanks, at least I'm warm." "Really?" Sean's enthusiasm returned; his hand moved inside her robe. "Yes really," she answered. *I know what he's trying to start; I don't want to have sex with him, but, oh damn these feelings of obligation.*

She allowed him to continue touching and kissing her; and she tried very hard to pretend that she was enjoying it but she just couldn't. The passion was gone and nothing would ever bring it back. Her body wasn't ready for him, and it hurt when he entered her. So all consumed with his own desires, he never even noticed that she did not have an orgasm. He kissed her softly, and lifted himself off of her; she watched him go into the bathroom.

This isn't the end of it, Sean will want to have sex again; but I have to get through this; I can get through this. Turning on her side, she curled up waiting, dreading his return.

Mark awoke suddenly, not sure why. He stretched, running his hands down his body, realizing that he was aroused. *After all these years; today I wake up with a hard on. Sabrina; she precipitated this.* He was annoyed with himself, having always been able to control his urges, but now, he quite liked this feeling, and he liked the way she made him feel. He pushed the thoughts from his mind and let his body relax. *Is she destined to be with me? Only time will divulge that answer. Please let her be the one. I don't want to be alone anymore.*

After a leisurely brunch, Sean finally got the guts to turn the conversation to the tour. "We had better start with the packing." "Sean, tell me again about this tour?" "It's like I said before; twenty-one days, eighteen cities and all on the east coast." "That's a lot of traveling, could be pretty chaotic." "Yeah it's gonna be a tough one all right, I know; I've done it many times before. Look, if you don't feel that you're up to it, then it's fine with me if you'd prefer to stay home."

Sabrina was temporarily speechless. *I can't believe that he is giving me a way out.* "If you don't mind then, the way I've been feeling for the last couple of days, well, I don't think I'd enjoy it very much." "Hey, your health is far more important. Charles will be here to take care of you; so don't feel bad about not being able to go." He pulled her up to hug her. "So how about helping me pack?" Sabrina agreed to that, and followed him back upstairs.

As she suspected, her day was not permitted to progress without having sex with Sean again; and again; and again. Packing took the better part of the day, because he kept coaxing her into bed; but still there was no satisfaction for her. She wasn't repulsed by him. She had lost her passion for him. All she thought about was the other women. *Did he make love to them the same way?*

By dinner time, she found it very uncomfortable to sit at the table. Her body was in pain, more than the usual discomfort that she experienced after having sex, but she never acknowledged it in front of Sean. Charles had made a special meal; a going away feast for Sean. She dispatched her meal with haste, wanting only to relocate to a more comfortable setting.

Standing against the railing on the deck, she sighed; she had missed the sunset, and that in itself was depressing. She glanced toward her house. *No lights are on inside the house, good. Mark is keeping our plan a secret.* Her mind drifted, thinking about tomorrow, her freedom; but they were quickly dashed when Sean surprised her by picking her up in his arms. "It's getting late," he said with a devilish grin. "Time for bed."

She was numb through the whole act of sex, and Sean never knew it. Finally exhausted, he rolled himself off of her; he was asleep within minutes. Sabrina turned away from him; her silent tears soaking through the pillow. *Why did he have to turn out to be such a jerk? It had all been an act, a come on, just so he could get what he wanted. Well, this time the story is going to have a very different ending.* Holding onto that thought, sleep came quickly to claim her.

Chapter 6

Sean was the first up; he had showered, dressed, and taken his luggage down stairs; all without rousing Sabrina. It was the first day that her affliction hadn't woken her prematurely. Standing beside the bed he watched her sleep.

How the sheet clings to her body. So peaceful, I hate to wake her, but I don't want to leave without saying good-by. She needs her rest. Maybe I'll just write her a note, that's too impersonal, too cold.

Sabrina stretched; Sean sat beside her. "Good morning, beautiful, how do you feel today?" he asked. She was about to speak, when she felt her stomach rise up in her throat. Scrambling past Sean she headed into the bathroom, for what had become a ritual.

What could be making her so sick? She isn't like this any other time of the day, just the mornings. I don't like to see her this way, but I don't know what I can do to help her either. For the first time in his life he was experiencing feelings of helplessness, but it didn't last long. His true agenda didn't have any room for those kind of feelings.

Sabrina soon returned to the bedroom; but she had to pause and lean against the bathroom door. Her body was weak, unstable. Realizing that something was wrong, Sean went to her. Feeling her knees wobble he instinctively picked her up and carried her back to the bed. Her body trembled as he held her.

"You're not getting much better," he said laying her down as he brought himself close to her to keep her warm. "Let me call the Doctor?" "No, Sean. No Doctor." "This has gone on far too long." "I'll be fine. I told you it always bothers me more in the mornings. I just need a few more minutes to rest; then I'll be fine. When do you have to leave for the airport?" "Soon." "How soon?" "Soon, like thirty minutes too soon. I really don't like it that I have to leave you here when you're not well." "You have to; your fans are counting on you; besides I'm feeling much better now." As she sat up, her stomach churned again.

I have to show him that I'm strong enough. I don't know what I'd do if he should change his mind and stay home.

"We do have time enough to have tea together," he said. He escorted her down the stairs. They sat quietly at the table, neither of them speaking. The tension between them grew stronger. Sabrina tried to ignore the knot that was developing in her stomach. Sean swallowed hard, pushing back the lump that was growing in his throat.

Why is it so hard to leave? I'm not ready to give her up just yet, but I can't force her to go with me. He began to think about Robbie. *She will know how to make me feel good. Even when she's mad at me I can still get her into bed. It won't be such a bad trip after all.* Charles appeared at the doorway. "Excuse me sir; but it is time for you to leave."

Sabrina stared blankly at Charles. *How cold his words are. His expression never changes, always solemn, this apathetic gray haired penguin who looks so naked without his starched black and white plumage. He never speaks to me or calls me by name. Is he afraid that he might slip up and use a forgotten name, one from Sean's repository of female conquests. Not to worry Charles, my time is over and you may carry on keeping Sean's sordid secrets.*

Sean casually nodded to Charles, who exited the house to wait for his employer at the car. Reaching across the table to Sabrina's hand, Sean held it tight as he got up from his chair. Helping her up, he embraced her shoulders. Still not speaking, they walked slowly through the house to the front door.

When they had reached the alcove, he stopped, positioning himself in front of her. Taking her face in his hands, he kissed her so tenderly that she succumbed to her tears. "Shhh, there is no need for tears. If you need me, just ask Charles; he'll know how to get in touch with me." They embraced; all the while her mind fought a raging battle.

I have to know. One way or the other, I have to know. "Sean, I, I love you." He brought her face back to meet his, kissing her again. Her eyes searched his face, hoping his response would be the one she so desperately wanted to hear; but all he said was the wrong words. "I know Sabrina." Kissing her again, he was in the car before she had time to fully process everything. As the car drove away, she could see him waiving to her; but he could not see the tears that were flooding over her cheeks. *This was my last effort to prove to myself that Mark was wrong about him. I have failed miserably.*

"They're gone," she said quickly, when Mark answered the phone. She never heard his response, for she had already hung up the phone. *She's really hurting and she shouldn't be alone.* He hurried himself to the car, to her aid. Expecting to find the front door unlocked, but instead it was wide open; he stepped in and called to her; no response. He visually scanned the down stairs for her before going up to the bedroom. As he neared, he could hear noises from inside; he called to her again. "I'm in here," she answered.

Mark located her in the closet, throwing her clothes into a suitcase, that teetered precariously on a chair. "How can I help?" he asked. Sabrina never turned around, continuing with her task with great force. "How could I have been so stupid? You were right. That son of a bitch! How could I let myself get so sucked in? Damn him; damn him to hell!" Taking her by the shoulders, Mark forced her to turn around. Her tears fell heavy, intensifying the anger and the sadness in her expression.

It distresses me to see her like this. She needs a friend. I so want to embrace her. Without warning, Sabrina concealed her face against his chest. Not astute in his ability to comfort, he put his hands on her shoulders. When her cries had turned to intermittent sobs, he released her. "Feel better now?" "Yes, and no. Christ, I don't know how I feel anymore!" "The sooner you get out of here the better it will be. Now, shall we proceed with a bit more organization this time?" He pointed to the over filled suitcase, piled high with an unruly mess of clothes. She frowned as she looked upon her creation. He smiled at her and she returned the gesture.

With much clearer thought, Sabrina packed up her things in a more orderly method. "That's everything," she announced, closing the suitcase. "What about these?" Mark gestured to the clothes that still hung in the closet. "Leave them! Sean bought them for me; and I don't want them anymore!" Without saying anything else, he picked up the suitcase and carried it downstairs.

Sabrina took another look about the bedroom and the bathroom, just to make sure that she had collected everything that was hers. She picked up Patches from the bed and went downstairs. Mark watched her, as she wandered from room to room, picking up the odd item that was hers; finally making her way back to the living room where he was waiting for her. "Ready?" he asked. Sabrina nodded her head, and followed him to the door. She stood for a moment just outside the threshold; taking one last look at what could have been. *Time to go home.*

Like a well-rehearsed play, Mark brought in the suitcases, Sabrina put them away. On his last trip into her bedroom, he planned on leaving his packages and letting her have some time to herself. They hadn't spoken at all since leaving Sean's house, and Mark was not about to push her into a conversation; at least not yet. Just being near her was more than he had imagined. Sabrina hadn't really noticed Mark coming and going; she was busy arranging her closet.

As he moved towards the door, he was halted abruptly when he heard her cry out. Going back to the closet to see if she was all right, he found her, with her hands braced against the wall, slightly bent over, a chilling look of pain on her face that scared him immensely. "What happened?" "It's my back; an awful pain in my back."

"Let me help you. Does it hurt you to walk?" "Some," she answered, pausing every couple of steps, as the pain increased and then decreased just as quickly. He finally got her to the bed, assisting her while she sat down. Laying on her side, she drew her knees up. "Looks like you've overdone it and pulled a muscle." "I don't think so; it happened the other night too, and I hadn't been doing anything. It must be a part of this flu or just plain old tension." "Is there anything that I can do to help?" "No, I, I can't ask you to," she stumbled over her words.

"I said anything, and I meant it; now tell me what to do." His tone, as his expression, were unyielding. She took another breath, embarrassed by what she was about to say. "It would help if, if you rubbed my back for a few minutes. There might be something in the bathroom cabinet that you could use."

Mark was already moving before she had finished her sentence; but he didn't go to her bathroom, he went to his bedroom. He was well informed when it came to muscle pain, and the cream he had in his room would help her.

She eased herself onto her stomach, with her arms above her head. Mark pulled a chair up beside the bed. His hands began to shake, as he folded her T-shirt up, exposing her back, but it wasn't enough, her shorts would have to be moved down around her hips in order to get to her lower back. Taking a breath, he tugged at her shorts.

Noticing the sweat on his palms, he wiped it on his jeans before dispensing some of the cream. With great care he moved his hand across her back. Her skin was warm and velvety beneath his hand. As he massaged, a curious sensation overtook him; his mind flashed onto bits and pieces of his reoccurring dream. They were incomplete images, merely glimpses. Like seeing something out of the corner of your eye, but when you turn to focus on it, it disappears.

There is something so very familiar about her; yet still so elusive. Is Sabrina the woman that has captivated my dreams for all these years? Is she the one that had caused me to forsake all others? If I could only recall that dream more clearly, I need more details.

The soul was elated; the barrier was crumbling. This body would respond to it and to the other. From this moment on the soul would control the heart inside this body, it would say and do everything that it told it. The other was weakening; the realization would come soon. It had waited this long for the revelation; it could wait a little longer.

With Sabrina peacefully resting, Mark stretched out on the sofa in the living room; his mind raced out of control. *If she is the woman from my dream, then I have to find out for sure, and nothing is going to stop me. The feelings that I'm experiencing are strong, solid; even when she isn't around me. She has to be the one that I have been waiting for. What else could it be?*

Mark thought back, to all of the women he had met in his life. *How they vied for my attention, my affection, but none of them had ever stirred any emotion in me, only her, only Sabrina makes me feel this way. I'm not losing my mind. The voices, the feelings; they weren't coming from my mind; they were coming from my heart.*

Icy fingers clenched around this new warmth, chilling him to the bone. *Oh God. What if this sickness isn't the flu? What if she's pregnant? What do I do then? I can't allow her to tell Sean about it; I know what Sean's solution would be, and that would destroy her. The best thing she could do would be to never tell Sean. I will be here for her, to help her cross that bridge.* He closed his eyes, his mind went blank; the sounds of the ocean surf carried him away; to her.

An intriguing aroma aroused him from his nap. He sat up, taking in a full breath; the sumptuous scent made his stomach rumble with anticipation. He followed the scent into the kitchen, where Sabrina busied herself at the counter. "Something sure smells good," he said. Sabrina wasn't startled by him, as she had heard his footsteps on the hardwood floor. "I hope it tastes just as good." "What are you making?" "The house specialty is all." She grinned at him from over her shoulder. "Did you have a nice nap?" "Yeah I did; a bit unplanned though. So how are you feeling?" "Fine; really good; you have the magic touch."

Maybe this time I do, but will I be able to take away her pain later, if my suspicions are right? She caught the serious glance that he sent her way. "I mean it; I feel fine. I have no more pain, but I did tell you that it would go away, just the same as the other night, so there is no need to discuss it any further. I'm famished; so make yourself useful and set the table please."

I can't get over the change in her; she's happy, or is it a mask, so I won't see how she really feels? She has to be hurting inside.

Complying with her request, he took the dishes to the table. Sabrina followed him with two bowls of salad. "The main course still needs a few minutes more, so we might as well start with this." She was like a jack in the box, up and down checking on dinner. Soon she began to return with bowls, containing mashed potatoes, peas and carrots and finally a casserole filled with pieces of steak covered with onions and gravy. A feast was laid before him. "Go ahead," she told him.

Eagerly he filled his plate, making sure he had something of everything before he started to eat. After a couple of bites he reached his hand across to her. "Pinch me," he said. "What?" "I must still be dreaming; I have never tasted anything so good." She blushed at the compliment. "Thank you." Trying not to stare, she occasionally stole a peak while he was eating. The expression on his face pleased her; and it pleased her more when he had a second helping.

I don't know how to thank him for everything he's done; but this is a start. He is such a mystery, and one that I definitely want to solve.

Contented, Mark leaned back in his chair. "That was the best meal I've had in a very long time; thank you." "You are very welcome." After his brief rest, Mark began collecting the empty dishes. "Leave them; I'll do them later," Sabrina said. "No way, I'll clean up, and you can just sit there and relax." His voice commanded her, and she obeyed.

It's quite nice that he's so willing to help. Such rare qualities he has, completely different from other men I've known. Even when I was married, I never got this kind of cooperation. Something tells me that I need to get to know him better. It's strange, once I met him, all of the fears that I had about him vanished. What is so familiar about him? I can't put my finger on it. Is it that I've seen him on TV, but had not really paid attention? She shook her head, trying to make sense of her thoughts. *Some fresh air should help.*

The sun was already beginning its journey down to the other side of the earth. Sabrina could see the lights inside Sean's house. *I wonder if Charles has phoned him, to tell him that I've gone? Who cares?* She turned her gaze back to the ocean, watching it gently creeping closer to the house.

It feels so good to be home, even though I haven't spent a lot of time here. It's still mine, at least for a while longer, and it is safe; now that Mark is here with me. A smile came across her face as the warm evening breeze moved over her. Without any warning her smile turned to a grimace. Pain surged through her back and into her stomach. She gripped the railing hard; taking a deep breath to cleanse herself of this torment. By her third breath the pain had disappeared; she took two more just to relax.

Mark had come onto the patio, and by observing her stance, he knew exactly what was wrong. "It's back again, isn't it?" he asked. "Yeah, but it's gone now." Hesitant, he lifted her face up; he saw no pain reflected in her eyes. Taking his hand in hers, she tenderly stroked the back of it. "I'm okay so don't worry." Her words were faint to his ears; but the sensation of her touch was strong, and loud in his heart.

Turning to look back out at the ocean, Sabrina released a heavy sigh. "Is anything wrong?" Mark asked. "Not really. I've just come to a decision." "What would that be?" "It's so beautiful here," she said softly, still staring out at the ocean. "I thought that this is where I was meant to be but it isn't." "What are you saying?" "I'm leaving. I've decided that I'm gonna go home. This was a nice diversion but it's not for me. I don't belong here." "Yes, you do." "No, I have thought about this a lot and I can't justify being here, unless you know of a reason why I should stay."

Confused by his own thoughts and desires, Mark pulled his hand away from hers, and took a step back. Sabrina was confounded by his action. *I've never had a man pull away from me like that. I guess my senses were wrong about him.* "Did I do something wrong? If I did, I'm sorry." "No, you didn't." "Then what? " "Not now!" his voice turned loud and threatening. *I don't understand what I've done to cause such a reaction from him, but if he doesn't want to be near me then I'll oblige him.* She ran from the patio and into her room.

Mark heard the slam of the bedroom door; his fist hit the railing with the same force. "Damn it!" *My emotions are so mixed up. I like the feeling of her touch. I wanted to hold her but no I had to pull away. I can't let her leave. How stupid could I be?* He paced back and forth along the length of the deck.

She deserves an apology, but how can I explain my actions, without exposing what I'm feeling? It's far too soon for her to know that; and what if she doesn't respond the way I hope? Could I handle it? How she confuses me, and excites me at the same time. He stopped his pacing; punched his fist into his palm, and headed into the house; to her room. *I will apologize, and let fate decide what happens next.*

Sabrina had given up on trying to figure out what she had done wrong; she was angry, and upset with herself. Sitting up in bed, she was watching TV when Mark knocked at the door. She hesitated; he knocked again. "Come in," she responded.

The sight of her in bed, the sheets pulled up, and tucked under her arms made him nervous; he turned his eyes downward. "What do you want?" she asked, careful of her tone. "Never mind; I'll talk to you tomorrow," he said turning to leave. "Mark wait; you came here to tell me something, and I would like to hear it," she tried to coax him back. He stood fast; his mind locked in combat. "Mark, come here, please." Her voice was so soft and tender.

Giving in, he turned around, walking towards her, every step an effort. Sabrina patted the bed beside her. "Sit down." Against his better judgment, he did as she asked, but faced away from her. She touched his hand quickly. "Hey, I'm over here," she said. When he made no attempt to look at her, Sabrina leaned slightly towards him trying to see his face.

"Are you embarrassed by this scene?" she asked. "A little." "Why?" "I shouldn't be in here especially with you, like that." "It's okay, really. Now please talk to me." Sabrina sensed his unease and to try and alleviate some of it she pulled the sheet up high around her neck and folded her arms across her chest. Shifting himself sideways, Mark brought his right knee up onto the bed. Sabrina's eyes widened; his shirt was completely unbuttoned. *He must have done that in the kitchen.*

As he moved, the opening grew wider, exposing his chest to her. The tattoo of the snake crawled over his shoulder and the head of the beast lay just above his collar bone. The detail was exquisite but it didn't hold her attention for very long. His body was far more intriguing. The muscles were not as defined as Sean's were, but they were far more powerful. A faint covering of red hair was barely visible against his pale skin.

She closed her eyes briefly, commanding her mind to return to the original quest. "So what did you want to talk to me about?" she asked. Mark swallowed hard; he lifted his head slowly. His eyes scanned over her shape, until he was looking into her eyes. "I need to apologize for my behavior. I had no call to snap at you like that and I am sorry." "I accept your apology. Now, tell me the rest." "The rest?" "Yes. I get this distinct impression that there is a lot more you want to tell me." "No, I can't." "Mark, I know there's something bothering you, and if you want to talk about it, I'm here to listen."

Even though her voice calmed and comforted him, he was still defensive. "I don't know what to do. You'll think I'm a deranged fool." "Well, you're wrong. Over the past few days I've come to value what you have to say, and there's nothing that you could tell me that would sound foolish." *She's trying to build up my confidence.* Reaching for his hand, she gave it a reassuring squeeze. Mark looked at her, his mouth opened but no words came out. Tightening her grip, she used her eyes to urge him on.

This is the most difficult thing I've ever faced. Getting beaten and bruised in the ring was one thing, but this terrifies me. I'm about to open my heart to this woman, and I'm so afraid that she'll plunge a knife deep into it. The dilemma was tearing him apart. *I've just got her to leave Sean, gained her trust; but to tell her this, she will think me a lunatic.*

Sabrina stayed quiet, but her expression begged him to speak. "This isn't going to be very easy for me," he began, rubbing the moisture from his hands onto his jeans. "All I ask is that you say nothing until I'm finished." She nodded her head; the anticipation was killing her, but she didn't let it show.

"You already know that I've led a solitary life for many years now, and I've never let myself get close to any woman. I've never wanted to, until now. For some strange, obscure reason, something I don't fully understand yet, you have awakened feelings in me. Sensations I've never experienced before. From the first time I saw you, and before, I was drawn to you. Thoughts of you have invaded my mind constantly. I don't understand what's happening to me; but I do know, that right now, all I desire, is to be near you, and to know you. Please don't leave."

He looked at her face. It was devoid of all expression. She tried to speak. "Not yet," he continued. "What I told you about Sean is the truth. It wasn't just a scheme to get you away from him. I know how he operates, and I just couldn't bear to see him hurt you; you don't deserve that. Maybe I'm just being selfish; wanting you away from him, hoping, that maybe, you and I could someday become closer. It wouldn't surprise me at all, if you told me to go to hell right now; and if that's what you want, then I'll leave tonight and never bother you again." He lowered his head, preparing for the worst.

Sabrina sat back, stunned by what he had said; she pulled her hand away from his. Mark looked up at her, waiting for the moment when she would cut his heart out, and throw it away. She sat up straight with her eyes fixed on his. *Here it comes.* He braced himself for the worst. With a swift, elegant motion, she lifted her arms up and placed them around his neck; bringing herself closer to him, her head resting upon his shoulder.

Mark felt paralyzed. *I don't know what I should do. Is this pity? Does she feel sorry for this naive attempt at self expression?* Feeling his hesitation, Sabrina whispered into his ear. "Hold me. Just put your arms around me, and hold me." He was elated at her request, but still cautious as he embraced her. *Is this her way of letting me down?*

Between her movement, and his, it caused the sheet to slip off down to her waist. He felt her breasts pressing against his chest; his heart pounded. Taking a bold chance, he began to caress her back. *She hasn't rejected me, but she hasn't said anything either. She must feel something for me, why else would she want me to hold her like this?*

Their embrace continued in complete silence; Sabrina wondering what she should do next. *Since Mark is so out of touch with women, maybe he doesn't know what to do.* Her hand slid down from his neck to his chest, and under his arm to his back. She repeated the motion with her other hand. The tenderness of her touch filled him with warmth, as he focused on her hands, softly gliding over his back. Yet he still waited for her to crush his heart.

Sabrina turned her head; her lips brushed against his neck, as she leaned back to look at his face. He watched with nervous anticipation, as she unconsciously wet her lips, then closed her eyes. *Is she signaling me to kiss her?* He leaned into her. Her lips quivered in anticipation. He kissed her ever so softly. He was very much inexperienced, but the feelings he had at this moment made it seem easy. She tasted so sweet; he kissed her again; this time with a new found hunger.

At that moment, Sabrina didn't want him to stop. She tasted the tenderness and the passion, much stronger than anything she had ever experienced before and she wanted more. She gently pulled him with her as she laid back against the bed. Realizing what she was doing, Mark released her, letting her settle back alone. Redirecting his gaze, he pulled the sheet back up, covering her semi nude body. She was confused.

"Mark what's wrong? I thought you wanted." It was so hard for her to find the right words. *His feelings were very clear; but why does he keep pulling away?* Mark looked at her again. "I do; I want to make love to you; you have no idea just how much I want that; but it can't be now." In her eyes he could see the caring individual that lived within. The understanding that radiated from her face made it easier for him to speak.

"You must understand that I have to be sure. After being alone for so many years, I need to know if what I'm feeling is right, and you need time to work through everything that has happened." Sabrina's feelings were all mixed up, but she understood what he was saying to her. Taking his hand she held it close to her heart.

"I do understand; and to be perfectly honest, I too, would like to get to know you better. It's hard to explain, but I have also been having these strange feelings when you're around, and even when you're not. I can't really explain them to you; at least not yet anyway. Know this; I am grateful for your honesty about Sean, and about yourself. Of everything, I value that most of all." "So, will you stay?" Mark asked cautiously. "Yes. I have a reason now."

She had spoken so softly to him, all the while holding his hand. Mark couldn't speak at that moment; he was so captivated by her. He freed his hand to touch her face. Instinctively she tilted her head so that her cheek rested in his palm. The feel of her skin was so soft.

How I want her, my body is more than willing. He was very aware of how uncomfortably tight his jeans had become. It embarrassed him, and he hoped that she didn't notice; but she had closed her eyes, enjoying the gentleness of his touch. "It's getting late, and you really need to rest," he said. Standing up, he turned himself away from her, hiding what his shirt could not. "We still have a lot to talk about; but it can wait."

He hurried down the hall to his room. Shutting the door, he unzipped his jeans, relieving the discomfort. God had outdone himself on Mark's height, making him a towering giant of nearly seven feet; but he had also given him the physique to go with it. That was the primary reason that he had abstained for so many years; because of his physical size, he had never been able to give a woman pleasure, only pain.

I desperately want to be with Sabrina, but I can't stand the idea that I might physically hurt her too. Taking a cold shower, he tried to get his body to relax and to clear his mind; but both endeavors were ineffectual. Sleep was just as useless; his mind clung to thoughts of her, how good her body had felt next to his. *Someday; someday she will lie beside me as my mate.*

When Mark left her room, Sabrina stretched and wiggled in her bed. She was elated that he had told her about his feelings for her. *But still, what exactly is it about him that makes me feel this way? Not even Will had been able to excite me this way, this goes far beyond anything I ever experienced with him, but there is so much more to Mark; more I need to know; and more I crave to learn.*

Her mind was flooded with questions, but it all kept coming back to the sensations she got when he touched her, and when he kissed her. She tossed and turned most of the night. Her dream had finally returned, but with only brief flashes of the man. Patches gave up his attempt to sleep by her side and continued his night on the chair beside the bed.

The days had elapsed too quickly; three weeks were just about up. Sabrina's morning vigil with nausea had passed and she was feeling a lot better now; thoroughly convinced that Mark had a lot to do with it. *He's so attentive, and always so considerate.* They had spent most of their time talking, really getting to know one another; yet still keeping some secrets. She didn't say it, but she thought often about Sean's return; it scared her.

The phone rang, late one night, Sabrina instinctively went to answer it, but Mark stopped her. "Let the answering machine get it," he said. She was puzzled by his reaction, but when she heard the voice on the answering machine, she understood. It was Sean. Sabrina listened to the angry voice. "Sabrina, answer the phone; I know you're there; now pick up the damn phone! I want an explanation. Just what in the hell is going on? Pick up the phone!" There was a long pause before he hung up; Sabrina was visibly upset. Mark wanted to comfort her, but she shrugged off his advances and walked away.

I'll allow her some time alone, before I make another attempt to talk to her. I haven't touched her, or held her since that first night, and I so desperately want to hold her now, to ease her pain.

He watched her, standing against the railing on the patio. *Even from here I know that she's crying. No more, this stops now.* He went to her; putting his hand on her shoulder; she shrugged it off. Reattaching his grip, he turned her around; she fought him. "Leave me alone!" "Not this time, I'm not going to let you torture yourself in silence."

He enveloped her in his arms and she melted against him. He could feel her tears, soaking through his shirt; he held her until she was ready to let go. "We need to talk about this, now." "I don't want to talk about it." "It has to be now," he demanded. He moved her over to a chair, and pulled another one up close in front of her. Spreading his knees, he trapped her in place. "Now talk to me," he said, in a much calmer voice. "I'm not letting you go until you do."

Sabrina sighed, and rolled her head from side to side, relieving the tension that was trapped in her neck. "That phone call really upset you. Why?" "He's so angry with me." "Why do you think that is?" "Because of the way I left; not telling him what my plans were." "You're wrong. Sean is pissed off because he's never had a woman walk out on him before. He doesn't know how to deal with it."

The next question on his mind turned his stomach, but he had to ask. "Do you have feelings for him?" "I did, or at least I thought I did; but Sean wiped that all away on the morning he left." "I don't understand?" "That morning, I told him that I loved him." "And?" "He had no response at all. Nothing. That's when I knew that what you had told me was all true; he only wanted me for sex, nothing more." "What will you do if the phone rings again?" "The same thing I as did now; let the machine answer. Why did it take him this long to try and contact me?" "Do I really have to give you the answer to that question?" "No. I guess he found someone else to occupy his time. What I have to figure out though is what I'm going to do when he comes home."

"That's easy, I've taken care of it; his tour has been extended for another week, and when he does get back, he won't get in here, I guarantee it." "You can't stay here forever; you have to work too." "Not for a while;

I took a month off to start with and I've already extended it to two months now, but I can extend it longer if I have to." "Why would you do that?" Sabrina asked. "To be with you," he said softly.

Finding a smile in her heart, she shared it with Mark. *He makes me feel so good inside.* Sliding herself forward in the chair, she sat on his knee. He was startled by her move, but willingly accepted her. He placed his hand around her back to steady her, but she had already anchored her arm around his neck. Her expression softened as he looked at her. It was a look that he hadn't seen before, and one that he couldn't quite figure out. She softly touched his cheek with her fingers; leaning in closer, hesitating for a brief moment before she kissed him. Mark responded to her, deepening their kiss.

He had longed for this moment. Her hand trailed down his neck and over his shirt, until she found his hand. Raising it up to her breast, she held it in place until he began to caress it. His kisses moved over her throat, to the top of her breast that showed above her tank top. The feel of his mustache on her skin made her shudder with delight. His soft kisses moved back up her neck, until he again found her lips, his tongue teasing at them before plunging deep inside her mouth. *I want him to make love to me, but I don't dare say it.*

As if reading her mind, Mark slipped his arm under her knees, and in one swift move, he stood up, with her held firmly in his arms. He carried her into the house, pausing only to shut the patio door. They kissed again and he continued on his course to her bedroom. She was so aroused with anticipation. *Tonight, he will be with me tonight.*

Pausing at the side of the bed, he lowered her down. Releasing her hold she eagerly awaited his body to be beside hers. He ran his hand over her hair and smiled at her; turned and walked to the door. She lifted herself up on her elbows. "Where are you going?" "Not yet," he said, closing the door behind him. Frustrated, Sabrina threw one of the pillows at the door before flopping back onto the bed. *Why does he tease me so?* She could find no logical answer for that question. *What is he waiting for?*

Trying to be quiet, she padded around the kitchen, still hurt, and frustrated over last night's events. *He must have his reasons; but damned if I know what they are.* She heard his bedroom door open and then close. He appeared in the kitchen, all bright and cheerful. "Good morning Sabrina."

"Morning," she muttered. "You had better get dressed." "Why?" "Because we're going out." "Where?" "You'll have to just wait and see," he said steering her out of the kitchen. "I suggest you put on a pair of jeans and some boots." "Well, I don't have any jeans, and I don't have any boots." "Well then, we'll just have to get you some; now get a move on." He gave her another less than subtle nudge.

She muttered and grumbled to herself the whole time she was getting dressed. *What is he up to now?* She returned to the kitchen. "I'm ready, I guess." "Great, then let's go." "Where are we going?" "Out. You've been cooped up here way too long. It's time you went out and had some fun." In her mind, she did agree with Mark. *I haven't been out of the house for quite a while, and a day away just might do me some good.*

Mark drove her car; usually she would have been nervous, not accustom to being a passenger; but with Mark, she felt safe. She only glanced at the speedometer once, and since he was keeping to the speed limit only helped to relax her more.

He pulled into a mini mall about thirty minutes from home. Sabrina hadn't noticed this one before, probably because it was so small, and there was nothing remarkable about it. Mark made her wait until he opened the door for her; he put his arm around her shoulders, clasping her to his side. They walked toward the few little stores that made up the mall. "A western store?" she asked. "Where else would you go to buy jeans?"

The strong aroma of leather permeated the store. It reminded her of when she was younger, when she worked at a stable just so she could be around the horses. Mark caught the attention of the young female clerk, standing behind a counter. By the look on the girls face, Sabrina knew that she had recognized Mark. She rounded the counter and bounded her way to them. Sabrina figured she was about twenty, and she wore the typical attire of tight blue jeans and a western shirt.

The clerk stopped only inches away from Mark, her eyes were wide and fixated on him, her voice filled with nervous vibration as she spoke. "Can I help you?" Mark deepened his voice when he spoke to her. "Yes, you can; the lady here is in need of a pair of jeans and boots." "Yes sir." The young girl directed Sabrina to the racks of jeans, helping her to select a couple of styles. Mark asked Sabrina what size shoe she wore, then picked out a pair of black cowboy boots for her to try on with the jeans.

He browsed through the store while she changed, but couldn't find anything that suited him, let alone fit him. There weren't many stores that carried a line of clothes in his size. Everything was either too short or too tight. Most of the time; when he did find a shop that catered to his stature, he would buy as many things as he could; just in case he never got back there for a while.

The clerk was beginning to bother him; she had followed close behind him as he toured the store. He hated being followed by fans; they never knew when to quit. He went back to the fitting room to wait for Sabrina. She peaked her head out from behind the curtain. "Are you ready for this?" Sabrina asked with a wide smile. "Come on out." Pulling the curtain back, she cautiously stepped out. Mark's eyes opened wide, and he smiled at her. "Wow!" "Is that good or bad?" she asked, turning around giving him the full view. "Good, hell it's terrific!"

Sabrina had selected a pair of black denim jeans, that fit her body so perfectly that they were like a second skin. Her top was once a western shirt, that had been turned into a button front halter top. The collar was still intact, but most of the back had been cut away, along with the sleeves. The front was cut and stitched in a way that made it lay flat against her stomach yet accentuated her breasts, it too, was black with bright red piping for trim. The black boots that he had selected completed the look.

"Are you going to say anything else?" she asked with nervous anticipation. Mark moved to her, placing his hands on her soft round shoulders. "Well?" She was still waiting for an answer. He couldn't speak; her beauty had taken his voice from him. All he could do was kiss her. She responded immediately; putting her arms around him, pressing herself closer to him. She could feel his heart pounding in his chest, in time with hers. Mark looked over to the clerk, who was standing with her mouth open. "We'll take these," he said.

It was difficult for him to tear himself away from her, but if he didn't, the clerk would have one hell of a story to tell her friends. Sabrina collected her things from the dressing room and went to the counter. The young girl began clipping off the price tags, as she rang the sale into the register. "There's one more thing you need," Mark interrupted walking away. "What else could I possibly need now?" "You need a hat to go with that outfit." She knew better than to question him. She followed and began trying on different hats until she found one that she liked. She held one out to Mark. "You need one too."

I don't really want one, but if it pleases her, then I'll do it. She giggled quietly every once in a while, when he tried on one that just did not suit him. Finally finding one that they both agreed upon, they took them back to the clerk; who had stayed put, only after Mark had glared at her not to follow them again.

He shooed Sabrina away from the counter while he paid. Not that he didn't want her to see how much he was spending, but because what he was really doing was adding to his order, a piece of silver jewelry from the glass cabinet under the register. He tucked it into the front pocket of his jeans so that she wouldn't see it.

The young clerk could only let her imagination fill in the blanks. Of all the articles she had read about the Warlock, none of them ever mentioned that he had a lady. A part of her was jealous. She had been to many wrestling events; specifically to see the Warlock, to feed her fantasy. Standing near the front window of the store, she watched them walk to the car. When they kissed again, she began to weep. Her fantasy was in the arms of another woman.

When Mark got in the car, Sabrina again questioned him. "Now will you tell me where we are going?" "No." Realizing that her quest was futile, she gave up and relaxed against the seat to watch the scenery. They drove up into the hills, away from the ocean, away from the traffic. The air turned warm and dry, and the plant life reflected the change. They had gone from lush greenery to a brown, dry grassland. Trees were few. Only the very large ones showed any signs of life.

They continued on this route for nearly an hour, when Sabrina began to notice evidence of human habitation amongst the desolate hills. Fences began appearing along the sides of the road, along with the odd mailbox. Mark turned the car off the road into a driveway. They passed under a large wooden archway, but she didn't have the chance to read what it said.

The driveway took them past fields of cattle, and along a border of tall pines. Buildings became visible in the distance. She could make out a large home, painted pure white, with bright green shutters and trim. To the far left of the house was an equally large barn, painted in the same colors as the house. Mark pulled the car along side the house. "Wait here for me," he said.

She watched him walk to the barn, disappearing into its shadows. She tried to be patient, observing the gently sloping fields that rose up behind the house. They were lush and green, with various arrays of shrubs, a rather stark difference to the scenery along the main road. The sound of footsteps nearing the car made her refocus. Mark opened the door for her and extended his hand. "Will you please tell me now what is going on?" she begged. Mark gave her a sly grin. "Mmmm, not yet. Come with me."

As they approached the barn, Sabrina detected the familiar scent of horses. They walked through the barn, passing many stalls, some empty and some not. She wanted to stop and look at the horses, but Mark urged her on. Exiting at the far end of the barn, they were greeted by a man, wearing faded jeans and an old dirty T-shirt. A tattered old straw hat sat atop his head. Sabrina couldn't determine his age, as the many years of outdoor work had weathered his face.

"Ready?" Mark said to the man. "Yes sir, everything is ready; just like you asked for." The man spoke with an accent that was unrecognizable to her. He directed Mark to the side of the barn, where stood two magnificent horses. Sabrina was filled with excitement. "We're going riding?"

"That bay there is for you ma'am." Sabrina didn't hear him; she had already neared the big bay gelding and was quietly talking to him while she stroked his neck. Mark's horse was a black gelding, slightly taller than the bay, but much heavier in frame. The man again spoke to Mark."Everything you asked for is in these saddle bags. You two have a nice ride and I'll see you when you get back." He never waited for an answer he just returned to his chores. "We can go as soon as you like," Mark said. "Oh Mark this is so great! How did you know that I liked horses?" "Lucky guess."

Leaving the barn, they kept the horses at an even walk up the hill, letting them get used to their new riders. Following the trails that led off from the top of the hill, every once in a while letting the horses run a bit, before bringing them back to a slow walk. They approached a split in the trail; Mark turned his horse to the right fork. "We have to go this way," he said. "Why? No, I know the answer; you'll see. Right?" He paid her remark no attention. She had given up trying to reason out his actions; but she was intrigued by how secretive he was being.

The trail was narrow, and she had to follow behind, keeping her eyes trained on Mark all the time. Watching everything from the way his legs gripped the horse to the way his body moved in the saddle. Slowly from one side to the other and now and then his hips would move forward then back. Every movement of his body unintentionally fueled her fantasies.

When the trail again widened, he stopped and waited for her to reach his side. "So where do we go now?" "There," he said pointing off to the right. Following the direction of his arm, her eyes fell upon a lake. Mark took the lead again, but they both let the horses maneuver the slope at their own pace. When the slope began to level out, Sabrina spurred her horse into a gallop and passed Mark. He immediately took up the chase, but because of her head start he couldn't make up the distance.

Sabrina was almost halfway around the lake when she decided that she had better stop. The horse needed the rest, and Mark needed to catch up. She had already dismounted and was walking her horse to the lake when he showed up. "Show off," he said, dismounting near her. "No! I was just having some fun."

After the horses had some water, they walked them for a little bit. "Let's go over there," Mark said, pointing to a large tree beside the lake. The shade felt good to Sabrina, after being out in the sun for so long. She tied her horse to a smaller tree, but still in the shade cast from the larger one. "Hungry?" he asked. "Yeah, just a bit; but I'll survive until we get home." "Don't need to," he said, lifting off the saddle bags from each horse. She didn't bother to ask; for she already knew the you'll see answer would be what she got out of him.

Leaning against the tree trunk, she watched him unpack the saddlebags. First out was a large blanket, which he spread upon the grass. "Sit down," he said. She obliged quickly. It had been a long time since she had been riding, and her body wasn't used to it anymore. She quietly acknowledged the slight cramp in her belly. *Riding in new jeans isn't comfortable.* Stretching out on her side, she continued to watch him pull things from the bags.

"So what all have you got in there?" Sabrina asked. "Let's see; I've got wine, fried chicken, potato salad and some fruit." "When did you plan all this?" "This morning, before I came to the kitchen." "You are unbelievable." He hid a shy grin from her as he continued to lay out their meal. He served up their feast, and they ate quietly, watching a pair of ducks that were drifting along the lake shore.

When she was done with her meal, she set her plate down and reached for one of the saddlebags. Mark's large hand stopped her from opening it.

"What do you want?" "You said there was some fruit in there; I was kind of hoping for a couple of apples for the horses." Mark lifted the bag up, and dug through it. Finding the apples, he tossed her two. Sabrina fed one to each horse before returning to her place on the blanket.

"Ready for dessert?" Mark asked. "Sure. What have you got?" "Let's see," he said, opening a container. "I've got some grapes, and some strawberries." "Oh now if we only had some whipped cream," she sighed, pushing her fantasy back into the abyss. He waived another container near her. "You really thought of everything." *I had to; you need to feel special.*

Sabrina cautiously moved herself closer to him. Taking a strawberry from the container, she dipped it in the thick cream. Lifting it to her mouth she swirled her tongue over the tip before taking a bite. Mark watched her every move, and she knew it. Her erotic actions were done solely to torment him. Reaching for another this time she directed it towards him.

She boldly teased him with it before putting it in his mouth. Traces of whipped cream lingered on his lips; she couldn't resist the temptation to kiss it away. He took her down onto the blanket beside him, kissing her with a great hunger. The weight of his body pressed against her, making it hard for her to breathe. Mark felt her labored breath, and rolled onto his back, pulling her on top of him, her legs straddling his hips. Their kisses became fevered, yet tender.

Sabrina poised herself up on her knees; she needed to catch her breath, but it also gave her the chance to move her hands over his shirt, feeling the strength of his body. She leaned back down and spoke softly, still breathless. "Make love to me Mark."

He pushed her back up, and elevated himself to a sitting position. "I can't Sabrina." "Why not? We know that we both have feelings for each other; I just don't understand." A tear traveled down her cheek; he brushed it away. "Please don't cry. I can't explain my actions to you yet; but I promise I will, soon. All I ask is your patience; and your forgiveness. I do care about you, more than you realize."

Working his hand into his pocket, he retrieved the piece of silver he had hidden there. He helped Sabrina into a sitting position beside him, and adjusted himself so that he could see her face. She noticed how his expression had changed, to one of seriousness. A deep line appeared in his forehead. His lips were drawn tight together, deep in thought.

I am so confused. We have become closer; but is this the right time? Taking her hand, he held it so tight that it hurt her. "Mark!" She freed her hand, shaking the circulation back into it. "I'm sorry," he said lowering his head.

Something is preying on his mind, and I need to know, but only if he's willing to talk to me. Sabrina ran her hand along the inside of his thigh. "What's wrong Mark?" "There is nothing wrong. In fact, everything is right, so very right. We've only known each other for a few weeks; but, I feel that I've known you forever. I don't understand it myself, but I can't deny what's in my heart."

"I'm not sure that I understand what you're trying to say." "What I'm trying to say, is that I want to be with you. I need to be with you. I want to be there when you're happy, when you're sad, and when you're hurting. I want to be with you every day, and God willing, every night; for as long as you want me."

Sabrina rocked back, biting her lip. She was absorbing every thing that he was saying, and still could not believe it. "This may not be the right time to be telling you this Sabrina, but you must believe me when I say that this is not some act. Everything that I've told you is the truth, and it comes from my heart, and my soul." He held her hand gently in his. "I have something for you. I would like you to wear this; as a reminder of my commitment to you, and so that you will have a piece of my heart with you always."

He cautiously began slipping the silver ring onto the finger of her right hand. Sabrina pulled it away abruptly; he felt his heart rip in two, but then she spoke. "If you truly mean what you say, then you should be putting that ring on this hand," she said, extending her left hand to him. "Are you sure?" he asked, his voice was shaking almost as much as his hands.

"I have never been so sure of anything as I am right now. I don't know why I'm so drawn to you; but my heart tells me that I never want to be away from you, ever. I admit that the first time I saw you I was terrified, but that was because I didn't understand what was happening, but now, now I understand and I can see so clearly. I want to be with you, Mark. I need to be with you."

She fought her tears as Mark placed the ring on her finger, and held her trembling hand as she looked at it. It was a heavy silver ring, with two gold hearts on top. *It is the most beautiful thing I have ever seen.* She bit her lip hard, trying to hold back her tears, but it was no use, they rolled freely down her cheeks; but this time they were tears of joy, not sadness. She fell into Mark's arms, holding him tight, afraid to let go for fear that it all was just a dream. Mark ran his hand through her hair, as he rocked her slowly.

I have found in her, the part of myself that has been missing for all these years. I feel whole again, renewed. She is teaching me how wonderful it is to love, and be loved. Nothing will ever take that, or her from me.

They stayed locked in their embrace for a long time. He noticed how even his heart seemed to beat in time with hers. He kissed her forehead. "I hate to break this spell, but we should be getting back," he said. Sabrina looked at him, her eyes pleading to him. He could not refuse; he nuzzled his face against hers and kissed her.

Now, more than ever, I want to make love to him, but his feelings matter to me. I won't coerce him into something he isn't ready for. Just to feel his arms around me will be enough.

She helped pack up the saddlebags and tie them onto the horses. They headed back to the stable slowly at first, but again letting the horses run whenever possible. Mark was ahead of her and didn't see her horse stumble. She didn't come off, but the sudden, unexpected lurch, made her lose her balance. She jammed her abdomen hard into the saddle horn. Momentarily without breath, she regained her seat and rode on, catching up to Mark. She didn't tell him what had happened, but slowed her horse, letting him walk the rest of the way back to the barn.

The pain in her belly burned with each step the horse took, and she was glad to be off of him. Mark put his arm around her as they walked back to the car; thankful of it, since the pain hadn't subsided any, and she was afraid that she might not make it back on her own. Staring out the window on the way home, she hid her discomfort from him; telling herself that it would go away soon, but it was a strange pain, sharp and stabbing, only sometimes, and then subsiding to a dull ache, only to return with sudden excruciating force. She felt every bump and pot hole in the road.

Choosing her steps cautiously as she entered the house, she walked right past Mark to her bedroom, thinking how good a shower would feel right about now. "You have some messages," Mark said, causing her to stop in the doorway. "I think we both know who they're from. Play them, or erase them; I really don't care. I'm gonna take a shower."

Mark detected a strange tone in her voice, but dismissed it as fatigue. He played the two messages on the answering machine; both of them were from Sean. He didn't sound as angry as the other night, but Mark could tell that he was still pissed off. On the second message Sean recited two phone numbers that he could be reached at. *She won't be phoning you.* He erased the messages. *Sabrina had the right idea; take a shower and get rid of this horse smell.*

Quickly stripping off her clothes, she looked into the mirror, observing the large red bruise that was forming just below her navel. A sudden, sharp pain made her double over onto the counter. It didn't last long, and when she was freed of it she started her shower. The pulse of the water against her belly made it hurt more, and she ended her shower sooner than she planned. She couldn't be bothered to towel off; choosing to wrap her robe around her, she went to sit on the bed. The pain was coming more frequently, like a wave washing over her; it made her nauseous and light headed.

I don't want to be alone; I need Mark; he'll know how to make me feel better. Staggering to the bedroom door; she had to lean against the frame, as another wave consumed her.

Mark had just come out of his room. He saw her leaning against the doorway. Her face was pale white, and reflected an expression of severe pain. He reached her just as her body began to slide down to the floor. Picking her up in his arms, he carried her into the bedroom and laid her on the bed.

Removing his arm from under her body, he saw that his shirt sleeve was soaked with blood. Fear and panic surged through his body as he dialed 911, demanding an ambulance. Sabrina was unconscious, but he still spoke to her, trying to bring her around. When she began to stir, she was immediately seized by another surge of pain. "What happened?" she asked, her voice weak. "You fainted. Why are you in such pain?" "I had an accident with the horse." "What do you mean?"

I don't understand. How could she have had an accident? I was with her all the time. Parting her robe, she exposed the bruise. Mark's heart was in his throat. *I know now what's happening to her.* "Rest; you're going to the hospital." She didn't have the energy to argue with him. Mark covered her as best he could, trying to hide the blood from her, but it wasn't easy. It had already soaked through her robe. He could hear the siren getting closer;

he left her briefly to let them in. She drifted in and out, but never coherent enough to understand the paramedics. She was bleeding heavily and the paramedics did what they could, but they weren't able to stop it. Mark rode with her in the ambulance. *She is going to need me now more than ever.*

The attending Doctor took her straight to an operating room. Despite Mark's pleas for information, the emergency room staff ignored him. He paced diligently in front of the doors that led to the surgical rooms; torn up inside with worry. Lifting his eyes upward he prayed silently. *Please, don't take her from me, not now.*

After an hour and a half of torturous waiting the Doctor emerged through the doors, he walked towards Mark and guided him to a seat. Doctor Maynard's face was expressionless, and that made a knot form in Mark's stomach. "How is she?" Mark was afraid to ask. "She'll be just fine; but I'm afraid that she lost the baby. Fortunately for her she was very early on, just over a month would be my guess. It may sound cold, but it was a good thing that this accident happened." "What do you mean?" "It wasn't a normal pregnancy; it was what we call an ectopic, which means that the baby was growing in the fallopian tube, not the uterus. She would have had to have it terminated anyway." "Will she be all right?"

"Oh yes, she will recover fairly fast, and there's no reason that she can't have more babies, but I would suggest that you wait a few months before trying again. I'm not saying that you can't have intercourse; just take precautions to prevent another pregnancy before her body is ready." "Can I see her?" "Sure, she'll be coming out of recovery in about thirty minutes. You can wait in the room that we have assigned to her, if you like. First, let me see if I can find you something else to wear." He pointed to the blood soaked shirt that Mark was wearing. Mark followed Doctor Maynard down the hall to a private room. Picking up a scrub shirt from a trolley he handed it to Mark.

The wait was just as tedious as before; during the thirty minutes Mark must have checked his watch at least twenty times. Finally, two orderlies appeared at the door, one at each end of a hospital bed. Sabrina looked so pale and fragile, covered up with thick blankets. Mark pulled a chair up beside her and reached under the blankets for her hand. *It's so cold.* He held it tightly between his hands. A nurse came in carrying a bag. "These are hers," she said.

Mark disregarded the woman's comment until she pulled a small envelope from her pocket and handed it directly to Mark. It was Sabrina's ring. He placed it back on her finger and kissed it. The nurse paid Mark no attention as she continued with her routine check; as she was leaving she spoke to him. "If you talk to her, she'll come around a lot sooner."

Mark stroked Sabrina's forehead and called her name. "Sabrina, it's Mark. Can you hear me? Wake up, oh please wake up." He bowed his head and swallowed hard; seeing her like this was tearing him apart inside. He felt a burning sensation in his eyes. It was tears. A sensation that he had not experienced before. Not as a child, and not even when his parents had died. He had never been able to shed a tear for anyone, or anything, until now.

It's her, she's making me come alive, for the first time that I can remember I feel real emotions. Sabrina's fingers moved in his hand; he called to her again. "Sabrina, wake up." Her head moved toward the direction of his voice; she struggled to keep her eyes open. "Mark. Where? What happened?" "Shhh, you're in the hospital. You had an accident with the horse; remember?" "Mmmm, I'm so tired." "You just rest now." His comforting words fell upon deaf ears.

He remained by her bed, keeping watch over her, never releasing her hand. The nurse returned every hour to check Sabrina's blood pressure and to take her pulse. On her third trip in, she spoke to Mark. "I'm sorry sir, but you're going to have to leave now. Visiting hours are long over." "I'm not going anywhere." "Sir you have to; it's hospital policy." The nurse's tone had become more demanding.

Mark stood up and ushered her out of the room. His size alone was incredibly intimidating, and when he spoke in a deep, commanding voice it unnerved her even more. "I told you that I'm not leaving her here alone. Do you understand?" "But sir, it's policy." "Your policy can go straight to hell." The nurse took a step back, poised ready to run, when Doctor Maynard appeared behind them. "What's the problem here?" Dr. Maynard asked. The nurse quickly recounted to him her conversation with Mark. "That's all right; he can stay. Now please return to your duties." The nurse hurried down the hall, glad that her shift was over, and that she wouldn't have to deal with him again.

Mark thanked Doctor Maynard for allowing him to stay. He replied by giving Mark some good news. "She should be able to go home tomorrow morning around eleven; but she is going to need some clothes, since hers were so badly soiled." "That's good; I can sneak away early in the morning and get whatever she needs." Mark was becoming anxious. He needed to be with her. Doctor Maynard sensed his agitation. "Well good night then." Mark didn't answer him; he returned to his seat beside her bed; quietly watching her, and holding her hand.

How I want to hold you in my arms, if only to tell you that I'm sorry. This is all my fault; if I hadn't taken you riding this would never have happened. Guilt smothered him like a blanket. *I caused this. I caused you to lose your baby.* A thought flashed into his mind, making him sit up straight.

She doesn't know about the baby; and maybe she never will. I won't tell her. I could just keep it a secret. It would only cause her more grief, knowing that she was carrying Sean's child. Anger burned in his stomach. *How could Sean be so careless? How could he do this to her?* Deep down inside, a small part of his soul was relieved that Sean's baby was no longer growing inside her. *If she's meant to have a baby, then it should be mine. Please let it be mine someday.*

He maintained his vigil all night, never moving from his seat, or away from her side. The late duty nurse was far more compassionate than the other one. On one of her trips in to check on Sabrina she brought Mark a cup of coffee and a blanket. He paid her no attention, as she set the cup down before him, and spread the blanket across his back. Exhaustion finally forced him to lay his head down on the bed. The nurse came back in and fixed the blanket around him, after she had completed her check of Sabrina. Admiring his devotion; staying with her all night; at least he was getting some rest too.

Mark was awakened by the sounds of the hospital coming back to life; orderlies and nurses moved about the hallway with trolleys of linens and medications. He checked his watch. It was not quite seven. *Plenty of time to go home, get her things, and be back before she is ready to leave. She will probably sleep for a while longer.* "I'll be back soon, my love," he whispered as he kissed her forehead.

The ride home in the cab was irksome. It didn't take any longer than if he drove it himself; but his anxiety made it feel twice as long. Patches was waiting just inside the door, Mark didn't see him until he heard the screech as he stepped on his tail. *No time to check on the cat, I have to get back to Sabrina.*

It felt strange to be going through her things, but he had to. *Her stomach will probably be sore, so she won't want anything tight around her waist.* He finally selected a sun dress. A sweater was on the chair; he took that too and a blanket to lie over her in the car, just in case she was cold.

With everything stuffed into a tote bag, he headed for the car; just as he was about to leave, the phone rang. He hesitated at answering it, but what if it was the hospital. He answered it on the third ring. "Hello." There was a long silence on the other end; he repeated himself. "Hello." "Mark? Is that you?" "Yeah who's this?" "It's Sean; and just what the hell are you doing at her place?" "That's none of your damn business." "Put Sabrina on the phone." "She's not here." "Don't pull that bull shit with me; put her on!" "I told you she's not here!" "Then where in the hell is she?"

The anger that Mark was feeling began to get the better of him and he began to yell. "She's in the hospital, you son of a bitch!" "Why? What's happened?" "Why should I tell you? You're nothing but a selfish, uncaring bastard! You treat women like dirt, and leave them when you've had enough of them!" "Mark you damn well better tell me what's going on!" "You want to know; fine, I'll tell you! She's in the hospital because she had a miscarriage! You dumb son of a bitch, you got her pregnant! That should make you happy; now you won't have to pay for her to have an abortion! You make me sick!" He slammed the phone down into its cradle. He was angry. Angry at himself for having told Sean about the baby; but it was done. *I'll deal with Sean later, right now I have to be with Sabrina; she is my only priority.*

The shock was immediate; the phone slipped from Sean's hand to the table. Mark's words echoed in his head. *Sabrina is pregnant? How?* He searched his mind for an answer. *How could she be pregnant? I always used a condom, so there wouldn't be any mistakes, or surprises.* He sat down hard in a chair, as he realized that he hadn't used a condom that first time they were together. He buried his face in his hands. *It wasn't the flu that she had, after all. It was morning sickness.* His heart weighed heavy in his chest. *I should go to her, but I won't be able to get out of my tour obligations.*

Reality hit him, like a kick in the stomach. *I had created a life; a part of myself grew inside her.* He had never really thought about being a father, giving up his wandering ways for a chance at a stable life, but now that chance was gone. *Will I be able to get her to forgive me, for not being there for her. Why was Mark there? Why had she gone home? Did she know? Did Mark tell her about the other women?*

A combination of pain and anger surged through him as he stood up; grabbing the chair he threw it across the hotel room. The chair exploded when it hit the wall, sending slivers of wood over a vast area of the room.

Robbie came out of the bathroom; a towel wrapped round her. "What the hell? Sean, what's going on?" "Get out!" "What!" "Get your things and get the hell out of here!" "But Sean." "I said to get out, now!" Robbie threw her clothes on, grabbed her few possessions, and ran from Sean's room. She didn't understand why he was so angry, but she knew that she had never seen such anger from him ever before, and it scared her more than anything.

Sean slammed the door shut behind her; he staggered to the bed and fell onto it face first. He thought about Sabrina, and what he had lost; but more importantly he thought about Mark. Convinced that he had taken her from him, that singular thought angered him more than anything else.

Mark made it back to the hospital just before eight thirty. Driving slowly and cautiously back to the hospital he tried to dispel his anger for Sean. He didn't want Sabrina to see that look on his face. He paused outside her room, taking a deep, calming breath, before he went in. He was quiet, just in case she was still asleep.

She was turned on her side, her back facing the door. Figuring she was awake; he set the bag down on the chair and leaned over to give her a kiss; she was crying. "Hey now, what's this?" "Go away; just go away," she sobbed. He went around the bed and pulled another chair up beside her. "Tell me what's wrong." He rested his hand upon her shoulder, she tried to shrug it off, but he wouldn't budge. "Tell me Sabrina."

Her tears ran heavy as she tried to speak. He waited patiently, caressing her shoulder for reassurance. Her words were torn apart by deep sobs. "The Doctor was in a little while ago; he told me that I." Mark finished her sentence. "He told you about the baby; didn't he?" Her lips trembled; he sat on the bed and took her in his arms. Sabrina held on to him tight; her cries were filled with pain.

I wish I could wipe away her pain, as easily as I wipe away her tears. If only I had been here, she would never have found out. Holding her, he let her cry, reassuring her with a gentle touch, rather than words.

Only when her sobs had silenced, leaving her body trembling, did he speak to her. "It's going to be okay. We'll get through this; together," he said in a calm, soft voice. Sabrina looked up at him. "How can you say that? How can you want me, knowing about?" "Whether you had carried this baby or not, I would still want you. My feelings for you are much stronger than you know." Mark paused briefly debating on whether or not to continue to say what he was thinking; he pressed on.

"I don't mean to be cruel; but in a small way, I am relieved that you lost the baby. For your sake, that is. Sean would have only pressured you into an abortion." "I didn't even know that I was pregnant, but you're right; it is better that it happened now, rather than later." Her tone had changed, she was coming to terms with her loss, and with the realization that Sean would have never accepted it.

Mark brushed his hand over her cheek. "How would you like to go home?" "Oh yes; I don't want to stay here any longer." "Do you think that you can get dressed, or should I get a nurse to help you?" "I think I can manage." "Okay then, I'll go and sign you out while you're getting changed," he said and passed her the tote bag from the other chair. "I brought you something comfortable to wear. I'll be back in a few minutes." "Before you go, could you untie the back of this for me?" She reached for the bows on her gown. "Sure I can."

His hands trembled, as he tugged at the bows. Having started with the lowest one, when he reached the top, he had to move her hair out of the way. It made his hands shake more, as he slid his hand along her neck, picking up her hair and putting it over her shoulder.

I have to fight these urges, to push this gown from her shoulders and hold her perfect body against mine. I want to be unbound of my shackles of fear, to embrace the power of love, but I must be patient.

Sabrina waited until she heard the door close before she slipped off her hospital gown; she put on her sun dress. *Mark was so thoughtful to bring this.* Her stomach hurt when she moved herself to the edge of the bed, forcing her to look. The bruise on her belly was a little larger than the saddle horn, and it had turned a bluish black, with purple around the edges. As she passed her hand over it, it stung, even under her own gentle touch. An overwhelming feeling of sadness washed over her; for the loss of her baby, and for knowing that Sean would only have made her get rid of it.

This is how it is meant to be. What kind of a man is he? How could he make a woman throw away her baby as easily as throwing away an old pair of shoes? She heard the door open again and quickly pulled her dress down.

"Ready?" Mark asked, moving himself in front of her. Sabrina poised herself to get up. "Definitely." He reached out to help her. "I can do it," she announced, trying to be strong. Sliding herself over the edge of the bed, she rested her feet on the floor for a moment while she thought out the best way to stand up. When she stood up, her knees went weak; she fell against Mark. Her body shook, as she struggled with the effort to stay standing.

A nurse had entered the room, pushing a wheelchair, just as Sabrina made her feeble attempt. "I see that I arrived just in time; you're going to be needing this," she said as she pushed the wheel chair over to Sabrina. "I can manage on my own." "No, sorry, it's hospital policy. No one walks out of here, every one gets a ride," she said patting the back of the wheel chair. Mark gave Sabrina one of those do not argue looks and helped her into the chair. The sudden bolt of pain that ran across her face stabbed him in the heart. She squeezed his hand until it passed.

The nurse handed Mark a small bottle of pills. "The Doctor wanted her to have these pain killers; the directions are on the label." The nurse pushed the wheel chair, while Mark went ahead to bring the car around to the door. "You sure have a wonderful man there. He stayed with you all night; never left once." "All night?" "That he did, and he gave the staff a bad time about it when they tried to get him to leave. Honey, that man sure loves you." Sabrina didn't respond; her mind clung to the last words the nurse had said.

It's apparently quite obvious, even to a total stranger, that the feelings that we share are strong.

Mark helped Sabrina into the passenger seat of the car; it took her a minute to seat herself comfortably. She pulled the seat belt across her, but kept her arm between it and her belly. The drive home was torturous; every bump in the road sent pain shooting through her body. She had given up on trying to sit comfortably, as the stopping and starting motion of the car had not allowed her to stay in one spot. Mark was very aware of her discomfort, by the way she gripped the armrest on the door. He tried to watch the road, and avoid any pot holes or bumps, but it was next to impossible, not everything was visible.

When they arrived home, Mark was quick to support her as they walked into the house. He let her set the pace, and never tried to hurry her. Patches was waiting inside the door, but ran away when he saw Mark. "What's the matter with him?" Sabrina asked. "He's mad at me." "Why?" "When I came home to get your clothes I accidentally stepped on him." "Don't worry; he doesn't hold a grudge; he'll come around soon."

They reached the bedroom; Mark held her arms while she eased herself onto a chair. He hadn't had time to clean up the bed sheets until now. Sabrina was shocked by the amount of blood. It made her stomach turn and made her remember that horrible night not so long ago. She had never seen the mess that was left behind then and was grateful that she never had.

Why do so many bad things happen here? I can't allow myself to be drawn back into that nightmare again. Mark is here now and I feel that only good can come from that from now on.

Mark pulled the sheets off into a ball on the floor and found clean linen in the closet. When he had finished making up the bed, he returned to help Sabrina over to it. He couldn't help noticing that distant look in her eyes. "Is everything okay?" he asked. "It is now." "I know it looks pretty bad but it really wasn't." "I wasn't thinking about this. I was just remembering the last bad thing that happened in here."

"Don't go there Sabrina. You have to put it all out of your mind so you can get the rest you need." "I have, thanks to you. I'm so glad you're here. I don't know what I would have done if you hadn't come into my life when you did." "You would have been fine, because I would have found you no matter where you were." " Thank you Mark." "So, where do you keep your night gown?" "Don't have one, and don't want one." "You've just had surgery; you need to keep warm." He left the room and returned with one of his T-shirts. "You can wear this. How would you like a nice hot cup of tea?" "That sounds really good." "Okay, you change, get yourself into bed; and I'll get a you a hot cup of tea."

He left the bedroom door part way open. *Just in case she needs me, I'll be able to hear her.* Sabrina changed and put on his T-shirt. *It has his scent.* She held it to her nose. She leaned back against the pillows exhausted; having made every move ever so carefully that her body had become tense, anticipating pain. It felt good to lie back; it took the pressure off of her stomach and her back. While Mark waited for the kettle, he turned the ringer off on the phone, and turned the volume down on the answering machine.

There is no need for her to be disturbed by anything; not until she's feeling better. Sean will try to phone again, and I'm not ready to deal with that yet. He fixed the tea and took it to her room; he thought she was asleep, by the way she rested against the pillows. Her eyes opened when he walked in. He handed her the mug and she took a long drink.

"You look tired." "I am," she said placing the empty mug on the bedside table. Hot or not, it tasted too good to linger over. "Why don't you try and get some sleep?" She agreed, and slid herself down in the bed until she lay flat; Mark made a move to get up. "Please stay with me," she said lightly holding his arm. "Please, I don't want to be alone right now." "I don't think it's such a good idea." "Please."

Her eyes pleaded to him, as she continued to tug at his arm. He lay down beside her, on top of the sheets. Carefully maneuvering herself toward him, she snuggled close. With her head resting against his shoulder, she passed quickly into sleep. Mark too, was exhausted and sore, from his restless night at the hospital; laying down was a welcome relief.

She looks so peaceful beside me. I want to put my arms around her, but I fear that it would press too hard against her and awaken her pain again. I have to be content with just being able to be with her, even if I can't touch her. It wasn't long before he followed her into the land of dreams.

Chapter 7

Sean found it increasingly difficult to keep his mind on his work; after learning about Sabrina. His performance in the ring deteriorated greatly; losing matches, that didn't go unnoticed by the owner of the company. Delusions had him seeing her face amongst the thousands of fans in the arenas; there one minute and gone the next. Scouring the crowds, he searched for her, ignoring his opponent.

He began declining all social contact with the other wrestlers in the company, and with Robbie. Being so all consumed with Sabrina that nothing else mattered anymore; except for the last day of the tour when he knew he would be returning home.

He had learned of Mark's extended leave of absence, and that worried him. His informants told him that Mark's leave had begun the day of the party and no one was certain of when or even if he would make a return. *Why then, why did Mark make that request then? He never takes time off. Why is he at Sabrina's? Did he persuade her to leave?* So many questions swirled through his mind like a tornado, but no logical answers came forth.

He was nearing exhaustion, as the tour neared its end. *At least I will have two weeks at home, to sort things out, before having to leave again. In a few days I'll be home, and I'll try and make things right with Sabrina.*

Brent and D'arcy both tried, on countless occasions, to get Sean to open up about what was troubling him, but each of them had met with Sean's anger, and gave up their inquiry. His friends were distancing themselves from him, yet he couldn't see it.

Sabrina was finally beginning to feel better. She had spent over two weeks in bed, primarily sleeping, her body recapturing its strength. Mark had been so attentive, and supportive; never pressuring her into discussing what she was feeling; about Sean, the baby or him; she wasn't ready yet. Whenever the sensations of sadness became to overwhelming for her, he was there, to hold her until it departed; staying with her at night, until she was asleep, then quietly slipping away to his room, but always returning before she awoke in the morning. He wasn't comfortable with staying with her all night, yet he had stayed, because it made her feel better; filling an unspoken need for both of them.

On this morning, Sabrina was awake early, Mark was not beside her, nor was he anywhere in the room. *I had my suspicions, and now they're confirmed.* Stretching out, she rubbed her back; it ached from being in bed for so long. It didn't take much for her to be convinced that a long, hot shower would do wonders, since she hadn't had one in days, as Mark had commanded her to stay in bed as much as possible; but no more. Pushing back the sheets, she sat on the edge of the bed for a few moments.

The pain in her belly was only a memory now. *Time to get on with life.* Carefully standing, holding the head post to steady herself, she felt a little wobbly at first, but that soon passed. She made her way into the bathroom, running her hand along the wall for guidance. She started the shower and pulled off Mark's T-shirt. Standing in front of the mirror, she scrutinized her bruise. It was still dark near the center, but had begun to fade to a yellowish stain around the edges. Running her hand across it, she felt no pain; her body had recovered quite quickly. The warm water was refreshing; she closed her eyes and let it wash away all her aches.

Mark crept into her room, as he had done so many times, but this time he was stopped in his tracks. Sabrina wasn't in bed. He went to the bathroom door; it wasn't closed tight; he could hear the shower running. *I'll give her a few more minutes; if she's not out in five minutes, then I'll go in to see if she's okay.* While he waited for her, he puffed up the pillows, stopping only to hold one against his chest. Her scent was strong on that one, sweet and pleasant to his nostrils. He clutched it tight as a whirlwind of fantasies spun in his mind.

The bathroom door moved; he tossed the pillow aside, and rose to move towards her; she waived him back. "I'm okay," she said. "You should be resting. What are you doing up?" "I can't stay in bed forever; besides, my back hurts from just lying around, and." "And what?" "I don't feel right about having you wait on me."

He met her in the middle of the room. His hands gently rested upon her shoulders. "I'm doing this for you, because I want to; I really want to." "But Mark." "No buts about it, just get comfortable with it, and enjoy it." His smile warmed her. She slipped her arms around his waist and tilted her head back to look at him. "I guess I can do that." She lay her head against his chest. *Her body feels so good against mine.*

"Would you like some breakfast?" Mark asked. "Yes, I would, but would you do something for me first?" "Sure, anything; you know that."

Sabrina looked up at him, her expression so soft. "Kiss me," she whispered. Mark was speechless at her solicitation, but very pleased. *She still wants me.* As he leaned down to her, their lips touched tenderly. She felt him try to back off, but she held her lips to his, desiring more of him.

When he broke free of her, he stood straight with his head held up out of her reach. "What?" Sabrina asked, feeling the tension building in his muscles. "I can't. It's not right." "What do you mean by that?" "It's not the right time yet; your body needs to rest; to recover." "I feel fine; my body feels fine. I have no more pain." "It's not time yet." "Damn it Mark; you keep saying that. When will it be time?" "Soon." "That answer isn't good enough anymore; I need an explanation. Damn it I need you. I need, I crave to feel your physical love," she pleaded with him for an answer, that held more detail than his customary noncommittal response. "I want to, and when the time is right I will. Just give yourself a little more time, okay?" His answer displeased her, and hurt her.

Why does he have to be so vague? The signals, I know he wants me. So why does he continually pull away from me, teasing me? She remembered that she had promised not to push him. *No matter how difficult it will be, I will honor that promise.* With his aide she walked out to the patio, where he left her while he fixed breakfast.

Standing at the railing, she watched the ocean. *So much has happened to me, but I can't deny the urge to run away, to leave this place forever. What started out to be my piece of heaven on earth, has turned into a living hell. My worst nightmares come true. It would be so easy to get in the car and disappear; to move on to someplace new and start over; or just go home.*

As strong as her feeling of running was, the one that made her stay was unmistakable. *How can I leave him now, now that I have found him? This man who makes me feel things that have been long dead, and forgotten. I want to be with him, in every sense of the meaning. I have to know if there is a possibility of a permanent relationship.*

Playing with the ring on her finger, she remembered the moment when he had given it to her; how happy they had both been. *Could he still feel the same way now, knowing about the baby? He has been so caring, or is it just a front, to help me get through this trauma.* Crossing her arms over her chest, she hugged herself. *How can I be sure? I have to know if this is real, or just another male mind game.* The tension in her neck was creeping upward; she closed her eyes, rolling her head from side to side, releasing the strain.

When she opened her eyes again, her gaze had settled upon Sean's house. *He will be home soon. How am I going to deal with that? He was so angry when he phoned. At least he doesn't know about the baby. That is one less problem to deal with and I'm not about to tell him. Having to confront him about leaving will be a formidable challenge; there is no need to make it worse.*

So caught up in her thoughts, she never heard Mark come on to the patio. He placed the breakfast tray down on the table; he could tell that she was not aware of his presence. Walking up behind her, he touched her arm; she jumped and turned at the same time. "Christ Mark, you scared me half to death!" "I'm sorry." He tried to hold her, but she pushed past him and went to the table.

They sat together, but very much isolated. In her mind, Sabrina played over and over an imaginary conversation, between her and Sean trying to put together a believable explanation for him, playing his role too, anticipating his reactions and responses. Mark could see that she was lost in thought and never tried to initiate a conversation.

What could she be thinking? Is she having misgivings about leaving Sean or is she questioning my commitment to her? I very much want to prove my love to her; but I've abstained for her own good. She's not ready, and I couldn't bear to hurt her, but I am hurting her, not physically, but emotionally. I'm rejecting her, by repeatedly giving her inadequate excuses. What can I do to let her know that I still need her; that I still want her? What can I do? His mind latched onto that question, searching for an answer.

The day dragged on tediously for both of them. Mark attempted several times to get Sabrina to talk to him, but she refused; preferring the solitude of her thoughts. That became very evident to Mark, for every time he lingered in her space she would move to another room, away from him. She went to bed without even saying good night; never asked him to stay with her until she fell asleep.

Feeling rejected and isolated in his bed, in his room; sleep evaded him. He tossed and turned all night long. *I have to regain her trust, and win her love; but how? How can I break through the wall around her, that I, myself have built to protect her.*

The sun began to slice through the curtains, sending golden fingers of light across the bed. An idea came to his mind. Picking up the phone; he dialed the number of the hospital, asking to speak to Doctor Maynard. Explaining to the switchboard operator that he had to talk to the Doctor now, as there was no way for him to call back. Mark told her Sabrina's name, and that his call was in reference to her. He waited, impatiently, as he was put on hold, abandoned in limbo, listening to the monotonous elevator music.

Maybe I should hang up, but I may not got another chance to do this. Fifteen minutes had passed and his patience was wearing thin. A voice on the phone snapped him back to reality. "Yes, this is Doctor Maynard. How can I help you?" "Yes, Doctor I wanted to ask you a couple of questions regarding Sabrina Scott." "Give me a minute to quickly review her chart." Mark waited, again. "Oh yes, the young lady that had the miscarriage. What did you want to ask?" Mark hesitated. *I know what I want to ask, but forming it into words is the hard part.*

"Doctor Maynard, how, how long should she wait before having sex?" "Well, as long as she isn't still experiencing any physical pain, I see no reason for you to abstain, but I must remind you to take precautions regarding pregnancy. Her body is not into a regular cycle yet, and probably won't be for about another month or so. I recommend that within two weeks you should be using some kind of protection regularly. Her body isn't strong enough yet to handle another pregnancy. Should she get pregnant too soon she will run the risk of having another miscarriage." "Thank you, Doctor Maynard you have been a great help." They exchanged their good-byes and Mark hung up the phone.

A wide smile shone from Mark's face, as if a tremendous weight had been lifted from his chest. *Finally, I can show Sabrina just how much I love her; and I will tell her too. I am going to make today a very special day for her, starting with breakfast.*

Mark slowed his pace as he passed by her room. *I can't afford to have her wake up too early.* He tried to be as quiet as he could in the kitchen, but his excitement made him shaky, causing him to lose his grip on just about everything he picked up. He cursed himself, for being so clumsy, even though nothing had hit the floor. He felt like a teenager again, preparing for his first date; nervous and anxious.

To be with her, tonight and always; but I'm still worried; she has become so apathetic. Does she not want me anymore? Have I stalled her off a little too long? I refuse to believe that. I'm more sure, than ever before, that she is the one for me. I'm meant to be with her, and no one else. Today, is not a day for thoughts of apprehension; today is for making it all up to her. To make up for my mistakes and all of the holidays she has missed.

Holidays; such a worthless, desolate word for people who are alone. They're just like any other day, nothing special. Like today, March 21st, my birthday. I've never had a purpose to celebrate, to feel joy, or give thanks; what was the point? Holidays are for families, and friends; and for lovers. I've known too many of those days. Those long endless days that only reminded me of my own desperate loneliness. Sabrina must have felt like that. She had never said anything about them. They all passed like normal days; but no more. Every day is a reason to celebrate, now that I've found her.

He placed her breakfast on a tray and took it to her room. Not bothering to knock, he opened the door and entered. She was awake, but still in bed. He startled her and she sat up, clutching the sheets tightly to her chest. "Good morning," he greeted her. A mumbled, 'Morning' resounded back at him. He placed the tray in front of her. "What's this?" "Breakfast," he smiled at her and left her alone. *What a nice surprise.* She looked over her tray of French toast with fresh strawberries. Trying to figure out his actions was a futile endeavor; she gave up and enjoyed her breakfast.

Mark had left her to make a couple of phone calls. Having come up with a few ideas, he wanted to make sure that his plan went smoothly. *All I want is to make her feel good again, that's all that matters. I'm not even going to tell her that it's my birthday today. This day is for her and only her.*

He met her in the hallway; she was carrying the tray back to the kitchen. "I'll take that," he said. She touched his arm briefly. "Thank you." "You're welcome." *She's speaking to me again, that's a start.* Following him into the kitchen, she stayed only long enough to get another cup of tea before she went out to the patio, to partake of the morning sun. Mark watched her from the kitchen.

She still looks so sad. She doesn't even bother to get dressed anymore, preferring the comfort of her robe over clothes. If my plan works, then she should return to her normal, vibrant self. The woman who drives my senses wild with desire. It has to work; it just has to. Even if we don't make love tonight it will be worth it if I can just get her to smile again.

Mark kept himself busy throughout the morning, making sure that he gave Sabrina her space when she needed it. He kept looking at his watch, the afternoon was upon them and the first part of his plan hadn't come to fruition yet; he went to his room to make a phone call to find out what the delay was. He had just picked up the phone, when he heard the doorbell; he smiled. *Now to stay in here and make her answer the door.*

"Mark, could you get that," Sabrina called. There was no answer; the bell rang again. Sabrina went to the door, hesitant to open it. She peered through the peep hole. A young man waited outside; holding a box. "Can I help you?" "I have a delivery ma'am." "You must have the wrong address; I'm not expecting anything." "No ma'am, the address is correct. This delivery is for a Sabrina Scott." Upon opening the door; the young man handed her a long, white box tied up with red ribbon. "Just a minute, I'll get my purse." "No thanks, the tip has already been taken care of."

Sabrina closed the door, carrying the box over to the couch, where she sat down with it on her knees. There was no card on the outside anywhere. She puzzled over it, not knowing whether she should open it. Mark came out of his room.

"Was that the doorbell?" he asked. "Yes, it was." "Who was it?" He was trying to keep his excitement contained. "It was a delivery boy, with this." She lifted the box up so he could see. "What is it?" "I don't know. I haven't opened it yet." "Why not?" "I don't know?" "You better open it; it's the only way to find out what it is, and who it's from." He bit his lip on that one, hoping that he hadn't given himself away.

Sabrina fumbled with the bow and finally got it off of the box. Mark had moved himself into the kitchen, but kept a close watch on her actions. She slowly lifted off the lid and gasped when she looked inside. The box was filled with red roses; their fragrance drifted up to her. A card lay on top of them; she picked it up, but hesitated before opening it. *What if, what if they are from Sean? I have to know.*

Her hands trembled as she pulled the card from its envelope. There was only one word written on it; Mark; tears welled up in her eyes. Picking up the box, she went to the kitchen. She stood hushed in the doorway, unable to find the words. Mark sensed she was behind him and he turned to face her. Seeing the tears in her eyes, he went to her. "Roses aren't supposed to make you sad," he said softly.

She laid the box on the counter, and put her arms around him. "I'm not sad, and thank you. I know what you're trying to do, and I do appreciate it." She hugged him, then picking up the box, took it to the sink; inhaling the fragrance of each rose as she put them in a vase. His attempt to cheer her up was succeeding. The vase was transferred to the center of the dining room table.

How beautiful they are, and how sweet he is for getting them. She remembered the significance of the color of roses. *White, like the ones Sean gave me, meant friendship, but red, like these, meant love. I wonder?* Pulling one from the vase she carried it with her to her room; laying it on the bedside table while she had a nap.

The doorbell rang again that afternoon; she didn't hear it. Mark was pleased that she was resting. He accepted the package from the delivery boy; who stood at the door in awe; he recognized Mark. Knowing that look, Mark shut the door before he was asked for an autograph. He liked the recognition, and admiration of his fans, but not always. Today he had no time for it.

Taking the package into the living room, he opened it as he walked. Having ordered three videos, he was curious about which ones they had sent. He had asked the clerk to make the selections for him, as his career didn't leave him the time to indulge in movies. He had tried to go to a theater before; but because of the constant interruption by fans, had never been able to see a movie in its entirety. He studied the movie titles; they were familiar to him, but he couldn't remember what they were about.

Making his way out to the patio, he stretched out on one of the lounge's, folded his arms above his head and smiled. *One more delivery to go and the plan will be complete.* He checked his watch. *Two hours until my next surprise gets here.* He stayed on the patio for only thirty minutes, the California sun was warm and he never allowed himself to stay in the sun for too long. For one, he never tanned, his fair skin only burned; and secondly, a tan would not be in keeping with his character. The Warlock was a part of the world of the un-dead, and a pale complexion only served to enforce his mystical appearance.

On his way back into the house he picked up the videos and took them to his room; he didn't want Sabrina to see them just yet. Sabrina was in the living room when he came out of the bedroom. *Damn. How can I get her to stay in her room until I'm ready for her to come to dinner? I have to come up with something fast, but what?*

"Did you have a nice nap?" Mark asked. "Yes, I did." "Ready for tea?" "Always." Mark went into the kitchen; he paced nervously, waiting for the kettle to boil. *How can I get her out of the way for the next hour?* Sabrina had been observing his actions from the doorway. "Is there anything wrong?" she asked. "No!" he snapped quickly. "I'm sorry," he apologized when he realized what he had just done. "It's okay; you obviously have something on your mind; I had no reason to ask." "No. It's not acceptable for me to speak to you like that. Yes, I do have something on my mind, but I just don't know how to say it."

She moved closer to him, but didn't touch him. "If you have something to say to me, then just say it." "I was hoping that; if you don't mind; you would go back to your room until dinner is ready." "Why?" "I don't think I'm ready to tell you that. Would you please do this for me, and not ask any more questions about it." His hands found her shoulders, while his eyes trained on hers. She was quiet for a moment, wondering what was going through his mind now.

"Will you?" he asked again. "I don't know what you've got up your sleeve; but yes, I'll do as you ask." "Thank you." She took another step closer to him. "That answer isn't good enough." Her arms encircled his neck, pulling him downward, while she lifted herself up on her toes to kiss him. Mark returned her passionate advance, but quickly pulled away. Sabrina sighed deeply. "I know, not yet."

She rubbed her cheek against his face. He had let his beard grow in. Not a full thick beard, but a subtle line that followed his jaw to his chin where it thickened a little and joined his mustache. It was a good look for him, strengthening his firm, square jaw and adding to his mystical sex appeal. She liked the bristly feeling of it against her skin.

Taking her tea she went back to her room where she could explore her fantasies in private. After she was gone, he let out a sigh of his own; his body felt like it was going to explode. The passion that he felt, let him know that she still wanted to be with him, and that made him feel very good. *Despite all the times I've pushed her away, she still comes back to me, just as hungry as before. I'll not push her away ever again.*

Time was passing faster. He set the table and prepared the dining room, making sure he was creating a romantic setting. Confident that everything was properly in place, he poured himself a cup of tea and went into the living room to await the last delivery.

Banished to her room, Sabrina sat on the bed. *This man is so mysterious, but so exciting. Guess I should dress for dinner.* Roaming through her closet, she picked up different outfits, then put them back. *I feel so much more comfortable in my bathrobe, but it might not be appropriate.* She continued to paw through her wardrobe, unable to make a decision. A thought came into her mind, she went to the set of drawers; opening the last one she retrieved a box. Inside was a brand new electric blue satin robe. *Perfect.*

Dropping her terry cloth one on the floor she slipped on the new one. The satin was cold against her skin; it made her nipples hard, and very pronounced under the fabric. Standing in front of the mirror she admired her selection. The satin had a way of clinging to her, accentuating her curves. The decision was made. *I'll wear this to dinner; it's comfortable, yet sexy. If this doesn't get his attention, then nothing will. I want so much to be with him; I'm tired of this game. If he won't make the first move, then I will have to.* Returning to her bed, she turned on the TV and awaited his call.

Mark's patience was wearing out; the delivery was late. He began his pacing again, contemplating another phone call. The pacing was halted by the ringing of the doorbell. Pulling the door open, he snapped at the delivery man for being late. The man, intimidated by Mark, began to apologize repeatedly. Mark took the parcels and received instructions on how to keep everything warm until it was to be served. Dismissing him abruptly, Mark shut the door and returned to the kitchen to carry out his instructions. He emptied salad into bowls and carried them out to the table, setting them atop the plates.

A simple breakfast or lunch he could handle, but a special dinner required outside help. He finished with the final touches for the room and then turned out the lights. *Perfect.* Standing back he admired his creation. *Now to get Sabrina.*

She had heard the doorbell, and had wanted to sneak a look from her door, but changed her mind. *He wants me to wait, then wait I will.* She concentrated on the game show that was on the TV, trying hard to ignore her urges of curiosity. Mark knocked on her door, but did not open it. "Dinner is ready," he called. "Coming." Sabrina took another look in the mirror, straightened her robe, and tightened the belt. *Now to see Mark's reaction.*

Opening the door, she could see that his back was to her, he turned when he heard the sound of the latch. His eyes widened as he felt his chin drop. "My God, you're beautiful." Sabrina felt a blush consume her body. *I've definitely got his attention.* With a crook in his elbow and her arm secured through it, he escorted her to the dining room. He stopped her at the doorway. She was amazed at the transformation of the room. It was illuminated by many candles, placed strategically around the room, and on the table. *How romantic.*

In her heart, she knew that he was doing more than just trying to cheer her up. *Maybe my wait is over?* She shuddered with anticipation. Urging her on, he seated her at the table, and took the chair opposite her for himself.

In candle light, she's even more beautiful. The glow of the flame brings out the golden highlights in her hair. The flickering shadows caressed her face. He couldn't tear himself away; especially from her eyes; they sparkled with such vibrance and life. He was completely captivated by her. *If she asks me to make love to her at this moment, I would without any hesitation. So many fantasies but I have to wait. Patience, just have patience.*

Her gentle touch against his arm brought him back. "This is so wonderful. Did you do all of this by yourself?" she asked. He nodded, putting his dream aside, as he lifted a bottle from a container beside his chair. "Champagne?" "Yes, please." He poured her a glass, and one for himself. Lifting his glass up, he made a toast. "To new beginnings," he said touching his glass against hers.

She blushed again, but this time he couldn't see it. They began their meal with the salad, not talking, but each of them thinking of the other; fantasizing. Mark excused himself, taking the empty dishes to the kitchen; he returned in a couple of minutes carrying two plates, covered by silver domes. She couldn't wait; she had to see what was hiding beneath.

Lifting off the dome revealed prime rib with roast potatoes. "I hope you like it," he said. "Oh I will. This is my all time favorite; and it's been a long time since I had it." He refilled her champagne, and discretely watched her from the corner of his eye. She savored every bite until her plate was empty. "That was so good." "Can I interest you in some dessert?" Mark asked. "Not right now; I honestly don't know where I'd put it." He filled her champagne glass again, before he left with the dishes. She liked champagne. Taking another sip, she held it in her mouth, the bubbles bursting against her tongue. Picking up her glass, she walked out to the patio.

Mark returned to the dining room and was surprised to find her gone. "Sabrina?" "I'm out here." He followed the sound of her voice. She stood against the railing, the wind flapping at the bottom of her robe. "This is almost a perfect evening," she sighed. "What do you mean by that?" "There is no sunset tonight," she said pointing to the heavy clouds along the horizon. "A spectacular sunset would have been a perfect addition to this wonderful evening."

The storm that was coming, sent blasts of cool wind ahead of it, as a warning; she shivered. "You shouldn't be out here; it's getting cold." "I'd like to stay for just a few more minutes." Taking a step sideways, she moved closer to him, but did not touch him, hoping that he would do something.

The signals were very clear to him but he had to begin the next phase of his plan. Taking her by the shoulders, he began steering her back into the house. "How about a movie, since the sun isn't cooperating with you?" "That would be nice, but there's nothing good on TV tonight." "That's okay I have some videos." "You didn't miss a thing, did you?" "I don't think so. Get yourself settled in your room and I'll get the movies." He watched her as she walked back to her room; his eyes admiring her beautiful form moving against the satin robe.

They had to watch the movies in her room, since that was were the VCR was located. He retreated to the kitchen, poured two cups of tea; taking them up to her before going to get the movies from his room. He paused for a brief moment outside her door; closing his eyes he offered up a silent prayer. *Please, let her love me. Let her be the one that I've waited so long for.*

Sabrina was already seated on the bed. She had pillows stacked up behind her for support. He immediately noticed that the lower portion of her robe had parted, exposing her leg and part of her thigh. He avoided staring at her, by fumbling with the videos then handed them to her. "You choose," he said.

She reviewed the titles and then handed her selection to Mark. He took it, turned on the TV and the VCR and pushed in the tape, before settling himself into the chair beside her bed. *How awkward he looks. That chair is not meant for someone so tall.* "Are you planning to sit there for the whole movie?" Sabrina asked. "For as long as I can anyway." "Come," she said patting the empty space beside her. "Sit here, with me." "Are you sure?" "Yes, I'm sure. You'll be a lot more comfortable. There are some spare pillows in the closet that you can use to put behind you." Mark found them and tossed them onto the bed; Sabrina fluffed up each one and set them in a stack beside her.

Sitting on the edge of the bed Mark slipped off his boots. *If nothing else, at least I'll be close to her for a while.* He pushed himself back and leaned against the pillows. "Now that looks a whole lot better," Sabrina said with a smile. She pushed the play button on the remote, then reached over and turned out the lamp beside the bed. The room went dark, except for the flickering glow from the television. "What are you doing?" Mark asked. "I'm just trying to make the room look more like a theater, or are you afraid to be alone with me, in the dark?" Her voice was low and seductive; he shook his head and folded his arms across his chest.

It's as if she knows what is on my mind. "Watch the movie," he ordered her, knowing that she had been watching him instead. She settled herself against the pillows, concentrating on the story that was unfolding on the screen.

They watched the movie intently, speaking only rarely. Sabrina jumped, concealing her face against his arm when a scary scene developed. She held tightly to him, peeking out carefully, to see if it was safe to watch again. Mark freed his arm from her grasp and put it around her shoulders, for security. She wiggled herself closer to him.

When the next fright scene appeared on the screen she hid her face against his chest. He liked having her against him, so soft and warm. The movie continued, but Sabrina kept her head resting against him, just in case she needed to hide again; but mostly because she wanted him to hold her.

Mark glanced down at her; in the commotion of her being scared, and moving over to him, her robe had loosened, falling partly open at the chest. *I have to try.* He slowly moved his hand down her arm, and back up again; using his fingers to gently tease her robe open even more.

Sabrina shifted and he returned his hand to her shoulder. She was aware of what he was doing, and she knew by moving again it would give him a better look at her. As she moved, her robe gapped open even more, exposing the top of her breast. It beckoned to him, this time he slowly moved his hand off her shoulder, across her throat and down to her breast.

He began to stroke it softly with his finger. Sabrina rose up; her breast filled his hand. *How firm and round it is, and so soft.* Holding his hand over it, he felt her nipple become hard beneath his palm. She abruptly sat up, pulling herself away from Mark, and his touch. "What's wrong?" he asked confused by her action. *She has been boldly asking me to make love to her; but now, she is the one pulling away.*

"Please don't. Don't tease me like this Mark." Mark touched her shoulder. "Look at me." She remained quiet. "Please Sabrina; look at me." She turned herself; her head lowered. He coaxed it upward, so he could see her eyes. What he saw in her blue eyes was such a deep sadness. "I'm not teasing; not anymore. I want to be with you; to make love to you; but only if you want to," he said as his hand brushed softly against her cheek.

"I don't want to pressure you into anything Sabrina and considering what you have been through both physically and emotionally it wouldn't upset me if you wanted to wait. I'm not looking for excuses I'm just concerned about you. I don't want to see you push yourself into something that you're not ready for, that your body isn't ready for."

She wanted to answer him but she couldn't; her voice had been momentarily stolen from her. "Oh Mark," she struggled to regain command of her voice. "From the first moment that you walked into this house I knew that I wanted you. That feeling hasn't changed. I understand and appreciate your concerns but I'm fine," her voice softened to a breathy whisper. "I still want you Mark. My body yearns to feel your love." Mark moved himself closer to her, kissing her lips softly. She responded hungrily, wanting more, so much more.

Laying her down upon the bed, his kiss deepened. His hand found her breast, gently caressing its softness. He moved his kisses slowly down her neck, making her moan softly; then continued across to her breast. Careful with his actions, and not wanting to appear to be too inexperienced, he gently teased at her nipple with his tongue. She shivered at his touch. Never had she been so aroused as she was at that moment; her body was on fire with flames of passion.

She began to work loose the buttons on his shirt, gliding her fingers over his body, stroking his chest, reveling in the power of his massive frame; but then she stopped suddenly. Something, an image, flashed in her mind. She pushed Mark away and sat up. He lay back on the bed, unsure if he should speak or not, her reaction confused him.

He bit his lip. "Did I do something wrong?" he asked. She looked at him with such a puzzled stare, but did not speak. Pushing herself up onto her knees, she straddled his hips, pulled open his shirt wide, and shut her eyes. From the look on her face, he could see that she was in deep concentration. *What is she thinking about?*

Her hands moved slowly across his chest, taking in every feature, tracing over every muscle. The light touch made his muscles flex uncontrollably; Mark could keep silent no longer. "Sabrina, what is it?" She bit her lip hard, as a single tear rolled down her cheek; she opened her eyes and looked at him. The way she looked at him was different; he couldn't figure it out; he repeated his question to her. A smile came to her lips. "Nothing's wrong Mark; in fact, it's right; so very, very right."

I know now, that he's the man that has invaded my dreams so many times. When I touched his bare chest it all came clear to me; no more fragmented visions; they all culminated with one single touch. Leaning down upon him, she kissed him. This epiphany ignited a new passion, an insatiable hunger.

Sitting back up, she reached for the tie on her robe to undo it. Mark stopped her. He wanted to savor this experience and prolong the inevitable for as long as possible. His movements were slow, and exciting; he untied the bow, letting it fall loose. Sliding his hands slowly over her shoulders, down her arms, pushing the robe away from her, exposing her entire beauty to him. Methodically, Sabrina worked at the button of his jeans, but could not release it. Her frustration was getting the better of her; wanting, craving their bodies to be together as one.

Sensing her anxiety, Mark took her down onto the bed beside him, loosening his jeans he slipped them off onto the floor. It was a relief for him, to have them off; he was in full arousal and the jeans made him very uncomfortable. Returning his attentions to Sabrina, he began again his pleasurable task of kissing her, and exploring her body.

He ran his hand down over her stomach and along the outside of her thigh. Reversing the action when he had reached her knee; now moving upward, along the inside of her thigh. She moved her leg, inviting him to touch her; she shuddered and moaned when he did, enthralled in ecstasy as he prepared her body for him.

She stroked his chest, moving lower and lower, until she found that special part of him. She gasped softly. *He's so big; I want him more than ever.* Mark had felt her touch and had heard her sudden, breathy gasp. He backed away from her slightly. "Do I scare you?" he asked. "If you want me to stop I will." "No, Mark," she whispered, still stroking him gently. "Don't stop. I want you."

Urging him onto her, she hungrily anticipated the moment when he would be joined with her. Still hesitant, he resisted, prolonging the pleasure of touching her body. When he could wait no longer, he supported his weight with his arms, not wanting the force of his body resting on her. With her legs entwined with his, her hands on his hips, she guided him to their destiny.

Mark watched her face for any sign of pain. *Whether I want to or not, if I hurt her, I'll withdraw immediately.* Seeing only the longing in her eyes, he kissed her again. Their kisses became deeper, more sensual, as their bodies moved slowly together as one. With each movement she took him deeper, and deeper inside. Slow, steady movements; each of them exploring the intense pleasure, and the passion that they were feeling.

The excitement was building; their bodies began to move faster. An intense orgasm ripped through each of them at the same time. Sabrina's back arched, her hands holding tight to Mark's back. She shuddered uncontrollably beneath him. Mark trembled with the ecstasy that he had never before experienced with such gratifying pleasure. *It is her. I'm sure of it. All those visions had been real. The pleasure she brings to me is real.* The waves of electric energy returned with an intensity far greater than when they first touched. This mysterious sensation charged their bodies with a fervourous power.

Her body held him tight, refusing to let him go, but when his arms could no longer take the strain, he carefully pulled himself away from her, falling onto his back. Sabrina snuggled against him, using her leg around his to keep her in place. They were both saturated with sweat; she felt a sudden chill and pulled the blankets up over them. Exhausted, more than she had ever been, and with Mark's warm body holding her tight, she soon was sound asleep in his arms.

He kissed her softly. *I know that I've fallen in love with her. I want to wake her and tell her, but my conscience won't allow it yet.* He tightened his hold on her. Her arm was across his chest; he felt her grip. In his mind, he made her a solemn vow.

I promise you, I will always protect you and keep you safe; and I will love you for all eternity. Tomorrow I will tell you; tell you that I love you;

but I also want an explanation for that strange behavior. What had made her act that way? Pushing it away from his mind, he thought it not worth worrying about tonight; he closed his eyes, content, and happier than he had ever been in his life. *I've found her, my heart led me to her and nothing will take her away from me.*

The souls rejoiced. The love expressed by the union of these physical bodies had reunited them. No longer were they adrift in a sea of humanity. Their love had stayed the course, returning them to again partake of their undying bond. Together they would grow stronger, teaching these bodies how to love and give them the ability to hear the unspoken needs of each other. The seeds of their destiny had been planted and like their love it would need to be nurtured carefully if it were to grow and survive the torments and trials of this life.

Sabrina was the first to wake; she still rested in Mark's arms. *To have slept so soundly, as to not move all night, held in the arms of a man that really loves me.* She listened to the methodical beat of his heart; her hand passed softly across his chest. *The vision that had permeated my dreams has finally come to be. I was meant to be with Mark. I'm sure of it. All those years of degrading torment were but mere memories now, I feel wanted, needed.* The loneliness, that had so often struck fear in her, had dissipated; pushed into the dark depths where it belonged.

Thoughts of last night still lingered in her mind. *How gentle he is.* Careful not to wake him just yet, she moved her hand down lower, over his stomach, not at all surprised when she encountered his already firm erection. Tracking its length with her finger, amazed at his size, cautiously she encircled her fingers around it, but they didn't meet. *How a man, so well endowed, could give me such pleasure, I don't understand. All I know is that I desire him again.* This insatiable hunger compelled her to continue her gentle strokes, feeling him grow even larger and harder.

Mark stirred when she teased at his nipple with her tongue; she kissed his cheek. "Good morning," she whispered. Mark stretched slightly. "Good morning." The sensation of her hand moving over him became very apparent. "What are you doing?" he asked. Supporting herself on her elbow, she looked into his green eyes with a smile. "What do you think?" She kissed him. Mark responded, pulling her onto him. His hands caressed her body, preparing her for him. Her sensuous kisses were soft against his neck; stimulating his skin and fueling his desire.

Pushing herself up onto her knees, she took him in, with delicate moans of pleasure. Taking his hand she urged him to sit up. Careful not to lose him, she maneuvered her legs around his waist, pulling herself closer to him, and forcing him deeper inside her.

The rapture that she brings to me is indescribable; she knows so much more about sex than I do, but I'm more than willing to learn. I crave to learn more, and with her as my teacher I can only imagine the pleasures the future holds for us.

Mark kissed her deeply. Her eyes became fixated on his, as they rocked slowly. *I want him to see the ecstasy, the desire on my face.* Her eyes closed briefly, as another intense orgasm gripped their bodies. They held each other tight, feeling each other shudder and tremble with the force of their wondrous pleasure.

Relaxed, and exhausted, she rested against him, nuzzling her face against his. "Sabrina I have to get up." He tried to move her but she refused; her body holding him securely in place. Lifting her head she looked at him, a smile on her lips, one eye brow slightly raised. "What?" he asked not understanding the look. She bit her lip. "You're already, up." She pushed her body down against his.

He smiled at her remark. "That's not exactly what I meant." Using his strength, he lifted her off and laid her down beside him. "We can't stay here all day you know." "Yes, we can. I know I'd like nothing better than to stay here and make love to you all day, and all night." "You won't be able to unless you eat something, to keep your strength up." "Oh I'm hungry, but not for food."

She reached out to him; he shook his head. *How can I refuse that beautiful pouting face?* Pressing his body against hers, he kissed her repeatedly. *I could easily make love to her again, but I won't. We both need a rest.* Mark rolled away from her and sat on the edge of the bed, pulling on his jeans. "Aren't you going to have a shower?" Sabrina asked. "Yes, I am." "Oh good!" She responded to him by running her hands up his back. Mark stood up. *If I stay any longer I won't not be able to leave.* "I'm going to have a shower, in my room; and you are gonna have one here."

She was slightly disappointed, that she had been unable to convince him. Wrapping her arms around herself, she hugged; she felt so good, so energized. Her shower would be quick but thorough. *Today I'll get dressed; after spending so much time in a bath robe, Mark deserves to see me at my best again.* She changed the sheets on the bed in record time; her motor in overdrive; wanting to finish her chores so she could be with him. *Nothing is going to bring me down today, or ever. Not if I can help it.*

Sean was finally on his way home. He fidgeted in his seat on the plane, his anxiety driving him. Several times he had gone to the phone on the plane and dialed her number, only to get the answering machine. *Why doesn't she answer the phone?* He never left a message. *I want to talk to her, not a damn machine. Only ninety minutes until the plane lands, and then another hour until I'm home.* He was tortured by his thoughts, about the baby, and about Mark being at her house. Anger burned in his chest when he thought about Mark being with her. Yet the one thing that angered him more, was the fact that she had left him

We may not have been together for very long, but it was supposed to be me that broke it off, not her. That's how it had always been. Eventually he would just get bored of having one woman around all the time, then he would move on to the next one.

It hurts me to know that she had walked out on me, before it was time. I wasn't done with her yet. What if Mark had seduced her? No, he had sworn himself to celibacy; everyone knew that. *Could something have happened to make him change?*

Sean made another attempt with the phone, only to slam the receiver down when he got the answering machine again. *Damn it; an hour to go.* The anxiety was building in his body with every minute that ticked by.

Mark and Sabrina enjoyed a leisurely brunch; it was difficult for her to keep from touching him, but she had to resist. Shooing her from the kitchen while he cleaned up, she went into the living room and put on a CD; the beat of the music took control of her body. With his chores complete, Mark returned to her, quietly watching the way her body swayed to the music, so sensual, so seductive. Watching her hips slowly roll from side to side turned him on; his heart began to beat faster.

Seeing him, Sabrina moved towards him, her body rubbing against his. "Dance with me." "I don't dance," he answered sternly, turning off the stereo. *I have to end this distraction before I completely lose control.*

"Hey, why did you do that?" "I want to talk to you about something very important."

He sat himself down on the couch. Sabrina, straddling his legs, sat on his lap. "No, fooling around; this is an important conversation." "One thing first," she said leaning in to kiss him. "Enough already," Mark said sternly. "I'm sorry; I just can't help myself. I like kissing you; among other things." She settled herself beside him with her legs crossed in front of her. "So what's on your mind?" she asked.

He held her hand, more as a support for himself; never having the opportunity to discuss sex with a woman before, it made him very uneasy. Taking in a full breath he began. "How do you feel today?" "Great, wonderful, happy, elated," she sighed softly. "Why do you ask?" "Do you have any pain or discomfort?" "No. I told you that my body was healed. The pain went away long ago, so I don't understand why you'd ask."

"I didn't mean that; I meant about last night, and this morning," he said with some hesitation. She realized what he was trying to ask her; she squeezed his hand. "You're worried that you may have hurt me; well, you can put that thought right out of your mind. You caused me no harm at all." "Are you sure? You're not just saying that to spare my feelings?"

"I admit that sex has never been a comfortable situation for me and for several days after I've always had to deal with the physical repercussions." "I did hurt you!" "No. Mark, if making love with you had hurt me, in any way, do you think I would have pursued you again this morning? For the first time in my life there is no pain."

He laid his head back against the couch, exhaling the breath that he had been holding. "That's why you abstained all these years; isn't it?" Sabrina asked. He nodded. She played with the strands of auburn hair that framed his face. "Until now, and I am so happy that you chose to break that vow with me." "I still have so much more to learn." "What more do you need to learn?" "I have to learn how to please you."

Sabrina sat herself across his lap, holding his face in her hands. "Oh Mark, you please me in ways that I can't even begin to describe." "How can you say that? You're so much more." "Experienced?" "Yeah." "Not really," she smiled, softly plying him with gratifying kisses as she spoke. "As long as you, follow your instincts, your heart, and your fantasies, you will never lack for creativity, or lust for love."

Giving in to her amorous advances, he pulled her closer, kissing her deeply. When she began to make a soft purring sound, he intensified the pressure. Needing to catch his breath, he released her, but held her tight. "See," she panted. "You know exactly what to do." The potency of his kiss left her debilitated; she laid her head against his shoulder.

When Mark picked up her hand, she opened her eyes; watching him play with the silver band on her finger. "What are you thinking about?" she asked. When he didn't answer, she looked up at him. There was a mystifying look on his face, one that she could not interpret; it distressed her. "What's wrong?" "There's something else I need to talk to you about, but before I do I would like you to clarify something for me."

Looking into his eyes, she could see the seriousness. "I would like you to tell me what made you cry last night; and I would like the truth." His insides were in turmoil. *I want to believe that she has been completely honest with me, or did I hurt her somehow, and she's just too afraid to tell me.*

Sabrina sat back, running her hand through her hair. *I never thought I'd have to tell my secret, but he has a right to know.* "Well?" Mark coaxed. "Okay, but in order for you to completely understand what I'm about to say, I'm gonna have to go back a few years." She tossed it around in her mind, just how to begin. Mark squeezed her hand, lending her some of his strength.

"I've never told anyone about this ever," she began. "So please bear with me." She paused for just a moment. "A long time ago, somewhere in my late teens I'm not exactly sure, I began having this dream, this vision; but never complete, only fragments. What I do remember about it though, is how vivid, and intense it was. Even long after I was awake, the sensations I had of touch, and of experiencing what was taking place, was so very strong, but not being able to see, or remember it, in its entirety was equally frustrating."

"What was your dream about?" Mark asked. "A man; but I could never see or remember seeing his face, but I could feel his body. That was the one thing that stayed with me, even after I would awake, and last night, when I touched you, really touched you, for the first time, I remembered. I knew that feeling, that sensation. Oh this sounds so crazy." "Tell me all of it," Mark urged.

She hesitated a moment to breathe before continuing. "When I touched you last night, all those sensations came back, so strong; and I made the connection. It was you; you are the man that has occupied my dreams for all these years. I knew it last night and as sure as I'm sitting here now, I know it to be true. Now, I've not been a nun all my life; I've had other lovers; but never, never did those feelings connect with any of them. At that exact moment last night, I knew that I was meant to be with you, that it was right. For the first time in my life, making love felt so very right."

A tear ran down her cheek. Mark brushed it away. "Now I can tell you," he sighed. "Tell me what?" "I also felt that we were meant to be together. I can't explain it. Like your dream, I too, have had strange feelings for many years now. When I saw you I wasn't sure, but when I touched your hand that first time I knew. I knew it in my heart; and I think, no, I know, that I've fallen in love with you." He waited for her response, hoping that it was what he wanted, but also fearing the worst.

Sabrina felt paralyzed. *I can't believe what I'm hearing; but it's exactly what my heart wants to hear. He doesn't think me to be crazy, he loves me, and I already know that I love him.* She leaned into him, kissing him passionately. "Make love to me," she whispered. He held her for a few minutes longer, before picking her up in his arms, and carrying her off to the bedroom. The years of searching were over; perseverance had brought them together, and opened the door to their hearts.

The afternoon passed slowly; time had no meaning for them today. All that was important was exploring their feelings, and giving each other pleasure, which they did with great tenderness. The world had stopped turning, leaving them lost together to explore their new found love. Sabrina had cuddled up beside Mark, her arm across his chest, holding on as if to never let him go.

Mark ran his hand over her arm. "How do you feel?" he asked still concerned for her physical well being. "Wonderful," she answered in a dreamy voice. "How about you, how do you feel?" "Tired, but otherwise I feel great. Actually, I've never felt better; somehow stronger, more alive than ever before. I never knew that great sex held so much power."

Sabrina pushed herself up and looked into his eyes. "Mark, this isn't sex. Sex is brief and meaningless; something you do to merely fulfill a physical need. This isn't sex at all; it's more, much more, this is." "Love?" he asked, completing her sentence. She hesitated with her answer. "I think so," she whispered. He pulled her close. "I don't think so; I know so. I do love you Sabrina." She kissed him tenderly. "And I know that I love you, Mark." She snuggled back down beside him, wrapped in the safety of his arms.

When Sean's plane finally landed at the airport, he was on his feet quickly, pushing his way through the others in first class, needing to be the first to disembark. Waiting for his luggage was worse; pacing back and forth, watching each bag that came along the conveyer belt. Ironically, he had been the first person off of the plane, but nearly the last to collect his luggage. Already pissed off with that ordeal, he went outside only to find that Charles wasn't waiting for him.

"Where the hell is he? He knew what time the plane was to arrive," he muttered to himself continually as he paced along the sidewalk. A few photographers tried to get some pictures of him, but he was quick to push them aside. When he was in the mood, he could be very accommodating to the press, and to his fans, but today, he wanted no part of them. *All I want is to go home.*

Charles tried to apologize for his tardiness, by offering up an explanation; but Sean didn't want to hear any excuses. He barked his commands to Charles, ordering him to drive faster. Charles complied, only to bring the limo back to the designated speed limit within a few minutes. A speeding ticket would only anger his employer more.

Traffic was light and they made good time getting home. Sean was out of the car before the engine was turned off, and was out of sight when Charles got out. He knew that Sean was headed for Sabrina's. He shook his head in pity when he thought about what Sean was going to encounter at her house.

Charles had seen Mark there, with Sabrina, and he had deduced that she had taken a new lover. It bothered him, that he didn't have the guts to stand up to Sean and tell him what he knew, but then again it wasn't really any of his business. Taking the luggage inside; he left it in the hall, and went to the open patio door, watching Sean stomp his way up the beach, every once in a while kicking a piece of driftwood out of his path. Charles returned to his duties when he saw Sean disappear around the far side of the patio.

Sean muttered and grumbled to himself all the way to Sabrina's; as he rounded the patio and walked up the path to the front door he tried to calm himself down. *There's no point in being angry with her right away; I just want some answers.* Stopping near the front door, he hesitated at knocking. He began pacing, sorting through the thoughts in his mind. *Calm, I need to be calm.*

Once he was sure of what he wanted to say, he knocked on the door and waited; no answer. *She has to be here.* He knocked again; still no response. He went back down the path, and up the stairs to the deck. Looking through the patio doors he saw no one. A light was on in the kitchen. *She must be home.*

He tried the door, it was unlocked; he slid it open quietly and went inside. He didn't call out to her, but instead walked to the kitchen; she wasn't there. Patches had strolled out of the bedroom and sat watching him. Sean spotted the cat and decided that she must be in her room; probably resting. *That has to be why she never heard me knocking.*

He walked towards her room; the door was not quite shut. Sean slowly pushed it open a little more; his eyes fell upon the bed, where Mark lay, Sabrina in his arms, the cotton sheet barely covering their nude bodies. His stomach tightened into a knot; the sight of their bodies so close together hurt him. His anger wanted him to yell out, but his gut told him to leave. He left the house as quietly as he had entered. Walking slowly along the beach until he came to a large log; sitting down, he released the tears he had been fighting back.

How could she? How could she turn to him? Of all people, why did she go to Mark? I thought we could have had something special; we created a child together. Why would she seek comfort from him? It was my baby, not his. I should be with her, comforting her. We shouldn't be apart, not yet. I could be faithful to her; at least I could try. Damn it, I have to get her back; I want her back. Nobody has ever taken anything away from me.

His thoughts were confused. *I do want her back; but only so Mark can't have her. I've beaten him in the ring before, and I will beat him at this. I'm not going to let Mark win, this time, or any time.* His mind was set and determined. *I will get Sabrina back, and if that means fighting Mark, then so be it.*

His mind created the thoughts, but Sean couldn't see that he was thinking of Sabrina as an object; like some toy one of the other boys had taken, without his permission. His own selfishness had been clouded by his anger.

Going back to his house, he phoned the wrestling organization to find out when Mark was scheduled to return. With all of the information written down, Sean compared it to his own schedule. Mark's tour dates and his coincided. *Perfect, just about two weeks until our first show together.* "Charles, pack my things; we're going back to Texas for a while. Try and get us on a flight out tomorrow morning." "Very good sir." Charles didn't pursue an explanation; he knew better than to question Sean's motives; he began preparing the house for their departure. Sean had disappeared into the basement, but Charles could hear the distinct thuds of fists hitting the punching bag.

Mark awoke with a start; Sabrina was still asleep beside him. *Something awakened me; but what? My senses tell me that something isn't right, but I can't figure it out.* He slipped away from her and pulled on his jeans; she didn't wake. Walking slowly through the house, he surveyed each room very carefully. *Nothing is out of place and the front door is still locked. So why does my gut tell me otherwise?*

Walking through the living room, he saw the curtain caught in the patio door. *Someone has been in the house; I'm positive, I was the last one to shut the door, and that is most certainly not the way I left it.* He opened the door and stepped out onto the patio, scanning in all directions for any sign of an intruder. No one was visible; he went to the railing, grabbing a hold of it tightly.

He was angry with himself, for not hearing someone moving about the house. *Sabrina's safety is at stake, and I let her down.* He lowered his head in shame, but then noticed the footsteps in the sand. Following the imprints around the patio to the stairs and then back to the beach; the trail led to Sean's house. *Damn it!* He smacked his hand on the railing. *That son of a bitch was here; in the house.* "Welcome home Sean; I hope you liked what you saw."

Mark began thinking about what might be going through Sean's mind, seeing them together; a small part of him did feel remorse. *This isn't the way I had planned for Sean to find out about us; but I'm relieved that it's done. Now I can deal with it. I wonder what his next move will be? I know *that Sean can be prone to sudden fits of anger, and I hope, that if it comes to that, that Sabrina won't get caught in the middle.*

The sudden loss of warmth had awakened Sabrina; she called to Mark but received no answer. Dressing quickly she went to find him. She spotted him out on the patio. She could tell his mind was somewhere else. Moving quietly across to him, she stood beside him without speaking. The wind whipped her hair against his arm; he drew her to him. Wrapping his arms around her, he held her against him. She laid her head back and stared out at the ocean.

I feel so safe, with his massive arms protecting me. Her hands trailed over his biceps, particularly over the tattoo of the snake that dominated his arm. The light touch on his skin made him flex his muscles and tighten his hold. Her hands slid over his forearms, pressing them against her. Contentment, that was the feeling they both had. Still quiet, Mark unconsciously began rocking her back and forth, his chin lightly resting atop her head. *I never expected to ever feel like this, with any woman; but Sabrina has melted away my reluctance, and has opened my heart to the power of love. I will be forever grateful to her for coming into my life.*

Sabrina watched the birds running along the shore, darting in and out with the movement of the tide. They fluttered their way down the beach. Her eyes followed them until her gaze fell upon Sean's house. A paralyzing fear consumed her; Sean was standing on the deck. Even at this distance she knew his eyes were fixated on her, and Mark. Breaking loose of Mark's hold, she ran into the house.

Mark knew what had upset her; he had been watching Sean, long before Sabrina noticed him. Straightening his stance, with his arms firmly crossed over his chest; Mark signified to Sean that he wasn't about to back down. *Sabrina is my woman now, and no one, not even Sean had better try to take her away from me.*

When Sean finally disappeared from view, Mark went to find Sabrina. She stood behind the couch; her arms braced against the back, her body trembling. He went to her, embracing her. "It's okay; don't let him get to you. You know that I won't let him anywhere near you." "I don't want to see him, or deal with him at all." "You won't have to; I'll make sure of that."

He reassured her, by gently rubbing her back. Sabrina looked up at him. "I only want one thing," she said. "What would that be?" "To be with you; for as long as you want me." "For as long as I want, eh. How does forever sound?" "Wonderful," she answered, laying her head against him. "So what do you want to do for the rest of the day? Since the afternoon is shot to hell, that only leaves us with the remainder of the evening," she said hoping his answer would be the one that she wanted to hear.

    A smile beamed across Mark's face. "What I want to do is hold you, kiss you, and make love to you." His voice was as compassionate, as was his touch. He guided her around to the front of the couch. Easing himself down, bringing her with him, he held her close, becoming consumed by his feelings. Their expressions of love sustained them until late in the night, foregoing even dinner for the gratification that their love offered them.

Chapter 8

The days slipped by with little regard for time or date. Days and nights rolled together unnoticed. All that mattered for Mark and Sabrina was that they were together; their love growing stronger. Talking was redundant. They had become so in-tune with each other. By merely reading expressions, or body actions, they knew exactly what they each wanted, needed, or felt.

An ethereal connection had formed between them. A bond so compelling and profound, as if they had been together forever, not just a few weeks. This eerie connection bewildered Sabrina, but how to approach the idea with Mark was even more confusing. She even entertained the notion that their souls had been together in some other time, to be again reunited, in this life. Reincarnation was not a frivolous thought, for she always believed that she had walked this earth before.

What an extraordinary revelation it would be to find out that Mark had been my mate in some other time. I wonder if he believes in it, or if he would consider regression hypnosis? If I don't ask, I'll never know. I'll talk to him when the time is right.

Another week was nearing its closure; Mark was becoming sullen, somewhat distant. Several times Sabrina had caught him looking at the calendar, counting days. Never questioning him, but she suspected that this ritual was a reminder to himself that he would have to return to work very soon. It was early on Friday morning when she awoke alone again. Mark was not in the bedroom or the bathroom; fear instantly knotted her stomach. *He has to be here. He wouldn't leave without telling me.*

With a sigh of relief, she located him in the kitchen, again standing in front of the calendar counting days. Walking up behind him, she slipped her arms around him as she kissed his back. "Good morning," she said. The silence was ominous. Moving around in front of him, she hopped up on the counter. His face was partially obscured by his long hair, but not enough to hide the serious expression beneath.

"Okay, it's time you told me what is so important that you have to keep counting days," she said. Mark still didn't speak. Taking his hands, she tugged him closer to her. Close enough that she could wrap her legs around his waist, locking her ankles together, binding him in place. "What is the matter?" she asked again, moving the hair away from his face. "I'm not letting go until you tell me what's going on."

Mark lowered his head and sighed, before looking back up into her eyes. "After you came home from the hospital, I called the Doctor and he told me that we shouldn't wait more than a couple of weeks before starting to use birth control." Sabrina remained quiet as he continued. "The time is up; and we have to decide on what method we want to use." Sensing his awkwardness, she smiled and kissed his lips gently. "That's really easy to answer," she paused a few seconds before continuing. "None."

"What do you mean none?" "None. I don't want to use any condoms, or pills, no diaphragm, no IUD, nothing." "Sabrina you don't understand, we have to use something, or you could get pregnant. The Doctor said that if you got pregnant to soon you could run the risk of having another miscarriage." "Mark, I do understand what you're saying," she said looking deep into his green eyes. "I love you so very much and I don't want to use any kind of birth control." "If you get pregnant it could be detrimental to the baby, and to you."

"I know you're concerned and I appreciate that. The thought of having your baby growing inside me would be the ultimate expression of the love we share, but if you're not ready, then I'll respect your wishes too. This is a decision that we both have to agree on." "Please understand me, I am thrilled that you would want to have a baby, my baby, but I will not jeopardize your health, you mean far to much to me. As much as I want to say yes, I'm not willing to gamble with the chance of losing you."

He held her tight, his emotions beyond words. "I love you, Sabrina. So what are our options since traditional birth control is out of the question?" "There are ways; but let me take care of that." She held on to him, hiding the conflict that was gnawing away at her.

Oh Mark, I hate having to lie to you. I am taking a chance with my health I know, but my body doesn't run on a regular clock and birth control pills won't correct it, they only make me sick. As for all the other methods, well, I just don't like them. I guess our future is in the hands of fate and whatever happens or doesn't happen is not for me to worry about anymore.

Sitting back, she held his face in her hands. "Can you tell me now, what else is bothering you?" "Nothing." "Mark, please tell me." "How is it you always seem to know when something is on my mind?" "We'll discuss that another time; now tell me." "I have to go back to work soon." "I figured as much. When?" "Sunday; and you're coming with me." His response was adamant, and he wasn't going to give her an opportunity to decline. Answers were beyond her. She had no intention of staying behind. He was a part of her, and being away from him would be torture. She held him close.

Working her robe loose, she felt his chest against her breasts; it excited her. "I love you," she whispered into his ear. His kisses were fervent, yet tender against her neck; his mustache tickled against her skin stimulating her desire. With her legs still wrapped around his waist, she worked open his jeans, pushing them down over his hips. Mark's height made it easy for him to make love to her where she sat on the counter.

As they relaxed into a lover's embrace, Sabrina spoke to him in a way that made his heart fill with joy. "If I do get pregnant, this time the child will have been created out of pure love." Her love filled his soul to overflowing, and excited his body even more.

After a quiet, leisurely morning, Mark persuaded Sabrina to go for a walk along the beach. It took some intense powers of persuasion on his part; finally he had to show her that Sean's house had been shuttered, indicating that he would be gone from here for quite a while. They wandered slowly along the beach, always in physical contact with each other. The wind blew warm off of the water, and brought with it that salty smell that she liked so much. She stopped and untied the ribbon that held her hair in a ponytail. The wind quickly whipped her hair about her neck.

Turning to Mark, she reached around his neck to undo the long braid that laid against his back. "Please don't," he said grasping her arm. "I like your hair loose." "I know you do, but the wind will only tangle it up in knots." "I'll brush it for you when we get back," she said, giving him that pouty look that always made him surrender.

He looked at that face, that beautiful face. "Oh hell, how am I supposed to say no to you when you look at me like that?" Sabrina smiled, and continue undoing the braid. The wind had ceased momentarily. She ran her hands through the long auburn waves. It gently framed his face, giving him a mysterious, dark look. "Now, that's much better. You look so sexy this way." With a remark like that he had no choice but to kiss her.

Resuming their walk they stopped now and then to check out sea shells that had become embedded in the sand. A large collection of driftwood logs lay off to their right, and by mutual agreement they headed towards them for a rest. Mark straddled one of the logs so he could hold Sabrina against him. She leaned back, his loving arms encircling her. The wind had eased to a light whisper, but still maintained its hypnotic effect. Sabrina began playing in the sand with a stick she had found. She drew out a heart, and in the center of it scribed their initials. His arms tightened around her waist, as he rubbed his face against her hair.

She turned her head around to look at him and at the same exact second without even making eye contact they both said "I love you." She giggled at how they both had the same thought at the same time; again; this strange phenomenon of saying the exact same thing at the same time, had been occurring more frequently over the past few days; and it fueled Sabrina's belief that they were truly soul mates.

"All right, now you have to tell me just how you do that," Mark said. "Do what?" "You know; say what I say; what I'm thinking." "I don't know, really." "You must have some idea?" There was a long pause between them until "I have a theory" they said in unison. Sabrina laughed a bit harder this time. "Damn it!" Mark replied, not angry, but confused.

"So what's your theory?" Sabrina asked, still grinning. "I'd like to hear yours first; mine is gonna sound pretty strange." "Well then you'll probably think that mine is completely off the wall." "Go ahead; I'm listening." Unsure if she wanted to even look at him during this conversation, she hesitated before finally turning herself around. Mark's eyes quietly begged her to begin.

"Let me say this first; no matter how strange this sounds, I have, in no way, taken leave of my senses." She wiped her palms across her legs, removing the evidence of her nervousness. "Well, I guess the direct approach is the easiest," she said before pausing to take a long breath. "I know you Mark. Not in the sense of what we have shared over the last few weeks; but, I feel like we were together in some other time, some other life."

Mark's head dropped; he shuddered from the chill that shot up his spine. "I told you it would sound crazy." "No, that's not it at all." "Then what is it?" Sabrina asked. "It's; it's just that I've had a similar feeling. Something inside of me keeps telling me that I've known you before. I've tried to remember if maybe we had met previously; but I couldn't put my finger on it. I just knew that there was something familiar about you.

Something that drew me to you, told me that I had to be with you; it goes much deeper than my dreams," he said glancing at her cautiously.

Sabrina squeezed his hand. "This is so weird; incredible, but weird." "Does this mean that we're both nuts?" Mark asked. "No, my love, not at all." Moving herself closer to him, she rested her legs atop of his. Mark put his arms around her for support. "You know what would be really neat to do?" "What?" "Regression hypnosis, to find out when and where we were together before." She felt him tense. "Or not." "Not. I don't want to know." "Why not?" "I don't want to know how or when we became parted. I'm happy that we're together here and now; and that's all that matters." "Okay, it was just a suggestion," she said slowly rubbing his arm.

I have upset him. Bringing him close, she comforted him. The feeling of his new beard against her throat made her burn with delight. Pushing away from him she stood up. "Race ya home." *I know it'll take him a few minutes before he's even able to get up, and that will give me the head start I need.*

Mark braced himself against the log. *I have to vanquish these stimulating feelings that are enflaming my body. It isn't easy, when all I can think about is her. It consumes me, every hour of every day. She must think that I'm making up for all those lost years, but that is so far from the truth. She turns me on. That all consuming desire to be with her takes control of me every time; and knowing that I'm giving her pleasure, and not pain, fuels that desire into a raging inferno.*

After a series of deep breaths, he was able go after her. Running wasn't an easy task for someone of his size, so he walked back to the house. As he started up the stairs to the patio, he picked up her shirt. A smile came to his face. *I know what she's up to.* Inside the patio door lay her shorts and across the living room her bra hung on a lamp. The anticipation was arousing. Entering the bedroom, he scanned it quickly, but didn't see her anywhere. Taking another step in, the door shut behind him.

Surprised by the noise, he turned quickly to see Sabrina standing behind him; she was completely nude; her beauty was breath taking, he moved to her. Impeding his advances she took his hand, guiding him to the bed. He tried to take her in his arms, but she resisted. Working diligently, she loosened the buttons on his denim shirt. Mark undone his jeans, and they fell away. "Lie down," she whispered. He complied with her request eagerly. She poised herself beside him, he touched her breast; she pulled away. "Not yet, I want to please you first this time," she whispered.

The seduction began with kisses to his neck; he touched her again; she pushed his hand away. With considerable difficulty, he laid his hands down beside him and permitted her to continue. Her lips teased at his nipples. Mark lay immobile; his eyes closed, his body surging with stimulating sensations every time her tongue touched his body. Down his chest, over his abdomen, her tongue trailed. His muscles tightened with anticipation, as she continued down lower, below his waist. Deliberately bypassing that part of him she dearly craved she kissed his inner thigh, before moving back to the base of his hard shaft. Drawing her tongue slowly up its length she delicately swirled it around its head.

His body shuddered with this new sensation. Her actions were painstakingly slow, and loving, careful not to hurt him as she drew her lips over his massive size. Reaching for his hand, she guided him to the warmth between her legs. When he touched her inside, her actions quickened. Instinct told her that he wouldn't be able to last much longer. She straddled him and their bodies came together. Their movements were in perfect harmony, gradually increasing speed to a frenzied velocity. As her orgasm built, she sat straight, driving him deeper in. Mark raised up his knees for her to brace herself against as her body began to shudder with the intense ecstasy.

Exhausted, but so very satisfied, she lay down beside him, pulling up the blanket. The dewy perspiration on her body made her tremble against him. He held her close, to warm her. "You are so incredible; I've never experienced anything like that before," he said. "What do you mean?" "What you just did to me, I've never." "Never?" "Never."

She hugged him. "I love you, and because I do, that makes it my job to please you, in every way." "I love you too Sabrina, with all my heart and my soul, and as for pleasing me, you do that every morning, when I wake up with you beside me, and every night when I go to sleep with you in my arms. You please me when you look at me; with so much love in your eyes; when you touch me and hold me. Every second, of every day you please me; whether we're making love or not. If anything, I should be the one learning how to please you more."

His words were tender, filled with emotion; Sabrina couldn't speak, but Mark felt her tears fall against his chest. "What's wrong?" he asked lifting her face up. "Nothing." "Then why are you crying?" "Because you love me. For years I've longed to hear those words from anyone, but to hear them now from you fills my heart beyond anything I could have ever imagined." "Oh come on, you've been loved by someone before." "No Mark. No one ever loved me."

To hide the pain that she suddenly felt Sabrina turned away from him. Mark carefully pulled her back to him. She covered her face with her hands but he gently eased them away from her face and looked deep into her eyes. "Who hurt you Sabrina?" "I can't. I won't go there. Maybe someday I'll be strong enough to tell you but for right now I can't. I just want to hold on to this feeling and to you for as long as I can."

With his fingers lightly touching her skin he caressed her face slowly. Leaning in close to her and with his deep voice now but a soft whisper he spoke to her again. "I meant what I said; I do love you Sabrina and I'll prove it to you every chance I get; starting right now," he kissed her softly, but briefly. "Come on and get dressed. We're going out." "Where?" "Out."

"Can I have a shower first?" she asked. He looked at the clock on the table. "Sure, go ahead." Sliding off the edge of the bed she stood in front of him, taking up his hands. "Only if you join me." "Only for a shower, and nothing more," he tried to make his answer firm, but he knew full well that it would be virtually impossible to resist her. They hadn't experienced a shower together.

Waiting for the water too warm, she hid her nakedness against his body, just holding him, listening to his heart beat. When they stepped in the shower, she restrained her urges to seduce him, touching him only to wash his back, concentrating on the tattoos on his arms. Besides the large snake that coiled around his arm there were many others, of demons and devils, witches and dragons and even a castle.

The meaning she couldn't ascertain, but the artwork was beautiful. The colors not bold and vivid, but subdued, giving just enough contrast to create the desired effect. His artwork adorned both arms, from his elbows to his shoulders, creating a story along the way, one that she fantasized over; her mind creating a tale of his past life adventures. Her concentration had worked, before she knew it the shower was over, she hadn't made any advances toward him.

Mark wrapped a towel around himself, and headed to his room to get a clean set of clothes. Sabrina was nearly ready when he returned. "Don't you think it's about time you moved your things into here," she said. "Not much point to it, since we're leaving on Sunday." She finished buttoning her blouse, nodding her agreement with his statement. "So where are we going?" she asked. "I thought we could go into the city for a while." She froze. *Los Angeles is not a place I really want to go.* Mark put his arm around her, seeing her hesitation. "It'll be fine; it's not as bad as you may have heard."

The drive along the coast highway was pleasurable for her; she hadn't ventured down this route before. With Mark driving, she had a chance to take in the scenery, enjoying the changing shore line. The houses had begun to disappear along the water front, but had increased along the hills opposite. Traffic was picking up too; she tensed every time Mark wove between cars. Trying to focus her attentions on other things, but she found herself returning to the traffic ahead. Mark noticed her unease when he caught a glimpse of her pressing her foot down onto an imaginary brake pedal. "Still not used to being a passenger?" he asked rubbing her thigh. "No, I'm not, but I guess I can get used to it." "It won't be much longer now."

She turned her attentions to the city that was opening up before her. The residential areas were now behind them, and rows of offices, and small shops took their place. The outskirts of the city were comprised mainly of one, and two story buildings, gradually increasing in size as they neared the downtown area. Streets were lined with tall palm trees, giving life to this concrete maze, that was congested with vehicles and people. *I prefer the solitude, and the slower pace of the beach house; too many rats in this race.*

Her mind was so absorbed in watching the activities on the street that she didn't notice that Mark had parked the car. She was startled by his touch. "Sorry," he said. She didn't wait for him to open the car door, but he was there, with his hand to help her out. Trying to pull him close, he resisted. "Just put your motor in park for a little while," he said trying to be firm with her, but her smile only made him laugh; he took her hand. "Come on."

They walked along the sidewalk, window shopping mostly. One store in particular caught her attention. *I want to go in there, but I can't take Mark.* They walked on, past two more shops, when Mark stopped. "I have to go in here," he said. "Sure, but if you don't mind, I'd like to check out a shop we just passed. I won't be gone long." "Okay, I'll be inside when you get back."

Sabrina took note of the store front, before heading back to the other shop. She glanced back; to make sure Mark was not in sight. She entered an adult store, for lovers. Browsing the shop quickly, she knew exactly what she wanted; she moved about the lingerie racks. *So many things to choose from; I don't want anything too far out, just something sexy.* A black outfit caught her eye; she took it from the rack. It was a two piece set; a long black satin robe covered a long black gown made of stretch lace. She held it up against her at the mirror.

The lace gown was cut low in the front, and in the back; an under wire form had been sewn into the bust area. With no second thoughts she took the item to the cashier and completed her purchase. *Our sex life doesn't need any boosting, but it will be fun to dress up, to drive him wild with desire.*

Returning to the shop where she had left Mark, she scanned the contents as she walked in; it was like a costume shop, but for wrestlers. Mark was talking to a man at the counter when she entered; he acknowledged her, and picked up his parcels. "Did you get a new outfit?" she asked. "Yes, I did," he answered. What he neglected to tell her, was that he had picked up one for her too.

"Can we go home now?" she asked. "Soon, I have one more stop to make first. What did you buy?" "Just something I needed," she answered with a smile. He put the packages into the trunk before opening her door. She didn't ask where they were going, but sat quietly, thinking about when she would wear her outfit. Just thinking about it, and envisioning Mark's reaction aroused her.

They didn't drive far when Mark again parked the car. The sidewalk was busier than the one before, but they walked on without taking much notice. Mark directed Sabrina into a jewelry store; complete with an armed security guard. "Have a look around. I'll be a few minutes," he said heading off towards a gentleman behind a showcase. Sabrina surveyed the jewelry cases. *The pieces are beautiful; but well beyond my budget.*

Mark caught her attention, motioning her to come to him. "I would like your opinion," he said, as she neared. "Sure." He was standing in front of a showcase of rings, men's as well as ladies. Two trays had been removed and rested atop the counter. "What do you think of these?"

"They're all beautiful," she answered, picking up a gold band, encircled with diamonds.

Holding it between her fingers she watched the light reflect off of the stones. "No. Which one do you think would suit me?" Sabrina put away the ring that she had been holding, along with her fantasies and looked over the men's rings as she was asked. "This one," she said, picking up one with a large single diamond. "Thanks."

She wandered away again, as another item in the store had caught her attention. *Why is he in here looking at rings? No, it couldn't be.* She pushed the thought from her mind. When she had turned away, Mark picked up the ring that had fascinated her. He handed it to the jeweler, after he put back the one that she had picked out for him. The man promptly put the trays away in the showcase and locked it up. He removed a small tag from the ring in his hand and Mark followed him to the cash register. Sabrina continued to look at the items in the showcases; the designs fascinated her, making her completely unaware of the transaction that was taking place behind her.

Mark soon returned to her side; taking her hand, he slipped off her silver ring. "What are you doing?" she asked. "Since we're here, you might as well get this one cleaned." His explanation didn't make much sense to her. He handed the ring to the jeweler, who departed into a back room. Sabrina rubbed at the empty place on her finger. "What's wrong?" Mark asked. "It just feels strange, not having it there." Mark took her hand gently. "Maybe this will help." He slipped the diamond band onto her finger.

Her eyes popped open wide in surprise. "Mark, you shouldn't!" "Yes, I should." "This is an eternity ring." "I know; and that's just how long I'm going to love you; for all eternity." Her lip quivered, feeling the tears well up in her eyes. "No tears," he whispered, bringing her close. Sabrina held him tight; her body trembled.

The jeweler interrupted their moment, when he handed Mark, Sabrina's silver ring. He put it on her other hand. "See, you still have my heart on this hand; and now all my love on the other." She had to kiss him; it didn't matter that they were in the middle of a store. "Shall we go home now?" he asked. "I need a minute; my knees are weak." "That's easy to fix."

Picking her up in his arms he carried her out of the store, past the guard, and all down the sidewalk to the car. The people on the sidewalk stared rudely as they passed by. The attention that they drew embarrassed her. Hiding her face against the hollow of his neck, she stole the opportunity to kiss him softly. Mark let her stand again when they reached the car, but she still kept her arms around him, her body pressed close to his. "I love you so very much," she said softly.

In the sunlight, he could see how the tears sparkled in her eyes, waiting for an opportunity to spill out. He brushed her cheek with the back of his hand. Fortunately, his dark glasses shielded his own moist eyes from her. *I have always dreamed of this moment, of when I would fall in love, but I had no idea that it would feel so good. I know that I should ask her the question that goes with that ring but I just can't. I know that we're meant to be together but we need just a little more time together. When I am free of my fears then I will ask her.*

The sun dazzled, and danced on the diamonds in her ring. *I want to tell him just how I feel, but none of the words that are rattling around my mind seem sufficient. The way I'm feeling is indescribable, beyond words. How this man; that I had only met a few short weeks ago, that had unnerved me so bad; would turn out to be such a sensitive, passionate, loving man. I have found my true soul mate, the man I would do anything for.*

Mark kept a close eye on her, knowing that she was far away in her thoughts, he touched her hand gently. His touch brought her back to the present. "Where does your tour start?" she asked. "Florida. Why?" "I was just curious. I was wondering, if maybe I should pick up something new to wear, that's all." "Sure, why not." He made a quick right turn with the car. "You want to go shopping, then that's what we'll do." "I didn't mean right now." "It has to be right now. When else are you going to get the opportunity? This is Friday afternoon, and we leave on Sunday morning." "You're right, as always."

He rubbed her thigh gently, forcing her to look out the window, and stop concentrating on his touch; at least for a little while. She had been watching the shops along the road, but didn't see any that appealed to her. Mark made another right turn and slowed the car down to find a parking space. Sabrina read the street sign as they turned the corner.

"Mark I really can't afford to shop here; there must be a department store somewhere nearby." "You'll never know unless you look, now come on." "Mark this is the most expensive street in this town." "So who said you were paying anyway." "You don't have to do this. I am very capable of buying my own things." "I know; but I want to. Everything I have is yours Sabrina, my heart, my soul, my love, and my money." "But Mark." "No buts about it; it makes me happy." Sabrina sighed, as she took his hand. *He never ceases to amaze me.*

The sidewalk was relatively quiet; not nearly as crowded as the other one. Tourists, armed with cameras, scanned the sidewalks, hoping to catch a glimpse of a celebrity. Mark and Sabrina moved about them unnoticed. Mark had his hair pulled back into a braid; his forehead concealed by a blue baseball cap. Dark sunglasses also helped to change the look of his face.

He directed her into one of the clothing stores, waiting patiently, while she browsed through the racks, only offering up his disapproval when she picked out something that was too conservative. *She has a body to die for, and it needs to be shown off.* Sabrina picked up a more sexy outfit; the expression on his face told her that he approved. The prices were not as bad as she had anticipated, and that let her make a couple more selections without feeling guilty.

While she was in the fitting room Mark's attention was directed to a black dress that hung against the wall; he envisioned her in it. It was made of some type of shiny black cloth that stretched. On the hem, and around the strapless bust, were wide bands of sequins. Motioning to the clerk, that had been helping Sabrina, he asked her if it came in Sabrina's size. The clerk nodded and retrieved one from the rack. She suggested a black lace shawl to go with it and Mark agreed. He hurried the clerk with the purchase, afraid that Sabrina might see what he was doing.

By the time she returned from the fitting room, the clerk had the dress and shawl neatly concealed inside a box on the floor beside her. Sabrina returned the items she didn't want and brought the others to the clerk. Trying to open her wallet was futile, as Mark had already handed the clerk his credit card.

Sabrina wandered about the store, while Mark waited for the packages. "Ready to go; or would you like to go to another store?" he asked, slipping his arm around her. "No, I'm ready. I don't need to do any more shopping for a while." Tired, from the excitement of the day, and the stuffy heat of the city, Sabrina was drained, physically and emotionally. Leaning her head back against the seat of the car she closed her eyes, intending to just rest for a moment, but the gentle motion of the car soon lulled her into sleep.

Mark awakened her with a kiss on the cheek; they were home. Her nap had been refreshing. She stretched when she got out of the car, bringing life back to her limbs. Mark had already gone into the house with all of the packages tucked securely under his arm. She admired her ring again, the sunlight catching every facet of the diamonds.

It must have cost quite a lot, but it really doesn't matter anyway, he had given it to me, that is the most important thing to remember. She made a silent promise to herself. *Every moment that I'm with him, I will let him know just how much I love him.* Her mind toyed with a few ideas while she picked some of the wild flowers that grew along the front of the house.

"Are you coming in?" Mark asked. He had been leaning against the wall of the entrance way watching her. She smiled and walked to him. "So what are you thinking about?" he asked, playfully trapping her in his arms. "Oh, just about how much I love you." *Her smile has a new radiance to it. I can actually see the love. It makes me warm inside; I am so privileged.*

"I am so lucky," he said. "As am I." Sabrina pulled herself back from him. "This isn't getting dinner ready you know." She made a move towards the open door, but was stopped by Mark's arm, still around her. "Why don't we go out for dinner? That's something we haven't done yet." "I don't know. I'm not really in the mood, but then again I'm not overly enthused about cooking either." "Great; I know the perfect place, and it's not that far away. I'll make a reservation."

The excitement in his voice is so evident; everything for him is so new and exciting. It's funny, how restricted our lives have been, mine by guilt and his by choice, but for me anyway it was all worth it. I survived all the degradation knowing deep down inside that he was out there waiting for me, waiting to love me.

She was still standing in the closet, very much undecided on her selection when Mark came in. "Our reservation is for seven thirty," he said. Sabrina nodded a mute response. He could tell she was having difficulty making a choice; he decided to tease her on. "So what are you going to wear?" "I don't know. Is this a casual restaurant, or a fancy one?" Sabrina asked. Mark shrugged, which was of no help to Sabrina. "Maybe I can help you decide," he said with a sly smile.

From behind his back he produced the box that he had kept hidden from her. "What's this?" "Open it and find out." She sat down on the bed, the box on her knees. Her hands trembled with anticipation. Parting the tissue paper she pulled out the lace shawl. "A little revealing isn't it?" She held it up it front of her. "There's more; just keep looking." Putting the shawl beside her on the bed, she continued to part the tissue until she revealed the black dress.

With no further regard for the box, she stood up; holding the dress up to look at it. The box tumbled to the floor, spilling the tissue about her feet. "Oh Mark, this is wonderful." Pleased with her gift, she reached for him, pulling him closer to her. Her feet stumbled over the box; she lost her balance, falling backwards onto the bed, taking him with her. The full weight of his body pressed against her with great force.

It was the first time that she had really felt his entire weight upon her. Mark lifted himself up quickly. "Are you all right?" he asked frantically. Sabrina took in a breath; their collision had knocked the wind out of her. "I'm fine." Slipping her arms around him, she urged him back down to her, but his resisting strength held him steady against her pull. "No, your body can't handle it; you know that I weigh three hundred pounds." "Yes, I know all that; but please, just for a minute."

Against his better judgment, he eased them both down against the bed, slowly settling his body against hers. He kissed her softly, focusing his attention on her breathing. When her breaths became evidently labored, he rolled over onto his back taking her with him. She rested against him, giving herself a moment to catch her breath. Mark rubbed her back slowly. "Are you all right?" "Oh yes; I'm splendid." She shifted herself upward to kiss him. "Thank you." He responded to her kiss, then lifted her off. "You had better get dressed. We only have about twenty minutes before we have to leave." Mark left her to get himself changed. She had slid over to the edge of the bed, where she sat until he had left the room; she rubbed at her breasts.

The sudden force of his body against mine hurt me slightly but I could never tell him; it would upset him. Picking up the dress she headed off to the bathroom. *I have to make myself look good for him.*

During her time at the beach house, she hadn't bothered with much make up; but for tonight, she would add a few highlights. Her skin was already taking on a rich California glow, but she attributed it more to how Mark made her feel, rather than the effects of the sun. A touch of blush on her cheekbones, some mascara and a thin line of color to brighten her eyes and the look was complete.

She slipped on the dress; the design flattered her figure. The stretch material hugged her waist and hips, and clung to her bust. She had never worn a strapless dress before, but very much liked the feel, and the look of it. The sequin border along the top twinkled in the light of the bathroom; she moved it about. Since it was stretch fabric she could wear it higher, and more conservative, or slide it down a little lower, and be more daring. She decided on lower. She brushed her hair, letting the soft blonde waves drape over her bare shoulders. Applying a soft pink lipstick to her full lips, she took another quick look in the mirror and went to find her shoes.

She was standing in the closet, adjusting her shawl, when Mark came back; he called to her; she didn't answer. Emerging from behind the closet door, she watched for his reaction. His eyes widened, his mouth fell open, but no sound came from it.

She moved to him slowly, placing her hand upon his chest. Through his black silk shirt, she could feel the beat of his heart increase. "How do I look?" she asked. Mark had to swallow hard before even attempting to speak. When he did regain command of his voice a soft, 'Oh my,' was all he could manage. Her hand glided slowly across the silk. "Do we still have to go out?" she asked softly. *Her voice, it's so sultry. I'm so tempted to say no.* "Yes. Yes, we do." He chased away the thoughts of making love to her right then. *I have to show some resistance, or we will never leave the house.*

On the drive to the restaurant he seized every available opportunity to hold her hand, or to steal a glimpse of her beauty, all the while smiling to himself. *I am so blessed to have found her.*

Sabrina had caught sight of his smile, but didn't comment on it; she knew he was happy, it transmitted in his touch. When he wasn't able to hold her hand, she let hers rest against his thigh, wishing that they could be closer together, but the bucket seats of her car kept them apart. *I can wait.* Casting her gaze out the window, not to look at the scenery, but to just daydream. *What an incredible lover he is.*

A soft, sighing moan escaped her lips, unnoticed by her own ears. Mark noticed it immediately. "Everything okay?" he asked. Sabrina rolled her head in his direction and nodded. Her face had a far away, dreamy look to it, with just a hint of a smile. *I know what she's thinking about; I've seen that look many times before, when we made love.*

Her hand began to roam over his thigh, even through the fabric of his pants, her touch ignited him, he fought off the feelings that were rising in his body. Safety, he thought, catching sight of the restaurant. "We're here."

Sabrina turned off her wandering mind to survey the restaurant's exterior. Details were hard for her to see, since it was now dark. The only lights were the dim, yellow lamps along the walls of the building. The front entrance was a shade brighter, but not by much. It illuminated enough of an area that she could see a valet standing at the curb, and behind him, a long line of couples waiting to get inside.

The valet was prompt. Reaching Mark's door before the car hand come to a complete stop. Another waited on her side, offering his hand in her aid. The line of patrons was directed away from the entrance by a series of gold braided ropes. As they passed, Sabrina could hear the whispers from the crowd, and saw the fingers, pointing rudely at them. *They must recognize Mark; and they did, at least, have the decency to keep their place.*

The interior of the restaurant was as dim as the exterior. Low light seemed to be the tradition in the finer restaurants. Brighter light would not have improved the scene any better, as the walls were done in a dark walnut paneling, and the floor in a rich red carpeting. The head waiter greeted Mark. "Good evening Mr. Cassidy; please, follow me." Sabrina figured him to be a man in his early fifties, but the low light made it hard to really tell. He wore a black tuxedo, immaculate in every detail, and a recognizable look of pride on his face.

They followed him through the center of the main dining room, past the other patrons. The tables were all adorned with candles and flowers, atop stark white linens. The reflections from the diminutive flickering flames, frolicked about on the crystal glasses, suggesting that they were mere spirits trapped inside the facets of the crystal.

Sabrina again saw the looks of recognition on some of the faces. A young woman rose from her seat and made an attempt to approach them, but she was quickly halted by a waiter. Sabrina tightened her grip on Mark's arm, keeping herself close to him; not for reassurance, but to make a statement; a statement of ownership. *He belongs to me, and I to him.* It only took moments to pass through the dining room, but the echoing silence made it last forever.

The waiter had stopped just ahead of them. He showed them into a private dining room. As soon as he had left, Mark noticed Sabrina relax against his arm, her fingers loosening their grip. He turned her around to face him. "In time you'll get used to the stares, and the whispers. It goes with the territory," he said.

He had left his long, dark auburn hair loose, the way she liked it. It brushed over the top of her breast that sent a tingle up her spine; she kissed him. "We came here for dinner; remember? Keep this up and we'll be asked to leave." He released her from his embrace. Sabrina bit her lower lip. "Okay, I'll behave; but when we get home," she cut off her own sentence, slowly drawing her hand across his chest as she moved away. *Heaven help me.* Mark sighed.

Their dining room was as dimly lit as the other sections of the restaurant, but it offered them a spectacular view of the ocean; the main dining room did not. A table, set for two, was poised near the balcony; the glass patio doors were open, allowing the gentle ocean breeze to permeate the room, taking great delight in taunting the flame on the candles.

Sabrina dropped her shawl over the back of one of the chairs and stepped out onto the balcony. At each side was a solid wood wall that protruded out beyond the railing; ensuring complete privacy for its occupants. The sun was long down, but Sabrina still took in the rippling reflections of the moon. Tonight it was as equally wondrous as a sunset.

Mark approached her, softly kissing her shoulder. She tilted her head inviting him to continue. With no hesitation he kissed her again, moving up her neck, stopping only to tease her ear lobe. Standing behind her, he began to feel like a voyeur, as he watched her chest heave upwards when he touched her; he straightened himself up.

Leaning back against him; she crossed her arms over her chest holding her shoulders. "Are you cold?" Mark asked, encircling her with his arms. "No." "Then what's the matter?" "This must be some kind of dream; the product of an energetic imagination," she said with a slight sigh. Mark turned her around. His face had a serious look upon it. "You're not dreaming; it's all real. I know you've been through a lot, in a very short time, and it must seem like something from your imagination, but it's not." He paused briefly to take her hand. "There is something that you can do, if you ever get the feeling of being lost in a dream. I want you to look at this ring, and remember that I love you, now and forever." He held her hand against his heart, until she embraced him as hard as she could.

They were so all consumed with each other that they never noticed the waiter arrive with their meal; not until they heard the door close as he left. "Ready for dinner?" "Sure," she answered politely, even though she would have preferred to skip dinner and go home.

She picked at her meal, not because she didn't like it, but because she couldn't take her eyes off of Mark. His hair, hanging loosely about his shoulders, the way she liked it, framing his face, giving him that dark, sexy look. His green eyes, so much more intense in the candle light. The combination of all these things made her blood afire with passion. Her mind locked onto the music that quietly filtered into the room, she knew the song and it made her desires even more intense.

Standing at his side, she urged him to get up. "Dance with me," she said softly. "I told you I don't dance." "Then hold me." Holding her was something he could do, and did, with no hesitation. Sabrina rested her head against his shoulder, and without thinking began to gently sway her body to the beat of the music. Unconsciously, Mark followed her lead, holding her, moving with her body. "So you don't dance, eh?" "This isn't dancing." "Close enough." Feeling her hands increase the pressure against his back, he leaned down and kissed her.

It has become so easy for me to read her. She wants more than what I can give her here. He cupped his hand over her cheek. "Let's go home," he whispered. Closing her eyes, she tipped her head into his hand; his thumb stroked her temple. "You didn't answer me?" "Promise me one thing first," she said. "What would that be?" "Promise me that you will always hold me like this, whether I ask you or not." "Of course I promise; always. Maybe I'm being a bit selfish taking you on tour with me; but I can't bear the thought of going even one day without being able to hold you, or touch you; or make love to you."

His fingers traced down her neck, across the top of her breast. His soft words, more than his touch, brought all her emotions racing forth. Seeing her lip quiver he drew her close. She calmed herself, listening to the rhythmic beat of his heart, feeling the gentle strokes of his hand on her hair.

Spreading wider, the opening in his shirt, she kissed his chest, moving upward until she found his lips. Mark was the first to break away. "We have to go home; now!" He said, his voice cracking from the tension. Sabrina knew that look on his face. He picked up her shawl and placed it around her shoulders. Hooking her arm around his, he directed her back out through the dining room. Some of the faces had changed, but the stares and whispers were still the same.

They went out to the curb to await the valet's return with the car. The line of couples waiting to get in had shortened, but not by much. The whispers were louder this time; but still, they refrained from approaching. The valet arrived with the car. Mark held her back a moment, whispering into her ear. "Shall we give them something to gossip about?" he asked, giving her a wink. With a grin she answered quickly. "Sure, why not."

Taking her in his arms, he kissed her with a powerful passion. She melted backwards in his hold. They both could hear the whispers grow louder; Mark increased his pressure on Sabrina. Releasing her, she took in a long breath. "Now we positively have to go home," she said with an almost nervous stammer in her voice.

Taking a brief moment, he surveyed the shocked faces of the crowd. Some whistled, while others looked away, ashamed by their display of affection. Satisfied, that he had achieved the desired effect, Mark got into the car. Sabrina had tried to sit quietly, waiting for him, but she could not control the tremors that made her hands and legs twitch without warning. Mark had excited her so much that her body was experiencing an intense anxiety reaction from not being able to have him. *Think of something else; just think of something else.*

Checking her watch again was meaningless, she had forgotten how long the drive was, and what time they left the restaurant. Searching the passing scenery for a glimpse of something familiar, but the darkness kept its secrets hidden from her. Her hands began to tremble again; she concentrated hard on making them stop. Mark noticed her rubbing her hands together. He reached over and touched her leg. "Are you cold?" "What?" She was startled by his voice. "You're shaking; are you cold? I can turn the air conditioning down if you are." "No. I'm not cold, very much to the contrary in fact."

Knowing that tone, he began to gently massage her thigh; pushing her dress higher each time. His hand pushed down between her thighs. She adjusted her seat allowing him more freedom of movement. He could feel the moist perspiration on her thighs. He had to keep his eyes on the road, but his mind was solidly focused on her, and the invitation she was presenting to him. He moved higher towards the source of the warmth; but then withdrew his hand abruptly.

"Damn it this isn't right! I'm not going to risk getting into an accident over it." Sabrina wanted to speak, to beg him to pull over, but that wouldn't be right either; they weren't kids. Both of his hands were now tightly gripping the steering wheel; she leaned back against the seat and closed her eyes.

Playing with the ring on her finger, she reran in her mind the moment that he gave it to her; it made her smile. *Steve never did anything as exciting as this when he proposed. He never even bought a ring, but Mark didn't propose, he just gave me this and told me he'd love me forever. Maybe someday, there will be a gold band to go with this. Sabrina Cassidy; I like the sound of that.*

Her fantasy continued, as she imagined herself marrying Mark. The type of wedding they would have, being with him forever, and to complete the fantasy a couple of children, one boy and one girl. The car came to a stop, and so did the fantasy.

She was out of the car, and waiting as patiently as she could, by the front door; urging him to hurry with the lock, but it was dark, and he was having trouble, since they had forgotten to leave the light on when they went out. Once inside she could no longer restrain herself. Pulling his jacket off, she threw herself into his arms. He scooped her up, carrying her to the bedroom. Their love making was intense, yet still tender, as if it was their first time, filled with all the mystery and anticipation.

Mark settled onto his right side with Sabrina's back molded against his body. His hand caressed the length of her body before he picked up her left hand. Raising it to his lips, he kissed her ring. "We have just consummated our relationship; and do you know what that means?" "What does that mean?" she answered without turning to look at him. "It means; that from this moment on, we belong to each other, forever, and nothing, or no one, will ever come between us." Sabrina waited a moment, expecting to hear until death do us part, but that was her fantasy taking over again. She pulled Mark's arm across her, holding it to her breast. "Forever; I like the sound of that." With a yawn she slipped back into her fantasy.

Chapter 9

The reflection, that stared back from the mirror, was rough and haggard. A far cry from the sexy, desirable image that was once Sean. Sleep had become but a vague memory, the deficiency showing in the dark circles surrounding his eyes, and in the deep lines on his forehead. He had been in an emotional whirlpool since walking in on Sabrina and Mark at the beach house. Confusion clouded his mind; his concentration was meager. Unable to keep his mind on his work, and it showed every time he got into the ring. Losing nearly every match that had been set up, now a threat of suspension, or even worse, being fired, loomed over him.

A fist smashed into the face in the mirror. Shards of glass showered into the sink. The pain of the cuts never registered in his mind, only the pain that seethed in his gut. Pulling a towel from the rack, he wrapped it around his hand as he went to the bedroom.

Falling backwards onto the bed, he tried to push away the thoughts that raced about his mind. He was obsessed with Sabrina, and with the two questions that taunted him over and over again. *Why did she not tell me? Why did she turn to Mark?*

Tightening his hands into fists, he pounded on the mattress. As consumed as he was with Sabrina, his ever growing, raging, hatred of Mark, was becoming the foremost thing in his mind. Anticipating the moment when they would meet, when he would have his opportunity to exact revenge upon Mark for taking her away. In the ring or not, it didn't matter, hurting Mark was the one, the singular priority.

Lifting his arms up, Sean noticed the blood that stained the towel on his right hand. Unwrapping it, he saw the small slivers of mirror that glistened through the blood still oozing from his knuckles. The pain still had not completely registered as he plucked the shards from his wounds. Blood trickled down between his fingers, dripping off onto his jeans.

"The next time I have blood on my hands, it's gonna be yours Mark, and your face is gonna look just like this. She won't want to be with a mangled piece of trash after I get through with you. Soon, you big bastard, very soon I'm gonna beat the crap out of you. They'll be scraping you off the mat with a shovel when I'm done."

Sean went back into the bathroom to clean up his hand. The water washing over it made it sting, but that only increased his level of anger.

With his hand bound in clean bandages he began sorting his gear for the show. *I have to be at the arena early, waiting for when Mark arrives.*

Oblivious to his fans, waiting in the lobby, Sean bulldozed through, knocking a couple off balance, causing them to fall to the floor. A barrage of verbal assaults bounced off of him like rain off a duck. An attractive young woman stood next to the big limo, waiting for her chance to get close to Sean. He saw her, but not her youthful beauty; all he saw was an obstruction. "Get out of my way, bitch!" he snarled.

The woman, stunned by his remark, stood firmly in her place. Sean took her by the arm, physically moving her from his path. "Hey!" she yelled, regaining her balance. Sean turned to look at her. He felt the burning sting on his face as she slapped him. He had no reaction.

"You son of a bitch!" she yelled at him, as he got into the limo. He leaned against the back seat, running his hand over his cheek, feeling the welts that grew larger. A few months ago he would have taken that woman into the limo with him, and he would have made love to her all the way to the airport; but now, pretty women, and sex, no longer fueled his desires. Even Robbie had abandoned him, after he refused her many advances.

I want Sabrina. To hold her body against mine, that's all that matters now, that and hurting Mark. Sean closed his eyes trying to relax, but it was no use; his mind, again, envisioned Mark making love to Sabrina. He shook his head, sending the vision back into the void. *I have to stay focused on the task at hand; selecting the exact time to execute my plan.* A faint smile appeared on his lips, as he remembered that the show was going to be televised.

Perfect, in front of all those people in the arena, and all the others watching on TV, what an absolutely perfect opportunity to beat the crap out of Mark. The whole world will get to see their favorite star get his ass beaten into a bloody hunk of meat. That's how it will work. I'll wait until that one moment when Mark is most vulnerable, and completely unprepared. His smile widened. For the first time in days a sense of calm washed over him; he felt relaxed and in control.

Chapter 10

Mark's internal alarm clock woke him the same way it did every morning. Sabrina lay close beside him, her arm still embracing his chest. Neither of them had moved all night and his back ached from having slept in one position. *She looks so peaceful, I hate to wake her, but we have a plane to catch in just a few hours.*

"It's time to get up," he whispered. Sabrina groaned her disapproval, turning over onto her left side away from him. He turned towards her, grateful to relieve the ache in his back. Gently pulling her hair away from the side of her face he began a slow, methodical journey of soft kisses up her neck to her ear. "We have to get up." "Not yet," she yawned. Searching for his hand she pulled it across her. Mark continued his kisses, knowing that it would keep her awake. "Come on," he implored her, nuzzling her neck. "Join me in the shower." That got her attention, she leaned back against him. "Now that's an offer that I can't refuse." He kissed her cheek again, before heading off to the bathroom.

He glanced over his shoulder, as she opened the door and stepped in to the shower. Still sleepy, she moved herself close to him; slipping her hands around his chest and laying her head against his back. His chest was lathered with soap; she delighted in gliding her hands over his slick body. Taking the soap from him, she ran it over his back with one hand, while the other she used to explore the sexy body before her.

So firm and smooth, so powerful, he makes me feel so safe. I don't understand this insatiable need to touch him and be touched by him. Why do I crave this unending physical contact? Kissing his back, she handed him the soap. "My turn," she said. He readily obliged her, washing her back first. Rubbing the soap briskly in his hands, to get a thick lather, he reached around her and began washing her chest; pausing briefly, to pay extra attention to her breasts as they slipped through his hand. The stimulation made her back up against him.

Knowing what she was doing, he ceased his caresses. "We can't do this; there's too much to do," he said. Sabrina turned to face him. "It's okay; could you at least hold me for a few minutes?" "I can't refuse that." He held her tight, while she rested against him. The warmth of the water, and the sensuous feeling of her sleek body against him, made it difficult for him to let her go.

I could easily give in to her invitation, but to hold her for a few more minutes will have to be enough. A strange feeling, almost a fear, flickered inside him; an uneasy feeling about this trip. *I get the feeling that somehow this will be the first true test of our love.* He hugged her tighter, afraid to let go. Dismissing his fear, he reached to turn the water off. "Not yet," Sabrina said, releasing him. "I need to wash my hair first. You go on; I'll only be a couple of minutes."

By the time she had completed her shower, Mark was finished his packing. She surprised him when she came into the bedroom. He hastily stuffed a bag into his suitcase and shut the lid. "Are you hiding something?" she asked. "No." "Then what was that?" "What?" "That bag you stuffed in there." "Oh that; it's a new costume, that's all." "Can I see?" "Not right now; you can see it tonight."

I hope that she won't pursue the issue any further. It's her costume, and I want to surprise her with it. Sabrina is a part of my life now, and I want her to be a part of my work as well. If she's at the ring with me, then I won't worry about her being alone. Picking up the case, he headed for the door.

"How about I make breakfast?" Mark asked. "Hold it right there! What makes you think that you can get away that easy?" Mark stopped. *Damn it, not convincing enough.* Sabrina stood before him, her eyes scanning his face. He waited nervously for the next set of questions. *What will I say, to get out of not telling her what I have hidden?*

Putting her arms around his neck, she pulled him to her and kissed him. Surprised by her actions, it took him a few seconds to respond to her. Satisfied, she relaxed her hold. "Now you can go," she said, with a smile. He watched her disappear behind the closet door; relieved that she hadn't grilled him about the mysterious bag.

As she dressed, she smiled to herself. *I know that he's hiding something from me, but then again, I too am keeping a secret.* She laid her new lingerie on the bottom of the case. *I'm not quite sure when, or where, I will surprise him with it, but I'm positive that it will be a night that he'll never forget. I love him so much, that pleasing him has become my only priority. He has done so much for me, and I'll do anything for him, as long as it makes him happy.* A smile beamed across her face when she heard his voice, calling her to breakfast. She called back, to let him know that she would be there in a minute.

Finishing her task quickly, but thoroughly, she closed the suit case and carried it out to the hallway. Mark greeted her at the kitchen doorway; a plate in each hand, but still able to give her a quick kiss as he passed by.

His tour itinerary was on the table; Sabrina read through it while she ate. Reading at breakfast had always been a ritual for her; it didn't matter if it was a newspaper, or a cereal box, she just had to read something, to get her mind functioning. The itinerary was for two weeks and listed ten shows, and three promo dates, thirteen days, with only one day off.

A somber mood came over her as she scanned the list again. *With all these shows the chances of meeting up with Sean are running pretty high. Can I handle it; seeing him again? How will Sean react, considering the way I left him? Why am I even worrying about it? I have no feelings for Sean anyway.*

Mark could see that she was somewhere, far away, and the look on her face worried him. "Are you all right?" he asked. Sabrina forced a partial smile, but avoided looking into his eyes. "I know that schedule looks pretty hectic, but we'll have plenty of time together." *I hope that's the reassurance she needs.* She just stared blankly at the paper.

Mark's senses were confused. *Something is bothering her; but what?* She didn't notice him get up, until he turned her head to look at him. He was kneeling beside her chair, which made them eye level to one another, and impossible for her to avoid his gaze.

"Tell me what's bothering you Sabrina." She touched his hand, searching for some of his inner strength. "Is it the schedule?" "No." "Then what's bothering you?" "I was just thinking. Is Sean going to be at any of these shows?" "I'm not gonna lie to you; he'll most likely be at all of them, but I don't want you to worry about it. I told you that we would deal with this together."

Her eyes glistened with tears. It broke his heart to see her cry, and to hold her was the only way he could think of to comfort her. "I love you so much, and I promised you that I wouldn't let Sean get near you ever again." He rubbed her back. Sabrina leaned back, wiping the tears from her face. "Mark, it's not so much me, but I'm worried about what he might do to you." "He can try all he wants. I've beaten him many times before. Besides, he should be able to understand, you've made your choice, and what you once had is now over. If I know Sean, he has probably found himself another lady, or he's gone back to Robbie."

I know that he's trying to settle my nerves, but deep inside, I know that there will be a confrontation with Sean, very soon, and it won't go as smoothly as Mark wants me to believe. He pulled her close again; hoping that he had banished her fears, but his own nagging doubts still prevailed.

Sean arrived at the arena very early; tossed his gear into the dressing room, and had taken a seat high up in the arena, watching the crew, as they set up the ring and the lighting. No longer able to control the frequent shifting in his seat, caused by agitation, and planning his assault on Mark; he rose and began pacing along the aisles. The pacing soon turned into a jog, then to a run. Up the stairs, along the corridors that encircled the arena; driven on faster and faster by his rage.

Oblivious to his surroundings, Sean rounded a corner and ran full on into Tony and D'arcy, hitting with such a force, that all three men were knocked off balance, like a bowling ball heading for a strike. Sean fell to his knees on the concrete floor. Tony hit the cement wall, and D'arcy was tossed across the hallway.

"Hey man, what the hell is the matter with you?" Tony snarled angrily. "Yeah Sean, what's up?" D'arcy added, dusting himself off. Sean stood up slowly, holding his knees. The pain that pulsated in them was intense, and it made him angrier. "Screw off!" he growled to Tony, as he limped away. "Sean, for Christ's sake, what is wrong with you?" D'arcy called to him.

Sean turned back, to face the two men, whom he had once called his friends. His face was red and hard deep lines that were carved into his forehead dripped with sweat. "I told you to leave me the fuck alone; got it! No more damn questions; just stay the hell away from me!" Getting no further response, Sean turned his back on his friends, limping away to his dressing room.

Tony and D'arcy were both stunned into silence by his appearance, but more so by his attitude towards them. "What in the hell is wrong with him?" D'arcy asked. "I don't know man; but it's been getting worse over the past few weeks, and I can't figure out why. He won't talk to anybody; and I'm afraid that if he doesn't smarten up soon he's gonna be out of a job." "That's for sure; I know the boss is pretty pissed with him." Their friend was in trouble, and they were both helpless. All they could do was to watch him dig himself deeper, and deeper into his own personal and private hell.

Mark and Sabrina made it through both airports completely unnoticed. There were no waiting fans or photographers. His return to the ring tonight was being kept a secret; as a special treat for the fans. Sabrina was glad to see the hotel; after being cooped up in the airplane for so long all she wanted to do was to stretch out on the bed and relax for a little while. She leaned against him, as they walked across the lobby.

Mark waited until the elevator doors had closed before he kissed her. "You keep doing that and you just might not make it to the arena tonight," she said. He was about to indulge in her sweet lips again, when the door opened. Taking her hand, he guided her to their room. The thought of being alone with her, in a hotel room, had begun to make his heart beat faster.

This is ridiculous. I have been alone with her; only somehow a hotel room offers up more illusions than being at home. They were seductive, a secret getaway from the real world. A stereotype created by generations of movies and cheating spouses. I don't harbor any fantasies, for she fulfilled all of them the day she came into my life.

He was about to follow her into the hotel room, when a voice called to him from behind. His first instinct was to ignore it, but the voice called again, more insistent. Mark turned to see Brent coming toward him. "Hey Mark, how have you been? You've been away a long time," Brent said greeting him with a handshake. "Fine," Mark replied. "Just getting in, are you?" "Yes, I just checked in a few minutes ago."

I really don't want to be having this conversation right now, but I can't be rude either. I hope that Brent did not see Sabrina. I don't want it known that we are together; not yet. His heart stopped, when he heard Sabrina's voice. "Are you gonna stand there all day, or are you coming in?" she called.

Brent's brown eyes widened when he heard the female voice. "You have a woman with you?" He was amazed, knowing Marks history. "This I gotta see!" Pushing past Mark, he entered the room. Sabrina was standing at the window, looking over the city. She turned around when she heard the door close. The recognition was immediate, and the shock settled in quickly.

"Close your mouth Brent," she said calmly. "It's not polite to stare." "Sabrina?" Brent stammered over her name. "Yes, Brent, it's me." "Oh man, I gotta sit down."

The room fell silent; Brent overcoming the surprise, Mark and Sabrina both anticipating the next question. Brent took a breath, rubbing his hands along his knees. "Man, Sean is sure gonna be glad to see you. He's been so." "I'm not here to see Sean," Sabrina announced, abruptly cutting him off. Brent looked first at Sabrina, and then at Mark. *I don't understand. If she isn't here for Sean, then why is she here at all?* "That's right Brent; she's not here to see Sean, because she's here with me," Mark said putting his arms around her.

The look of shock intensified on Brent's face. *What do I say?* His mind tossed around many thoughts. *Should I tell her how messed up Sean is; or congratulate them?* He looked at his watch. "I gotta go," he announced. *I'm taking the coward's way out, but I need time to adjust.* Sabrina stopped him at the door.

"Please Brent, please don't tell Sean, or anyone, that I'm here with Mark. The truth will be told when the time is right, but that decision is up to Mark and myself, and I hope that you will respect that." "I give you my word. Your secret will not be told by me," he answered. The feeling of her hand gently squeezing his only aided in securing his promise.

Once free of their room Brent rested against the wall in the hallway. *Sean is gonna go ballistic when he finds out. I will keep my promise; not so much for her, but for myself. I don't want to be on the receiving end of Sean's anger. The best thing I can do would be to avoid them all; at least until the dust settles.*

With the door securely locked, Sabrina braced herself against the frame; her insides quivered uncontrollably. Mark came to her; she turned, and sought the comfort of his arms. Her inner turmoil radiated outwards, making her body tremble. Mark held her tighter. "It's gonna be all right. Brent will keep his promise; so don't worry." Her silence reflected his own fears, about coming face to face with Sean. *I've been dreading this, knowing how hard it would be on her.*

"We don't have to be at the arena for a few hours yet; why don't you go and lie down for a while," he said. Lifting her face upwards, in her eyes he could see the exhaustion, the stress of worry. "Will you come with me? I need you near me right now." Without answering, he picked her up and carried her to the bed. Laying her down, he took his place beside her. She slid her back close to him, her head resting on his right arm, while clutching his other arm to her chest.

Damn it she's crying. She hides it well, but those are tears dripping onto my arm. "It's gonna to be all right; you'll see. I promised you that we would deal with this together, and I won't let you down, ever." Mark moved closer, resting his leg across hers, reinforcing the vow that he would always protect her and keep her safe.

When Brent arrived at the arena, his mind was still in turmoil over having to keep quiet about Sabrina and Mark. Confusion reigned over the situation. *Sabrina doesn't want me to tell Sean, but he must already know? That would explain his behavior over the past few weeks; or would it?* He shook his head, as he walked to the dressing room, contemplating the events of the past weeks.

The barbecue at Sean's, that was when I saw her the last time. Then Sean went on tour, and she didn't come with him. His eyes widened. *That's also when Mark took his leave of absence. That's it! When Mark canceled his tour, that's when Sean started acting crazy. He has to know about them; it's the only thing that makes any sense.* His heart sank, as he thought about tonight, and the inevitable confrontation that would take place. *I've witnessed Sean's anger before, and I feel sorry for Sabrina. She's about to get caught up in the middle of the madness.*

Mark still held Sabrina in his arms. She had cried herself to sleep, but it wasn't a peaceful sleep. Her slumber was tortured, by sudden body tremors, and mournful sighs. *It tears me apart, to lie beside her, knowing she's being tormented by Sean, even in her dreams. The one place that I can't protect her. We have to leave for the arena very soon, and waking her, would at least, free her from this silent persecution.*

Calling her name, he summoned her back to him. As she turned to him, Mark raised himself up on his elbow, allowing her more room. "Feeling better?" he asked. She nodded, and stretched, bringing her arms about him, insisting that he come to her. His resistance was futile. He leaned down to kiss her. Their lips met with eager passion. Mark pulled back, and knelt beside her; taking her hand he helped her up to him. Her face had regained that warm, loving glow. "Have I told you today, just how much I love you?" "Yes, you have, but you can tell me as often as you want," he answered.

She couldn't help but smile. *His openness always makes me feel good.* "We have to get going," he said. With his hand extended, he helped her up. A brief touch on her shoulder, and he went to prepare his gear for tonight. Sabrina went to the bathroom, to wash away the evidence of her tears. When she returned to the bedroom Mark was waiting for her. "I have something for you," he said, handing her a long black robe. "What's this for?" "I'd like for you to wear it to the arena."

Her expression changed, her smile curling up one side of her mouth. "And what would you like me to wear under it?" she asked. "What you have on is fine." *He completely missed my advance. I'll wait a couple minutes more, to see if it has a delayed effect.* No luck.

"So why do I have to wear this anyway?" Sabrina asked. "So you won't be recognized." She played with the sleeves, that dangled well below her hands. "A bit big don't ya think?" "No, that's the way it's supposed to be, and when we get to the arena you'll have to put the hood up."

Reaching around her, he pulled the large hood over her head. It covered part of her face, forcing her to look down at the floor, in order to see anything. "Perfect." "Oh come on; I can't see a damn thing." "That's the whole idea; if you can't see properly, then no one will be able to see you." "Now I understand," she said pulling the hood back. "So where did you get this?" "I had it made for you. Remember that costume shop in Los Angeles? It matches the one that I wear." "You are so amazing."

After trying several, unsuccessful attempts to free her hands, she gave up and put her arms around Mark, sliding her body against his. "Are you sure you want me to wear clothes under this?" "At least for now," he grinned. Their attempt to kiss was halted by the ringing of the phone. Breaking himself free, Mark answered it. Upon hanging up, he announced that the limo was waiting.

Sabrina shuddered, as a cold chill raced up her spine. The more she thought about going, the more unsettled she became. She jumped when Mark touched her shoulder. He put his arm around her, keeping it there, all the way down the elevator and into the limo.

She was quiet, but her mind worked in overdrive. *How will I deal with Sean, but more importantly, how will he react to Mark?* That one thing worried her the most. *Will Sean be able to accept my being with Mark, or will he lash out in some way?* Mark's arm around her only offered her comfort on the outside; it couldn't reach the trembling soul trapped within.

The anguish was sensed by the other. This would be the first test of their bond in this reunion. They would have to be strong for one another and allow the real love to conquer this dilemma. The bond was indestructible, it had healed the pain of many indignation's suffered through time and it would restore their commitment now.

During the drive Sabrina had kept her hand resting on Mark's leg, but now, with the arena coming into view, her idle hand unconsciously began rubbing against the rough denim of his jeans. The closer they got, the harder she rubbed. The limo passed through the entrance gate; her hand formed into a fist.

Mark stroked her hand, trying to relax her, but the more he tried, the more she tensed beside him. "You really don't want to be here, do you?" he asked. "I don't know. I am nervous about tonight; but, on the other hand, I don't want to be away from you either." "I love you Sabrina, and that's all you need to remember."

The limo came to a stop inside the arena. Through the tinted windows she could see the crew, diligently working at their assigned jobs, unconcerned with the presence of the limousine. "Ready?" "I guess so," she answered with some reluctance. He started to pull the hood up over her face. "Wait a minute," she said. "What is it?" "Something I forget to do earlier." She kissed him deeply, leaving him drained and weak. "Whoa," he exclaimed, catching his breath. "This is not exactly the right place to start this; but if you come with me, I just might be able to help you forget all about your worries." The devilish smile on his face made her blush.

Pulling her hood up; she followed him from the car. Having to look down made it difficult to maneuver, but with his arm around her shoulders traversing the corridors was easier. She had no idea where in the arena they were, and after walking for a few minutes they finally stopped. Mark had released his arm from her. She was afraid to move, in case she tripped, or bumped into something.

Mark's black boots came into her field of view; he was standing in front of her. "Lift your head up," he told her. She complied readily. He made an adjustment to her hood, allowing her to see properly. "There, if you wear it like that, then you will be able to see, and still no one will see your face." "Oh yes, this is much better." They were standing inside the dressing room; she spotted the mirror on the wall. She played with the hood, making sure that she could adjust it, without his help. She smiled to herself, pleased with her accomplishments. She had mastered the sleeves, and now the hood.

Mark sifted through his bag, sorting out his costume for tonight, but still keeping his surprise for her well hidden. A knock came to the door; Mark motioned to Sabrina to replace her hood, before he opened the door. Through the shadows of her disguise, she saw a middle aged man enter the room. She recognized him as the owner of the wrestling organization, but could not recall his name. The two men shook hands, and the look on his face indicated to her that he was very pleased to see Mark. She listened to their conversation.

"Am I glad to see you back on tour again Mark. It's been too long; your fans have really missed you." "It's good to be back." "Who's this?" "A new part of the show; and that's all you need to know right now." "Okay Mark, whatever you say. All of your gear is here like you requested. I had it staged near the entrance." "Good." "Is there anything else you need?" "No, just keep it the way we discussed and it will work out perfectly." "That's all been taken care of. You're set for the beginning of the second hour, right after intermission." By the time this man had left, Sabrina's mind was filled with more questions.

With the door closed and locked Mark turned around. Sabrina was standing alert with her arms folded across her chest and a pensive glare sent his way. "What do you mean, that I'm part of the show?" she asked. He motioned her to sit down on the bench; he sat astride it facing her. "I'm waiting for an answer," she demanded. "I'm sorry, for not saying anything about this earlier, but I wanted it to be a surprise. I didn't want to scare you. I love you, and I want you to be a part of my life forever; that means personally, and professionally. I want you with me always, every where I go." *I can't stay mad at him; I love him too much.*

"So, what exactly do you have planned?" she asked. "I would like for you, to come to the ring with me; wearing the robe of course; and portray a disciple of the Warlock." "What would I have to do?" "The plan is for you to accompany me to the ring, and when I tell you to, you would remove my robe, exit the ring and wait for me until the match was over."

He lifted her hands to his heart. "By having you at ringside I wouldn't worry about you being alone, here, in the dressing room." "No one will know who I am?" "No one; I promise." She contemplated the offer. "If that's what you really want, then I guess it's okay," she answered.

"It's not what I want; it's what I would like," he said, taking her in his arms. "This is what I really want." Tonight his passion was forceful. Pulling open her robe, caressing her body; his tongue plunging deep inside her mouth. His kisses moved across her face and down her neck; touching on a sensitive spot that made her shudder. "Oh Mark, make love to me, right here, right now." He didn't answer; he wanted her just as much as she wanted him.

Fueled by his passion, and not rationalizing his actions, he tore at her shirt. The power of his hands ripping it wide open. The sound of cloth ripping sent Sabrina's mind flashing back to that horrid day, when she was attacked.

Through Mark's aggressiveness, she began reliving the whole event. The terror surfaced and she fought back. Freeing herself from him, she ran across the room to the door, frantically trying to undo the lock, but could not. Sliding down to the floor she was shaking uncontrollably; her knees pulled up to her chest covering her nudity.

Mark was distressed by her reaction. "Sabrina, what's the matter?" She never answered him, for she couldn't hear him. Getting up, he noticed the piece of torn material in his hand. His heart was ripped from his chest, as he realized what he had done. Kneeling by her side, he called her name. It took several moments for her to hear, and recognize his voice. When she did, she thrust herself into his arms crying hard. "Oh baby I'm sorry. I'm so sorry." Tears streamed down his face as he held her. In his mind, he was beating himself up, over the pain he had caused her.

In one obtuse moment, of unbridled passion, I made her relive that terrifying day. It had taken her a long time before she had opened up to me, and told me about that day, with all of the horrific details.

As I listened to her unburden herself and tell me what that malefactor had done to her, my mind made the connection. The description of the physical trauma that she had suffered coincided with the night that I was awakened with the pain in my chest and the cut on my lip. I couldn't tell her about my experience, as I didn't fully understand it myself. We hadn't even met then, but it confirmed my belief now that our souls were bound to each other. Each of us pledged to one another centuries ago, destined to find each other time after time. That's the only explanation I can come up with to justify her pain manifesting itself in me.

No matter how well she tries to hide it, I always know what she's feeling. Sometimes the sensations are delayed by a few hours, but they always appeared. Even when she had the miscarriage I could feel her pain. Not nearly as intense as what she went through, but I knew exactly where her pain was. That's why I have to protect her. I can't bear to feel her suffer in any way.

I had put it all out of my mind. She had told me that she had dealt with her feelings, and had moved on, but her scars weren't healed yet, and it is my fault for clawing them open again. I wouldn't blame her if she rejected my love and companionship. She will need time to trust me again; but I will wait, no matter how long.

Repositioning herself in his embrace, Sabrina wiped the tears from her face. She could see the sorrow on his face, and the faint trace of tears in his eyes. "Sabrina I'm." Her fingers pressed gently against his lips, stopping him from saying anything else. She took another moment before speaking to him.

Mark agonized over what she would say. *Anger will be her most logical response and I'm prepared for that.* He was not prepared for what she did say. "You have nothing to be sorry about," she said, in a calm voice. "Yes, I do! It's my fault, what I did. I made you remember. If I had kept control, then this would never have happened. I don't know what came over me. I have no explanation for what I did, but I am truly sorry for hurting you."

He was very much surprised to feel the softness of her lips against his cheek, instead of the burning sting of her hand. Something he felt he deserved more than her tenderness. Reaching for his hand, she held it to her bare breast. "What came over you, and me, is called passion, pure unadulterated passion. Yes, it is the first time that we both have been so aggressive, and I was not prepared for the outcome. I love you, with all my heart; and I know that you would never intentionally hurt me. I really thought that I had buried that day forever; but obviously not."

"We're going home. Screw this show, and the tour; I'm taking you home." "No, Mark, the last thing I need is to be locked away with my thoughts. I want to be here. I need to be here, now, with you. I need something that I can be involved in, something to keep my mind busy, but we are going to have to be careful." "What do you mean?" "I mean, that when we make love, it will have to be slow and caring; not aggressive and forceful, not for a while anyway." "Maybe we should just abstain."

Sabrina felt her eyes moisten with tears. "Don't you want to make love to me?" The very words were being choked in her throat. As soon as he had said it, he realized that he had hurt her, again. "Of course I want you; I love you. I just thought that maybe you should take some time." "No. I don't want to even think about not being able to make love to you. I need your strength; your love, now more than ever." She kissed him; pushing his shirt open; their bodies came together. Leaning back in his arms, her eyes beckoning him to come to her, as he eased her down. "Are you sure?" he asked. "Yes, I'm very sure."

Looking into her blue eyes, he could see the love radiating from them; it warmed his soul. She cradled his face in her hands, tenderly drawing him closer to her, until she was able to kiss him, yet detecting some resistance from him. "What's wrong?" she asked.

Mark's eyes drifted to her bare chest. Her breasts were so round and perfect, her nipples hard and inviting. For the first time he saw the faint, tiny scars left from her attack, his gut tightened into a knot. Sabrina repeated her question. Mark sighed. "This just isn't right. It's not the right place. You deserve comfort, not the cold, hard floor of a locker room. We don't have to stay until the end of the show; we can leave right after my match."

Pushing herself up, she leaned against the wall. "If you feel better about waiting, then we'll wait. As long as you're happy, that's all that matters to me." Mark brought her to him. "You know, that's just part of why I love you so much. No matter how bad you hurt, or how inconvenienced you get, you still put other people's feelings before your own. Your compassion for others is remarkable, and I promise you, that tonight, all of your needs are going to be fulfilled completely."

"Maybe, maybe not." "No, damn it! There are no maybes about it. Tonight you and your needs will come first. You will always come first. My career, my life, they're meaningless unless you're happy and safe. I would quit this circus in a heartbeat if it meant I was able to stay with you and do nothing but tend to you and your needs."

He stared at her intently, causing a deep grove to form along his forehead. "Oh Mark, the one thing I could never fault you for is caring. I don't know why I am so privileged to have you in my life but I am grateful for each and every day. I cherish everything you do and say. I love you."

Moving her hand gently across his forehead she smoothed away the worry lines before she softly nuzzled her face against his. "I have a surprise for you, back at the hotel," she whispered, her sultry voice was fanning the flame inside him. "Surprise!" he said suddenly, getting to his feet. "I have a surprise for you."

Taking off his shirt, he put it around her and helped her up. "What have you done now?" she asked following him across the room. Mark kept quiet as he pawed through his bag. Finding the package he handed it to Sabrina. "What is this?" "Open it and find out."

I like getting presents. When I was younger presents were only received on birthdays, and Christmas. Never did I receive anything just because somebody felt like it, but Mark is different, and if he had picked this out for me, then it has to be great.

She quickly opened the package to reveal the shiny black garment within. Holding it up, she gazed upon the long black gown. "Well, what do you think?" he asked, his anticipation was overflowing. "It's beautiful; I love it." "I had it made to go with the robe." Sabrina stared at him with a puzzled frown. "So tell me, what is the point of my wearing this under the robe, if it's not going to be seen?" "Yeah it will; it'll be seen by me." "Oh you are so bad; so very, very bad," she said as she kissed his eager lips.

Restraining myself isn't easy, but I know that I have to; for her. "I have to start getting ready, and so should you," he said holding her away from him. "There's a room over there that you can use." She didn't understand why she was being sent away but she respected his wishes. Collecting her things, she gave him a quick kiss before she left the room.

I hate to exclude her, but I need the solitude to prepare myself for the match. Performing the same ritualistic routine before every show; carefully laying out his costume in the order that he put it on. Mark focused his attentions on his opponent's strengths, and more importantly his weakness. He had the advantage tonight, he knew whom he would be facing in the ring, but his opponent did not. It was important to Mark, and to the fans, that his return be kept secret. Since tonight's show was being televised, it would electrify the crowd and really get them pumped for the second half of the show.

It hadn't been an easy road for him over the years; he had been injured several times, the tattoos covering the scars on his arms. Liking the look of the body art, he continued to get more and more tattoos, until they had nearly covered both arms. He had become addicted to the ink, and the art. It had become a symbolic statement of his life; tortured by personal demons.

Looking at his arms in the mirror, he tried to find an appropriate spot where he could have another tattoo placed, one that symbolized his union with, and his love for, Sabrina. *I can't hide it on my chest, or my back; it has to be visible, a declaration for all to see, of my devotion to her. Maybe I could persuade her to get one as well, but I won't pressure her into it.*

Sabrina fixed her hair, and touched on some make up. *I want to be sure that I look good for Mark.* Stripped down to her thong, she stood looking at her reflection in the mirror, liking what she saw. Holding the gown up against her, she noticed that it had considerable stretch to it. Wiggling and pulling, she finally got the dress in place. It fit were it touched, but it was comfortable.

Being strapless, she moved it about until it rested low on her breasts. Across her stomach, sewn in red and silver leather strips was the symbol of the Warlock; the letter W, made of four silver swords. The blades of which, turned from silver to red part way down, making them appear as if blood were draining from them.

The dress had two slits in the front, that ran from the hem at her ankles, all the way up to her hip bones. *Good thing I wore a thong.* The back hem of the dress was much lower than the front and dragged upon the floor behind her. *I feel sexy, very sexy; with this outfit I could make love to Mark and never have to get undressed. I'm glad that I have the robe to wear over top, wearing this alone, in front of people, would make me so nervous.* She wrapped the robe around her and fastened the Velcro down the front. She quietly opened the door; Mark didn't see her, but she watched him intently.

He was dressed in black tights, and a long sleeve black shirt; his long hair loose, and wet around his shoulders; the sight was an instant turn on. *His powerful form so perfectly defined by his outfit.* It made her shudder. Mark was beginning to tuck in his shirt as she came up behind him.

"Can I help?" she asked slipping her hands around his waist, moving them slowly down the front of his tights. He seized her hands before they moved to low. "No, but thank you." She was standing directly behind, and that made only her arms visible to him in the mirror. "Let me see how your outfit looks," he said turning around. "What's with the robe? Doesn't the dress fit?" "Oh it fits." "Well then, let me see."

With a smile, and a hint of a laugh, she began undoing the Velcro tabs. "I should have some music to go with this," she chuckled. "I can fix that." Moving to a panel on the wall he pushed a couple of buttons and music filtered into the room. "Is that better?" Mark asked. She snickered to herself. *Even though we're alone, I'm still embarrassed.* "I'm waiting," he said, folding his arms across his chest, his face lacking any expression.

Sabrina closed her eyes for a moment. The music permeated her brain, the beat taking control of her body. Keeping her eyes trained on Mark as she undone the robe, watching his reaction; she slid the robe around her shoulders, exposing one and then the other. Mark had moved closer to her, but still his arms were folded, his expression solemn. Frustrated, that she hadn't even raised a smile from him, she dropped the robe to the floor. "Oh to hell with it!" Still facing Mark, she put her hands on her hips, glaring back at him, a sarcastic tone in her voice. "Well!" Mark's jaw fell open, his arms limp at his sides; he had to sit down.

Pleased with his reaction she moved closer to him and raised her foot up onto the bench beside him. Raising her leg up made the dress fall away from her thigh. "So what do you think?" Sabrina asked. Mark swallowed hard, forcing his heart back into his chest. "My God; it's even better than I imagined." "Then it meets with your approval?" "Very much!" Sabrina lifted his hands. "Come here," she said softly.

His knees felt weak, but he managed to stand, holding her against him for support. His tights were thin, like her dress. She could feel him pressing against her, hard. "Would you like me to wear this back to the hotel?" she asked, wetting her lips, in a sensual way, that made him crazy with desire. "Would you?" Was all he could say.

She could feel his heart beating fast. Sliding her hands down his back she brought him even closer; biting at her bottom lip, waiting for him to make the next move. He kissed her, a long, passionate, lover's kiss, that made her spine turn to jelly. "You're really gonna make me wait, aren't you?" she asked breathlessly. "I don't want to; but I have to; it's nearly time for my match," he explained, letting her go. Mark had no sooner said it, when there was a knock at the door. A faint voice on the other side called, "Fifteen minutes," and then there was silence again.

Mark picked up her robe and place it around her. "It's show time." "I'm still not quite sure what you want me to do?" "It's really easy. My music will begin playing; you go through the curtain and take a few steps onto the platform. Stop and wait; I'll follow behind in a few seconds. Then proceed down the ramp to the ring, but not to fast. If you turn to your left you will see a set of stairs; climb them to the ring, enter and wait for me. There might be some pyro set off, so try not to panic; it won't be near you. Once that's over with, I'll tell you when to help me with my robe. Take it and leave the ring at the opposite corner. Wait there until the match is over. That's all there is to it."

Butterflies swarmed in her stomach. "That's all; I don't know if I can remember it." "Sure you can. It's not like you haven't been out there before." "I know, but." "Don't worry; you'll be fine." Another knock at the door, "Five minutes," called the mystery voice. Mark picked up his robe. It was black, with a bright red lining, and his Warlock symbol emblazoned on the back. She watched as he fasten it around himself; her stomach was in knots. "You'll be fine," he reassured her.

She couldn't tell if the butterflies were causing her nerves to be on edge, or whether it was her intuition. *There is still something about tonight that just doesn't sit right.* Mark paced the length of the dressing room, waiting for the knock at the door, to let him know that it was time, but he was actually trying to walk off the foreboding feeling that gnawed at his gut.

Sean had hidden himself in the shadows, near the stage entrance. With all of the excitement of the show, no one had noticed him disappear into the darkness. *Mark's turn is coming up soon, and I'll be ready for him.* His heart pounded with the anticipation. *I have waited a long time for this.* He ran his plan over and over in his mind. *I'll let Mark get into the ring; let him have his few seconds of glory, and then I'll strike. This isn't going to be a wrestling match; this is going to be an all out fight.* Sean wiped the sweat from his hands and waited.

Brent paced around the backstage area; he had been unable to find Sean, and every one he asked said that they hadn't seen him. *I know he's here, but where damn it, where? It worries me to think about what Sean might do, when he finds out that Mark is here, with Sabrina. I know I said that I didn't want to get involved but I just can't stand by and watch. There is gonna be an explosion of anger tonight and I can't sit back and watch Sabrina get caught in it. The way Sean has changed over the past few weeks makes me think that there is more to this than just a failed relationship, and with Mark in this mix now, I don't even want to think about how extreme Sean could get. I've seen his anger before and when he's like that no one is safe.*

Tony and D'arcy emerged through the curtain; they had been paired together for a match. Brent motioned to them. "Have either of you guys seen Sean lately?" "No man. We haven't seen him since early this afternoon," Tony answered. "So what's up?" "Nothing I hope," Brent replied, still scanning the backstage area. "Look I can't go into details, but I need you guys to hang around here, and keep your eyes peeled for Sean. If you see him, we gotta stop him from going to the ring during the next match." "Why?" Tony queried.

Brent became more agitated with the questions. "Look I don't have time for this bullshit! If you see Sean, we gotta stop him from doing something really stupid. I'll explain it all later, then you'll understand. Just trust me."

The entrance music for the Warlock began to play. "Hey, Mark's back," D'arcy announced. "Yeah, there he is," Tony pointed down the hall. "Where? Where is he? Did you see Sean?" Brent snapped at them, his eyes darting back and forth. "No, we didn't. Christ, would you lighten up!" D'arcy barked. Tony continued to point. "Who's that with Mark?" "Beats me; new twist to the act probably," D'arcy offered. The three men watched as Mark, and his companion, walked past them, towards the curtain. Tony and D'arcy focused on the monitor, while Brent continued his visual search for Sean.

From his unseen vantage point, Sean saw Mark approach the curtain. He barely noticed the robed figure that walked with him. The screams from the fans in the arena were deafening. Mark passed through the curtain and the noise intensified. Sean was numb to it. His adrenaline rush blocked out all but his own rage. Sean knew Mark's ring routine very well, and he had already selected the exact moment when he would strike. As Mark entered the ring a series of pyro explosions went off. The smoke drifted in Sean's direction, offering him the ideal cover.

Leaving his hiding place, Sean moved along the side of the ramp, that stretched from the entrance stage to the ring. His movements were unnoticed by even the fans. From his new vantage point, he watched, as Mark's attendant helped to remove his robe and then leave the ring. Mark faced his fans on each side and then, turning his back, acknowledged the fans at the end of the ring. Sean's heart pounded; his moment was here. Jumping up he ran as fast as he could to the ring, sliding in under the bottom rope.

Catching Mark completely by surprise, Sean's forceful punch in the lower back sent Mark rushing forward into the ropes. Turning around quickly, Mark expected to see his opponent. "Sean, what the hell are you doing?" "As if you didn't know, you son of a bitch! You got balls, trying to take her away from me!" Sean began throwing more punches. Mark was still unprepared as Sean's fist landed hard on his face. In seconds, the two men were locked in mortal combat; much to the delight of the fans.

Tony, D'arcy and Brent had been watching the monitor, until they became distracted by a fight that had broken out near them between two other wrestlers. Trying to pull the fight apart caused them to ignore what was happening in the ring.

Sabrina was frantic. Sean's punches had been striking Mark with cruel voracity, and now rivers of blood streamed over his face from open wounds on his cheek and forehead. She looked toward the curtain. *No one's coming to stop this!* Climbing back into the ring, she tried to pull Sean away from Mark, but her size hindered her attempts. Sean wielded another blow and Mark staggered backwards. In an act of desperation, Sabrina stepped in front of Sean, using herself as a shield.

Brent heard the screams and cheers from the fans; but it didn't sound quite right. Turning to the monitor, he saw Sean grab Sabrina, tossing her aside like a rag doll. He took off running towards the ring, calling to Tony and D'arcy to follow him. Sabrina had barely hit the mat when Sean was back to attacking Mark. Dragging herself up, she made another feeble attempt to pull Sean away, but it was useless; she didn't have the power. Sean pushed her aside again.

Brent hit the ring, followed closely by the other two. It took their combined strength to pull Sean back, and restrain him. He struggled wildly, but they held him fast. Sabrina crawled to Mark. His face was smeared with blood, as were his hands. He rested against the ropes for support; his breathing labored from the bruise on his ribs.

"Are you okay?" she asked, frantic with worry. Mark nodded, to winded to speak. Sabrina rose and turned to Sean, her robe still intact, the hood still concealing her face. She stared at Sean, as he struggled to break free of the arms that bound him; all the time still screaming at Mark. "You son of a bitch, I'll teach you! You don't mess with me you fucking bastard!"

I've heard enough! Without a second thought, she raised her hand and slapped Sean across the face. The force spun his head sideways. "What the hell are you doing?" he yelled, spitting blood from his mouth. Raising her hands to her head, she pulled the hood back. Sean's expression of anger dissipated. "Sabrina?" "Yes, Sean, it's me." "I knew it; I knew that you'd come back to me!" Tears glistened in his eyes. Sabrina kept her voice steady, even though inside she was quaking. "No Sean, you're wrong, very wrong. My life is with Mark, not you."

That wasn't what he wanted to hear. He struggled again. Freeing one arm, he grabbed at her, catching only her robe as she stepped back. "You're mine!" Fearful of him, Sabrina pulled away quickly. Her robe came undone, she was free of his grasp.

A volley of whistles emanated from the audience, as she was exposed to the world. Sabrina paid it no attention. She was at Mark's side; her arm around him; helping him to stand up. D'arcy and Tony muscled Sean out of the ring, still screaming and fighting. "This isn't over you bastard; I'll get you!" Brent picked up Sabrina's robe and offered his assistance to Mark; who took it without resistance.

The paramedics were waiting for them when they cleared the curtain. The shock of what had happened was beginning to set in; Sabrina began to shake. Brent wrapped the robe around her; resting his arm across her shoulders for comfort. The paramedics wiped away the blood on Mark's face, and dressed his wounds. Sean's blows had produced several wide cuts on his forehead and jaw, not bad enough for stitches, but effective enough to make Sabrina feel ill. Her heart was breaking to see him hurt, and in pain. *All I want to do is to hold him and have him hold me.*

"Better let the medics have a look at you," Brent said. "What? No, I'm fine." "I don't think so; you were limping," he replied, signaling one of the paramedics to them. Seeing the paramedic go to Sabrina made Mark squirm in his seat. He wanted to go to her, but they weren't finished with him, and he was unable to see what they were doing to her.

Sabrina conceded to Brent's request; her hip was hurting more than she wanted to admit. Looking down, she could see the large, red area that covered her leg, from her hip to mid thigh. Through the red, the beginning of a bruise was forming. The paramedic determined that other than a bad case of mat burn she would be fine. He handed her an ice pack to put on it.

Mark implored the paramedics to hurry up with what they were doing. *I have to be with her.* With the last bandage in place he pushed past them. She fell into his arms, holding him tight, hiding her sudden burst of tears. Her body trembled violently against him. He hugged her tighter. "Let's get out of here," he said. Sabrina pulled back slightly, wiping her face. "Please; I don't want to be here anymore." "I'll go with you," Brent interrupted.

Mark looked at him somewhat confused. Catching the glance, Brent tried to explain. "Look man, Sean's already gone, but he's staying at the same hotel, and just in case the guys can't keep him in control, that's why I'm offering to go with you." Mark nodded his acceptance of the offer. *At least I have some allies.* They didn't need any unexpected confrontation, given Mark's weakened condition; the results could be disastrous.

The hotel room was a welcomed sight. Sabrina disappeared into the bathroom, but quickly returned, wearing a bathrobe. Mark grabbed a beer from the small fridge, and tossed one to Brent, before asking Sabrina if she wanted one. She readily accepted, and drank nearly half of it before stopping for a breath. The entire event had upset her. *I know that alcohol isn't the answer, but it does in a small way help to settle my frayed nerves.*

Careful of her hip, she eased herself onto the couch, tenderly rubbing her hand over the sorest point. Mark took a seat beside her. Bruises were becoming visible around the bandages on his face. His lip was slightly swollen and grazed. She carefully kissed his cheek. He put his arm around her. *I need her close to me tonight.*

"How do you feel?" he asked. "I'm fine; a little sore, but otherwise fine," she kept her leg covered. "What about you?" "I'm good. I know it looks bad, but it isn't. Believe me; I've had worse." Sabrina snuggled against his shoulder, but cast her gaze to Brent, who was sitting across from them. "Would you mind telling me just what the hell happened tonight!"

It seems as if she's demanding me to give her a reasonable explanation. Brent shifted in his seat; very uncomfortable with her question, and unsure of how, or where to begin.

Trying to avoid her eyes, he became locked onto Mark's. "She asked you a question," Mark said. Brent felt Mark's eyes burning into him. "Oh man, you're really putting me on the spot. I didn't want to be the one to tell you, but considering what happened tonight, I guess I really don't have a choice."

Brent got up and began pacing in front of the window. "Over the past few weeks Sean has, well, changed. He's not the same man that we all knew. He's become sloppy in the ring, incredibly rude, and angry towards everyone. He won't talk to, or associate with any of us. He's become a recluse; and nobody could figure out why."

Stopping briefly, he observed Sabrina's face for any indication that she understood what it was he was trying to say; her face was blank. Brent took a deep breath and continued. "Since Sean refused to talk to any of us, I tried to figure it out on my own, but only after I saw you together. I had to go all the way back to when Sean first started bringing you to the matches, Sabrina. He was so happy then, full of life, and he was unbeatable in the ring. Then, after the barbecue, when he returned to the tour and you didn't, because he said you were ill, that's when he started to change."

Again he paused, searching for some sign of recognition; but again he saw nothing. "Now, we all know that Sean is, well, a collector, of women, and he doesn't stay alone for very long; but when he came back, not even Robbie could hold his attention for very long. I didn't give it much thought; but when you, Mark, took that leave of absence, that's when I think Sean put it together. Somehow, he must have confirmed his suspicions about you two, and that pushed him over the edge completely. His only goal, right now, Mark, is to take you out anyway he can." Brent sat back down, awaiting for their reaction.

Sabrina laid her head back and stared at the ceiling. "It's all my fault," she sighed. "No, it's not," Brent said, quickly cutting her off. "Sean is like a spoiled child. He doesn't like to lose; in the ring or out." "If I had only sat down and told him that it was over, maybe this would never have happened."

"No way; it would never work. Look, I've know Sean for a very long time, and I know for certain, that he would have reacted the same way," he paused to carefully select his next statement. "I don't mean to be cruel Sabrina, but you were just another temporary plaything for him. What's pissed him off the most, I think, is that you dumped him, and not the other way around. He has never had a woman walk away from him before; let alone walk into the arms of one of his rivals."

Mark stayed quiet, listening to what Brent had to say. *I know the real truth, and I pray, for Sabrina's sake, that it will never have to be told. It's a relief to have Brent reaffirm everything that I've all ready told her about Sean.*

"So what you're saying is that Sean is gonna come after Mark every chance he gets," Sabrina said, the sound of distress in her voice was very evident. Brent was about to continue when Mark cut him off. "If Sean wants a fight, then he'll get one. It seems quite obvious that he's beyond talking. So if he wants to settle this in the ring, then so be it."

Sabrina clutched at him firmly. "No! I don't want you to fight him and risk getting hurt!" "I love you; and I will fight for you. If that's what it will take to make Sean understand, then I have no other choice." No longer able to restrain her tears; and with nowhere to run, she fell upon the bed, hiding her sobs in the pillow. Brent moved towards the door. "I gotta go; she needs you man. Just so you know; Tony, D'arcy and I, well, we'll watch your back, and hers, if you need us." Mark extended his hand to Brent. "Thanks man, I appreciate it. We both do."

D'arcy and Tony had stayed with Sean, finally getting him calmed down enough, that he had stopped his pacing and yelling. Sean's jaw hurt from where Mark's fist had struck him. He could feel the swelling with his fingers. D'arcy had never seen Sean so angry, or so violent as he was tonight. *Risking another outburst, I've got to find out exactly what's going on.*

"Sean, I would like you to tell me what the hell is going on with you. You look like hell, and lately your attitude towards everyone really sucks. So what gives? Why did you attack Mark?" Rising suddenly, Sean moved right in front of D'arcy. "Why don't you go straight to hell!" Sean yelled. Tony quickly intervened. "Damn it Sean, if you don't snap out of this you're gonna lose your job." "It's none of your fucking business!"

D'arcy grabbed Sean by the arm, spinning him around. "You made it our business, when you pulled that stunt tonight! Christ, Sean you could have really hurt him." "That was the whole idea! That bastard is gonna pay for what he's done!" "What about Sabrina?" Tony added. "Did you plan on hurting her too?"

Sean stopped his pacing again. Remorse flooded his body. "Of course not! I would never hurt her." "Well, you did," D'arcy added, making the reality of his actions set in even further. Sean sat back down, his face in his hands. "Is she hurt very bad?" "I honestly don't know," D'arcy answered. Sitting down beside Sean, he had to force himself to stay calm. "Sean, I don't know what has happened between you two, but from my observations, Sabrina has chosen to be with Mark and you're gonna have to accept it." "I'll never accept it. Not until I have all the answers."

"Answers to what?" Tony asked. "I need to know what he did to her; to make her betray me; to lie to me. I need to know why she didn't tell me about," Sean stopped himself, his grief overwhelming him. "Tell you about what?" D'arcy asked. Sean began pacing again. D'arcy again prodded him for an answer. "What didn't she tell you?"

"She didn't tell me that she was going to have a baby, my baby! I have to know why she didn't tell me!" D'arcy and Tony were both stunned by Sean's announcement. "Sabrina's pregnant?" "Not anymore, she lost the baby and she didn't even tell me," Sean said, slumping onto the couch. Silence permeated the room as the trio reflected on the contents of the conversation.

The sound of Sabrina's muted sobs broke Mark's heart. He sat down beside her, rubbing her back; lost for the right words to comfort her. Sabrina turned over, raising herself up. He pulled her into his arms, cradling her against him. "I love you Sabrina." "I don't want you to fight Sean," she said, her eyes pleading with his. "Maybe if I talk to him, I can make him understand." "I don't think you should do that. He's obviously not in control of his actions, and I don't want you to get caught up in a situation that you might not be able to handle." "Then what are we going to do? It will be next to impossible to avoid him, since he's obligated to the same tour as you."

"That is not something you need to worry about; right now you need to get a good night's sleep. We will deal with Sean one day at a time; together." He pulled back the sheets on the bed. "Now get into bed." "What about you, aren't you coming to bed?" "In a minute, I want to wash up first." Sabrina's robe fell to the floor. Mark tried not to stare, but the bruise on her hip covered a large area. She saw the look. "It's not that bad, really," she said.

He continued on his way to the bathroom, his mind working hastily. *This problem with Sean is far from over; but protecting Sabrina, is the only priority, at any cost.*

Slipping into bed beside her, he snuggled up close. Offering his arm, as a support for her neck, his other hand glided over her silky body. Remembering his promise, to make her feel special tonight, but after the events of the evening, it would be best for both of them if they abstained tonight. Sabrina flinched when he touched her hip. "It still hurts?" "Just a bit," she answered, pulling his arm around her like a blanket. "I still think that I should try to talk to Sean." "I'll hear no more about it tonight; just go to sleep and forget about it." He kissed the back of her head, securing his hold on her, and silently declaring his oath to keep her safe.

The tour progressed slowly, taking them on a weaving pattern through the eastern states; fortunately, without any further incidents with Sean. Mark had arranged with the owner to have all of his future schedules altered, so that there wouldn't be any chance of a conflict with Sean, but the owner had all ready taken care of that. Sean had been suspended for causing the fight. He still traveled with the company, but he was denied access to any of the arena's during his suspension; being kept occupied with autograph sessions and promo stops.

Mark had always been a loner. Keeping to himself when he was on tour, and even now, he didn't make many exceptions. Being with Sabrina was the only company that he needed. The other wrestlers knew from experience that it was a hopeless venture to try and engage him in a conversation, so they kept their distance. Only on rare occasions, did he associate with them; but only when his own loneliness had become unbearable.

Sabrina had settled into a routine with Mark and was becoming more at ease in the ring. The fans had come to accept her; and inside, she secretly liked the cheers and whistles that were sent her way. Mark never said anything about it; as far as he was concerned she was there for safety. Keeping her close to him, close to the ring was the only way he could protect her. Their unique and special bond was growing stronger with each passing day.

Chapter 11

The schedule of show dates became tighter, as one tour led into another. Mark and Sabrina had been on the road now for nearly two months, without a real break and not enough time in between shows to go home for a good rest. Yet they still managed to find time to do things away from the confinement of hotel rooms and arenas. It wasn't easy to blend into a town that was promoting a show, but they managed. Stealing precious moments together, like a walk in a park, or even a little shopping, all was time well spent.

During the course of the tour, the show landed in Boston. Mark and Sabrina had arrived a day early, which gave them the opportunity to get away from the city for a while. Driving along the coast brought them to the town of Salem; a place that Sabrina had secretly desired to visit.

Walking around the old buildings and museums was a delight. Exploring the history of this town was equally intriguing as it was mystifying. Their journey took them away from the busy main streets, into an older section of town, where they came upon a very old house, weathered by time, yet it still had presence. Demanding that all who gazed upon it did so with reverence; and fear.

The iron gate squeaked in the wind, its mournful cry chilling. The land around the house was dead, barren and empty. Nothing but death and hatred grew behind the stone walls that surrounded this dark fortress. The darkness around this house was guarding the secrets that were contained within, forbidding those who stopped to gaze upon it, from learning the truth. The real truth that was secretly guarded, not the truth as recounted by history books.

Strange feelings came over Sabrina, as she stared at this relic. The whispers kept telling her that she had been here before, but this was her first visit to the town. The gloom, and despair, that emanated from this edifice unnerved her.

This house gives off an intense feeling of death. I can feel the waves of sadness. It must be my imagination, tricking me; making me hear sounds. The mournful cries of women tormented and tortured, the unearthly sounds of unspeakable acts of unending horror, done in the name of justice, and truth, and in the name of the Church.

They had returned in multitude. The voices of the old ones who refused to move on, taunting Sabrina's mind, making her relive the agony and the pain once again. They had always been with her, the voices of the past, but she had learned to force herself to ignore most of them, but they always came to her with a purpose, even if she didn't understand their persistent pleas.

She could no longer ignore them this day; the sounds screamed in her head, the souls of all those tormented women, crying out for redemption, calling out to their God for mercy and salvation, to at last bring a swift end to this misery.

I know nothing of the history of this house, or do I? Have I been here before? Had my soul once been trapped within the walls of this dark, menacing fortress, only to be finally freed, when death came to release me from my tormentors? But there was little comfort in death, not in this place.

The pain still lingered deep in her soul, traveling with her to each life. This was a memory that would not be abolished by time, or by love. It was forever to be a part of her past, her present and her future.

Mark had left her standing near the gate, while he wandered over to read a monument that stood nearby. When he turned, to call her to him, fear overcame him. She was still standing at the gate; her hands were drawn up in front of her. Partly bent forward, she rocked slowly, weeping in despair. There was a look of hopelessness on her face. He went to her, taking her hands. Her wrists were red, from where she had been unconsciously rubbing them. *It looks as if she has been bound by ropes.*

It took him several minutes to bring her back to him. She never spoke, but clung to him for protection. He never questioned her about the incident, afraid of what he might learn. *Somehow she is bound to this town, and not in a pleasant way. I can wait for her to tell me but I don't really want to know.*

I'm so grateful that Mark didn't press me for answers; I have no answer to give. The feelings, so strong and unnerving, have to be carefully sorted out before I can even begin to understand them myself. They became clearer that night, haunting her dreams, making her reject Mark. Leaving him alone at her side, unable to help her, as she relived the agonizing moments of that time in vivid detail.

The tour began taking them back in the direction of California, and home. *We've been gone so long. I feel so guilty for having left Patches at a kennel. I wish it would end soon and I could go home to the beach house; back to the silence and the solitude. The lease will need to be renewed soon, and a decision will have to be made, as to whether I continue to lease it month by month, or give it up completely.*

The choice is so hard. Mark has made no mention of his plans after the tour ends. I wish that I knew where I stand. Will I continue to be a part of his life, or will he let me simply disappear into the shadows? I know that he loves me, he gave me a ring, but is it a real commitment? She cogitated over it many times, but no clear answers sprang forth.

The tour had finally brought them back to Las Vegas, a full day before the show, giving them each enough time to recover from the jet lag, but rest was not on the agenda for her. Sabrina's energy level soared the minute the plane landed. She tried to maintain mastery of her excitement, but upon arriving at their hotel room she could no longer contain herself. She loved the excitement of Vegas, and she wanted to be out in it. Rushing to Mark, she knocked him off balance; they both fell upon the bed, her legs tightly embracing his hips.

"What is with your today?" he asked. "We're in Las Vegas; the city that never sleeps, where fun and excitement await you at every corner." "You sound like an ad for this place." "Oh Mark, I want to do something, something different, something daring and exciting. You've been here before; take me somewhere, please." "Sabrina we just got in and I'm a bit tired." "Oh please, just for a little while."

Mark pulled her down onto her back, pinning her in place with his long leg. "I would much rather stay here, and play," he said, toying with the buttons on her blouse. "There's plenty of time for that. We don't have to be out long, and then we can come back here and play all night." Her voice was hot and sexy and it made him weak. *She knows just what to do to control me.*

"Okay, okay, you win." "Oh thank you," she answered beaming with excitement. He rolled away from her, to the other side of the bed, where he picked up the phone. "What are you doing now?" "Well, you said that you wanted to do something really different; daring and exciting. Well then, that is just what you're gonna get." "What is it? What's your idea?" "No questions; you'll have to just trust me." The excitement was unbearable;

waiting as patiently as she could while Mark made his phone call; listening for any clue as to what he was planning.

"Hey man, it's Warlock. Not bad; listen, can you hook me up for later today. Sounds good; I'll be bringing someone with me. Good, see you then." *I learned nothing from this one sided conversation, but it doesn't matter anyway.* "You ready?" he asked. Bubbling with anticipation she bounced into his arms. "Sure am," she answered. He spun her around. "You won't forget this day," he said. "And you won't forget this night either," she said softly. Her eyes sparkled with love, resisting her was impossible. He kissed her, and she melted against him.

In the lobby, she scanned the casino; eager to play. Sensing her anxiety Mark parked her on a stool in front of a slot machine. "Don't go away; I'll be right back," he said, handing her two rolls of quarters. "Where are you going?" "I need to take care of something. I won't be long."

She played intently, only stopping briefly, when a machine in her row paid off. Her own luck was not as favorable. She was down to her last five quarters when Mark returned. "How are you doing?" he asked. "Not so good, but I think I figured out why." "You just realized that these things are rigged," he smiled. "No silly; I mean that I didn't have you with me. Hey, it works for you, when I'm with you in the ring, so why wouldn't it work for me now."

Mark shook his head. *There is some truth to what she says, my career has been on an upswing since she has been with me.* "Oh come on; I've got enough for one more play. What could it hurt?" She bit her lip and pouted; that look he could never refuse. "Why not," he conceded.

Leaning over he kissed her hard, his arm supporting her, as she leaned back. Licking her lips, their faces still close together, she looked into his eyes. "I don't know about this machine, but I can guarantee that you're gonna get lucky tonight." "Play the game; we have to get going soon."

Mark straightened up. Sabrina took his hand and deposited her coins. Squeezing his hand tight she pulled the arm of the slot machine. The wheels spun wildly. *I can't watch.* One by one she heard the wheels stop and lock into place. When the last one locked she felt Mark squeeze her hand, but before she could speak her ears were flooded with the loud sound of bells. She looked at the tray, but no coins had dropped out. *It must be another machine.*

Mark grabbed her into his arms. "You won!" Her eyes darted back to the machine. In the window, perfectly lined up, she saw three red number sevens. The lights on the top of the machine flashed; people began touching her with pats of congratulations, and hopes of getting some of her luck.

Mark kept a tight hold on her as the gaming attendant verified her win. "Congratulations Miss, you've won $5,000. Would you come with me please." They followed the man to the head cashier, where her win was verified, and authorized for pay out. The cashier counted out five packets of one hundred dollar bills. Sabrina was still overwhelmed. "What am I going to do with this? I didn't bring a purse." Mark asked the cashier for a zippered pouch. "We can put it in the hotel safe for now," he said, holding open the bag. She stuffed the bundles inside; taking some of the bills from the last packet and jamming them into her pocket. "You don't need that." "Yeah I do. I just might want to but something for my good luck charm," she said.

They stopped at the front desk and signed the pouch into the safe. "We have to get going," Mark announced. "Where are we going now?" "I don't know if it's going to be as exciting as this was, but I'm sure gonna try." He hooked her arm around his and escorted her out to the front of the hotel. No valet greeted them.

"Where is the car?" she asked. "There isn't one; we're taking that," he said, pointing to a motorcycle that rested near the curb. A rush of tingles covered her body as she eyed the magnificent machine; from the glistening chrome tail pipes to the elaborately painted gas tank. "You are truly incredible. How did you know that I always harbored a secret desire to be on the back of a bike?" "Come on, wrap your legs around and see how it feels."

The invitation is just too tempting. She curled her leg around Mark. "It feels pretty good to me." "Not me, the bike," he said, smiling at her imaginative flair. Still clinging to his side, her lips graced his neck with a kiss. "I still prefer your raw power between my legs over any machine." "Later; now get on the bike."

She waited for him to get on first. Then sliding in behind him, she cuddled up close locking her fingers together over his belt buckle. "There's still something missing in this picture," she said. "What would that be?" "I don't think my attire really goes with this bike." "What would you like to be wearing?" Mark asked even though his imagination had all ready provided him with an answer.

"Oh, I think something in black leather would do quite nicely." "I think I can fix that," he answered just before he started the bike. The twin exhausts exploded like thunder as he revved the engine. The sound attracted much attention as it echoed off of the building. *Mark has made so many of my dreams come true, and these unexpected surprises always thrill me.*

They toured past all the major casinos, stopping now and then to watch some of the outdoor performances put on by the larger hotels. It was hot in Vegas, it was only the beginning of June but summer seemed to be all year round, and the breeze created by the motion of the bike helped to cool her down on the outside. Mark turned the bike off of the main street and pulled up in front of a shop that catered to the biker crowd.

Walking into the store they were greeted by two sales people. A man with the stereotypical biker look, black jeans and a Harley T-shirt, stretched tight over his rotund belly, scruffy long graying beard and a multitude of tattoos. The other clerk was a woman, in her early twenties, not overly pretty, but a tremendous figure. She was dressed similar to the man but only her clothes fit much tighter, showing off her ample figure.

"Can we help you?" the woman asked. "Sure can; my lady needs an outfit. Something in black leather, and it's gotta be sexy; very sexy," Mark replied. Sabrina blushed as she turned to him. "Mark!" "Hey, don't look at me like that. You wanted the outfit, but I get final approval." "Come on girl," the young woman said, taking Sabrina's arm. "I've got the perfect outfit for you; one that will show off that terrific body of yours, and will most definitely please your man."

Mark wandered about the shop while he waited for Sabrina. He found a new jacket for himself, and surprisingly, a pair of jeans. His wait for Sabrina took forever. Finally the young woman returned from the back room; she looked straight at Mark. "She'll be out directly. She's a bit shy I think, but man, let me tell you that you had better grab hold of something, because when she does get out here, you're gonna be blown away."

Mark didn't know what to think. *Could it be possible for her to look better than she already does?* "Come on girl; get your ass out here; your man's waiting."

Sabrina took a deep breath. *I feel so awkward; but so sexy.* She stepped through the curtain, her eyes steadfast on Mark for his reaction. He was poised against the counter when she entered. His eyes widened at the sight before him, his heart pounding loud in his ears. She was wearing a pair of black leather chaps, with a black leather thong. A silver buckle lay against her belly, just below her naval; her shapely waist completely exposed.

Moving his eyes upward, he looked over the black leather halter top, that laced up the front. *It looks as if it's too small, since the laces don't allow the leather to meet.* Through the interwoven laces he could see the soft curves of her breasts; her hard nipples pressed against the cold leather.

His racing heart had begun to calm, until she turned around to give him the complete view. At that point he gripped the counter to keep himself standing. The chaps were cut away at the seat. Her firm, shapely buttocks framed by the leather. "Hey man, you better start breathing or we'll have to call the ambulance," the young woman said, giving him a slap on the shoulder.

Mark was breathless at the sight. Sabrina walked slowly toward him, her high heel boots clicking on the tile floor. "Does this meet with your approval?" Sabrina asked. Mark swallowed hard. "Oh yeah," he answered, pausing to take another breath. "We'll take it, but she's gonna need a jacket to go with it."

The young woman handed Sabrina her old clothes, and went to get a jacket that matched the one Mark had picked out for himself. Sabrina rifled through her jeans pocket and put her money on the counter; Mark pushed it back to her.

Not this time. Turning Mark to her she kissed him. He couldn't help giving in to her, the feeling of her body compressed against him, the fantasies that swirled in his mind consumed him. While she kept Mark occupied, Sabrina pushed the money back to the man behind the counter. The transaction was complete before Mark even knew what had happened.

Inside he was annoyed at how she had been able to trick him so easily, but he never let it show. *I know he's upset with me. His silence says more than he realizes. It makes me feel a whole lot worse.*

She watched him store the parcel into the saddlebags on the bike; when he was done she took his hands. "I'm sorry Mark; I just wanted to do something for you. You do so much for me; always buying me things. I needed to do this for you, because I love you." "I love you too, and taking care of you, and your needs is what I want to do. It's my job to provide for you."

Sabrina put her arms around him. "I love you so much. So, do you want to go back to the hotel and play?" Her sexy tone touched him deep inside, but he had to refrain. "Not yet," he said, getting onto the bike. "We have one more stop to make first." Sabrina got on behind. The bike seat was warm from the late afternoon sun. It took her a couple of tries before she could sit comfortably.

The sun was beginning to go down; the lights from the casinos beckoned to potential patrons. The outdoor displays of erupting volcanoes, and medieval tournaments attracted many people, who were just now coming back to life, after another hot day in the desert air. Mark stopped the bike along a side street that was dominated by adult entertainment stores. "What are we doing here?" Sabrina asked. "You'll see," Mark said taking her hand.

As they walked along she observed the reactions of the people they passed. Men whistled at her, while she heard some of the women call her unpleasant names. *Jealousy. They don't have the body, or the guts to wear this, so all they can do is insult someone who can, and does.*

Mark opened a shop door, the windows were painted black, nothing on the outside offered her a clue as to what was inside. She followed Mark in. They had entered a tattoo parlor. A man came out from a room at the back of the small shop. "Warlock, man it's good to see you again," he said, shaking Mark's hand. "It's been a while hasn't it. Harry, this is Sabrina. Sabrina, Harry. He's done all of my body art." "Nice to meet you Sabrina," he said, extending his hand. Sabrina shook it, surprised by how cold it was, but more intrigued by the tattoos that covered both of his arms, and parts of his hands.

"So Warlock, what can I do for you tonight?" "Well, Harry, I need something that will represent my love for Sabrina; but its gonna have to fit in with all the others." "And the lady, what would she like?" Harry was looking at Sabrina, but she was still processing what Mark had just said, and hadn't fully heard what Harry had asked. Mark gave her a nudge. "Harry asked you what tattoo you want." Without thinking, Sabrina blurted out her answer. "I want the mark of the Warlock." Mark was pleased with her answer. Harry directed them into a private room and seated them both.

Sabrina was suddenly struck by what she had said. *Getting a tattoo frightens me, but I can't back out now.* "I'll do yours first, Sabrina. Where do you want it?" Harry asked. She looked to Mark for an answer. "Shoulder,"

Mark said. She slipped off her jacket, while Harry made a quick sketch of the symbol. He prepared the area of her arm, and applied the transfer to it. Sabrina jumped when she heard the sound of the electric needle start up. Mark moved his chair in front of her and took her hands in his. "Look only at me," he said, in a calm, soothing voice.

She squeezed his hands as the needle began piercing her skin repeatedly. The stinging bite soon eased to a mild burning sensation. Within thirty minutes it was all over. Harry cleaned the area again and covered it with a bandage. Trading places with Sabrina, Mark settled back into the chair and waited for Harry to begin. Harry had no need to apply a transfer to Mark. He could do his free hand, as Sabrina was going to be the model.

After some time Sabrina began to fidget in her chair. "You can get up if you like," Harry said. She excused herself, and walked back out into the front of the parlor to look at all the tattoo patterns along the walls. *So many designs; some simple and others ornate and bold.* She rubbed at her arm below the bandage; it burned a little.

Over the buzz of the needle, she could clearly hear Mark's and Harry's voices. "Nice ass," Harry remarked. "Yeah," Mark replied with a smile. Harry's curiosity was getting to him. "So who is this lady anyway?" "She is the one and only love of my life Harry, the one and only." "Sure took you long enough Warlock; but you picked a good one." "Sure did, I've waited for her for a very long time, and it was well worth the wait." "Good for you; it's about time you thought about settling down, focusing on your personal future and not so much on your professional life." "I've been doing just that Harry. My future is right out there; with her."

Sabrina wandered back to the little room, and leaned against the doorway. The conversation quickly shifted direction. "You got your tickets for the show tomorrow?" Mark asked. "You bet I do; ringside, as always." "Great, then you'll get to see both of us in the ring." Mark smiled over at Sabrina. The look on her face suggested to him that she had heard their previous conversation. "There we go, all done." Harry wiped the area of Mark's arm with disinfectant and waited before putting on the bandage.

Mark always liked to see his new piece of art before it was covered. He went to the mirror. "Sabrina, come and see." She was amazed at what she saw. Harry had recreated her image onto Mark's arm. He had drawn her wearing the leather outfit, and even included the Warlock tattoo on her arm. Every detail was etched with such precise perfection, from the strands of hair to her hard nipples against the leather top, everything as perfect as a photograph.

"This is incredible," Sabrina said. "Harry is the best, no doubt about it." Bringing her closer to him, Mark looked at her with a slight smile. Sabrina saw the gleam in his eye. "What now?" she asked. "I was just wondering if there might be something else you would like to have done." "I don't need another tattoo yet." "I wasn't referring to that," Mark said, his smile growing slightly wider. "Then what?" "A piercing perhaps?" "Any suggestions as to what I should have pierced?" Sabrina asked. Without answering her, Mark stroked the tip of her breast with his finger.

The shock of his action jolted her spine erect and with wide eyes filled with astonishment she stared up at Mark. "We need to have a serious conversation," she said, trying to be stern but she couldn't shed her smile. "About what?" Mark asked. "About all those thoughts that are hiding in the dark corners of your mind." "They're not hiding; they're screaming to be let out." Pushing away from Mark, she headed for the door. Mark exchanged hasty good-byes with Harry and ushered Sabrina back to the bike. She leaned against him. "Now we're going back to the hotel, right?" she asked. "Most definitely."

The hotel was alive with patrons when they returned; the lobby and casino crowded with people. Mark deliberately kept their pace slower than normal as they passed through the masses. He was watching the reactions from the people as they looked at her. When they were finally alone in the elevator, Sabrina couldn't restrain herself any longer. By the time they had reached their floor, she had his shirt unbuttoned, and had loosened the belt on his jeans. Mark searched his pockets for the room key, when he finally found it and opened the door; they nearly fell into the room.

Sabrina was too preoccupied to notice the changes in the room. She was pushing Mark's jacket off as she backed into the room. "Oh good, it's here," he said, looking over her shoulder. "What's here?" "My last surprise of the night." She turned around quickly. Laid out on the table, was a light buffet, complete with champagne, but what caught her attention the most was the large bowl of fresh strawberries, and another bowl of whipped cream. A multitude of fantasies flooded her mind and she wanted to play them all out.

For a moment she slipped away from him. He watched her intently and could only imagine what was going through her mind. With her eyes closed and her head slightly tilted to one side, her tongue slowly licked at her full, sensuous lips. She emitted a soft breathy moan that turned his blood to fire. "Tell me what you're thinking about?" he asked as he nuzzled her ear. "I can't tell you yet, but you could get me a drink."

After a sip of champagne, Sabrina took his glass and set it on the table beside hers. Moving close to him, she kissed him tenderly, all the while pulling off his shirt. "You made me feel very special today; now it's my turn to make you feel special," she said guiding him to a chair. He began undoing the laces of her top; it fell away to the floor.

Her physical excitement, combined with the cool breeze from the air conditioner, hardened her nipples. Mark reached for a berry, then dipped it in the whipped cream. As he raised it toward her, he deliberately brushed it against her breast. The sensation of his tongue against her skin sent shock waves of ecstasy through her body. "More," she begged. Mark readily gave in to her less than subtle command, fulfilling both of their secret desires.

I like fore play, knowing that the inevitable result will be one of exemplary pleasure. During our time together he has become very skilled at knowing what to do to make me crazy with desire.

Mark worked loose the buckle on her chaps and they slid down her legs. She stepped out of them and kicked them aside. Mark began playing with the ties that held her thong in place, but before he had a chance to get them undone she sat astride his powerful thighs.

Dipping a berry in the cream, she teasingly fed it to him; slowly kissing away what remained on his lips. At her silent command, he raised up his hips, while she unzipped his jeans, freeing the power within. With her arms around his neck, their bodies pressed against each other; they kissed. Long, slow, passionate kisses. Mark caressed her body, carefully loosening the ties of her thong. Sliding it slowly off of her made her moan. He made a move to get up with her. "No, stay here," she whispered. Unable to wait any longer, she lifted herself up and took him in, moving slowly, letting him see the pleasure on her face.

They both enjoyed the slow, gentle pace of making love. The feeling of their bodies joined together as one, as their hearts and souls were joined, for all eternity. Sweat glistened on their bodies, as they approached their much anticipated climax. Mark supported her back, as the ecstasy made her arch away from him with waves of electrifying tremors.

Exhausted, she lay against him, her head resting on his shoulder, her hot breath panting against his neck. Mark reached for his shirt, beside the chair, and put it across her back, inadvertently bumping her shoulder. "Ouch!" "I'm sorry; it'll be better tomorrow," he said, kissing the top of her shoulder. "How does yours feel?" "It's okay; I don't even notice them anymore," he answered.

Sabrina snuggled closer to him. "So tell me, why should I get a nipple piercing?" she asked. "Forget it; it was just a stupid idea." "No, your suggestion had a purpose; I saw it in your eyes. Now tell me." "Forget it, really. Your body doesn't need any more improvements." "Excuse me?" Sabrina asked as she leaned back. Taking his hands she held them to her breasts. "These are real Mark; no implants or surgery." "Really?" Mark asked, astounded that such perfection could have occurred naturally. "Really," Sabrina answered as she lay back against him. "And as for your request, I will take it into consideration. This has been the best day; thank you." Before Mark could reply, a knock at the door stopped him.

"Who is it?" Mark called. "It's Nick. Mark, I need to talk to you." "Give me a minute." Nick Mannetti was the owner of the wrestling organization. "What does he want?" Sabrina asked, slipping her arms into Mark's shirt. Mark zipped up his jeans. "I don't know. He doesn't usually make personal visits." Sabrina rummaged through her bag, looking for a pair of shorts. "Come on Mark," Nick called impatiently. "Yeah, yeah, I'm coming."

Mark waited by the door until Sabrina was reasonably dressed. Nick pushed his way into the room. "What the hell took you so long?" Nick asked. He spotted Sabrina and the clothes scattered wildly about the floor. *Damn it I've intruded on their intimacy.* "Oh! Oh I'm sorry," he blushed. "I really am sorry, but this just couldn't wait until tomorrow."

A man in his early fifties, Nick was strong in his stature, and very well groomed. His black hair perfectly styled, with not a single hair out of place. A man that flaunted his wealth and success, from his manicured nails, to his rich cashmere suits. Having always been a successful business man, it was only a few years ago that he started this wrestling company, on a dare really from other business people he knew.

His company was still by no means the world wide success that he had dreamed of but it was gaining popularity within the confines of North America. Nick was driven to achieve and his methods were not always on the level. He could be pleasant and understanding when the mood struck but he also had a darker side that liked to create volatile situations amongst his wrestlers. For Nick the bottom line was making money and sometimes people got hurt because of his greed.

Sabrina quietly stared at this man and it made her uneasy. *I don't trust this man, even though I really don't know him that well. I've heard from Brent, that Nick could be very underhanded if it suited his purpose. What does he have planned for Mark?* He paced nervously about the room until Mark finally broke the tension.

"So what the hell is so important Nick?" "Mark we've got a bit of a situation. Sean is demanding that I authorize a match between you two." "No way," Sabrina jumped in. "Sean is looking for revenge. All he wants is to injure Mark." Her agitation made her tense. Mark put his arm around her. "It's okay," he told her. "We both knew that this was inevitable. Sean isn't going to back off no matter how long we try to drag this out." "I don't want you fighting him; and that's exactly what it's going to be an all out fight." "I hate to add fuel to this," Nick interjected. "But Sean has asked for a no-holds barred match."

"Mark this isn't going to be the solution." "Maybe not, but it will be great for the ratings," Nick added. Sabrina glared at him, tears burning her eyes. "How dare you say that? You'd risk Mark's safety just for the ratings! You heartless bastard!" Pulling away from Mark she locked herself in the bathroom. "Well, Mark, what's your answer?" Nick continued to push. Mark's feelings were torn. *I don't want to cause Sabrina any distress, but I have to deal with Sean.*

"Come on Mark I gotta know tonight, right now." "All right, damn you! You got your match; but on one condition. You guarantee me that Sabrina will have two body guards while I'm in the ring with that bastard."

"You got it Mark. You know I've never pried into what's going on between you and Sean, but you got to admit that this feud is going to make for a great show, and one hell of a future story line." "Yeah, yeah whatever, but just so you understand, this isn't gonna be like any other match. Sean is out to inflict pain, and draw blood." Mark paused, moving closer to Nick, stabbing at his chest with his fingers. "And that's exactly what he's gonna get back!"

The intense look in Mark's eyes struck fear in Nick. *Have I done the right thing, forcing this match? Am I setting up my two top stars for major injury? The fans would love this brawl, and the ratings would sky rocket.* Nick brought himself back to reality. "Great, it's set then. I'll see you tomorrow night. Try and get there early; we need to get a couple of interviews in before the show starts."

When Mark slammed the door shut behind Nick, he turned to the bathroom door. *No, she needs some time alone.* Going back to the table he picked up his glass of champagne and downed it in one swallow. The glass hit the wall, exploding into a shower of fragments. His anger had taken control of him for a brief moment. Ashamed of his actions, he fell onto the bed, taking slow deep breaths to wash away the horrible feeling; and to pray for Sabrina's forgiveness, and understanding.

With a wide grin on his face, Sean hung up the phone. *I got what I wanted. Mark in the ring in a no-holds barred anything goes match. I will show Sabrina that I'm the better man, that I'm the one that she should be with.*

Relaxing back into his chair he closed his eyes, remembering their time together. The one thing that was first, and foremost in his mind, was the sex. *We were good in bed, good enough to have created a life.* His heart carried that burden heavily.

Why didn't she tell me she was pregnant? Mark must have poisoned her mind. He probably told her that I wouldn't be tied down by any one woman, but if she had only told me, I would have done the right thing. I could have made a commitment. He tried hard to convince himself that it was possible. *I could learn.* His frustrations built up to the point where he was about to explode. As a release he kicked the coffee table, sending it tumbling across the room. *Mark will feel that anger tomorrow night.*

Sabrina jumped when she heard the door slam, and again at the sound of breaking glass. Giving up her seat on the edge of the bath tub, she splashed water on her face at the sink. Drying her face, she could see, reflected in the mirror, the large wet tear stains that covered the upper part of Mark's shirt. She tried to dry them with the towel before leaving the bathroom.

Mark was laying on his back on the bed; his arms folded across his face. Sabrina scanned the room for the broken glass. Spotting the twinkling shards against the wall she went to Mark. Sitting down beside him, she placed her hand on his chest, waiting for him to make the first move.

Slowly he moved his arms away to look at her. *Her eyes, she's been crying. It makes me sick to see her upset.* "You agreed to the match, didn't you?" "Yes, I did," he answered. "I wish there was some other way to resolve this." "I know, but Sean isn't about to back off, until he either gets what he wants, or accepts the fact that it just isn't going to happen." "What do you mean, gets what he wants?" Sabrina asked.

Mark pushed himself back against the headboard. "He still wants you. He's never felt the rejection of a woman, and he can't handle it. In his mind, your relationship isn't over, because he didn't end it, and he's blaming me for what happened." "That's ridiculous. All you did was open my eyes to the kind of man he is. I made the choice to leave." "I know that, and you know that, but Sean thinks that I pulled you away from him; that I destroyed your relationship, and he also blames me for." "For what?"

I never wanted to have to tell her the truth, but by letting my emotions run wild I've opened that dreaded door.

Sabrina edged closer to him. In a sudden burst he pulled her into his arms, holding her so tight that for a moment she couldn't breathe. "Oh God, Sabrina, I love you so much. I've waited all my life, all eternity, for you; and all I want to do is love you, and protect you." She could feel his heart racing.

Wiggling free of his hold she leaned back. In his eyes she could see a deep sadness, it worried her. "What's wrong Mark?" "There is something that I need to tell you, and I'm afraid that it's going to upset you. I had hoped that you would never find out, but I knew that it couldn't be kept a secret forever."

"Mark you're scaring me. What is it that you have to tell me?" She paused to touch him tenderly. "Whatever it is we can handle it, together. Our love is strong, and can, and will, survive anything." He drew on her love, for the strength that he needed at that moment. "Sean knows. He knows about your pregnancy, and about the miscarriage." He awaited her reaction.

Sabrina closed her eyes, taking a deep relaxing breath. *I'm relieved that my secret is no longer hidden.*

To Mark's amazement a tiny smile graced her lips. "I'm glad he knows. Now we can deal with it properly, and move on with our life." "You're not angry with me; because you must know that he found out about it from me." "Mark I'm not mad at you. I know you better than you think and I'm pretty sure that it was an accident. You probably let it slip out during a moment of increased emotions. Am I right?"

Her soft touch smoothed away the worry lines on his face. He buried his face in her shoulder and she continued to comfort him. "I don't want you to worry about it anymore. This will pass, and Sean will eventually come to understand that we are together now and forever."

Pulling away from him, she straightened herself. "Speaking of us; we seem to have forgotten that tonight was ours, and I for one am not about to give it up," she said wandering over to the table. "We still have some champagne; but we'll have to share." "You have it." "No, we have to share, because I want to make a toast," she said, pulling him up to his feet. "What do you want to toast?" "I offer a toast to our love. May it continue to grow stronger; and may our union someday be blessed with the creation of a new life." Taking a small drink, she handed the glass to Mark. His smile had returned, and that made her happy.

Setting the glass back down, she pressed her body close to his. "How about we dim the lights, get in to bed, and watch a movie?" Her voice had started out soft and sexy, and ended perky. Mark readily agreed and they were soon cuddled together under the blankets. She tried to concentrate on the movie, but her mind wandered.

Now that I know what's bothering Sean, I know exactly what I have to do. Mark won't like it, but if my plan works, I just might be able to stop this battle between them. Entwining her leg with Mark's she cuddled closer to him. "Tired?" "Uh huh," she murmured dreamily. Mark kissed the top of her head, turned off the TV, and secured his hold on her. "Sweet dreams my love," he whispered to deaf ears.

Sean arrived early to the arena. He had to see Nick and sign the contract for his match tonight. The arena was bustling with roadies, hauling in equipment; Sean walked towards the ring, that was still under construction. He took a seat a few rows back. He had no need to plan his performance for tonight. It needed no rehearsal, no choreography; just pure raw emotion. *If I get hurt so what? If Mark gets hurt, all the better, he deserves it.* Checking his watch it was time to find Nick. *Still enough time for a workout before the show.*

Finding Nick was easy; he always stayed around the back stage area, supervising the setup. "Sean, good to see you," Nick called, walking towards him. "Yeah right. So where is the contract?" "Right this way," Nick said as he directed him to a make shift office. The contract lay on the table; Sean picked up a pen and signed. "I suggest that you read that first." "Why? It's just a contract." "Sean there are some conditions that have been added." "Yeah, like what?" "Like you are forbidden to go anywhere near Sabrina, under no circumstances are you to approach her, or try to engage her in a conversation at any time during this event."

"That's bullshit! Mark put you up to this didn't he! You spineless son of a bitch! You're gonna let him tell you what to do! Bullshit! I'll do what's right for me!" Sean's anger exploded; he threw the contract at Nick. "Sean I'll only say this once; you break the conditions of this contract and you'll pay the consequences; no one else, just you." "Fuck you!" Sean yelled and stormed from the office. Nick straightened himself, running his hand across his hair, smoothing it back into place. A smirk was beginning to grow on his face, broadening his already square jaw.

Well, that should make for a very interesting night. I'll let him think that it was all Mark's idea, but it wasn't. Nick enjoyed stirring the pot, so to speak. He liked the outcome when he played one wrestler against the other. This was not a normal match; the winner would be decided in the ring tonight, not in a contract, like all the others. Anger consistently made for a better match; and the fans always loved it when two guys went at each other hard and fast; and if blood was drawn, they liked it even more.

This war between them could become a very profitable story line for the company; if only there was some way of getting Sabrina more involved in it. I need to find out the history first, before I can make plans for future shows. Whom can I ply for information? Tony and Brent would be the two most likely subjects. If anyone knew anything it would be them; now to get them to open up; voluntarily of course. Nick's smirk broadened into a full smile; he was pleased with himself, at just how manipulative he could be.

Mark made several attempts to coax Sabrina out of bed, to go to the gym with him, but he finally conceded that he was fighting a losing battle. He knew that she always slept more when she was upset.

It's so tempting to stay with her; to crawl back in, beside that warm, sexy body, but I have to be prepared for tonight. I have to be alert, both physically, and mentally, and a long workout at the gym is the only way I know to achieve that; right after I make one very important stop first. I can't tell her yet, but when the time is right and I'm completely free of my own fears then I'll tell her and our world will be right. I've made her wait too long already.

"So what are you going to do while I'm at the gym?" Mark asked. "I thought I'd do a little shopping. There are a few things that I need, and I'd like to get a special gift to send to an old friend back home." "Would you like me to arrange for a car to take you?" "No. I can manage. If there is nothing close to the hotel then I'll just take a cab." "Make sure that you're back by three, so you can have enough time to get ready for tonight."

Picking up his gym bag, he headed to the door. "Hey, aren't you forgetting something?" Sabrina queried as she tried to hide her smile. "No, I don't think so," he answered, looking at his bag. "Come here," she summoned. He sat beside her, a silly grin on his face. "So what have I forgotten?" "Don't be such a smart ass." She put her arms around him to kiss him. Mark patted her hip. "See you later; and have fun shopping."

He's gone. "Oh Mark, I wish that I could tell you everything that I have planned for today, but you'd only stop me." Turning over, she picked up the phone; asking the switchboard to link her to D'arcy's room. Sabrina knew by the gravely voice that answered the phone that she had awakened him. "D'arcy I'm sorry, this is Sabrina." "Sabrina, is everything okay?" "Yes, fine. D'arcy I need you to do me a huge favor. I would like you to arrange a meeting with Sean for me." "That's not such a good idea." "D'arcy please, I have to do this. Please help me. Arrange it for one this afternoon, in your room; but do not tell him that he's coming to see me."

The long silence worried her. "Please, please say you'll help me." "Okay, but it goes against all my instincts, but understand one thing Sabrina, I will not leave you alone with him." "Agreed, I was going to ask you to stay anyway. Thank you so much; I'll see you just before one then." Hanging up the phone she bounced out of bed. A feeling of dizziness shrouded her; shrugging it off as getting up too fast, she continued on to the shower.

Making a brief stop at the front desk Sabrina retrieved some of her winnings. *I have to get something very special for Marion's birthday.* Leaving the hotel, she walked down the sidewalk, peering into shop windows until she found one that looked promising. Browsing through the shop she found the perfect gift, a beautiful crystal bowl, rimmed with gold. *Marion will like this.* Holding it up to the sunlight, she watched the light dance about the crystal, casting prisms of vivid color onto her arms. She arranged for the store to pack it securely and have it sent by courier to Marion's address.

Sabrina had just put away her wallet when the wave of dizziness overcame her again; she wilted to the floor. As her eyes fluttered open she saw the blurred face of a young man hovering over her. The smell of ammonia burned her nostrils. Her head was in a fog, but she could see that the young man was wearing a uniform. *A policeman, no, he's a paramedic.* She could see the medical symbol on his collar.

"Miss, can you hear me?" "Yes, but please don't yell." She tried to sit up but couldn't; she was being restrained. Panic set in as she looked about, finally realizing that she was in an ambulance, and her restraints were those on a stretcher. "What's going on?" Sabrina asked. "You passed out, and we're taking you to the hospital." "No, I'm fine. I don't need to go to a hospital, really; I'm okay." "I'm sorry miss. You need to see a Doctor." Sabrina laid back, giving up the argument. *He's only doing his job, and this dizziness does worry me.*

The hospital was no different from any other; everything was clean and bright, and smelled of antiseptic. The paramedics transferred her into the care of an emergency room physician and his staff of nurses. The questions they bombarded her with quickly became annoying. What's your name? Do you know were you are? What day is it? Sabrina could no longer keep her frustration in check.

"Look I'm fine. I haven't eaten anything today and that's why I passed out, simple as that. Now when can I leave?" The Doctor, whose face was obscured by a green mask, glared at her, and the bad attitude she displayed. "Ms. Scott, please relax," his said, his voice was arrogant and commanding. "We need to run a few tests to make sure that there is nothing wrong." "Please can you just hurry up. You can call me at the hotel with the results." "We'll see."

I have to stay calm and rational, but time is ticking by fast. I have to get out of here soon. "I can tell you exactly what's wrong. It's called stress, and coupled with the fact that I've been too busy to eat today, that's what made me sick."

Reasoning has made no head way with the Doctor. Maybe I should try a harsher approach. "Now look, I have to be back at my hotel by one for a very important meeting! So take some blood, give me a sandwich, and let me out of here!" The Doctor shook his head, as he tried to concentrate on his instructions to the nurse.

Sabrina became more angry at being ignored. "Damn it; listen to me! If I'm not released from this place by twelve thirty I'm going to leave anyway! So can you get this show on the road!" Having relayed his instructions to the nurse, and hearing enough from Sabrina; the Doctor left the room. "Where the hell is he going in such a hurry?" Sabrina demanded an answer.

The nurse moved to Sabrina's side. Her expression was calm, as was her voice. "Look honey, you're not the only patient in here; and he really doesn't need to be here while I take care of your tests. Now is there someone I could call for you? You might feel better with a friend or family member with you."

Sabrina lay back on the bed. "No. My man doesn't need to be bothered with this. He has a very important show to prepare for, and having him here, would only throw his edge off." "Oh, so you're in show business?" "Sort of; actually it's sports entertainment; you know, wrestling." *Damn it, I've said too much, but no one would know who I am anyway.*

The nurse stopped what she was doing to look up at Sabrina; her mouth had dropped open slightly. "What?" Sabrina asked, catching the look. "You're her, aren't you? The one who works with the Warlock?" "Yes, that's right." "Oh my husband is going to be so thrilled when I tell him. He watches wrestling every chance he gets, and now and then I watch it with him. This just makes my day," she said, her excitement overflowing. "Well then make mine and get me out of here soon." "Sure thing honey; I've got all the blood I need, and you need to make your contribution," she said handing Sabrina a plastic jar. "You fill this up while I raid the lounge for something for you to eat."

Sabrina was back, sitting on the bed when the nurse returned. "I hit the jackpot," the nurse said laying the tray down before her. The tray contained a carton of orange juice, milk, a ham sandwich, some carrots and celery, and a yogurt. "Looks like a feast," Sabrina said, opening the juice. "Everything your body needs right now honey." Sabrina wasn't really hungry until she saw the food, in her haste to eat she had to keep reminding herself to slow down.

The nurse continued with her routine, taking Sabrina's blood pressure and checking her pulse. "So how does it look?" Sabrina asked, licking up the last of the yogurt. "Great, you're just fine." "So can I get out of here then?" Sabrina had her fingers crossed. "Well, in my opinion, I see no reason for you to stay. I'll go and get the Doctor, and convince him that you're well enough to be released." "What about the test results?" "They will take a couple more hours, but there should be no problem. We can call you at the hotel later; and don't worry; it will be good news." The nurse gave her a wink as she left the room.

Settling into the back of the cab, Sabrina checked her watch. *It's twelve fifteen, still plenty of time to get to the hotel and to D'arcy's room before Sean.* She tapped her foot every time the cab stopped at a red light. *Relax, there's no need to rush.* The cab ride took only twenty minutes, but it felt like hours.

She hurried through the lobby, and up to D'arcy's room. He was two floors above her room, so there was no chance of running into Mark in the hallway. Instinctively, she checked both directions of the hall as she exited the elevator. Finding it clear she proceeded.

Hesitating outside his door, she listened for the sound of voices, hearing none she knocked lightly. D'arcy opened the door. "Cutting it close aren't you?" "Oh man, I've had one hell of a morning," she began, taking a seat at the table. "And don't even think about asking me about it. Oh, by the way, I would like to ask you for one more favor, if that's okay." "Sure, why not." "Could you use your influence to get two ringside tickets for tonight?" "Yeah; but Mark can get them too." "I don't want Mark to know," she said handing D'arcy a piece of paper. "Have a courier take them to this lady at this address." D'arcy took the note and read it aloud. "Nurse O'Brien, Vegas General Hospital, ER Dept. Sabrina what's going on?" "Please D'arcy no questions." "Okay, whatever you say."

D'arcy went to the phone. Sabrina relaxed back into the chair. Her nerves were on edge and it twisted her gut into knots. Waiting was not one of her strong points. When he hung up the phone, D'arcy was about to sit down when there came a knock at the door. He put his hand on Sabrina's shoulder. "Are you absolutely sure that you want to go through with this?" he asked. "No, but it's what I have to do." Another knock echoed across the room. "Answer it," Sabrina said. As D'arcy headed for the door, Sabrina moved to the window, hugging herself tight when she heard the door open. The sound of Sean's voice sent a chill up her spine.

"Okay I'm here. So what's so damned important?" Sean pushed past D'arcy; but hadn't noticed Sabrina. Taking a breath, she turned around. "Hello Sean," she said, her voice quivering on every syllable. Sean stopped in his tracks. His eyes locked onto her. In total shock his mouth moved, but no sounds came out. He forced himself forward to her.

"Sabrina, I've missed you." His arms locked around her; his embrace was awkward. Her body tensed at his touch. He attempted to kiss her but she pulled herself free. "Sean please, we have to talk." She sat down at the table, Sean in the seat across from her. D'arcy quietly moved into the bathroom. *He's left the door open, that makes me feel better, even in this difficult situation.*

"So what do you want to talk about? If you've been wondering if I missed you, you're right. Would I welcome you back; definitely," he rambled nervously. "Sean please, this is important. I want you to back off Mark." *This is not how I had planned to start this conversation.* Her abrupt, direct words angered him, and it showed clearly in his face.

"Damn him! He deserves to be beaten for what he's done; taking you from me!" "Sean, stop it! Just sit there, shut up and listen to me!" Sabrina was angry as well. Sean leaned back, surprised by her forcefulness. "The first thing that you need to understand is that Mark did not take me away from you; I made the decision to leave. Mark only agreed to help me. I left you because I didn't like the way things were going. Yeah, we had some good times, but I wasn't in love with you. Your lifestyle was not something that was comfortable to me." She paused to remind herself to maintain control of her emotions.

"Sean, you are the kind of guy that needs women around him; but not the same woman all of the time. I didn't fall in love with Mark right away; but when I did, I realized that he is the man that I've been waiting for. He fills my heart and my soul."

She took a moment to try and read his expression; she saw nothing. "I will always be grateful to you, for being there for me, when I was attacked, but Sean it won't go any farther than that. There is no one person to blame for this; it's just the way it worked out. Please understand; I am sorry if I have hurt you, but we were not meant to be together." Finishing her statement, she leaned back in her chair; the knots in her stomach tightened as she waited for his response.

The silence gave her a chance to really look at him. *How he has changed. He looks so much older, his blonde hair now flat and dull, his unshaven face, covering deep lines about his mouth, and his eyes, so dark and tired.*

Sean had heard every word she had said, it pierced his heart like a dagger; but all he saw was her beauty. "My God Sabrina, you're even more beautiful." "Damn it Sean. Did you hear what I said?" "Yeah I heard, but I don't believe it! He's poisoned your mind; you've been taken in by his smooth talk!" "No, Sean, I am very much in love with Mark. It's real, and it's forever." "But Sabrina, what we have is special, special enough to have created a child together." "Damn it Sean, my getting pregnant was an accident, and you know it! You never had sex without a condom, except that one time; and I never knew I was pregnant until I had the miscarriage!"

He smiled at her. "We had great sex didn't we?" "Oh for Pete's sake Sean; give up this ridiculous quest; open your eyes. I'm staying with Mark, no matter what!"

Anger didn't seem to register with him, maybe pleading would. "I beg you; stop this match tonight. I don't want to see either you, or Mark get hurt. So please, please let it end." "I can't and I won't! I will fight to win you back!" "And you'll lose! I will not leave Mark, ever. I had such hopes of being able to make you understand, but I see now that it's hopeless. I will accept you as my friend, but nothing more."

Sean stood up hastily. The chair toppled backwards hitting the floor with a thud that startled Sabrina. Bracing his arms on the table top Sean leaned toward her and she instinctively leaned away, just in case. "Then you better hope that Mark has good medical insurance, because he's gonna need it, a lot," Sean scowled. He left the room like a cyclone, leaving behind him a wake of destruction and a growing wave of fear.

Sabrina put her head in her hands and sighed heavily. D'arcy knelt down; comforting her as best he could. "Don't worry; we'll take care of you and Mark, and I'm sure that if I continue to talk to Sean long enough it just might sink in." Sabrina hugged him. "Thank you." She looked at her watch.

"I have to go; Mark will be back soon." "I'll walk you down; just in case Sean hasn't left yet."

Chapter 12

The room is empty; Mark is still out. The maid has been in to clean, and make the bed. All of our clothes are neatly laid over the back of a chair and the broken glass no longer glitters against the wall. Everything is in order; except for my talk with Sean.

Sabrina began to question her actions. *Did I do the right thing, or just make it worse? Maybe once he's had time to think about our conversation he'll understand, but he's not the same man that I knew. I know that he's upset and angry and I don't want to think about how extreme he could get if he refuses to let this go.*

Worn out from mental exhaustion, she lay down on the bed and was soon asleep. Her rest was deep, but fitful. Her dreams kept her moving, kept her reenacting her conversation with Sean. She wasn't aware of Mark sitting down beside her.

"Hey sleeping beauty, it's time to get up," he whispered softly into her ear. Her body jumped. Awake, but only semi alert, trying to focus her eyes on the face above her. Her first fear was that it was Sean. As her vision cleared, Mark's face became more visible. "Oh Mark, you scared me."

She sat up to hold him, shivering in his arms. "You're cold," he said as he pulled the bedspread around her. "I guess I fell asleep before I had a chance to get a blanket." His warm body felt good; she snuggled in closer. "That's the quickest way to get sick." "I know, but I was just so tired." "Did you have a busy day? What all did you do while I was gone?"

She mulled it over in her mind. *I can't tell him about the visit to the hospital, or the meeting with Sean.* "So, what did you do today?" he asked again. She decided to tell him about her shopping, but before she could the phone rang. "I'll get it," she said, trying to squirm free of the blanket. "It's okay I got it." He kept her firmly bound in his cocoon. "Hello," he said, then a long silence. He turned his eyes to her. "Yes, just a minute."

Cupping the phone in his hand, he looked at her with a questioning glance. "It's for you; a woman. A Nurse O'Brien. What's going on Sabrina?" "Nothing important, I'll tell you later." She took the phone from his hand, but before she answered she broke free of the blanket, and slid up against the headboard; suggesting to Mark that she would appreciate some privacy. Mark understood her actions, and set to unpacking his gym bag in the hall closet.

"Hello," Sabrina answered quietly. "Ms. Scott, this is Nurse O'Brien. I just had to call and thank you for the tickets. My husband is so thrilled to have ring side seats. You have to tell me; was that him, the Warlock, that answered the phone?" "You're very welcome, and yes it was." "Oh my husband isn't going to believe this. I can't believe how excited I am." "You'll have a great time." Sabrina paused, afraid to ask the next question.

"Is there anything else?" "Oh my yes; I am sorry; I almost forgot. Your test results came back." "So what's the verdict?" "As I told you earlier, it's all good news." Sabrina quietly sighed to herself. "I had my suspicions, but I needed the test to confirm it. Congratulations Ms. Scott." "For what?" "You're pregnant, isn't that just wonderful."

Sabrina went quiet for a moment, trying to absorb what she had just heard. "Ms. Scott?" "Yes. Are you sure?" "Positive, the test never lies. You're going to have a baby." "Well, thank you for calling." "Oh you are most welcome. Good-by Ms. Scott and congratulations again to both of you." "Yes, good-by."

Hanging up the phone, Sabrina drew her knees up to her chest, hugging them tight to her. She felt warm all over. *A baby, we're going to have a baby!* She could hear Mark going through his suitcase in the hall closet. *How do I tell him? When? It has to be a special moment.*

Mark had kept clear of the room while Sabrina was on the phone, but not hearing her speak anymore was his own signal to go back to her, to find out what the call was about. Sitting beside her, he started in on the interrogation. "So what was that call about, and who is Nurse O'Brien? Did something happen to you today?" "Gee, so many questions, I haven't seen you all day," she said, pulling herself up onto her knees, slipping one arm around his neck, the other inside his shirt.

Mark easily gave in to her advances, enjoying the sweet taste of her lips. When her kisses intensified, he realized what she was doing and he held her back. "Okay, enough! You're avoiding my questions." "But this is much more fun." "Damn it Sabrina! I know you're hiding something, now tell me what it is," he said sternly, scolding her. "Maybe I will and maybe I won't." "Sabrina!" "Okay! You don't have to yell. I was just having a little fun." *I know that I'm pushing his patience to the limit. I will tell him; some of it anyway.*

"After you left this morning, I went out to do my errands, nothing spectacular, just a little shopping." "I know that. I want you to tell me why a nurse is calling you?" "She helped me out this morning, and being that I was in such a good mood, I arranged for her and her husband to get tickets for tonight. She just called to thank me."

Mark got up and began pacing. "I don't buy it! I know you to well, and I know that there is more to this story that you're not telling me!" He stopped his pacing to look into her eyes. "You know, it really bothers me that you feel that you have to keep things from me. I love you, and that means sharing everything; not keeping secrets from each other."

She felt herself succumb to the guilt that he was putting on her. A feeling she hadn't had since her mother. She felt degraded and insignificant. The feelings filled her eyes with tears. *I've hurt him, and he's hurt me, but all I want is to hold him.*

He embraced her, knowing that he had made her feel bad. "Mark I'm sorry; it's just that I didn't want you to worry about me. You have to stay focused on tonight." "To hell with the show tonight, you come first, no matter what. Now please, tell me the truth." "Okay; but first you have to understand that I am okay."

Mark gently massaged the tension in her shoulders, before taking her hands in his. "Go ahead," he said in a calm voice. Taking a deep breath she began. "The morning routine you already know. I rushed out of here shortly after you; so intent on shopping that I forgot to eat breakfast. I did my shopping, got dizzy and passed out."

His grip tightened on her, but he didn't interrupt. "Well, the next thing I remember is waking up in an ambulance on the way to the hospital. That's where I met Nurse O'Brien. She was so nice to me; getting me something to eat, explaining the tests." "What tests?" Mark interrupted. "Don't worry. They were just routine tests to make sure that there was nothing wrong, other than the lack of food. Anyway, they kept me there for a little while and agreed that I was okay, so they let me go."

"Then why did that nurse phone you?" "As I already said, she was so kind, and her husband is a fan, that I thought I'd show my appreciation. She called to thank me for the tickets; and to give me the test results." "So, what are the results?" Mark asked the question but his gut didn't want to hear the answer.

Pulling away from him, Sabrina pushed herself farther back on the bed. *This is not how I wanted this to go. He won't let up until he knows everything.* Mark was at her side, his hand on her knee. "Sabrina, please tell me. What did she say?" "The tests were all okay, but one of them did show something." "For God's sake what did they find out?" Hearing the panic in his voice only served to intensify her own mixed emotions.

"Mark, I didn't want to tell you like this. Not with everything else that's going on. I wanted to wait for a special time and place. What I have to tell you could effect what happens to you tonight. It could throw off your edge, and I'm afraid that you could get hurt because your mind isn't on the match." "I don't care. If I have to, I'll cancel tonight. You are much more important to me," he said, choking on his words as a single tear rolled down his cheek.

The sadness that shrouded his face, caused her great despair. "There's no need to be sad," she said kissing away the tear. "But the way you've been talking. You've been preparing me for something terrible; haven't you?" "Oh my love; it's not terrible; nor sad or mournful, and I'm sorry if I have led you to believe that." "Then tell me and ease my mind."

The unexpected sigh made her straighten herself. "What are you waiting for?" Mark grew impatient. "I don't know! This isn't easy for me. This is not how I wanted to tell you." "Then stop searching for the right words, just say it; I can take it." "I love you so much Mark, and that love has been sanctified." She paused to share her smile with him. "I'm pregnant." "What? Really!" "Yes. Your baby is growing inside me."

With one swift movement, he picked her up in his arms and spun her around wildly, before laying her back down on the bed, kissing her passionately. "I love you. Oh thank you God," he said, his voice was filled with excitement. He laid his hand on her stomach; she moved it a little lower. "There; that should be about right."

Unzipping her jeans, his hand touched her bare belly, caressing it gently while they shared soft kisses. Sabrina tried to pull him down to her but he resisted. Rolling onto his back, he pulled her on top of him. "We need to be extra careful; my weight could hurt you, and the baby." Just saying the word made his body tingle with excitement. "You could never hurt me; and I tell you right now I will not even entertain the thought of abstaining." She had already undone the buttons on his shirt. "What I want more than ever is for you to make love to me right now."

They celebrated their love slowly, carefully and passionately. Mark held her close, his hand resting on her belly. "Thank you," he whispered. "You're welcome; but for what?" "For you, for bringing such joy into my life. For so many years I was an empty man; convinced that I was destined to be alone, but then you came into my life. You showed me what it was like to love, and be loved; and now you have given me this wondrous gift, this ultimate expression of love. I never knew that it was possible to feel this good."

She had lifted herself up, watching his face light up, as he talked. "I take it that you like my news?" "Like it. I love it; and I love you, Sabrina, so very much." He pulled her to him. "How do you feel?" Mark asked. "I feel fine. Do you understand why I didn't want to tell you like this?" "Not really. It's such wonderful news." "I know, but I had this vision of how it should be. You know, romantic, someplace special." "We're together and nothing is more special than that." "You're right. It is the best news ever, no matter what the setting."

"Do you have any nausea or cravings?" Mark asked. "No, my stomach's fine, but now that you mention it, I do have a craving." "What is it? I'll get you whatever you want!" Sabrina put her arms around him. "I have only but one craving, and that is for you. I crave your body next to mine; your lips kissing me, but most of all, I crave you making love to me, making me feel so special." "I think that I can take care of that craving." He began to kiss her cheek, then her neck and on to her shoulder. She leaned back, inviting him to kiss her chest. Their passion was building again, but was crushed by the ringing of the phone.

"Damn it," Mark muttered, reaching for the frustrating noise. "Yeah what?" "Mark, it's Nick. What in the hell are you still doing at the hotel?" "That is none of your business." "Well, it is my business when one of my stars is late for a show." "What?" "Get your ass over here ASAP. You've got thirty minutes before your first interview!" "Yeah, yeah, we'll be there." There were no good-byes, just a click as Nick hung up the phone.

"I take it we're in trouble?" Sabrina asked. "Ah screw him. We've got lots of time to get there. Besides he'd understand. I'm sure he remembers the moment when he first found out that he was going to be a father." "Maybe we shouldn't say anything just yet." "Why not?" "I just want to be sure that everything is all right with the baby. I know I could still be at risk, getting pregnant so soon after what happened before. I just want to be absolutely sure before we spread it around."

"That's fine, I can understand your fear and I do respect your wishes. We will keep it our secret for as long as possible." "I love you," she whispered softly. Mark smiled and handed her a robe. "We can grab a quick shower at the arena." "Together?" she asked. Mark surprised her from behind, holding her close to him, his hands on her belly. "Yeah, just the three of us."

I could stay in his arms forever, but time doesn't allow it today. "We have to get dressed and get out of here, or Nick is really gonna be pissed off," she said stepping away from his embrace. "You're right; but I can't help myself. I'm just so excited." "Well, put your excitement to use and get your pants on."

Sabrina was dressed before Mark, and had started checking her bag to make sure all of her costume was there. She picked up her new leather outfit to put it away, when she stopped, smiling to herself. "Mark, how about I wear this tonight?" "I don't think so." "Why not? Before too long it's not even gonna fit anymore, and besides you make me wear that robe." She cast a pout in his direction, knowing what it would do. "Okay, you can wear it. Now, can we go?" "You bet." She stuffed the outfit into her bag and was about to toss it over her shoulder. "No you don't," he said, taking it from her. "No more lifting or carrying for you." "I'm not crippled." "No, you're not; you're just pregnant," he smiled widely, consumed by a new inner warmth.

The limo pulled into the back of the arena and stopped. The driver was out and opened the door in seconds. While Mark retrieved their bags, Sabrina began a slow walk down the ramp to the arena doors. *I hope that my conversation with Sean will have some effect. Maybe he'll reconsider his plan of action for tonight.*

She was still lost in her thoughts when Mark called to her to wait up. Pivoting around to see him, a rock rolled under her foot and she fell to the pavement. Mark saw her ankle twist sideways, and watched helplessly, as her body impacted with the pavement. He was still too far away to catch her.

His heart pounded like thunder in his ears as he knelt down beside her. "Are you hurt? Do you have any pain?" His questions came fast and fearful. "No, I'm fine. Just help me up." Locking his arms under hers, he lifted her straight up, keeping hold of her while she reoriented herself. "Are you sure you're okay?" "Yes, I think so, other than feeling a bit silly." "Hey, what's going on?" Brent asked, trotting down the ramp behind them. He had only seen Mark lifting Sabrina up. "She fell." "You okay?" "Yes, I'm fine."

She went to take a step; the pain in her ankle made her grab for Mark. "You're not okay," he said bracing himself against her. "I guess I twisted my ankle." She held her foot off of the ground to keep the pain at bay. "Get one of the medics to look at her," Brent suggested. "That's not necessary; all I need is some ice and I'll be fine," she insisted. Her words were met by a swift action from Mark. He picked her up into his arms. "No arguments, remember?" His eyes fixed upon hers with deep intent. "Brent could you grab the bags I kind of got my hands full." "Sure thing; you get her into the dressing room and I'll go and get the medics for you." As they entered the arena, Sabrina became very aware of the stares they were receiving. She hid her face against Mark's neck to conceal her embarrassment.

The dressing room, at this arena, was much different from the others. The floors were carpeted and were furnished not with cold wooden benches, but rich leather sofas. Mark set her down carefully, making sure that her ankle was elevated on a couple of pillows. Brent appeared at the door, with two paramedics behind him. They immediately began assessing the extent of her injury; while Brent stowed their bags on a shelf behind them.

"It's just a sprain. We can tape it up and leave you some ice packs," the medic said. "That will be fine," Sabrina answered. "It's going to be painful for a while; if you like I could give you something for the pain." "No! No drugs!" Mark bellowed. "She can't have anything like that; she's pregnant." "How far along are you?" "First trimester, I think." "The pain killers would not have any effect on the baby, but if you can handle it without, you're much better off." "I think if you just tape it up really good it'll be okay." The medics finished their job and left quietly.

Both Mark and Sabrina hadn't noticed that Brent was still in the dressing room; until he spoke. "Congratulations you two." Sabrina jumped hard, as did Mark. Both were startled by the unexpected voice. Brent wandered over to them, extending his hand to Mark, and shaking his firmly. He then leaned down and kissed Sabrina's cheek. "This is great news." "Yes, it is; but we want to keep it quiet for a while yet." "Okay, but I really don't understand why you'd want to keep such good news a secret, but if that's what you want then I'll play along." "Thanks man," Mark responded, giving him a pat on the back. "I gotta go; I'm one of the first one's up tonight. Good luck tonight Mark, and congratulations again to both of you."

Mark was grateful for the peace and quiet once again. "You sit here and rest; I'm gonna get ready." "Wait a minute; I have to get ready too." "I think you should pass on tonight." "No way! I am not letting you go out there alone tonight!"

Standing up, she eased her weight down on her ankle. It burned at first, but gradually she became more tolerant of it. The tape helped to support her ankle, and she felt confident enough to take a few steps. *I have to ignore the pain. I have to prove to him that I can be a part of tonight's show.*

Mark waited for her to falter, but she didn't. *There's no point in trying to change her mind. She can be as stubborn as me.* He busied himself with sorting out his costume and hers, while she continued to force herself to walk. "Ready for your shower?" she asked. "Yeah, and you?" "Most definitely; but I'm going to need your help." "How is that?" "Well, it's going to be kind of difficult to shower while standing on one leg. I don't want the tape to get wet." "Okay, I'll shower first, and then I'll help you."

As soon as he was out of sight she sat back down, placing an ice pack on her throbbing ankle. *Please let it feel better soon.* Mark called to her from the shower. *Damn he's fast.* She hobbled her way in, dropping her clothes as she went. Pulling the curtain back, Mark helped her in, leaving her bandaged ankle dangling outside the curtain. He had stepped behind her so the water could wash over her. Grabbing the shower rod helped with her balance. She could feel his body pressing against her, supporting her.

His gentle kisses on her neck helped to relax her even more. Reaching around, he began rubbing the soap into a thick lather, massaging it over her body, taking extra time to play with her breasts. He liked the way they slipped through his hands. He washed her belly and down her legs, bringing his hand back up between her thighs. She leaned into him. "Not fair; I am at a disadvantage." "Sorry." "Don't be sorry; we'll just have to wait until later, that's all." He turned the water off and wrapped a towel around her, pausing briefly to rub her belly. "Do you think Brent will keep our secret?" she asked. "I really don't know; but I hope he will."

Brent wandered through the corridor towards his dressing room; his mind still processing the news. *Mark is sure one hell of a lucky man. To have found a woman like Sabrina, and now to be having a baby with one of the sexiest women on the planet, bloody incredible. From the very first time*

I'd seen Sabrina, I had entertained the hope of getting to know her; once Sean was done with her, but that will never happen now.

Even though he had been married for several years, it didn't stop him from taking a lover while on the road. His wife never traveled with him. She hated what he did; but she liked the money that he brought home. They never had children, and that bothered Brent a lot.

I want a family, a son, to carry on my name and my career. But his wife refused to give him a child as long as he was mixed up in wrestling and as a result they had begun to drift apart. Many times he had considered divorcing her, but he could never bring himself to do it. In a small corner of his heart he still loved her; considering they hadn't been intimate for over two years. He still hoped that she would one day come around to his way of thinking. He kicked a garbage can in front of him, sending it rolling and crashing along the hallway. *Damn it, if Mark could find someone like Sabrina then so can I.*

Tony poked his head out from behind a door, curious about the noise. "Yo Brent, what the hell is the matter with you?" "Nothing. I've just come to the realization that my life sucks." "What do you mean?" "For the first time I can see things more clearly, and you know what; as soon as I can tomorrow morning I'm gonna call my lawyer and start divorce proceedings." "Why? You've been married for so long; why now?" "Look man; my marriage is a farce. All I got is a woman that has my name; I got no kids. Christ we haven't made love for over two years. I'm just tired of this bullshit. I want a family, and I want a wife who loves me, and what I do for a living."

"Whoa, what brought this on so suddenly?" "Aw, I was just with Mark and Sabrina. To see them together, so much in love; that's what I want; and I'm sure as hell not getting it from that bitch I married." Tony couldn't get over the change in Brent; but there was one statement that had really amazed him. "How did you get into Mark's dressing room? No one ever gets in there." "Sabrina fell on the way in, twisted her ankle. I brought their bags in for them." Brent paused for a while. His mind grasped onto the potential difficulties that Mark's match could pose for Sabrina.

She doesn't need any crap from Sean. He turned back to Tony. "You know maybe we should be around when Sean confronts Mark tonight. Just to make sure that Sabrina doesn't get caught in the middle." "Yeah, I guess." The two men turned their attentions down the hall, and to Nick, who bellowed at them as he approached. "Why in the hell aren't you two dressed? Do I have to baby-sit every one of you guys? Get back to your dressing rooms. We have a show to put on, or have you forgotten?" Brent rolled his eyes as he looked at Tony. "I said move! Now!" Nick yelled again. Tony disappeared into his dressing room; Brent slowly moved along the corridor. *Bastard.*

Sabrina dressed in the shower area; Mark in the main dressing room. Respecting his privacy before a match, allowing him the solitude while he prepared himself. Making use of her time alone by resting her ankle on the bench, the ice packs numbing the pain. *Fortunately, the chaps and boots will conceal the white tape; and if I concentrate very hard on trying not to limp, maybe no one will notice.*

She heard the knock at the dressing room door, and then Nick's voice. He was loud, and she detected anger in his words. "What in the hell is going on? I have to find out from one of the crew that the paramedics were in here. I don't want to hear that you're injured. Taped or not, you are going on tonight."

Mark turned around, annoyed by Nick's intrusion on his privacy, but more so by the tone in his voice. He approached Nick. Mark towered above him. He knew that his size, and strength was intimidating to Nick. "So what if the medics were in here? And just for your information they were here for Sabrina, not me, you selfish bastard." "Well as long as you're not hurt, that was my only concern," Nick's voice quivered. Sabrina was leaning against the doorway of the bathroom. "Gee Nick, thanks so much for your concern," she lashed out sarcastically.

Surprised by her, Nick turned to face her; his mouth dropped opened. Sabrina could see his eyes grow wide, as he surveyed her from head to toe. With a slinky step she moved towards him. "What's the matter Nick; the cat got your tongue?" Nick's lips moved together several times before he could finally manage to speak. "Oh my," the words escaped his lips in a stutter. "Do you like my outfit?" "Oh yes; I like it very much." "Well, if you like this view, then you are gonna love the whole view."

Giving Mark a wink she turned around. She heard Nick gasp. As she turned back around he had slumped down onto a sofa. Mark stepped to her side; he put his arm around her. "So what do you think about my girl now?" Mark asked. Nick swallowed, the initial shock had worn off; he was more composed. "Sabrina, you have the sexiest body that I have seen in a very long time." Sabrina leaned up against Mark, to conceal her blush. Nick stood suddenly, his eyes wide with excitement, and a big grin brightened his face. "You have to wear that tonight. It's perfect. The fans will go crazy." His excitement made him pace, only because he could think better when he was moving.

"I am wearing this tonight; under my robe." "No, we have to come up with a way to get you out of that robe. It's perfect Mark. You know how Sean is, and the sight of her, dressed like that, will distract him enough for you to get the upper hand. It's absolutely perfect." "Look Nick, Mark doesn't need my help in winning a match. He's very capable of winning all on his own." "You're not seeing the whole picture here. This could be a whole new angle for the Warlock."

Sabrina stared at Mark; he was as confused as she was. "Okay Nick," Mark prodded. "Explain it." "Okay. Sabrina, you've always been coming to the ring in a black robe, usually with a black dress underneath. The fans have accepted you as the hand maiden of the Warlock. Now it's time to give them the Sorceress, the sexy vixen of evil, the temptress, the seductive collector of souls for the Warlock." "There is no way that I am gonna start something like that. Mark tell him he's nuts!" Mark didn't answer her right away; he was thinking over what Nick had suggested.

"Mark!" "You know; it's not such a bad idea. I've been wondering myself how you could become more involved." "See, even Mark agrees with me." "I don't believe this. Mark you're not thinking ahead," she said staring into his eyes. "Even if I did agree to do this, I won't be able to do it for much longer."

Nick looked at first one, and then the other. "What do you mean?" Nick asked. Sabrina raised an eyebrow as she looked at Mark. He took her hand and nodded; she turned back to Nick. "I'm pregnant." "Well isn't that wonderful news. Congratulations; and don't worry; we can work around it. I really think that this could be a great new story line for the Warlock. Please say you'll do it."

She could detect a faint hint of begging in Nick's voice. Searching Mark's face she could see his answer. "Well, if you think that it will help Mark's career, then I guess I would have to say yes." "It'll be great; you deserve some of the spotlight too," Mark said hugging her tight. "This is going to be a great idea. I'll send the costume designer down to take a look at your robe and the make-up gal to add some effects to the look," Nick interjected.

Checking his watch, Nick made a motion to leave. "Mark I'm gonna need you for that interview soon. We can use that first slot to begin introducing the Sorceress. Congratulations again on your baby, if there is anything that you need just ask," he patted Sabrina's hand. "Nick, could you," she hesitated. "Could I what?" "Forget it," she said turning away. "Mark we have to get going." "Give me a minute," he said.

Nick headed for the door and waited for Mark to join him. Mark took Sabrina in his arms, sliding his hands over the soft round curves of her ass. "I love you," he whispered, before turning to accompany Nick.

Catching her reflection in the mirror, she ran her hand over her flat belly. "Not much longer and the whole world will know about you little one." *I was going to ask Nick to keep our news a secret, but so what if everybody finds out now. Maybe this will be the one catalyst that will make Sean back off; make him realize that I'm not going to go back to him.* Her ankle was beginning to throb again. She put the ice packs back on while she awaited the arrival of the make-up artist and the costume designer.

Sean had returned to the arena late. After his blow up with Nick and his confrontation with Sabrina, he had gone to the bar, to settle his nerves with a few drinks. The arena was already packed with fans, their chants echoing louder and louder within the concrete walls. He had become numb to their screams over the years; and even more so now. His mind was focused on one singular thought, blocking out all outside distractions.

As he wandered through the corridor, to his dressing room, he had to pass the area that had been set up for interviews. His steps halted, freezing him in place momentarily. Standing in front of the cameras was Mark, unprepared and vulnerable. Seizing his opportunity, Sean lunged toward him. *Why should I wait until we're in the ring?*

Sean caught Mark entirely off guard, sending him backwards into a metal gate. Mark's face was engulfed with pain as his back impacted with a steel pipe. Sean continued his rapid blows to Mark's injured ribs. Nick, who had been conducting the interview, ordered the cameraman to keep filming the assault. Mark recovered some ground and struck Sean, sending him reeling backward; but only for a second; he was right back at Mark, his fists striking even harder than before.

D'arcy was on his way back from the ring, and saw the brawl between Sean and Mark. Grabbing Sean from behind, D'arcy pulled his writhing body off of Mark. It took all of his strength to hold him back. "Mark get the hell away from here!" D'arcy yelled. Mark pulled himself up slowly, and hesitated, he wanted to retaliate on Sean, but D'arcy pulled him farther away. "Go on, now!" "Yeah, go on; run away! You can't hide forever you bastard! Tonight I'm gonna end your career!" Brent had also heard the fracas, and came to D'arcy's aid. The two of them dragged Sean back into a dressing room.

Mark was hurt; his ribs ached with every breath he took. The medics tried to get him to come with them, but he refused, walking right past them towards his dressing room, and Sabrina. Being with her would make him feel much better.

D'arcy and Brent barricaded Sean in a dressing room. His rage still boiled, as he turned over tables, and threw chairs about the room. "Looks like we're gonna have our hands full tonight," Brent said to D'arcy, as they watched the tantrum continue. "Yeah, but the priority is Sabrina, and keeping Sean away from her," D'arcy added. "That's for sure. She doesn't need this bullshit; not in her condition," Brent said, softening his voice to a whisper. "What do you mean?" D'arcy asked.

Brent realized that he had just opened up Pandora's box. "Damn, I'm not really supposed to tell, but I guess it would be okay to tell you. Sabrina is pregnant." "Christ, are you sure?" "Yep, I got it straight from her tonight." "Maybe that's why she came to see Sean today." "What?" "Yeah she had me set up a meeting in my room. Man she did everything but get down on her knees to get him to back off Mark, and make him understand that she wasn't coming back to him, but she never said anything about a baby."

Brent and D'arcy were able to speak more freely, as Sean had gone into the shower. They took a few moments to absorb the events of the day. "Man, Sean is gonna go ballistic when he finds out," D'arcy said. "Yeah, but he's not gonna hear it from us, is he?" Brent added. D'arcy nodded his head in agreement. *Telling Sean about Sabrina's baby is not a task that I want to undertake.*

Mark rested briefly against the doorway to the dressing room. *I have to hide my pain from Sabrina.* He tried to take a deep breath, but the sharp pain in his side stopped him short. He held his side until the surge had passed. As he opened the door, he was greeted by her bright, smiling face, but watched as her expression turned to one of deep concern.

"What happened?" she asked. "Nothing. The interview just took a little longer than planned." "Don't lie to me." She touched his face, then showed him the blood on her fingers. Mark licked his lips, tasting the blood on his tongue. His lower lip oozed slightly from where Sean had hit him.

He lowered his head, ashamed that he had lied to her. "I kind of ran into Sean." Sabrina held him tight. He flinched as she applied pressure to his ribs. "You're hurt, aren't you?" "Not really." "Bullshit!" She frantically pulled his shirt up to expose the red area around his ribs. The sight made her ill. "Can you sit down?" she asked helping him to the sofa. "I'm gonna get someone to look at this." "No, it's fine." "Mark you could be seriously injured. I'm going to get you some help."

Going to the door, she opened it a crack; calling to one of the technicians that was moving some equipment. Hearing her shaken tone, the technician sprinted down the corridor, to find the paramedics. Going back to Mark, she stood beside him; cradling his head against her breast, stroking his hair. "This has got to stop. You are in no condition to wrestle tonight, and Sean is out to injure you." "I can't turn back now. If he wants a fight, then that's what he's gonna get." "He's crazy, over the edge. There's no telling what he could do, or what he's capable of," she said as she sat down beside him.

Mark turned to her, his arm holding his side as he moved. "If I don't do this tonight, it's only gonna postpone it to another night. I've never backed down from a challenge before, and I'm not going to start now."

"You have more to think about than just yourself, and I don't want to raise this baby alone." "It's because of you, and the baby, that I have to do this. Sean has got to understand that it's over between you, and if that means beating some sense into him then." "Shhh," she laid her fingers against his lips. "No more talk, just promise me that you'll be careful. I don't know what I'd do without you." He brushed away the tear that rolled across her cheek. His lips touched hers with such softness, as to melt away her fears.

Their quiet moment was abruptly shattered as the paramedics opened the door, without knocking. Sabrina stepped aside, while they checked Mark's injuries. The pain expressed on his face, when the medic touched his ribs; hurt her deeply; making her turn away. She moved away from the sofa, pretending to be busy with arranging the rest of their wardrobe. She became very uncomfortable when she caught one of the paramedics looking at her. She grabbed for her robe and sneered at him.

Mark refused their requests to take him to the hospital, and at his command they began wrapping tape around his ribs. As soon as they were done he dismissed them harshly. Sabrina watched as he carefully got to his feet, holding his side as he straightened. The tape covered a large area of his body, from just below his chest, to a couple of inches above his navel.

"Does it hurt much?" she asked. "A little; but the tape is more annoying." She saw the goose bumps that covered his skin. "You're cold. Come here." Opening her robe, she invited him in. Wrapping her arms, and her robe around him, she held him close. Her body was warm, and soothing to him. He held her tighter, her silky hair, cushioning her head against his chest.

"I wish that this was all over and that we were at home," she sighed. "Soon. After tonight only two more shows, and then a week of peace and quiet." A knock on the door distracted them. "Fifteen minutes," the mystery voice called. Sabrina carefully tightened her hold on Mark. *If only this was all just a bad dream, but I know it isn't. I'll have to be strong for both of us.* "It's gonna be okay," he said, trying to alleviate her tension as well as his own. Reluctantly, she let him go.

It'll be impossible to persuade him to not go on; but at least I'll be with him. Mark struggled with his shirt. The tape pulled as he lifted his arms up. "Let me," she said. Easing his shirt over his head she smoothed it over his back and began tucking it into his tights. Working her way around to the front, she ran her hand softly down his chest, pushing the silky fabric across his abdomen and low into his tights; searching for that part of his body that she craved so much.

Mark grabbed her arms. "Later," he said pulling her off of him. "I'm sorry I just can't seem to help myself." She came around to face him, biting her lip. "I think I've turned into a nymphomaniac." Mark laughed; it hurt, but he had to. "Now that's a real good one, a pregnant nymph." Taking her back into his arms, he pressed her hips firmly against him.

"If you describe yourself like that, then what would be the male version?" "Hmmm, let me see in one word, a stud. A gorgeous, virile, sexy stud is what you are." "You know; you are really bad." "I know; but you're to blame." "Well, after the show this stud is gonna take you back to the stable for a roll in the hay. You have given me a wonderful gift today and tonight I want to give you something." "I don't need anything Mark." "Yes you do. When this is all over tonight, and our problems are all put away, I want to give you a gift that you've waited too long to receive." "What is it?" "You must have patience for just a little longer, but I hope it will please you." Their lips met with electricity, making her shudder with the sensation.

Another knock at the door. "Five minutes," the voice called. Mark stroked her cheek; he hadn't noticed until now how different she looked. The make-up artist had turned her into a goddess. Her eyes were more vividly defined, making them jump out; to him, she had become the ultimate in sexuality and seductiveness. It would be a long night, waiting until they were back at the hotel.

"Time to go," he said picking up his robe. "You just keep having those naughty thoughts, and when we get to the ring the fans are going to love you." She was still nervous, about her new role, but more so about Sean.

At least my ankle has stopped throbbing; more likely it's merely the adrenaline rush that has overridden the pain. The music for the Warlock began to play. The arena became deafening from the screams of the fans. Sabrina took a quick glance around, fearing that Sean would launch a sneak attack, but other than technicians, the only person she saw was Tony. He smiled and winked at her; it gave her a good feeling.

Mark made his move through the curtain. Sabrina followed a few steps behind. The fans screamed his name, reaching out for him as he made his way to the ring. Mark moved very slowly, and methodically, as if he was oblivious to the masses that tried to touch him. He climbed the three steps to the ring and entered. Sabrina waited on the top step until Mark parted the ropes for her to enter.

Losing herself in the moment, in the mystical rhythm of the music, instead of coming around to face him, like she usually did, she slid her arms under his, and began caressing his chest, as she undid his robe.

The fans erupted as she sensuously glided her hands over his body, slowly removing his robe. Taking it, she tossed it to a waiting ring attendant. Mark had now turned to face her, keeping his mouth fairly rigid as he spoke to her. "Very good, now it's your turn, you sexy thing."

The music still played. Sabrina moved her body close to his, not close enough to touch, but enough to give a good effect. Her body swayed to the beat of the music. Mark grabbed the front of her robe with both hands and in one swift movement he tore it wide open. Pushing it back off of her he let it drop to the mat. She kept her eyes locked onto Mark's. She could hear the volley of cheers, and whistles, and cat calls from the audience. Stepping closer to him, she moved her body up and down against his side as she gyrated about him. The noise in the arena grew louder.

An announcer had entered the ring with them. He approached Mark for an interview. The music lowered until it was gone. "Warlock, if I may. I was going to start out by asking you about this match with the Guardian; but I think our fans would really like to know more about this gorgeous woman." As he said it there was another barrage of cheers from the fans. He held the microphone up to Mark, awaiting an answer.

Sabrina seized the opportunity to play with this man. Leaving Mark's side, she began teasing the announcer with soft strokes of her hand, as she rubbed her body against him. *He's visibly wary of me; whether it's an act, or not, I can't tell.*

Mark kept an eye on her antics as he spoke. "This is not an ordinary female. This she devil is the Sorceress, the evil seductress of the darkness." "So what does she do for you exactly?" the announcer asked. That question brought on more whistles from the audience. "As you see, she has been branded with the mark of the Warlock, making her loyal to my commands. What she does, is increase my powers, by supplying me with the souls that she has collected from her unsuspecting victims." The announcer made it appear that he was nervous with her advances. He backed off, and so did she. Returning to the side of her master, she again began caressing his body.

The announcer regained his composure and returned to the interview. "Now Warlock, about your match with the Guardian, this war has been brewing for some time now. What exactly is going on?" "The age old battle between good and evil, but tonight, Guardian, your soul will be sacrificed to the Warlock, to burn in hell for all eternity. Darkness and evil will reign triumphant tonight."

Mark ended the interview by walking away. The announcer left the ring as Sean's music started. Mark held open the ropes for Sabrina to step through. Her hand softly glided across his, as she went to the stairs and descended. She paced along the side of the ring, waiting for Sean to make his entrance, dreading this confrontation.

Sean burst through the curtain at a run toward the ring; he slid in under the bottom rope, was on his feet and attacking Mark in mere seconds. Mark was prepared for him this time. He pushed Sean away, sending him across the ring into the turnbuckle. Sean retaliated with a running kick that sent Mark crashing to the mat; pinning him down with repeated blows to the face and chest. The referee shouted at him to stop using his fist, but Sean ignored him. This was a no-holds barred match. Mark used his strength to throw Sean off of him, giving himself enough time to get back to his feet. Sabrina continued to pace; her stomach in knots, feeling each blow that struck Mark.

This is the worst match that I've ever witnessed. Mark's trying to keep his actions to wrestling moves, but it's so hard. Sean is doing everything against the rules. Even with a no-holds barred match, there was still supposed to be some degree of professionality.

Sabrina didn't notice Tony, until he touched her arm. "This has got to stop!" she said loudly. Tony could plainly see the despair on her face. "It'll be okay; look." Sabrina followed his gaze to the other end of the ring, where stood Brent and D'arcy. "This won't get out of hand," he tried to reassure her. "We won't let it." *I'm already convinced that this fight is out of control, and if they wouldn't stop it, then somehow, I'll have to.*

Sean had not seen her at ringside. His rage blinded him to everything but Mark. For a moment Mark had the upper hand; he had been able to mount an assault on Sean; and after many blows, he sent Sean headlong into a ring post. It took him a moment to steady himself. His shoulder burned from the impact with the steel post. Sean took the opportunity to slide out of the ring; he saw Sabrina and moved to her. Tony stepped in front, blocking his advance.

Sean advanced closer. Tony shoved him away. Mark was behind Sean. Catching him, he hurled him against the steel steps. Mark climbed back into the ring, lingering in the corner, nearest to Sabrina. The distress on her face worried him. He extended his hand to her. She reached for him, but could only touch his fingertips.

Tony had left her side, as he saw Sean grab a metal chair before climbing back into the ring. He reached for him, but he was just inches from his grasp. Mark felt the movement of the ring. *I guess Sean's back for more.* He winked at Sabrina and turned to defend Sean's next attack. Sabrina could only watch in horror as the scene in front of her unfolded, in slow motion.

Mark turned around as Sean raised the metal chair high above him and swung hard, hitting Mark in the head. The sturdy giant fell backward onto the mat, like a giant tree that had been cut away from its roots. The ring shuddered as Mark's body impacted with the mat. Sabrina looked on in shock. Sean still held the chair in his hands, a large dent in the seat. Mark lay motionless, but that didn't stop Sean from striking him again with the chair, once more in the head, and another blow to his hip.

Sabrina panicked, and climbed onto the edge of the ring. "You son of a bitch!" she yelled at Sean. Sean dropped the chair and went to her. "I told you; I'm the better man! I'm the one you should be with!" Without even thinking, she raised her hand and slapped his face. His head spun to the side with the impact.

She looked past Sean to Mark. He had moved. She watched him sit up. Blood streamed down his face. She felt sick. Slowly Mark got up, motioning her to get away from the ropes, and Sean. Sean turned back to Mark, pleased with what he saw, but it still wasn't enough. He lunged toward Mark. Mark caught him, but he could not see him. The blood had run into his eyes, blinding him. Mark kept his hold on Sean, and mustering all of his strength, sent him hurtling backwards.

Sabrina had turned to get down, but she wasn't quick enough. Sean's body impacted hers with great force, sending her face first to the floor below. She never had a chance to put her arms out to cushion the fall. She hit hard and passed out. The cement floor around the ring was covered with thin foam mats, but they served no purpose in protecting her.

Tony was at her side immediately, calling her name. When she didn't respond to him, he yelled at one of the ring attendants to get the paramedics. Brent and D'arcy had both seen Sean run into Sabrina. They both hit the ring; grabbing Sean, holding him back.

Sam had been watching from the backstage area. He yelled for the paramedics as he burst through the curtain. In seconds he was in the ring. Pulling off his T-shirt, he gave it to Mark to wipe his face. As he wiped away the blood, Mark's vision became clearer. He saw Sean being detained, then he saw Sabrina. Her limp body laying face down on the floor, the paramedics were administering oxygen to her. Mark went into a rage, lunging at Sean. His large hands finding Sean's throat, squeezing hard. Sam tried to pull him free, but he could not get a firm hold. "You fucking bastard!" Mark yelled at Sean. "This is all your fault!"

Sean writhed and struggled, as his life's breath was being choked out of him. Tony came to Sam's aid and the two of them finally released Mark's choke hold. Sean coughed and gasped for air. "Son of a bitch, you're fucking crazy!" "I'm crazy!" Mark lunged at him again. "If you've hurt her so help me I'll kill you!"

Sam and Tony managed to keep Mark from getting another hold on Sean, but they couldn't stop the knee that connected with his groin. Sean doubled over with the pain. Brent and D'arcy dragged him from the ring. Mark stepped over the ropes and jumped to the floor to be with Sabrina. Pushing the paramedics aside he knelt down. She was still unconscious, and could not hear his voice, or feel his touch.

"Let them do their work," Sam said, tugging at Mark's shoulder. "She'll be okay." "Go to hell!" Mark snarled. The paramedic handed Mark a thick gauze pad. "You're bleeding on her," he said. Seeing the red droplets against her skin, Mark took the gauze and held it to his forehead. He felt so helpless, watching the paramedics work on her. *God please, let her be okay.* They lifted her onto a stretcher; her arm dangled down at her side. Lifting it up, Mark laid it across her belly. His heart was breaking, thinking about the baby, hoping that the fall had not injured it.

The paramedics wheeled Sabrina out of the arena and into a waiting ambulance; Mark climbed into the back with her. Tony and Sam watched as the ambulance left the arena. The sound of the siren echoing off of the concrete pillars. "I sure hope that she's okay," Tony said. "It would be such a tragedy for her; for them both." "What do you mean?" Sam asked. "Oh man I guess that you don't know either." "Know what?" "Man, Sabrina and Mark just found out that they're going to have a baby." Sam was momentarily speechless; Tony's news gave him a sick feeling in his stomach. "All we can do is hope and pray that nothing goes wrong," Tony added, giving Sam a pat on the back.

Brent and D'arcy had dragged Sean into his dressing room. The blow to the groin had made it difficult for him to walk. D'arcy began pacing about the room; his anger getting the best of him, he walked over to Sean and gave him a shove. Sean wobbled backwards into a chair.

"You stupid son of a bitch!" D'arcy yelled. "She told you; no, she begged you to back off; but no, you and your God damn ego wouldn't listen! Now look at what you've done!" "I didn't cause her to fall!" "I don't give a shit! If you had damn well listened to her and given up this hopeless pursuit none of this would have happened!" "I'm not giving her up; she belongs with me!" "For Christ's sake Sean, open your fucking eyes, Sabrina is not going to come back to you; she's in love with Mark!" "No, she isn't; she's just caught up in the illusion!"

D'arcy's patience was shot. *I have to make Sean understand, once and for all.* "Good God man, what planet are you on! They are in love; everyone can see it." "She's not in love with him!" "I don't believe you. Are you that fucking blind? Sean, she is having his baby; and if that isn't love then I don't know what is." Sean was rocked by the announcement. "What?" "Yeah, you heard me; she's pregnant, with Mark's baby, and there is no way in hell that she's gonna come back to you, ever. Got it?"

Frustrated with talking to a wall; D'arcy grabbed Sean by the shoulders. "Has it sunk in yet? Has anything I've said seeped into that piss ant brain of yours? If it has, then you will give up this hopeless crusade. Christ Sean, you should be happy for her; she's found the love, that you and I both know, you're not capable of."

Brent pulled D'arcy away. "Let him be for a while; he's got a lot to think about now." D'arcy couldn't deny Brent's request. He rocked his head from side to side, snapping his neck into place. "I just hope that he heard what I said." "He heard you man; he heard you," Brent answered, following D'arcy out the door. Sean didn't even notice them leave; he sat slumped in the chair, D'arcy's statement echoing in his brain. The one and only line that kept swirling about, louder and louder, was D'arcy telling him that Sabrina was pregnant, with Mark's baby. Sean leaned forward, putting his face in his hands, he began to weep; painful sorrow filled tears.

Sam was only minutes behind the ambulance. *I'm not quite sure why I'm going, but after what Tony told me, I feel that I should be there.* As he entered the emergency room, Sam began to realize just why he was there. He could hear Mark's commanding voice, intimidating the staff; demanding that they do something for Sabrina, and rejecting their pleas to have his own wounds tended to. Sam followed the noise until he found them. Mark was at Sabrina's side, and in the way of the Doctor and the nurses.

He put his arm on Mark's shoulder. "Come on Mark let them look after her." "Screw you; I'm not leaving her!" "Look man, if I have to, I will knock you out and carry you out of the way myself; and you know that I can do it." "I can't leave her." Mark was trying hard to hold back his tears. "I have to stay." "I know Mark; but they can't do their job properly while you're here; and you need to have yourself looked at. Come on, I'm sure they can put you next door; so you can at least see her." Sam felt Mark ease up; he watched as Mark leaned forward and kissed her forehead. With the help of a nurse, he guided him into the next cubicle.

The nurse began closing the curtain that separated the two rooms. Sam motioned her to stop. Mark sat on the edge of the bed; his head was pounding. The nurse started to clean the blood from his face; checking to see the extent of his injury. She stepped in front of Mark, blocking his view of Sabrina. "Move, damn you!" he snarled. She jumped and stepped to the side.

Everything about Mark intimidated her, from his immense size, to his looks; to his commanding deep voice. She didn't want to make him mad. She finished cleaning the area of the wound, and handed Mark another bundle of clean gauze. She told him to keep it on the wound, while she went to find a Doctor.

Mark watched Sabrina's face for any sign that she was coming around. *There's nothing, no movement at all. She looks so frail laying there. I feel so helpless; and guilty.* No longer able to control his emotions, tears rolled freely down his face. Sam did the best that he could to comfort his friend. "She's going to be okay." Mark was unable to answer him.

The nurse returned with a Doctor. He had a brief look at the wound and began to stitch it up. It only took him a matter of minutes. Mark was oblivious to the length of time, or to the pain; he wanted to be with Sabrina. Sam had to thank the Doctor, on Mark's behalf, as he was not aware that he was done, or had even left the room.

"Hey man, how do you feel?" Sam asked. "How do you think I feel? The woman I love is lying there unconscious; and nobody is telling me a damn thing! So how do you think I feel?" Mark's voice increased in volume as he spoke.

Hearing the unsettling tone from Mark, the Doctor who was attending to Sabrina, came over to where Mark was. Mark was anxious for news. "How is she?" "She's stable for now." "Then why hasn't she woke up?" "That's due to the concussion." "What about the baby; is the baby okay?" Mark asked. The Doctor took a brief pause; his face seemed to lose all expression. Mark read the worst into it. "That's what I need to talk to you about." "Oh God, there is something wrong isn't there? Is she gonna lose this baby too?" Mark was ill with worry; his stomach churned. He tasted the bitterness of bile in his throat.

"Calm down Mr. Cassidy; I never said anything like that. Now tell me what you meant by lose this baby too?" "She had a miscarriage a few months ago; and the Doctor told her that she would have to be very careful if she got pregnant again." "How far along is she?" "I don't know; we only found out about it today." Mark choked back the bitter taste in his mouth, as the Doctor continued. "Okay; then what we need to do is an ultra sound to see what's going on in there."

The Doctor retreated to the other cubicle and gave instructions to one of the nurses, who quickly left the room. Mark fought his tears. "She just can't lose this baby; not now, and not like this." Sam sat down beside him. "Man have I been out of the loop too long," he said, hoping that Mark would enlighten him. "I'm sorry Sam, but I'm not in the mood to rehash all of that; not right now."

I have to concentrate on Sabrina. It didn't bother me when she lost Sean's baby; but this is different, this is my baby. Our love created this life. Now, to be faced with the possibility of her losing it; on the same day that we found out, it would destroy her, and maybe even our relationship.

The nurse returned to Sabrina's room pushing a machine. The Doctor waved at Mark to come to him. "It will take a couple minutes to get her prepared and then I can show you your baby," the Doctor explained. The nurse picked up a pair of scissors and made a move to cut away Sabrina's chaps. "Don't do that," Mark spoke harshly to her. "I'm sorry sir, but I have to remove her clothing." "I'll do it. Just don't cut it," he said pushing her aside.

His hands trembled as he undone the buckle. He had undressed her before, but never like this. Folding the chaps away from her, he managed to slide them off and lay them on a chair. Her thong was even easier; the leather ties came loose at his touch. Before he took it off, he pulled a sheet up, over her body. "Do you need her top off as well?" "No, not yet."

The lights were dimmed in the room, as the Doctor set up the machine beside the bed. Mark moved a chair over to Sabrina's bedside; he slipped his hand into hers and squeezed it lightly. The nurse folded the sheet down, exposing Sabrina's belly. She squeezed a gel onto it, and the Doctor began moving a thick wand around on her belly. From where Mark sat he could not see the computer screen, that the Doctor was watching so intently.

After several minutes, Mark could no longer stand the tension, he had to know. "Well, what's the verdict? Is the baby okay?" The Doctor looked over at Mark, and for the first time during this ordeal; he saw him smile. "Everything looks fine. The baby appears to be unharmed." He paused for a moment, letting Mark absorb the news. "Would you like to see your baby?" The Doctor turned the screen slightly so Mark could see it.

The image is so fuzzy. I don't see anything that looks like a baby. The Doctor moved the wand around and stopped; he pointed to the screen. "See there, that's the heart." Mark was amazed as the image on the screen pulsated with life; he was overwhelmed with emotion. *If only you could see this Sabrina.* He gave her hand another gentle squeeze.

The Doctor moved the wand again, this time Mark could see the whole baby; its head, arms, and legs all clear on the screen. "Sam. Sam, come here." Sam came around from behind the curtain. "What is it?" "Look Sam; that's my baby." "Well, I'll be," Sam answered, staring at the screen. He had never seen anything like it before either.

"Is it a boy or a girl?" Mark asked. "Well, that I can't tell you, for two reasons, one being, that the baby just isn't quite in the right position to see and second, I don't believe in telling parents what they are going to have. It takes the mystery out of the pregnancy." Mark had to be content with the answer. *In a way I do agree with the Doctor; it will be much more fun waiting to find out, rather than knowing now.* Mark continued to watch the screen; all of a sudden he noticed that the baby's heart had stopped beating; he panicked. "What's wrong? The heart stopped."

"Nothing's wrong; I just froze the picture for a moment." "Why? Did you see something wrong?" "No. I just thought that you would like to have this," he said handing Mark a sheet of heavy paper. Mark took the paper and looked at it. In his hand he held a picture of the baby. Tears overflowed in his eyes. "Thank you," he stammered. "We're going to have to move her up to a room soon," the Doctor said, turning off the machine. "The nurse will help you to remove the rest of her clothing and get her into a gown." "When will she wake up?" "I don't know. I wish that I could give you a better answer, but I can't. Just keep talking to her." The Doctor left the room.

Mark leaned over Sabrina and gave her a soft kiss. Mark was alone, with Sabrina, and his thoughts. He found it hard to speak to her. He comforted her as best he could, with soft strokes on the cheek, and gentle pressure on her hand. *I will wait for you, like I've waited all these years.*

Chapter 13

Three long arduous days had passed and still Sabrina had not awoken from her involuntary slumber. Stirring very slightly, but it was never enough to bring her back. Mark had not left her side once; sleeping in a chair, or pacing around the bed. Talking to her had become easier, and once he started he found it hard to stop.

Nearly sick with worry, he was becoming very disheartened. The Doctor offered him no acceptable explanations; but Mark perceived that her well-being was in jeopardy the longer she remained in this state. The nurse's were more forgiving, offering up more reasonable, understandable explanations that he clung to for emotional support.

This repose is her body's way of healing itself; it offers me some comfort; but I won't feel whole again until she's awake, and with me. I long to hold her in my arms again, to feel her body next to mine.

Tony had cleaned out their hotel room, and had brought all of their luggage to the hospital, before he had to leave with the tour. Nick had been in, to tell Mark to take as much time as necessary. Little by little, all of the guys had stopped in to see him, and to offer their well wishes for Sabrina. Mark had little or nothing to say to any of them; and they never stayed very long. Brent had been in every day; several times a day. He never instigated a conversation with Mark, just sitting quietly, waiting with him.

Today, when Brent arrived, Mark was still perched in a chair next to Sabrina; he couldn't help observing that Mark had not changed his clothes. *He's still wearing all his ring gear.* "Hey, Mark, any change?" he asked, touching him on the shoulder. Mark stretched in the chair. "No. No change." Brent walked around to the other side of the bed he was appalled at the sight. "Christ Mark you look like hell. Why don't you take a shower and put on some clean clothes?" "I won't leave her."

"Man, you're exhausted; go take a shower. I'll sit with Sabrina, and if there's any change I'll get you immediately. Come on man, you don't want her to see you like this; do you?" Mark stroked Sabrina's hand slowly. "I can't leave her." "Yes, you can. I'll be right here with her. Mark you need to take a break; you're not gonna do her any good if you get sick from exhaustion." "Okay; a shower does sound good." He kissed her on the forehead. "I'll be back soon." Picking up his travel bag he went into the bathroom.

Brent took up Mark's seat beside Sabrina; gently patting her hand. *Even lying in a hospital bed, you're still an exquisite creature. Mark is so lucky to have you. I want that same kind of life someday.*

Brent had stayed behind in Las Vegas to start his divorce proceedings. He was anticipating that his wife would give him a formidable challenge about it; but this morning, his lawyer had called to tell him that she had signed the papers with no quandary. She had accepted his bounteous offer of the house and a large cash settlement, alternatively to regular alimony payments.

If I had only known that she would accept so eagerly, I would have done it much sooner. With the papers signed, and the agreement made, there was no need for them to go before a judge; they were divorced; with the exception of waiting the few weeks for the final papers. *I am a free man now; but I'm not about to rush out and find a woman right away. I can play the field, but I am sure about one thing I want a woman like Sabrina. A graceful, caring, loving woman who will stand by me, and someday give me a child.*

He sat back in the chair, when he realized that he had been stroking her cheek while he envisioned his fantasy. *In a way, I'm envious of them, and of the relationship that they have. Many times I've wished that it had been me that had caught her attention, but on the day of the party at Sean's I was far more interested in getting drunk. I had deliberately avoided the opportunity, and I do regret it; but someday I will find that special woman.*

The shower had done Mark a world of good. In the solitude he had wept, praying for her expeditious recovery. Feeling somewhat revitalized yet still emotionally wearily; the evidence he could plainly see reflected back at him in the mirror. Dark, deep circles rimmed his green eyes, and three days of not shaving made him look even worse. He rummaged through his bag until he found his shaver, and an elastic band.

Combing his wet hair back, he hastily wove it into a long braid, securing it with the elastic. He shaved the stubble from his face and trimmed his beard and mustache. His momentum began to accelerate when he realized that he had been away from her for too long. He pulled on a pair of jeans and a shirt; leaving it unbuttoned as he left the bathroom; giving the tape around his ribs time to dry. The ribs didn't hurt any more; now if only the inner suffering would heal as fast.

"Any change?" Mark asked. "No, sorry." Brent noticed the tape. "How are the ribs?" "Not that bad. I'm gonna leave the tape on for a few more days." Mark was at Sabrina's side; leaning over her, he gave her a soft kiss. "What's this?" Brent asked, holding up the ultra sound picture. Mark smiled. "That my friend, is our baby's first picture." "Really?"

Mark saw the baffled look on Brent's face. He went to where he was seated, took the picture, and handed it back to him. "You had it upside down," Mark said. Brent scanned the image again. "I'm sorry, but I just don't see it." Mark took the picture back. "Here; this is the head, there's an arm, and that's a leg," he said, outlining the picture with his finger. As soon as he pointed it out, Brent could see it more clearly. "Wow, this is incredible." "That it is Brent. You know I never knew that I could be so happy. She's transformed my life; made me complete. There isn't a day that goes by that I don't give thanks for having found her." "You are blessed Mark." "Yeah; but so are you. You're married; you know how it feels to be in love." Brent lowered his head, walking toward the window.

"Brent, what's wrong?" "There's something you should know. I'm not married anymore; that's why I'm still here in Vegas. I'm kind of between homes right now." "Oh man, I'm sorry; I had no idea that you were having problems." "No, nobody did. I kept my home life to myself; what little of it there was." "So what are you going to do now?" "I'm not sure yet. I guess the first thing to do is to find myself a place to live. I can't survive in hotels forever; but I don't know where I want to settle."

Mark let his gentler side show. "Why don't you come and stay at my place in Texas? As soon as Sabrina is well enough, that's where we're going. She doesn't know it yet." "No, I'm not gonna be a burden on you two; you need your privacy." "Ah hell man; there's plenty of room." *The offer is too good to pass up.* "Thanks Mark; I do appreciate it."

Their conversation was abruptly halted; Sabrina stirred in her bed. Mark sat down beside her. He leaned in close, calling her name softly. "Sabrina; come on baby wake up. Sabrina, can you hear me?" Her eyelids fluttered. "Come on baby, wake up; you can do it," he urged. Sabrina blinked several times, her eyes adjusting to the light. Her mouth moved as she tried to speak. He leaned in closer to her; her voice was weak and faint. "Baby," she whispered. Mark looked into her eyes. "The baby is fine." He placed her hand, and his, upon her belly; his tears momentarily blinding him to her beauty.

Brent had left the room in search of a nurse; he returned promptly, but remained outside the door. *The nurse needs to check on Sabrina's condition, and my place isn't in there with them.* Mark appeared at the door; the nurse had excused him, much to his dismay. Brent could see that this revelation had changed Mark, his wide smile had wiped away the many days of no sleep.

"See, I told you that she would be okay," Brent said. "I know you did, but I still worry about her." "Why? She's gonna be fine; isn't she?" "Yeah; but it took me so long to find her, that I just want to protect her from anything, and everything that might hurt her." "You can't wrap her up in a cocoon, or keep her locked away. It's just not right. As bad as you want to keep her safe, you have to be able to let her have her freedom." "You're right."

"Mark, listen, you know you can count on me, and the other guys, to keep a watch over her too." "Thanks for all the support." Mark felt a need to unburden himself. "I've never been one to have a lot of friends; and that's my own fault; but it's good to know that you, and the others, have been so supportive lately." "Don't mention it. You and Sabrina are a part of this business. That makes you family; and a family takes care of its own."

The nurse came out of the room. Mark took her arm before she could get too far. "How is she?" "Still a bit groggy, but otherwise she's doing very well. She will be weak for a while; so don't push her too hard." "Can I see her, or do you still have things to do?" "No, I'm all finished for now; and I do believe that she is waiting to see you," the nurse responded with a smile. Mark was eager to return. "Come on Brent the lady awaits." "No, you go on and be with her. I'll come back later." *I can't intrude, not now.*

Mark didn't waste any time, or give Brent a second chance; he entered the room and was quickly at her side. Sabrina lay with her eyes closed; the head of the bed was slightly elevated. To Mark she still looked so frail and vulnerable. "Sabrina," he called, softly stroking her arm. She opened her eyes and smiled at him; her fingers searched for his hand. "How do you feel?" he asked. She licked her lips. "Thirsty," she answered. Her voice was cracking from the dryness.

He poured out a glass of water and held it while she took a long drink. "Feel better?" "Still thirsty." He went to refill her glass, but she gestured him to stop. "Would you like some juice instead?" Mark asked.

She shook her head no. Reaching her trembling hand to his face, her fingers traced over his lips. "You," she whispered.

Leaning down to her, he kissed her tenderly. He had waited so long for this moment that he had to focus his attention on being gentle with her. Her arms found their way around him trying to pull him closer but between her own weakness and his resistance she could not. "Not yet," he said quietly.

Her voice returned to its normal quality the more she spoke. "How long have I been here?" "Three days." "It feels much longer than that." "What do you mean?" "My back hurts," she said, squirming trying to relieve the pressure. "If you can turn onto your side, I'll rub your back for you." "How can I say no to that offer?" With Mark's help, she rolled onto her right side. Folding the sheet down to her waist, he loosened the cloth bows of her gown. The knots had left deep red indents in her skin.

He located a bottle of body lotion on the table next to her bed. "Where do you want me to rub?" "I don't care, anywhere, from my neck to my waist." Mark smoothed the lotion over her back and began to gently rub away her tension. "Oh that feels so good." He felt her muscles relaxing as he worked. She yawned deeply. "Still sleepy?" "Mmmm." He put the lotion away and got up from the side of the bed. She reached for him. "Don't leave," she said, looking at him over her shoulder. "I'm not going anywhere. I'll still be here while you sleep." "Hold me," she said even though her eyelids were fluttering to stay open.

Somehow she found the energy to wiggle closer to the edge of the bed. "There's room for you." *How can I say no to her, I've been waiting a long time to hold her again.* Kicking off his boots, he carefully laid himself down beside her. She lifted herself up enough for him to slide his arm under her neck; cradling her against him, his arms holding her securely. *It feels so good to lie down, but it feels even better to have her in my arms again.* Within minutes he relaxed into a deep sleep.

Brent had gone to the cafeteria, to get himself something to eat; taking his time, giving Mark and Sabrina the privacy that they needed right now. *I'm glad that she's going to be okay; but I hope that Mark doesn't seek some sort of revenge against Sean, even though it really wasn't Sean's fault that she fell. Mark couldn't see when he sent Sean into the ropes, causing* him to collide with Sabrina. In all my years in this business, I've never seen such a volatile situation as this one.

There had been occasions, when wrestlers were pitted against each other, but it was only a story line. One that was finely rehearsed and choreographed; and it was only done to boost ratings, or ticket sales. Never had anything gotten so personal. I don't know the whole story, as to why she left Sean, and I'm not sure that I really want to.

His thoughts carried him slowly back to Sabrina's room. From the doorway he could see Mark's body lying beside her. The vision of them together made him warm inside; but still painfully lonely.

The nurse was coming out of the next room. Brent stopped her. "Do you have a spare blanket?" he asked. "Yes, but why?" Brent pointed into Sabrina's room. "He can't do that!" "Yes, he can, and you're not going to disturb them, are you?" He had to hold her back from entering the room. "It's against policy." "Screw your policy; now get me that blanket!" His tone had turned harsh. The nurse didn't like being intimidated but she also didn't want to cause a scene. She went to get the blanket.

Brent went quietly into the room. Unfolding the blanket, he laid it over them. *Mark is so tired it will take a lot to wake him at this point.* He spread the blanket over his back, and went around to the other side of the bed to straighten it over Sabrina. With his task nearly completed, he felt something touch his hand. Looking down he saw Sabrina's fingers creeping over his hand. Her eyes fluttered open long enough for her to look at him and smile. He returned the gesture and tucked her hand back under the blanket. She was back asleep before he left the room. On his way out Brent stopped at the nurse's station, advising them all that they had better keep their distance from her room, for a few hours at least.

Returning to his hotel room; Brent called Nick to let him know that Sabrina was awake, and to tell him that he also needed some time off; to straighten out his divorce. An audacious lie, but he didn't care. He finally tracked down D'arcy at his hotel in New York. "Yeah she's awake and doing really good. The baby is fine too," Brent said. "That's great news; Mark must be relieved." "He sure is. He's finally gonna get a good night's sleep."

There was a short pause between them. Brent had run out of things to say and D'arcy fumbled with the questions in his mind. "So, what's up with you? I've been wondering why you stayed behind in Vegas, instead of moving on with the tour. Is anything wrong?" D'arcy asked. "No, there's nothing wrong; in fact, I've never been better." "Then why did you stay?" "Well, you see; I'm getting a divorce." "What!" D'arcy yelled into the phone. "Christ, what brought this on? You've always been happy, being married. So what happened now?" "I'm not going to go into details, but I haven't, or rather we haven't, been a happily married couple for quite some time now; and by mutual agreement we decided to put an end to this farce once and for all."

"So what are you going to do now?" D'arcy asked. "First, I have to decide on where I want to call home and as for the rest, it will all fall into place eventually. I don't plan on being alone for the rest of my life you know." "Well, don't let Robbie find out; you know that little tramp is just itching to get her claws hooked into one of us." "Yeah, I know; but you got to admit she is good in bed." "I mean it man. Don't get mixed up with her; especially now. Give yourself some time and space before you jump into the sac with any woman." "Don't worry D'arcy; I already know what kind of woman I want, and Robbie sure as hell isn't it. Listen I gotta go. I'm gonna stick around Vegas for a couple more days, so I'll keep you posted on how Sabrina's doing."

Brent said his good-byes and hung up the phone; he sat quietly for a moment; yet restless. *It's still too early to go to bed.* "I need a drink, to celebrate my freedom." He headed off downstairs to the hotel lounge. Taking a seat at the bar, he ordered a beer and began playing with the video poker machine in front of him, but paying more attention to the people that were seated in the lounge, looking for someone to keep him company tonight.

Like so many other nights on the road he felt lonely, he needed the companionship of a woman. His appetite for sex had always been good, but tonight his urges were even stronger. He discretely scanned the room again, by way of the mirror above the bar. Not one single woman was to be seen. All of the women in the bar were with someone. He downed his beer and ordered another.

What's the use? Who am I kidding? I'm never gonna find anyone even close to Sabrina; besides this isn't the place to find a woman like that. Man, Mark is sure one lucky son of a bitch. He continued to play with the poker machine, and consume more beer, for onto nearly two hours; until the bartender cut him off. Being even tempered, even when he had been drinking, he accepted the bartenders ruling and carefully headed back to his room. The casino had thinned out. Only the die hard gamblers still remained, poised in front of their slot machines, as if glued in place. His vision was poor, as he wove his way through the casino to the elevators.

Boy did I drink too much or what? The elevator went up, and so did his stomach. He swallowed hard, trying to keep it down. When the elevator doors finally opened he hurried down the hall to his room, the key slipped from his hand and he dropped to his knees to find it. Finally getting the door open, he crawled inside, into the bathroom. His stomach turned inside out, and so did his emotions. He passed out on the floor, tears glistening on his eyelashes.

Mark was the first to wake, surprised to see the sunlight filtering in through the blinds. *I didn't realize that I was really that tired, but I guess my body knew it.* Sabrina was still nestled in his arms. *She feels so good. I can still remember the first time that I held her like this, how soft and warm she was. I loved her then, and even more now.* She moved. *She's waking up.*

"Sabrina," he called softly. She stretched slightly, pulling his arm tighter against her. "Good morning," he said as he kissed her head. "Morning," she murmured. Mark tried to move his arm so that he could get up; she held fast. "I have to get up." "Stay with me," she said, her voice was still groggy. "Sabrina, I really have to get up," he persisted in his plea.

She released her hold and he carefully rose from her side. Pulling the blanket up around her, she compensated for the sudden loss of his body heat. Drifting back and forth between the veil of sleep and awake, she was still aware of what went on around her. She heard Mark come back from the bathroom and she pretended to be asleep.

"Okay, your turn," he said rubbing her hip. "I know that you're awake, because you don't usually smile like that when you're sleeping." "You caught me," she said, peeking at him through one eye. "Sure did, and I'm never gonna let you go either." She rolled onto her back and stretched. She was beginning to feel all of the aches and pains in her muscles. Whether from the accident, or from laying in bed for so long, she didn't know which.

"Come here," she said holding her arms out to him. Leaning down to her, she surrounded him with her arms, while he slid his under her back. He kissed her, lifting her upwards, until she was sitting. "Come on; you should try and get up," he said. "I don't really want to." "Do you want to get out of here?" Mark asked. She nodded her response. "Then you have to demonstrate to the Doctor that you are well enough to go home." *As usual he's right. I hate hospitals, and the sooner I can leave the better I will feel.*

She slid her legs over the edge of the bed. Mark didn't push her to fast; he knew that it would take her a bit of time to get herself adjusted again; he let her sit there for a little while. "Want to try standing?" he asked. "I guess." She wiggled over to the edge of the bed, until her feet touched the floor.

She hesitated; afraid to try this alone, afraid of falling. She grasped Mark's arm tightly, before lifting herself up. Her knees wobbled. She felt weak, lightheaded. He put his arm around her, holding her tight against him. "You're okay; I won't let you fall." Grateful of his support, she took a step, and then another. He kept a firm hold on her. He helped her walk around the bed and into the bathroom. With each step, she felt herself becoming steadier, and stronger.

When she called to him, he burst into the room. "What's wrong?" "Nothing. I'd like to take a shower but I can't get the seat to fold down," she said, pointing to the fold away seat in the shower stall. Adjusting it for her, he started the shower, regulating the water to the way she liked it. While he was busy with the shower, she leaned against the sink and brushed her teeth. Her arm trembled as it supported her. *I'm not quite as strong as I thought I was.* "Anything else?" he asked.

Taking a step, unaided, she fell into his arms. "Could you help me with this gown?" Sabrina asked. He smiled and guided her to the shower. Undoing the ties, the gown fell away to the floor. He couldn't help running his hands over her body, as he helped her into the shower, easing her down onto the seat.

I want to be in there with her, if for nothing else, than to just hold her. "Enjoy you shower; I'm gonna get you a clean gown. I won't be gone long." "No, wait. I don't want another hospital gown. I have one in my bag," she announced. He looked at her puzzled. "I saw our luggage in the corner of the room; it's in the small bag, on the bottom." "Call me if you need me; I'll be right outside the door." He shut the door, but didn't latch it, just in case.

Sabrina sat for a little while, leaning against the shower wall, enjoying the feel of the warm water on her body, washing away the stiffness;

her strength slowly beginning to come back to her. *I wonder if Mark found the gown? What he must be thinking?* It made her smile. *This is not exactly the place I had planned for him to see it; but those hospital gowns are so uncomfortable, and sleeping nude is forbidden. I can't believe that I had forgotten about it. Mind you we have been so busy lately. Oh well, surprises don't always have to be a prelude to sex.*

Mark opened the door. "You okay?" "Uh huh. Did you find the gown and robe?" "Yeah, I found it," he answered, examining the black garments in his hand. The water stopped running. "I'm done." He laid the garments across the corner of the sink, picked up a towel and handed it to her in the shower. She dried herself; while still seated on the bench. Wrapping the towel around her, she asked Mark to help her out. He handed her another towel, but kept his hands on her waist while she dried her hair.

The towel dropped to the floor and Sabrina carefully turned herself around to face Mark. "Feel better?" he asked. "Not quite." "What's missing?" Without answering him she lifted herself up, kissing him on the lips, a lengthy, satisfying kiss. "Wow, I guess you are feeling better," he said, catching his breath. "Mmm, but that's only because I know how much you love me. Now let me get dressed." "I don't think you're steady enough yet." "I have it all figured out."

Reaching down to his hands, she pulled them back to hold her waist. While he steadied her, she picked up her gown and slipped it over her head. The lacy material brushed over his hands. He moved them, one at a time, to let it fall over her body. He gazed, in awe, upon her reflection in the mirror. The black gown clinging to her damp body, giving her sensuous curves astounding appeal. Yet she still looked so colorless against the dark fabric.

"What do you think?" Sabrina asked. "It's beautiful. You're beautiful," he answered as his eyes scanned in every inch of her. "But it really isn't appropriate for the hospital." "So what? If I have to be here then I'm gonna be comfortable," she insisted. "Okay, I won't argue; just put the robe on." "Agreed." "Come on; your breakfast is getting cold," he said escorting her back to the bed. "You had better go and get something to eat too," Sabrina said. "I don't need anything." "Bull. I'm not going to be the cause of you getting sick; now go and get some breakfast," she was intent. Like a scolded boy, being sent to his room, Mark unwillingly accepted his banishment, and departed for the cafeteria.

Brent had spent a long time in the shower, trying everything he knew to alleviate his hang over. Brushing his teeth repeatedly but he could not get the taste of stale beer out of his mouth. He took some aspirins, to stop the pounding in his head, and dressed very slowly. Sudden movements made him dizzy with nausea.

I haven't felt this bad in a very long time; and I promise that I will never do it again. He picked up his gym bag. *A good workout should help me to feel better; but first I'll stop by the hospital and see Sabrina.*

The hotel casino was bustling with patrons, as he skirted around the lobby, to the parking lot. A young couple cuddled together on one of the benches. *Someday I'll know that feeling again.* He tried not to stare as he walked past, but their open display of affection was hard to ignore. He remembered how much like them he was, when he was first married. It saddened him. *All those hopes and dreams seemed a life time ago, but now I have a second chance; to make new dreams, to plan a new brighter future, if only I could find someone as loving as Sabrina.*

Leaving the hotel, he was blinded by the bright Vegas sun; he fumbled for the sunglasses in his pocket. The dark lenses soothed his sore eyes, and enabled him to see clearly without squinting. The sun was just beginning to climb up into the sky, but it was already hot and dry. The air conditioning in the rental car was a welcomed relief during his drive to the hospital.

He had become very familiar with the streets of Vegas; he had been here several times before, and nothing changed very much in the downtown area. Casino's opened and closed, but all the major landmarks stayed the same along the strip. Accidents were a common occurrence along the strip, which was always busy with tourists, who didn't know where they were going. So to avoid the congestion, he had learned to parallel the main streets.

By taking the side streets, he was at the hospital in only a few minutes. The corridors were quiet. Visiting hours were still a long time off, and the nurses, busy with their routine duties, didn't even notice him.

Arriving at Sabrina's room, he paused and then knocked before entering. She looked up and greeted him with a smile. His heart skipped a beat, as he stared upon this blonde beauty, wearing the sexiest black night gown he had ever seen. "How are you feeling today?" Brent asked. "I feel a lot better, thanks. Please sit," she said, patting the bed beside her. He accepted her offer and took a seat.

"Where is Mark?" Brent asked. "I sent him to get something to eat." Sabrina turned herself sideways, so she could see him better. His sunglasses hid his eyes from her, as he admired her body; but mostly he was fixated on her breasts. "Why are you wearing the shades?" she asked, breaking his concentration. "Is it that bright in here?"

Brent took them off and put them away. "Rough night?" "What do you mean?" "Your eyes, they're so bloodshot." "Well, let's just say that I've had better nights and leave it at that." "Okay, none of my business. Oh by the way, thank you for last night," she said placing her hand lightly on his thigh. Her touch turned him on. He could feel his jeans becoming uncomfortable.

"I don't understand?" "The blanket, that was such a sweet gesture; thank you." Leaning over, she kissed his cheek; part of her lip touching his. He came to full arousal, trapped beneath the denim of his jeans. He pulled his shirt across himself, hiding the evidence. "Don't mention it," he replied, his body pulsing with adrenaline.

"So how long do you have to stay here?" Brent asked. "Not much longer," Mark answered from the doorway. Brent was startled by his unexpected return, but it was just enough to bring his body back to its normal state. Sabrina extended her hand to Mark as he approached. He took it, allowing her to pull him into her. Brent got up, offering his seat beside Sabrina. She wasted no time in wiggling herself over to Mark, and into his waiting arms. He cradled her backwards to kiss her; Brent turned away.

"So are you going to elaborate on what you said a moment ago; or just tease me?" she asked, slipping her fingers between the buttons on his shirt. "I ran into the Doctor." Mark paused, taking a better look at Brent. "What happened to you?" "Oh he didn't have a very good night," Sabrina answered. "So tell me, what did the Doctor have to say?" "He said that you are doing so well, that he feels that you can go home." "Today!" "No, I'm sorry, not today," he said stroking her cheek.

Her expression of joy was dashed as he spoke; she lowered her head to hide her feelings. Mark raised it back up. "You didn't let me finish. I said you couldn't go home today, because I couldn't get us on a flight until late tomorrow morning." Her face brightened. "Do you mean it? I can go home tomorrow." "Yes ma'am, by tomorrow night you'll be at home, in your own bed."

As she kissed him, he could feel her pressure pushing him back onto the bed. "Hey, stop!" he scolded her. "You can't be doing things like that. For God's sake Sabrina, you were injured; your body hasn't completely recovered yet." She was stunned by his tone. The unexpected angry tone had hurt her; her lip quivered as her tears rushed forward.

All I wanted was to be held by him. My body is too stiff and sore to think of anything else. Realizing what he had done, he held her tight. "I'm sorry I yelled at you. I worry about you; I just want you to be safe. You've got someone else to think about now." He placed his hand on her belly, as she wiped her face with the back of her hands. "I have something that I think you'd like to see," he said. Reaching for the bedside table he opened the drawer and took out the picture. "The Doctor gave this to me when they brought you in. It's our baby."

Mark handed her the picture, watching her face as she looked at it. He could not detect any emotion, until her tears started again. "What? What's wrong?" Mark asked frantically. Sabrina lifted her eyes to meet his; her tears flowed in rivers; but she didn't speak. Through the glistening dew, he could see the joy, and the love in her eyes; he held her close. "I love you Sabrina."

Brent had left the room; unaccustomed to seeing so much emotion from a woman. He found the vending machines and got himself a cup of coffee. *Maybe this will help me to feel better.* He was about to get himself another one when Mark found him.

"How is Sabrina?" "Better; she's taking a nap," Mark answered, sitting down beside Brent. "Man these emotional swings are hard to take." "This is just the beginning my friend; you've got several more months to go," Brent said giving him a pat on the shoulder. "This is all still so new to me. Finally finding my soul mate, and now finding out that I'm gonna be a father. I feel like I'm on a roller coaster."

"You're not having second thoughts are you?" Brent asked. "No! It's just that with everything that's going on; this damn mess with Sean. I'm just glad that Nick agreed to give me unlimited time off right now. It's gonna give us the time we need to adjust, and to make sure that she's well enough to go back on the tours."

"You know Mark you're a very lucky man. You have a beautiful woman who loves you unconditionally, and a baby on the way. Man your life couldn't get any better than that. Just don't go overboard on trying to protect her." "You're right, and speaking of lucky, I would guess from the looks of you, that you didn't get any last night did you?"

Brent stretched to alleviate the kinks in his body. "No, all I got last night, was drunk." "You're trying too hard. You just got divorced; give it some time; you'll find someone." "I know. Ah enough of this, I have to get my stuff packed and figure out where I want to go." "Hey I told you you're coming back to my place. Besides I've already made your reservation; and who knows, you just might meet someone in Dallas," Mark said with a grin. "Make sure that you're back here by nine in the morning." "Sounds good, give Sabrina a hug for me and I'll see you later."

Mark watched Brent walk down the hallway and disappear around a corner. He returned to Sabrina's room and took his seat beside her bed. She was still asleep; the picture lay beside her, her fingers touching the edge of it. He watched her sleep; the gentle way her breasts lifted when she inhaled, and slowly lowered as she exhaled; her eyes darted beneath their lids. *She's dreaming, of what I wonder?* He relaxed back into the chair.

I hope that you won't be mad at me, when you find out what I've done. I told you that we were going home; but what I neglected to tell you is that we're going to my home, in Texas, not yours in California. When we left on this tour, I told you another lie, that I had arranged for a house sitter, but what I actually did was have my caretaker come up, pack up you things, your cat, and your car, and have it all sent to my place. I haven't been home since I first met you. I hate to deceive you like this, and I promise that I will tell you everything before we leave.

Two states away, the results of Sabrina's recovery had reached Sean, at his home. After his confrontation with Mark, and then D'arcy, Sean had taken some time off from the tour. For the past few days he had locked himself away in his house. He hadn't eaten properly, or slept very much. Wanting to be alone, he had dismissed Charles, and turned the phone off. Only the answering machine fielded the outside world. Spending most of his time thinking about what D'arcy had told him; it consumed him to the point that he had forsaken showering and shaving, and even changing clothes. Sean was relieved to find out that Sabrina was okay. Nick had tried unsuccessfully to reach him by phone, and had resorted to sending him a telegram.

No matter how many times he had replayed D'arcy's conversation, it was still hard for him to believe it. *Maybe Mark lied about her having a miscarriage? Maybe she still carried my child, not Mark's. That has to be it.* He repeated it over, and over, until he had convinced himself that it was the absolute truth. Now he began planning his strategy for getting her back.

With his workout completed, Brent showered before leaving the gym. His hangover had lessened considerably; only a slight, dull headache still persisted. *Strange, how I've been able to move about the crowded gym unnoticed. It always seemed that there were fans every where, but not today. No one has bothered me for an autograph or even a conversation; and I would have welcomed either. It's a strange feeling to not be noticed by anyone. The one day that I crave some attention; I get none. Maybe it was like Mark had said; I'm just trying too hard. That's it, just relax and things will happen when they are supposed to.*

When he arrived back at his hotel, he packed up his luggage; leaving out a clean set of clothes for tomorrow's trip. It was still early in the afternoon, and he was getting restless. Watching TV had not been a favorite past time, and going back to the hospital would only be an intrusion. *What to do?* He looked out the window of the hotel room. *What can I do for the rest of the day?*

Even in the bright sunlight, the lights from the casinos still sparkled. "Why not?" Playing in the casino for a while seemed like a good idea. He put on a baseball cap and his sunglasses; obscuring his identity, just in case.

He moved about the casino unnoticed by the patrons. They were too involved in their games to people watch. Not finding a game that appealed to him, he left the hotel and wandered down the street to the next one. The carnival atmosphere at the next casino made him feel like a kid again. He bypassed the slot machines and headed for the arcade. Tossing basketball's through a hoop was easy for him, and to the attendant's astonishment he kept winning. The prizes were stuffed animals, and Brent played until he had won the largest Panda bear. *Sabrina will like this.*

Unknowingly, he had attracted the attention of a young woman; standing against the corner of the game behind him, watching him win; but mostly just watching him. From her vantage point she could only see the back of him, but she thought him to have such a nice ass, that the rest of him had to be just as good. Taking a breath she made her move. "Aren't you the lucky one," she said, leaning against the game facade. "Your girlfriend is sure gonna love that bear." Brent was startled by her; he took a long look at her, before he spoke.

Standing beside him was a young, very attractive woman. Long blonde hair laid against her ample breasts. A tight tank top showed off her narrow waist, and her tight shorts outlined her curved hips. He stopped himself from staring. "No, this is for a friend of mine, and her baby." "She's a lucky lady to have such a friend as you. My name is Laurie." "Hi, I'm Brent." The exchange of introductions was made with the usual pleasantries. Brent asked her if she would like to play a game, and she accepted.

As they played, both Laurie and Brent became more relaxed with each other. He had already begun thinking about getting her into bed; and unknown to him, Laurie entertained the same thought. They played the afternoon away, until Brent's stomach rumbled, reminding him that he hadn't eaten yet today. He asked Laurie to join him for an early dinner. Without hesitation, she accepted his offer. They ate and drank. Brent was getting anxious. He wanted her, mainly because she reminded him of Sabrina. It didn't take much coaxing for him to get her up to his room. He kissed her, and undressed her, as he maneuvered her to the bed. Her willingness made it easy for him to make love to her.

His mind fantasized that it was Sabrina that he was making love to, and that brought out his hidden passion. At the moment of complete ecstasy, he kissed her neck, and whispered into her ear. "Oh Sabrina." Laurie pushed him away and got up. "If I had known that you were just using me to fulfill your fantasy over this Sabrina woman, I would never have gotten into bed with you," she said, pulling on her clothes hastily. "Man, you are one fucked up son of a bitch."

Brent heard the slam of the hotel room door; he lay back on the bed, pounding his fist against the mattress. "Stupid! You're a damn stupid fool!" *How could I let my fantasy surface like that? Being with them in Texas is going to be difficult. I will have to carefully guard my emotions, and my feelings towards her, or I will undoubtedly make an enemy of Mark. I can still have my fantasies, but she will only be a friend, and never anything more than that.*

Mark had stayed with Sabrina all night again; but despite her pleas, he remained in his chair, telling her to get her rest. It was difficult for him to stay away from her, when all he wanted to do was to hold her, but reminding himself that it was only one more night, helped to reduce the strain of his longing.

Sabrina was a lot more mobile in the morning. She had showered and dressed without any assistance from Mark, but still found herself sitting down every once in a while, just for a brief rest.

She sat on the edge of the bed, impatiently waiting for the Doctor to bring in her discharge papers. Mark sat beside her, holding her close. "Don't worry he'll be here soon," he said. "I know; it's just that I want so much to go home. I need to go home. I need to be with you again, to make love to you." As she spoke, her hand caressed his powerful chest. Mark had the same feelings too. "That will all depend on what the Doctor has to say. If he says that we should wait, then that's exactly what we will do. As difficult as that may be, it is for your own protection."

He could see by her expression, that it was not an answer that she wanted to hear. "I know it's hard to think about, but we have to think about your health, and the baby's." "Hold me then." "That, I can do." Taking her against him, he began gently rocking back and forth.

I have to tell her, putting it off will only make it harder, for both of us. "I have to tell you something, and I don't want you to get upset." "Go ahead I'm listening," she said, snuggling closer. "Well, when I said that we were going home, I didn't tell you which home. We're not going back to the beach house. We're going to my, no, our home, in Texas." He waited breathlessly, for her response. She lifted her head. "As long as we are together, it doesn't matter to me where we live." Relieved that she was not mad, he hugged her tight.

Brent knocked at the door before he opened it. "Okay to come in?" he asked, peering around the door. "Sure it is," answered Mark, waving to him to come in. Brent entered, the panda bear under his arm; he walked to Sabrina and presented it to her. "This is for you and the baby." Sabrina's face was illuminated with a broad smile, as she took hold of the giant bear; she hugged it tight. "Oh he's wonderful!"

Sliding off the bed she put her arms around Brent, kissing his cheek. "Thank you so much." "You're very welcome." He was becoming lost in the splendor of feeling of her body pressed against him. Their brief intimate moment was cut short as the Doctor walked in. "Ready to go I see," the Doctor said.

"Oh yes I am!" "Well, I need to complete a brief exam and then you can get on your way." The Doctor helped Sabrina back onto the bed. Brent left the room to wait in the hallway. The Doctor's exam was thorough but brief. "All done," he said as he folded over the flip chart. "You can leave just as soon as you're ready."

Mark neared the bed. "Doctor, I have one question for you before you leave," he hesitated, still uncomfortable with the subject. "What about sex; should we wait for a while?" "Well, in my opinion, there is no reason for you to abstain. The baby is doing very well, as is his mother." He paused, to look first at Sabrina and then Mark.

"I would however recommend that you both explore alternative positions." His eyes became fixated on Mark. "By that I mean, ones that will lessen your weight on her, and minimize the depth of penetration. As the baby grows, traditional positions will become uncomfortable, and awkward for her, and judging by what I've seen so far, this baby is going to be very big." "Thank you," Mark said, shaking his hand. Without any further discussion the Doctor left.

"Get me out of here," Sabrina announced loudly. Hearing her voice, Brent returned. "Need a hand with your bags?" Brent asked. Mark was quick to respond. "Yes, please, because I'm gonna have my hands full right here." He picked Sabrina up into his arms. "I'm not crippled you know; I can walk." "Yeah, so what's your point?" "So my point is, you don't have to do this." "Enjoy it, and stop squirming."

Mark carried her out of the hospital, to the rental car that Brent had waiting for them. As they drove to the airport, Sabrina suddenly remembered the money that she had won. "Mark, did you get the money from the hotel?" "Yes, I did. I had a courier bring it over. It's in the side pocket of your bag there." She settled back, to take in the scenery along the way; scanning both sides of the street for a certain store. When she saw what she wanted, she asked Brent to stop the car in the next block.

"We have a plane to catch," Mark reminded her. "I know; I'll only be a minute," she answered, getting out of the car. Mark opened his door to go with her. "No, I can do this by myself," she said pushing the door shut again. The two men watched as she entered an adult store. "What in the hell is she up to now?" Mark spoke aloud, but the question was meant only for him. Brent didn't dare to comment on Mark's question. His own fantasies answered it for him.

Within minutes she had returned to the car, carrying a brown bag. "So, what did you find to buy in there?" Mark quizzed, his curiosity not staying hidden very well. "That's for me to know; and you to find out later." He knew by her devilish grin that she was up to something; he shook his head and turned back to watch the road.

Before they sent their luggage through at the airport, Sabrina squirreled away the brown bag inside her suitcase. The airport was very busy with travelers; fortunately, all of them too busy to notice them. They were the only people in first class on the airplane. *It's quite nice to have the full attention of a flight attendant. It's uncommon.* It didn't take her long to figure out that the flight attendant was a devoted fan.

Ignoring the frequent visits from this uniformed female, Sabrina rested herself against Mark for a nap; her new bear clutched tight in her arms. Brent dismissed the woman, in a way he was quite harsh with her. "Can't you see my friend is tired? We will call you if we need anything!" *So many people looking out for my interests, it's a good feeling.* Sabrina took it with her into her dreams.

It seemed that only minutes had passed, when Mark gently awakened her. "We'll be landing soon," he said. She slowly straightened up; rubbing her neck, trying to work loose the kink from sleeping the way she did. Mark saw the discomfort on her face, and aided in massaging her neck. He leaned in close to her ear. His mustache tickled as he spoke. "How about a back rub when we get home?" he whispered to her in a low sexy voice. Sabrina looked at him, shaking her head no. Mark was confused by her response.

Leaning into him, her lips pressed against his ear; her breath hot, her voice a soft whisper. "You can start with my back; but I want a full body rub." She spoke slowly and in between each word her tongue teased at his earlobe. A warm flush came over him, and with each lap of her tongue an electric shock raced through his body. She moved her tender kisses across his cheek to meet his lips. "Is it a deal?" she asked. He felt completely debilitated. *She knows exactly what to do to make me give in.* "Yes, it's a deal," he finally answered. She kissed him again, to seal their agreement, then settled back in her seat; a devilish smile on her face, and Mark's hand firmly in hers.

Brent could only imagine what had just transpired between them; but looking at Sabrina it was obviously something that pleased her immensely. Mark, on the other hand, had a blank 'what the hell did I do' look. *Whatever it is, that she's planning, it means that I'll be spending the evening alone, while they go to bed early.*

A limo was waiting for them outside the Dallas airport. The driver took care of the bags, while the three of them relaxed in the back seat. The drive took them just over an hour outside of Dallas, past rambling estates and ranches. Sabrina took it all in, from the oil derricks, to the substantial herds of cattle. Everything was so immaculate and invigorating; the lush green fields, surrounded by white fences.

The limo turned off the main road, passing through a large double electronic gate. "This is it," Mark said. "Home." Sabrina peered out through the tinted windows. They were traveling along a black top drive, passing paddocks with horses, and others with cattle. "This is yours?" "Ours," Mark corrected her. "It's not much, but it's all paid for."

The driveway took them up a small incline and when the car broke over the hill Sabrina had her first look at the house. It was a sprawling rancher style house, painted bright white with blue storm shutters; a warm, inviting home. On the far right side, was a separate building that she recognized as a garage, by its wide blue doors. To the left of the house, set much farther back, was a barn, it too, reflected the colors of the house. Beyond the house, through the stand of trees, the land gently sloped upward to a hill. She could only imagine what was beyond.

They came to a stop, near the front door, that was guarded by two large pillars. A middle aged man appeared from between the pillars and opened the limo door. Mark stepped out first and turned back to help Sabrina. Brent had already exited from the other side. "Sabrina; this is Jim; he runs this place for me. Jim, this is Sabrina, the mistress of the house." Sabrina accepted his welcome, but felt a little strange at being called the mistress. *It has some sense of permanence, but it feels like the wrong word. Our relationship goes much deeper than that; I don't regard myself as just a paramour.*

Dismissing the remark she discretely took stock of the man before her. Estimating him to be in his late fifties, but it was hard to tell through the leathery, weather worn face. *He looks like a typical cowboy, with his plaid shirt, blue jeans and worn out old boots.* Beneath his beat up straw cowboy hat, she could see the traces of salt and pepper hair, neatly trimmed above his collar.

Jim walked with a slight limp, courtesy of a riding accident many years ago, but it in no way hindered his strength; and that was very apparent to Sabrina, as she watched him load up all of their bags, and take them into the house. "I'm gonna go and get myself settled," Brent said, following Jim inside.

"Would you like a tour; or wait until after you've had a rest?" Mark asked. "Tour first, please," she answered quickly, slipping her arm around Mark's waist. They walked slowly towards the barn. "This place is enormous." "Not really compared to some of the other places around here, it's only a hundred and fifty acres."

Why? In all the time that we have been together, why had he not said anything about this place? I understand that he's a very private person; maybe he just had to be sure about us first.

They walked through the barn; she stopped to pet one of the horses. "Are they all quarter horses?" Sabrina asked. "Yes, but how did you know?" "I love horses; remember?" She turned to Mark, her sudden excitement resounding in her voice. "Can we go for a ride?"

His expression turned serious. "I don't think that's such a good idea. Remember what happened the last time you went riding?" "That was just a freak accident. Please can we go." "No! No riding, not right now anyway. Not until you see a Doctor, and he says it's okay."

Mark pulled her close to him. "I'm not going to let you take any unnecessary chances with this baby." "Okay, you win, no riding, but if you can't find me, I'll be out here, spoiling these beautiful beasts." "Should I be jealous?" "Of course not; you're my first priority for special treatment," she said pulling his hips into her. "Want to go up to the hay loft and fool around?"

Mark couldn't help smiling at her care free attitude. "What am I gonna do with you?" "Make love to me," she said softly. He encircled her with his arms. "I love you so much." "Then kiss me; and let me love you. Let me give you the pleasure that you deserve."

Her kisses were a tender distraction. Her hands glided over his body, lingering at the front of his jeans. "No," he strained to say. "Shh; let me love you; I need to love you." Mark was mesmerized by her, as she led him into an empty stall, and closed the door. He reached for her. "No; you can't touch me," she said pinning his arms beside him.

Continuing her tender kisses, she gently pushed him back, against the wall, unbuttoning his shirt. Her touch was delicate against his chest. His muscles tensed when she stroked his stomach. She could feel his manhood growing harder, while she worked his belt loose, and guided the zipper open on his jeans. His heart pounded with eager anticipation.

She slowly moved her kisses down his throat to his chest, using her tongue to draw out a path. Mark had closed his eyes. His mind and body reveled in the sensuous feelings that she transmitted. Her kisses had reached the top of his jeans. His body tensed. He felt her fingers slip inside, freeing him from his confinement. He shuddered, as her tongue glided over him. Her motions were deliberately slow; prolonging the rapture. He was so aroused by this wondrous sensation; he could not maintain control any longer. She held him tight, taking all of his love, until there was no more for him to give.

His body relaxed against the wall, and she released him, retracing the path of her kisses back up his body. His chest heaved, as he panted from exhaustion. "Did you like that?" she whispered into his ear. "Oh, yes," he panted. Laying her head on his shoulder, she wiped the perspiration from his chest. When his breathing returned to normal, he let go of her. "We had better get back to the house, before they come looking for us," he said.

He left his shirt unbuttoned, as they walked back to the house. The steamy expression of their love, combined with the dry Texas sun, left him overheated. Sabrina kept her arm about his waist, leaning into him as they walked. He directed her around to the back of the house. A large serene pool stretched almost half the length of the house. Brent and Jim were seated at a table a few feet away, under the protection of a canopy, safe from the hot sun.

"Where have you two been?" Brent asked, with a silly grin, knowing full well, by Mark's appearance, that they had found some time for intimacy. "Oh we were just checking out the stud in the barn," Sabrina said biting her lip. Jim had removed himself from the table to get two clean plates; he heard Sabrina's remark. "What? There's no stallion out there." "Oh yes there is," she answered quietly. Jim came to realize what she was talking about, it embarrassed him to hear her talk like that, since he was very much old fashioned. He retreated to the house.

Sabrina took a seat at the table and began picking at the fruit platter in front of her. She scanned the other dishes, green salad, vegetables and fruit. "What's with all the rabbit food?" she asked. "That's my fault," Mark answered. "I told Jim that you're pregnant, and that you need to eat healthy meals." "Mark, I'm pregnant, not on a diet!"

Jim had returned to the patio and jumped into the conversation. "Excuse me, Mr. Cassidy, but when my Mrs was expecting she didn't eat like this either. She had some powerful cravings and it didn't hurt her, or our babies. Now ma'am, you just let me know what you want and I'll make sure that you get it. That baby is just telling you what it needs and you listen." "Why thank you Jim, I appreciate it very much," Sabrina answered. "In your honor," Jim continued. "I've planned a good old fashioned Texas barbecue."

"That sounds good," Brent cut in. Mark remained silent. Sabrina could tell that he wasn't pleased with the direction of the conversation. "Hey, it's okay," she said squeezing his hand. "Well, it appears that I'm outnumbered," mark answered somewhat sarcastically. Getting up from her seat, she relocated herself to Mark's lap. "You're not outnumbered; Jim is just passing on a little advice from his own experiences. This is fine for now; but even I don't know when, or even if, I'm gonna have a craving." She lifted his face, making sure she had eye contact. "If you want to set out the menu's, that perfectly all right with me. Okay?" "Okay." She hugged him and whispered into his ear. "This is all new to me too."

Jim had returned to the table with a pitcher of lemonade. "Now look at that, Mr. Cassidy, it sure is nice to have a woman in this house." He gave Mark a wink before returning to the house. He stopped momentarily at the doorway. "Ma'am, there's somebody here who really wants to see you."

Sabrina was completely perplexed by Jim's remark. She looked at Mark, who offered no answer, only a smile. A familiar sound made its way to her ears; she perked up, listening. Faint, but yes familiar. She followed the sound into the house, out from under a chair came Patches. He ran to his master, rubbing around her ankles until she picked him up. "Oh Patches." She cuddled him as he purred and nuzzled at her face. "Oh I missed you so much."

He had missed her as well. He didn't like his new home; despite Jim's efforts to befriend him. "Couldn't get him out of the bedroom," Jim said, watching the reunion. "He just stayed in there all day and all night.

Managed to pull your jacket onto the floor though; guess he recognized your scent." "Oh you poor baby," she talked quietly to the cat.

Mark stood just inside the doorway watching her; she wavered slightly, bracing herself against the back of a chair. He was at her side in a heartbeat. "You need to rest; I'll take you to our room and you can have a nap before dinner." She kept a hold on Patches, as Mark took a hold of her, escorting her up the stairs. For a rancher style house, she was surprised that there was an upstairs.

Pausing halfway up the staircase she let Patches go and leaned into Mark. He could feel her weaken, and picking her up, carried her the rest of the way. She didn't even have the energy to look at the decor of the house. The excitement of the day had drained her terribly, and a nap was welcomed. Mark walked into the bedroom and kicked the door shut; but not before Patches had slipped in. He wasn't going to let his master out of his sight.

Mark lowered her onto the king size bed and sat down beside her. "I told you not to overdo it; but you wouldn't listen," he spoke sternly. Sabrina ran her hand over his chest. "You did like it; didn't you?" "You know I did; but you have to take it slow, no more energetic, romantic outbursts, at least for a few days."

She pouted briefly. An idea popped into her head. "Would you get me that brown paper bag from my suitcase?" He retrieved the bag and handed it to her, unopened. "If I have to stay here and rest, will you stay with me, for a little while?" "I'll stay, but only if you promise to rest." "I promise. A little rest, and a little light reading, that's all, cross my heart." *I'm not quite sure if I should believe her; but if it means keeping her in one spot for a while, then I'll stay.*

"So, what's in the bag?" he asked. Sabrina opened it, and removed a book. "I heard what the Doctor said this morning; and I thought that this might be of some help." She held up the book for Mark to see. He read the title aloud. "The Encyclopedia of Sexual Positions." It embarrassed him to say it. She turned herself to look at him. "I don't want to miss a day without making love to you; and you heard the Doctor as well, as long as we're careful, and creative, we won't have to abstain."

Snuggling close against him, she began perusing the book. Each page was filled with photos, and explicit directions for each position. Mark was even more embarrassed. *I've never looked at anything like this before.*

I've never even bought a men's magazine. He relaxed slightly, the more they looked through the book, and talked about what they were seeing. *It's for her that I'm doing this, and that makes it tolerable.* They had only glanced through a portion of the book when it slipped out of her hands; she drifted sleepily in Mark's arms. Carefully, he laid her down and pulled the blanket up from the foot of the bed.

Brent had given up on seeing them for a while. He had seen the closed door of the bedroom, as he passed by on his way to the guest room. He busied himself with unpacking; sorting his clean clothes from the dirty ones; but even that task was tedious. "Ah the hell with it," he said picking out his swimsuit. "A few laps in the pool should help."

Diving into the pool, he attacked the water, slicing through it with a determined strength, a strength not born of anger, but of frustration. Brent repeated lap after lap, until his arms ached from the abuse; it was all he could do to pull himself up the ladder. *Being here is going to be one of the hardest things for me to do, watching them together, and myself, alone. I have to go back to work, that's the only solution. Tomorrow I'll call Nick and get put back on the tour. At least there, I might find some sexy lady who would be eager to spend the night with me, and put an end to this lonely feeling.*

Sabrina awoke to the sweet smell of charcoal, as it drifted in the bedroom window. Looking at the clock, it indicated to her that it was after six. *I hadn't planned on sleeping so long.* Reaching back to where Mark should be, she found only the emptiness. Patches was curled up beside her.

Rolling onto her back, she surveyed the room. It wasn't overly large, since the bed took up most of the space. A large chair, a desk and an armoire were the only other pieces of furniture in the room. A couple of western pictures hung on the wall above the desk, and another above the bed. The room was very modest, not showy at all. The walls painted in an off white, and the carpeting a dark sand color. *Better go and see what the boys are up to.*

She took her time in getting up. She still hadn't regained all of her vigor that she was used to. She made her way into the bathroom to freshen up; the size of the room took her by surprise. *Everything must have been custom built for Mark's size.*

To the left of the door, was an extra large shower stall, constructed with the shower head in the ceiling not the wall. Next to it, stretching along the wall, was a deep soaker tub, big enough for two. Across from the shower were the sinks; they were higher than normal as well, the top of the counter being the same height as her waist. The one thing that really caught her attention was the hot tub at the far end of the room, partially enclosed by a glass block wall and window. She dipped her hand into the water, grinning to herself. The soft meows from Patches snapped her out of her fantasy.

Descending the staircase gave her the opportunity to observe the living room, with its rustic pine furniture and Navaho print blankets. A truly western theme prevailed everywhere. The room wasn't flashy, or posh, but comfortable; functional and earthy. The living room and the dining room were all part of the one large room, that was the center of the house, and from its sides, doors and hallways led to other areas of the house.

Through the French doors, beyond the dining room table, she could see the three men. Jim tended the barbecue, Mark at his side, and Brent relaxing on a lounger. Each of them had a beer in hand and were involved in some serious conversation.

Making her entrance onto the patio, she went straight to Mark. His expression softened at the sight of her, welcoming her into his arms. His shirt was still unbuttoned, allowing her to slide her arms around him. She kissed his chest before seeking his lips.

"I missed you. I'm not used to waking up alone anymore," she said softly. "You were sleeping so sound; and besides we do have a guest, but don't worry, I'll be there every night, all night." She kissed him again, deeply and passionately. "Excuse me Mr. Cassidy; would you like me to put the steaks on now?" Jim asked, knowing he was interrupting their moment. "Hungry?" Mark asked her. "Starved." "Well then slap that beef on the grill."

Sabrina relocated herself to a chair beside Brent. For a moment she allowed herself to look at his body, it was the first time she had seen him without a shirt. *Wow. I never would have guessed that he was this powerful. The muscles in his chest are so pronounced and those abs, such perfect definition. Even his tan is flawless, but I wish he didn't shave his chest. I wonder what it would look like? Enough, I still prefer Mark's body, but it doesn't hurt to look now and then.*

Clearing her mind of its lingering thoughts, she turned her eyes to Brent's face. "You're awful quiet," she said leaning over to him. "I was just thinking." "About what; or is it none of my business?" "No, I was just thinking; no, more like envying, you and Mark, and your relationship. It's special; perfect." "Hey, why should you be envious of us, you're married." "Not any more; that's why I stayed around Vegas."

Sabrina was shocked by his announcement. "I don't believe it! What happened?" "It's hard to say; but we both agreed that our marriage was going nowhere, and the only logical solution was a divorce. She accepted the settlement; signed the papers and three days later, I'm a single man again." Sabrina moved herself to his lounger and hugged him. "I'm so sorry Brent." "Don't be sorry; it was over a long time ago." He liked the feel of her against him; letting her hold him longer than he should have.

"So what is this?" Mark's voice boomed. "Are you trying to steal my woman from under my nose," he added with a laugh. Sabrina turned to scold him. "You knew, about Brent's divorce, didn't you; and you didn't think to tell me." "Hey don't blame Mark; you had enough to think about without my problems clouding the issue." "Yes, that's partly true; but you're our friend and friends have to be there for one another. They don't let them go through something like this alone," she said, hugging him again. "If there is anything that we can do, just ask." "You already have. Mark has graciously allowed me to stay here until I find my own place, but I still think that you two should be alone." "Nonsense. If Mark said that you can stay, then that means he wants you to stay, for as long as it takes."

Mark had stayed silent, pleased to see Sabrina taking charge. *It means that she's feeling better.* He rubbed his hand across her shoulders. Jim announced that dinner was ready. Sabrina rose up, taking Brent's hand, until he stood beside her. She slipped her arm around his, and her other one around Mark. The two men escorted her to the table.

Sean had been reinstated into the tour, but used all of his free time to hone his skills, and watch videos of Mark's matches. Returning to the ring more focused, and more violent than ever before, winning all of his matches, despite Nick's arrangements for him to lose some. Each day he marked an X on his calendar; counting down the days to when the tour would end in Dallas. He had learned of Mark's retreat to his home in Texas;

and that there was an end of tour party scheduled to be held there. The guys had tried to keep it quiet, but Sean had overheard them talking.

I won't be on the guest list, but that isn't going to stop me from being there. It's been a long time since I was at Mark's home, but sneaking in would be easy. There are no security cameras, no major fences, no obstacles to slow me down. Once inside I'll wait for just the right opportunity to get Sabrina alone and if I can't get her to listen to me, then I'll have to take her away. Away from Mark's influence. Picking up his pen, he went to the calendar. *Only five more days to go.*

Dinner was barely over when Mark excused himself from the table. Having been away from home for so long there was a good deal of paperwork for him to catch up on. Brent disappeared into the house to make a phone call leaving Sabrina alone at the table. Jim was about to clear away the dishes but he couldn't be rude and leave her there by herself. Pouring himself another cup of coffee he reclined back in the chair pondering over how to begin a conversation with Sabrina.

Sabrina stretched and leaned forward resting her arms on the table. "That was a terrific meal. Thank you Jim." "You're very welcome ma'am. So, should I be calling you Mrs.?" Jim asked as he glanced at the ring on her finger. "No," she sighed softly to herself. "Ah don't you worry, he'll ask the question." "I don't know Jim." "He will," Jim said as he patted her hand gently. "Ya know ma'am, I've been with him a very long time and you are the first woman that he has ever brought home. You've changed him." "How's that?"

"Like I said, I've been here a very long time and this is the first time that I have seen him really happy. You've given him a lot. Ya know, this old house just may turn out to be a real home now, thanks to you. So don't you worry ma'am; he'll ask." " How can you be so sure?" Sabrina asked. "I know love when I see it ma'am." Giving her a soft smile, Jim excused himself and took the dishes into the house.

Sabrina sat back in her chair and played with the ring on her finger. *I wish it were true. I want him to ask me but in all honesty it doesn't really matter either way. I just want to be with him and to love him for as long as he wants me.* She quickly put away her daydream as Mark came back out to the patio.

Jim followed close behind Mark as he came to collect the last of the supper dishes. "Would you be needing anything else?" Jim asked. "No Jim, we'll be fine," Mark answered, dismissing him for the night. Brent leaned out the patio door to say his good nights and was gone before anyone could respond to him. Mark and Sabrina were alone on the patio.

A cool breeze drifted down from the hill. It made Sabrina shiver. Moving his chair closer to her, Mark rubbed her arm to warm her. The sun had begun to set, casting eerie spectral shadows across the yard. In the distance the lone, mournful howl of a coyote could be heard; making the approaching darkness more ominous. Mark could see her uneasiness. "Would you like to go inside?" he asked. "Yes, yes I would," she answered quickly.

She watched intently as Mark locked the doors. Her nerves settled slightly as he checked each one. "What would you like to do now, watch a movie perhaps?" Mark asked. Sabrina went to him, needing to be held; her body trembled. "Hey, what's wrong?" "I don't know Mark; just hold me." "Do you feel okay?" "I feel fine." "Then what's making you shake like this?" "I really don't know. Maybe it's just being in this house; it's all so new and unfamiliar." She paused to look up at him. "Can we just go to bed? I really need you to hold me." He rubbed her back, detecting the tension in her muscles. "I know what you need," he said. "What would that be?" "Come with me and I'll show you."

Putting his arm around her shoulders, he guided her upstairs to the bedroom, past the desk and the bed, into the bathroom. "You can choose, the shower, the tub or the hot tub." "Hot tub," she said remembering her daydream. Mark turned on the jets, and the water began to bubble vigorously. He dimmed the lights to create a more relaxing mood; and with the flick of another switch soft music permeated the room. She scrutinized his behavior. "It was part of the house plans," he responded to her silent question. He helped her to undress. Stealing the opportunity to touch her silky skin then helped her into the tub. She relaxed against one of the jets waiting for him to join her.

Mark settled himself opposite her. "Come here," he beckoned. She moved across to him; he turned her around so that she sat between his knees. Pouring water over her back, he gently massaged, pushing her tension down her neck, and out over her shoulders. It didn't take long for her to relax. Her arms limp against his legs; her head tilted to the side. With no resistance, he laid her back against him. "How do you feel now?" "Much better, thank you." "Can you tell me now what bothered you so much; and don't give me that bull shit about the new surroundings. I know you to well, remember?"

"I'm not sure, exactly; it's just a feeling that came over me, a feeling that something is going to happen." "Like what?" "It has to do with you and Sean. Damn it; I wish he would understand!" Her anger made her tense again. "Shh, enough about Sean, we have our own life to think about," he said resting his hand on her belly. "You're right; it's probably nothing anyway. No more thinking about Sean tonight, or any night." She relaxed back into his arms, to enjoy his touch. Yet the feelings still crept back, no matter how hard she tried to ignore them.

The water softened Mark's hands; his touch was gentle against her belly. Rubbing slowly from side to side, yet moving gradually upward until he reached her breasts. She heaved up under his touch; her body wanted him, needed him. She guided his hand down to her thigh, and with his soft touch and the turbulence of the water her body opened up to him. His slow, rhythmic motions brought her to the brink of ecstasy, but she had to have all of him. Turning around, kneeling astride him; she took him in. Her sexual cravings had intensified and Mark had come to know just how to satisfy her.

Through the misty veil of ecstasy, Mark recaptured the fantasy that he had envisioned so long ago. *It's real; she's real; bringing my every fantasy to vivid life. It's no longer just an illusion produced by a lonely imagination; she completes me, makes me a whole man. She is the woman I've waited for, searched for; and the woman I'll fight for. Fate had brought us together, and love will keep us together, forever.*

Tired and weak, Sabrina lay back in his arms. "You should go to bed; it's not good to stay in here for too long," he said. Mark got out first, wrapped a towel around his waist and then helped Sabrina out. Her foot slipped out from under her; she felt the sting of a pulled muscle deep in her groin. Mark had a firm hold on her so she wouldn't fall, but he never noticed her slip. She dried herself slowly, the towel absorbing more than she rubbed. The pain was taking more of her attention than she liked.

Mark had already turned the bed down when she entered the bedroom; he sat on the edge waiting for her. When she appeared, he stood up, letting her get in first; he followed, pulling the sheet over them and turning out the light. The moon light, beaming in through the skylight above the bed, soon took away the dark shadows, bathing the room in a soft blue gray hue. Sabrina lay on her back, massaging her sore muscle; undetected by Mark. She finally turned on her side, drawing her knees up. It lessened the pain and made her more comfortable. Mark put his arm over her and held her close.

I must keep this discomfort to myself; it would only make him worry, and besides a strained muscle is nothing to worry about. It'll be gone by the morning. She tried to convince herself of that.

Chapter 14

The searing Texas sun made the days insufferable. It wasn't until late afternoon that a soothing breeze would commence, making the heat more tolerable. Sabrina confined herself to the comfort of the air conditioned house; only venturing outside when the breeze intensified.

The irritation she was experiencing had not gone away, and frequently it would become unbearable; stopping her in her tracks, snatching her breath away. She had become accomplished at keeping it well hidden from Mark, even when a few intense moments occurred while she was with him, usually while they were out walking. She would stop, pretending to watch the horses until it had passed.

Brent had stayed on, but had kept pretty much to himself. Spending the days working on his tan, or perusing real estate catalogues. Sabrina had tried on numerous occasions to engage him in a conversation, but her endeavors were ineffectual. His responses were kept concise and candid, and didn't let her queries proceed any further. *He's probably still adjusting to his divorce.*

Mark had been with her constantly, with the exception of when she took a nap, attentive and always thinking of her before anything else. The calendar, on the desk in the bedroom, showed the tour schedule. The last day, marked with a red circle, was Dallas; the day after tomorrow. There was still a strange feeling about Sean, and the trepidation that came with it made her cold. Trying to ignore it seemed ineffectual as it returned during quiet times to gnaw at her.

Two days ago Mark had begun receiving phone calls from Nick. *I know that they trouble him; but getting him to talk about them, that would be on his own time.* So far, Nick had phoned only once a day, usually late afternoon. *Any time now.* Sabrina looked at her watch. The phone rang; she smiled at her uncanny timing. Mark picked up the cordless phone and walked to the far end of the patio; far enough away so no one would hear him. *I don't need to hear the discussion, his demeanor, his facial expressions, tell me everything. No more. No more secrets.*

When the conversation ended, he tossed the phone into a chair, and headed across the yard. Sabrina went after him. When she caught up to him, he was seated on a bench under the shade of a large oak tree. She sat down beside him, weaving her arm around his and taking his hand, quietly waiting, giving him the opportunity to speak first. When he didn't speak, she took the lead.

"Okay, no more silent treatment," she said, her voice was firm and determined. "I want to know what Nick said to you." Mark remained silent. "Mark, either you tell me, or I am going to call Nick myself and find out what's going on." "You don't have to do that," he answered with a sigh. "I'll tell you. Nick wants me to make an appearance at the Dallas show. I keep telling him no, but he's insisting." "So, why can't you go?" "The only reason he wants me there is to encourage this conflict with Sean, and I don't want any part of it."

"Let's look at this objectively; or at least try to. This difficulty with Sean isn't going to go away on its own; is it?" "No." "He wants you signed into a match to determine who is the better man; right?" "Yes, but that's all old news." "I know; just bear with me. Now, would this appearance be a boost for your career?" "Probably." "Then, in my opinion I think that you should do it. I want this to be over too, and prolonging it sure isn't helping." "I know but this way just isn't right, and who's to say that even when I beat him, he still doesn't let it drop."

"That is a chance we need to take; but then there's always my solution." "That would be what?" "Let me talk to him again. Not alone; but with Brent and D'arcy, and just maybe between the three of us we can bring this to a reasonable end." "I don't like that idea at all; and you know my reasons." "So, will you go to Dallas?" "I guess," he reluctantly conceded. "Will you come with me?"

Sabrina had to really think hard about that. "No. I think I'd like to stay here. It might be easier on you, if I stayed out of Sean's sight right now. You're not booked in a match are you?" "No, but I still have to be there for the entire show, so Nick can play out his agenda. I wish that you would change your mind and come with me." "No, I'm going to stay here, this time. Besides Jim's here, so what trouble could I possibly get into."

Mark hugged her close to him. "It's gonna be so strange being there without you." "Hey, it'll be okay. It's only an afternoon show, and it's not like you're thousands of miles away." They discussed her decision no further that afternoon, but sat quietly embracing, enjoying the shade of the big oak tree, and watching the horses running in the fields.

Such a peaceful place this is, just like the beach house, secluded, away from the everyday world, a place to dream of the future, and to strengthen our bond.

After dinner Mark and Jim planned out the menu for the party while Sabrina relaxed in a lounger, watching Brent do a few laps in the pool. "Why don't you come in for a swim?" Brent asked her, as he leaned upon the edge of the pool. "No thanks, maybe later," she answered. Brent splashed a little of the water at her before returning to his swim. *I would like nothing better than to go for a swim, but this damn irritation has now become a dull perpetual cramp in my side.* She rubbed at it cautiously, hoping to soothe it away.

As Mark approached, she halted her discreet massage. "Is there anything else you think we might need?" he asked handing her the shopping list. She took it, barely glanced over it, not even reading what was on it; and handed it back to Mark. "It seems fine." "You didn't have time to read all of it." She stood up carefully, resting her hands on Mark's chest. "I'm sure it's fine. You know what these guys like better than I do."

I can see in her eyes that something's bothering her; they don't have their usual brilliance. "Are you all right?" Mark asked. "Yeah, just a little fatigued. I think I'll go up to bed." "I'll go with you." "No, it's okay; you and Jim have a party to plan. Oh, try to include Brent; he seems so distant lately."

Mark gave her a light pat on the ass as she walked away from him. A sudden twinge in his side made him rub his ribs. *I guess I took the tape off too soon.* Dismissing the subtle annoyance, he returned to the kitchen to talk to Jim.

She ascended the stairs gradually each step was uncomfortable. Stopping part way up to rub her side, she checked to make sure that Mark wasn't watching her. The bedroom was a welcomed sight. Her side ached terribly; demanding that she lay down. Stripping off her clothes, as she approached the bed, she left them in a trail across the room. She never noticed the tiny stain of blood that had seeped through to her shorts.

Crawling into bed, she first lay on her back, but that offered no deliverance from this torment. Turning on her side, she pulled one of the bed pillows in close to her stomach. Drawing her knees up she at last found the relief she so desperately needed. With the pain held at bay, she soon fell asleep. For how long she wasn't sure, she heard Mark enter the room.

Remaining motionless, fearing that the pain would return if she moved, she heard him pick up her clothes and take them to the laundry hamper. He was trying to be quiet, but his footsteps fell heavy even upon the carpeted floor.

He was unhurried in his movements, as he got into bed beside her; not wanting to disturb her. Moving close to her, but he did not touch her. She could feel the warmth of his body. She awoke several times that night, from the urge to move, or from missing Mark's arms around her, she didn't know which had disturbed her the most.

Mark was the first to wake in the morning; not at all surprised to see that Sabrina still lay in the same position as the night before. He kissed her shoulder, and gently pulled her onto her back. Startled by the movement, her body tensed, waiting for the return of the pain. Detecting nothing, she opened her eyes. Mark's face hovered above her. He supported himself on one elbow, his other hand resting across her waist.

"Good morning," he said. "Morning." "Are you feeling better?" "Yeah, I guess I just needed the extra sleep." "Are you sure? You were awake quite a few times through the night. You're sure that there's nothing wrong?" "I'm sure. You know you worry too much." "Because I love you; that's why I worry about you; you're far too important to me."

His words brought a lump to her throat. *I want to tell you about this damnable pain, but you would insist that I see a Doctor, and I have had enough of Doctor's.* "How about a shower?" Mark asked, nuzzling at her ear. "You go on; I'll be there in a minute." He left her to go to prepare the shower. She went to stretch, but caught herself before she had gone too far, pausing to stroke her belly instead.

She listened as the shower started, then heard the door close. *I better get up. What actually inspired her was the opportunity to be with Mark. Since that last time, I've not made any advances toward him, and he has made none to me. Despite my primal craving, the act of sex just hasn't come into play. I've been going to bed earlier than him, and I guess that he's not pushing the issue because I've been so tired. Perhaps it was his own injury that made him refrain. That strikes logical; but he didn't abstain when he was injured before. This is too much to think about for this time of the morning. If I don't get up now, I will be showering alone.*

Brent had already finished his breakfast by the time they came downstairs. Jim had excused himself to go and prepare their meals. Sabrina took a seat across from Brent and picked up a glass of orange juice. He surveyed her from the corner of his eye. *Her complexion is so pallid.*
"Are you okay?" Brent asked. "Yeah. Why do you ask?" "Well, you've been going to bed pretty early and I was just wondering if you were feeling okay." "I'm fine and I really don't care to discuss this anymore!" her voice was slightly raised, and very stern. Brent kept silent, caught off guard by her unexpected attitude.

Mark had wandered over to the table. The tension was easy to detect. "What's going on?" he asked. "Nothing!" Sabrina answered. "Damn it I'm sick of this! Christ I'm not made of glass! I had a bad day yesterday, big fucking deal. I don't need to be treated like some fragile piece of art; I won't break!" Brent and Mark both stared at her speechless. Mark had never seen such an unprovoked irrational outburst from her before.

Standing up quickly, her chair toppled backwards, upsetting her even more. She hurried away from the table and disappeared around the corner of the house. Mark made a move to go after her, but Brent blocked his path. "Give her a few minutes," Brent said. "There is obviously something wrong, and I have to find out what it is." Mark tried to step past Brent. Brent held him in place. "Yeah man, there's something wrong; it's called hormones. I've seen my sister go through a similar stage when she was pregnant, happy one minute, sad the next and man, a real short fuse. Her body is changing and her hormones are in turmoil. Just give her a few minutes alone, and then go after her."

Brent's explanation makes sense. Sabrina's erratic behavior has to be connected to her pregnancy, and the stress over Sean isn't helping either. Mark calmed down enough that he could sit. He kept checking his watch and looking, hoping to see Sabrina return on her own. *It's hard to wait like this, but Sabrina needs some time, to sort out her feelings.*

She had gone to the barn, half walking and half running. Driven on by her tears, and the shocking reality of what she had done. Finding an empty stall, she went in and sat down on a bale of straw. Her vision was blurred by the rush of tears that streamed endlessly down her cheeks. She wiped them away only to have them return just as heavy. Her mournful sobs guided Mark to her. He paused in the doorway, his heart breaking at the sight. Sabrina rocked slowly back and forth as she hugged herself.

The look of despair on her face is more than I can bear. He knelt in front of her. "Sabrina," he called softly. Through the deluge of tears she opened her eyes, seeing Mark before her only made them fall heavier. Wary of how she would react he slowly extended his arms to her, she thrust herself against him and held tight. The force caught him off guard, but he kept steady. Her grip on him was tight enough that it became difficult for him to breathe. Her tears rapidly soaked through his shirt.

Staying quiet, he held her, rubbing her back, waiting for her to calm down. As her sobs subsided, she began to speak. "I'm sorry," she whispered hoarsely. "Hush, you have nothing to be sorry about," Mark answered calmly. Sabrina altered her embrace, but wasn't ready to let go.

She had never known the feeling of comforting arms about her until she met Mark. Her family was not one for physical expressions, and many times she had thought of how situations could have been resolved if they had just hugged. A silent, yet powerful gesture that let you know that you were loved, that you didn't have to feel alone.

As her body slowly stopped its heaving against him, her arms relaxed. The muscles trembled from being kept taught for so long. Mark loosened his hold on her and drew back. Her cheeks were flushed, her eyes puffy and red from crying.

"I'm so sorry," she repeated her apology. "Sorry for what?" "For my inexcusable behavior, I had no reason to yell at you, or Brent." "You have a perfectly good excuse; it's called being pregnant; and these hormone based mood swings are just something that we're both gonna have to get used to." "When did you become such an expert on pregnant women?" "Since I talked to Brent, he said his sister experienced the same thing."

"Does it get any better?" "Yeah; as your body adjusts it should ease off, but in the mean time I don't want you to feel bad if you yell or cry uncontrollably. Just know one thing, that I'm going to be with you, through all of it, no matter what." The way he spoke touched her heart and her tears fell again. He kissed her and held her close. "Always remember that I love you Sabrina."

After several more minutes, she was able to pull herself away from him, she had, for the time being, managed to gain control of her emotions; she rubbed her neck. "Headache?" Mark asked. "Yeah, from shedding too many tears." "It could also be from the fact that you haven't eaten anything yet today." Mark stood up, bringing her with him. "Come on let's get you some breakfast."

The pain returned, sharp and stabbing at first, then easing off. *I must have irritated it with all the crying.* Keeping this sudden resurgence hidden from Mark, she leaned heavily against him as they walked back to the house. Brent was still seated at the table; the newspaper spread out in front of him. Sabrina let go of Mark, walking towards Brent alone. *I know what she has to do, and she has to do it alone.* Unhurried, she used the time to find the right words. She approached Brent and stopped beside him. For a moment her mind went blank. Brent stood up to face her.

"Hey," he started to speak. Her fingers touched his lips preventing him from going any further. Taking a deep breath she began. "I'm sorry Brent; I had no cause to lash out at you. You've been such a good friend and I hope that my behavior hasn't jeopardized that friendship." "No need to apologize Sabrina, I understand what you're going through, and there is no need to worry about our friendship; it's still very much intact."

Putting her arms around his neck, she hugged. Brent returned the gesture, by hugging her waist. As his arm brushed against her side she flinched away from the source of the irritation. "Are you okay?" he asked quietly. She tried to think of an answer. "Yeah, I'm just a bit ticklish there, that's all."

Who is she trying to convince, me or herself? I detect the hesitation in her response. It makes me wonder what she's hiding and why.

"Hey, what's this?" The sound of Mark's voice surprised them. "I turn my back for five minutes, and come back to find my woman in the arms of another man." His voice was light, a wide grin accompanying his statement. Sabrina returned his smile with one of her own, and took a seat beside Brent. Mark presented her with a bowl of fruit salad. "What's this, more rabbit food?" She tried not to sound disappointed. "This is just the beginning Jim will bring out the rest in a few minutes," Mark reassured her.

The sweet aroma of bacon frying drifted from the open kitchen window. Her stomach growled with anticipation. She devoured the fruit to appease the hollow rumblings. Jim arrived with two plates, just as she finished off the fruit. He set one in front of her, and the other in front of Mark.

She was hungrier than she thought, and the eggs, bacon, toast and potatoes quickly vanished from her plate. Picking at Mark's breakfast, he finally conceded defeat and pushed the plate to her. "Now that is a pleasing sight, eh Mr. Cassidy," Jim said with a smile. "Pleasing for whom?" Mark answered. Sitting back in his chair; he folded his arms across his chest. "Here now, old Jim won't let you go hungry. I'll be back directly with yours."

Brent and Mark both remained quiet as they watched Sabrina methodically devour her breakfast, again. *I've never seen her eat like this before. It's amazing that she can eat so much. When she was pregnant before she didn't eat like this, she couldn't, but now, pregnant with my baby, she has the appetite of two men, and no sign of morning sickness.* Sabrina took a napkin and wiped her mouth.

Mark leaned over and kissed her; the sweet smoky flavor of bacon still on her lips made him kiss her more deeply. "Feel better?" Mark asked. "Oh yeah; even my headache is gone," she said leaning back in the chair. Jim returned with another plate, which he set down in front of Mark; who again offered it to Sabrina. "No thanks; I think that I've had enough." As she reclined, she stretched her legs out under the table. The pain reminded her that she shouldn't do that. Sitting up straight again, she tucked her elbow against her side.

"So, Brent, are you going into Dallas tomorrow?" Sabrina asked. *I've got to take my mind off of this pain, that's now cutting right through me.*

"Yeah, Nick booked me in a match with D'arcy. Are you going to be with Mark during the interviews?" "No, I'm planning to stay here, and maybe help Jim with the party preparations." "No, you won't," Mark cut in. "Jim has already hired extra staff for that." "Then what can I do?" "Rest, is what you can do."

He could clearly see the disappointment on her face and rubbed his hand across her shoulders. "I just don't want you to be all worn out before the party even starts. You can help Jim a little bit; but you have to make sure that you take a nap before I get home. Okay?" The warm smile, that he loved so much, returned to her face.

"Now if you gentlemen will excuse me, I'm gonna walk off some of this breakfast," she announced by standing up; picking up a couple of apples from the fruit bowl. "Taking a snack?" "No! I thought I'd go over to the horse paddock, and see if I can make a couple of friends."

With no further rebuttal, Sabrina walked away from the patio. Still keeping her arm pressed against her side until she was no longer in Mark's view. Once she had gone around the end of the house she began to rub at the pain, wishing that it would just go away. By the time she reached the paddock it had intensified, she grabbed the fence for support. Clearing her mind, she began a short series of deep breaths; forcing herself to relax with each exhale.

Mark had excused himself from the table, and had joined Jim in the kitchen, to go over the final details for the party. Feeling at loose ends, Brent decided to go for a walk. *Maybe I can get Sabrina to open up.* Taking his time, not wanting to give her the impression that she was being followed. As he reached the driveway he could see her at the paddock, leaning against the fence, her head down. His gait quickened, as did his pulse. Sabrina heard the click of footsteps approaching.

Fearing that it was Mark, she straightened herself, and looked over her shoulder toward the sound. The sight of Brent eased her fears. *I still have to hide this pain, even from him. I can't risk him finding out, and then informing Mark.*

Brent reached her side, resting his arm on the top rail of the fence, gazing at the horses. *How do I begin a conversation, without being overly bold, or abrupt, about the topic that's on my mind.*

"They're not too friendly today," she said. "Did you whistle to them?" Brent asked, relieved that she had spoken first. "I can't whistle that well." Brent released a couple of short whistles. One horse took notice and meandered towards them. Sabrina held out the apple, enticing the sleek gelding closer to the fence, until she could touch him. Rewarding him with the apple, she stroked his muscular neck as he munched. "I take it that you like horses." "Very much, and I like to ride too, but Mark won't let me."

She treated the gelding to the other apple. "I can understand why he won't let you; he's just being careful." "Overprotective is more like it, he won't let me do anything anymore." Brent detected a hint of frustration in her voice. "Is everything okay?" he asked. "What do you mean?" "With you and Mark?" "Of course it is; there are no problems there. I know he's just being cautious; but I'm just not used to all of this attention."

Brent hesitated before continuing. *I have to ask; it's now or never.* "What about the baby?" Brent asked. Sabrina went quiet for a moment. "The baby's fine, why would you ask that?" "It's just that I've noticed a few things." "Like what?" "Well, you seem to be a bit uncomfortable at times, like you're in pain." The knot in her stomach tightened, as she stared into Brent's eyes. *I've been so careful at hiding it. How could he know?*

"Oh that, it's nothing; just a pulled muscle." "Are you sure? Maybe you should see a Doctor about it?" "Now that's exactly why I've kept it to myself, Mark would want the same thing, and I'm telling you I don't need to see a Doctor, and it's nothing that Mark should know about." "Why shouldn't I tell him? I'm sure he'd understand." "No, he wouldn't, and you're not going to tell him. Are you?"

Damn it I've made her angry. It's very evident in her face, and in her voice. "Okay, just calm down; I'm not going to interfere, but I am going to say one more thing before we end this conversation, and that is, you should see a Doctor, just to make sure that you, and the baby, are okay." He turned away, leaning back against the fence.

I am such a jerk. Sidestepping closer to Brent, she took his hand. "I'm sorry that I got angry. I do appreciate your concern, but I'm fine, and I don't need Mark to worry about me. He has enough on his mind, with this damn problem with Sean. He doesn't need my problems to add to it," she said squeezing his hand. "Can you understand why I've kept this quiet?"

Brent sighed as he tilted his head toward her. "Yeah, I understand, but you should still tell him, maybe after the show tomorrow." "I had planned on doing just that, if it's not improved, but I'm sure it will be all over with by then," she said leaning closer. "Thank you."

Sabrina kept his hand securely in hers, even though they no longer spoke. She stared at the horses, while he stared into a void. *I've agreed to keep her secret, but it distresses me more than I like.* He was returned to the present when he felt her let go of his hand. "I'm going back to the house; I'm a bit tired," she said. He watched her begin her slow journey up the driveway; she stopped and rubbed at her side. Within seconds he was with her, wrapping her arm around his. She leaned into his strength all the way back to the house.

The sun had begun to set, as the plane landed at the Dallas airport. Heat waves, left over from the day, still radiated off of the tarmac. Sean stared blankly out the window, seeing neither the waves, nor the bright glow of the setting sun. The sharp slap of a hand on his shoulder turned his attention away from the window. D'arcy and Tony loomed above him. "Come on man get a move on," D'arcy said, gesturing at Sean to get up. Tony took the tote bag out of the overhead compartment, dropping it onto Sean's lap. They were the last to leave the plane.

Sean lagged behind as they made their way through the terminal. D'arcy had given up at trying to hurry him along; his words fell upon deaf ears. Sean's mind was somewhere else. Still alert enough to avoid obstacles that crossed his path, but lost, consumed, with thoughts of Sabrina. D'arcy was pacing impatiently beside the rental car, as Sean finally exited the terminal. He was tired, and waiting for Sean annoyed him. "Move your ass for Christ's sake!" D'arcy yelled. Sean ignored the remark. *My goal, my prize, awaits me tomorrow, and everything else is redundant.*

Sabrina was awakened by Mark's kiss on her cheek. "Are you coming for dinner, or are you going to stay here and sleep?" he asked. *I've slept away another afternoon, but it seems to be the only way to escape the pain.*

Long shadows, created by the setting sun, had begun creeping across the patio as they sat down at the table. The wind whispered through the leaves on the trees. Sabrina gazed about at the ominous shadows amongst the yard, and at the approaching clouds. It made her shudder, that in turn sent a piercing pain through her lower back. She kept her composure as it eased, and then disappeared.

"There's gonna be a storm tonight," she said looking back up at the sky. "What makes you say that?" Mark asked. "It's a feeling that I have; I can't really explain it. Since I was little, I always seemed to know when a storm was coming; and this one, is gonna be a really good one." Mark put his arm around her shoulder. "This isn't storm season; besides, the weather report said nothing about a storm tonight." "I'm not wrong Mark; you'll see."

By the time dinner was over, the wind had picked up considerably, sending collections of leaves across the patio in a frenzied dance, only to be trapped by the water of the pool. Looking out into the darkness, she could barely make out the shapes of the trees. The wind howled, as it forced its way through the branches, stripping away the leaves. The pain ripped through her like a twisting knife. She closed her eyes.

The familiar faint odor of an electrical charge infiltrated her nostrils; she stood up quickly. "I'm going in the house, and I suggest that you both come with me." Her urgency was very noticeable. Taking Mark's hand, she pulled at him to get up as she reached out to Brent. "Please, please, come inside; now!" She was more frantic.

There was only a few feet between them and the door, but it seemed to take forever to get there. They were no sooner inside when a bolt of lightning struck the ground beyond the hill; and with it came a thunderous report that made the house shudder. The windows rattled as if being rapped upon by multitudes of spectral hands.

Sabrina pressed her face against Mark's chest, holding onto him. "I told you," she whimpered. Another burst of lightning illuminated the sky. "Incredible," Brent mumbled, amazed at her prediction. Mark enveloped her in his arms. "You never cease to amaze me." Sabrina held tight, shielding herself from the next barrage of thunder claps. It made her tremble with fear. *I hate storms like this, as much as I hate knowing when they're coming.*

She stayed attached to Mark, as he guided her to the sofa. She jumped every time the lightning flashed. "You really don't like this, do you?" Mark asked. "No, I don't," she answered, obscuring her face, so that he could not see the reflections of pain that burned through her.

Brent could see her tense, and then relax. *I don't believe that her actions are all due to the storm, but I've promised her that I wouldn't say anything, despite how loudly my conscience begs me to speak.* Rising from his chair, he could no longer watch her torment. "If you will excuse me, I'm going to go and sort out my gear for tomorrow." Mark acknowledged him with a nod. Sabrina gave him a quick look, as another flash illuminated the room.

Finally alone, Mark lifted Sabrina's head up and kissed her. "Maybe we should do something to take your mind off of the storm?" he said in a soft voice. She felt his hand lightly glide down her throat, across her chest and stop, cupping her breast. Another flash, she lurched forward, forcing his hand hard against her. "Make love to me," she whispered in a voice that reflected the tremors that tormented her body on the inside.

Cradling her in his arms, he carried her up to their bed. *Making love will take my mind off of the storm, and maybe off of my pain as well.* The lights were off, but for a few seconds the bedroom became bright, as the lightning flashed outside the windows. Mark felt her anxiety. Trying to help her relax, he slowly kissed and caressed her body.

Endeavoring to lose herself in his affection was ineffectual. Her skin had become very sensitive; his touch burned against her. Her breasts ached when he touched her. She wanted to pull away from him, but she couldn't. The discomfort she felt was minuscule, compared to how much she wanted him, and needed him at that moment.

Lying down on her side, she coaxed him to lie beside, and behind her, persuading him to try a new position from the book she had bought. Continuing to kiss her shoulder and neck, his hand explored her body, and drew her closer to him. She eagerly awaited the moment when their bodies would become one. Mark too, experienced the anticipation, but he kept his eagerness at bay, allowing them both to fully experience this new sensation.

At the precise moment that he moved into her, her body succumbed to an intense orgasm, but what he didn't know, or see, was the intense pain that accompanied it. She felt her body contract around him, as the waves of pain cut her in half. She arched her back, searching for relief, but it didn't come.

Her body continued to pulsate with alternating waves of pleasure, and pain, as Mark moved inside her bringing himself to climax. The pain finally ceased when he withdrew; she fell limp from exhaustion. "I love you so much," he whispered, kissing her cheek.

The storm outside had intensified. The lightning flashed every few seconds, and the thunder rumbled without end. Sabrina pulled the sheet up, to cover her eyes. "Come here," Mark said turning her over. "I'll protect you." She rolled over to face him, entwining her leg around his, hiding her face against his chest, as another pulsating pain stabbed through her. Fear made her cling tighter to Mark. *This is more than just a pulled muscle. I should tell him, but I can't.*

Mark held her tight. *I admire her strength, but I also like moments like this, when her feminine insecurities allow me to be her strength, and her protection. I never knew that loving someone could be so wonderful; and nothing will ever change how I feel about her.*

Sean had scarcely slept all night; his mind raced endlessly, hour after hour, filled with fantastic revelations of Sabrina, and of his growing fury for Mark. The sunrise was a gratifying sight. *My wait is at long last over, today I will end this ordeal with Mark, and get Sabrina back, one way or another. I'm not scheduled to meet Mark in a match today, but I know that he's slated for promotional interviews, to boost the upcoming pay per view that we are contracted to.*

This is the paragon of all settings. Mark won't be expecting me to make a move, and that will be the ultimate in perfection; I can strike, incapacitate Mark, get Sabrina, and be far away before anyone realizes what has taken place. He felt good, and a rigid workout at the gym would only serve to make him feel even stronger. He grabbed his gear and went down to the hotel gym.

Brent was up early and quietly went downstairs for a swim. The air was clean and fresh after last night's storm. The sweet scent of wet grass drifted through the air. He took a deep breath and stretched. Out the corner of his eye he detected movement, Sabrina was curled up in one of the lounge's. She looked ghastly pale against her white robe. Wandering over to her, he sat down. She was startled by his unexpected presence. "Good morning Sabrina." "Morning," she answered, rubbing her eyes.

I can't restrain myself anymore; my concern for her overrides all other feelings. "Are you okay?" "Yes." "Excuse me, but I really don't believe you; you look like hell." Sabrina didn't answer him right away.

I can't tell him that I was kept awake most of the night by this nagging pain. This annoying pain, that paralyzes me, and then disappears, only to sneak up on me when I least expect it. "The storm, it kept me awake."

I'm not sure if I should believe her. The expression on her face suggests that it's more than just the lack of sleep, but I don't want to interfere. I hope she trusts me enough to confide in me. "If you say so, but I still don't believe you." He tried to get her to make eye contact, when she wouldn't he got up. "I'm going for a swim."

She watched him dive into the pool and swim to the far end. With great force she gripped the arms of the lounger as another wave of agonizing pain seized her. Brent had stopped at the far end of the pool, he had turned around, glancing toward her, he knew that she was in pain; he also saw

Mark come through the patio door. "Morning Mark," he called, warning Sabrina of his presence.

Mark waived to Brent as he walked to Sabrina; leaning down, he kissed her. "Good morning beautiful." The delicate kiss on the head wasn't satisfactory. Grabbing his hand, she yanked him down onto the seat, thrusting herself upon him. Somewhat surprised by her sudden action, but he consistently welcomed every opportunity to hold her. When he felt her tears drip upon his neck, he instinctively began to rock her. "What's wrong?"

She didn't respond immediately, but he could feel her clutch his shirt more firmly; permitting her to hold onto him a little longer before he freed himself. "Hey, what's with this?" he asked, cradling her face in his hand, coaxing her with his eyes to answer. "I wish," she began, only to pause to look into his green eyes. "You wish what?"

"I wish that you didn't have to go today." "Then come with me, and we won't have to be apart." "No! I don't want to go this time; and I don't want you to go either. I'm being selfish I know, but there's something about today that just doesn't feel right." "You're just tired. I know you didn't sleep much last night. Look, nothing is going to go wrong today; I'm only doing promo interviews. No matches; and you know that. You'll feel a lot better after you get some more rest; and you'll have all afternoon to do that."

Sabrina forced a smile and nodded. *He's probably right and I have no right in trying to make him stay.* "When do you have to leave?" she asked biting her lip, anticipating the answer. "Not for a while." He knew his vague reply wasn't satisfactory. Suddenly his face brightened. He sat straight, smiling. "But until I do have to leave, you're going to have my complete undivided attention; come on." "Where are we going?" "For a walk, and for the next little while, you and I are going to be the only people in the world." "I'm not dressed; and we haven't had breakfast." "So?" He picked up some fruit from the basket.

Placing his arm about her shoulders, he steered her across the patio. "We'll be back in a while," he called to Brent as they passed the pool. Brent watched them walk across the lawn, on into the trees. An inkling of jealousy churned in his gut. He shook it off and went back to doing his laps. Anything to take his mind off of the turmoil he was inflicting on himself.

Sabrina deliberately shortened her steps as they walked up the hill. Since she was in bare feet, and the soft grass had given way to rough, uneven terrain, she didn't want to step on a sharp rock. The grass thickened again as they neared the top. The trees had thinned out, allowing the earth to reap the benefits from the sun. She hoped that their trek was close to being over. She had forced herself to continue, even though the pain begged her to stop. Mark could feel her slowing. "Almost there," he said giving her a reassuring hug.

They finally topped the hill. It was the first time Sabrina had been up here. She stopped to survey the view. Behind her was the house, that now seemed so unpretentious and before her stretched a seemingly endless pasture, spotted with a few large trees. "So, what do you think?" Mark asked. "It's great. How far back does it go?"

Releasing his hold on her shoulder, Mark pointed out what boundaries he could. Taking special note to show her where the small lake was. Sabrina leaned against him, as she followed his hand. The lake wasn't visible to her, but she estimated its size by the dense growth of trees around it. "Does this remind you of anything?" she asked. Mark looked at her; his forehead became deep with lines as he thought. "Remind me of what?" "Of that wonderful day when we went riding." She waited for his response.

It only took seconds. He brought her close and kissed her eager lips. He remembered. With his arms securely around her, he lowered her down upon the soft grass, bringing himself down beside her. With outstretched arms, she welcomed his passionate kisses. "I love you," she said softly. His cheek brushed against hers, as he supported himself up on one elbow, to gaze upon her. "Don't stop," she begged. "I love how you kiss me; and touch me. I need that; I need you, to have you near me always."

Mark felt a lump in his throat. It was his heart. It made his eyes cloudy. *Her love is so pure, and it has touched my very soul.* "I will always love you; now and forever. You are my life, my soul, my reason to be." He kissed her again, with more passion. After several inviting heaves of her chest, he slipped his hand inside her robe. She moaned softly. "Do you want to make love here, or go back to the house?" Mark asked. "Neither; I'm quite content on just doing this," she answered.

To her surprise, his expression turned very solemn. "Did I give the wrong answer?" she asked. "No." "Then what's on your mind?" Mark repositioned himself up on his arm. "There's something I need to do for you. Something that I've put off for far too long." "Oh Mark, there is nothing you have to do for me. You have given me more than any woman deserves.

I have your love, and that's all I will ever need." "Hush a minute." He hesitated, to take a deep breath, and to ease his quaking body.

"I want. I would like. Now don't say anything right away you'll need to think about this." He took another breath. His heart raced. "What I have to do, or rather what I would like to do, is make you my wife; Sabrina, will you marry me?" He quickly avoided her eyes, afraid of what her answer might be. *It would break my heart if she says no.*

Sabrina felt her heart skip a beat, followed by a rush of warmth that covered her entire body. She touched his cheek, to make him look at her. "Mark, you know I love you." His heart braced for the answer that he feared. "And I don't need to think about my answer. Yes, I'll be your wife." His heart exploded with joy. He leaned down to her, nuzzling his face against hers.

"There is one thing I need to know," she continued. Mark sat back. "Anything, I have no secrets to keep from you." She took his arm, as an aid in sitting up. *He didn't keep secrets from me, but I am keeping one from him. I want to tell him, but now just isn't the right time.*

Mark silently urged her to ask her question. "Would you have asked me if I wasn't pregnant?" "Of course," his answer came quickly. "From the first moment that I met you, I knew that I wanted you as my lover, and as my wife." He picked up her hand. "When I gave you this ring, I wanted to ask you then, but I was too afraid. Afraid that you would say no. Sabrina I love you and the fact that you're pregnant has no bearing on the timing of my question. When we were in Vegas I was going to ask you that night after the show but circumstances changed that. I made my decision that morning before I even knew about the baby."

They sat quietly for a long time; she held his hand in hers, unconsciously stroking it with her thumb. "So, do we keep this a secret, or tell everybody we know?" Mark asked. "I don't know. What do you want to do?" "Well, I say that we keep it relatively quiet; until the party tonight; then when everyone is here we can make our announcement." "That sounds fine to me; I trust you to use your own judgment," Sabrina said.

Mark took her in his arms. The sudden twisting motion brought on another surge of pain; she held tight to him until it had passed. Mark checked his watch and sighed. "I hate to spoil this moment, but it's almost time for me to leave," he said. Helping her up, he kept her close to him as they made their way back down the hill to the house. The pain stabbed through her again. This time she doubled over from its searing effect. "What's wrong?" Mark asked.

No matter how desperately I want to tell him I can't. "I stepped on something," she answered, rubbing at her foot. *A bold lie, but I have to take the chance. To cause him any worry now would be unscrupulous.* "I can't have that," he announced. He picked her up and carried her the rest of the way, setting her down when they reached the patio.

Brent was coming through the door. "I was just about to come and get you; we really have to get going," he said. "Yeah, I know," Mark answered. "I'm already packed." He turned to Sabrina. "Will you walk me out to the car?" His answer came as a smile, and a hug. Brent walked ahead of them, stopping only to pick up the two bags near the front door. He took them out to the limo and tossed them inside.

Mark stopped just outside the front door; he held Sabrina ever so gently, stroking her hair. The longing in her eyes was hard for him to tear away from. He kissed her deeply. "You get some rest, and before you know it I'll be home again; and then we can celebrate this special occasion properly," he said, a wide smile brightening his face. She could still taste him on her lips, as she watched him walk away and get into the limo.

The car slowly disappeared down the driveway. *I have the urge to run after it; to tell him that I'm not well. To persuade him to stay here with me today; but I can't move, frozen in place by another crippling rush of pulsating agony.*

Mark agonized over leaving her behind, but she was insistent on staying, and he knew better than to force her. He stared out the back window at the figure that still waited by the front door. When she was no longer visible, he turned, and rested against the back of the seat. An indescribable, unfamiliar feeling churned in his stomach. He dismissed it as nothing more than hunger pains. A vision of her came into his mind; he began to smile as he thought about her being his wife; his eternal mate.

Brent caught the strange look on Mark's face. *It's uncommon for him to smile, but even this is different.* "So what's up?" Brent asked. "With what?" "Well, you look like the veritable cat that ate the canary. So what's going on?" Mark's smile widened. "Well, Sabrina said I could use my own discretion, and I have to tell somebody; but you have to keep this quiet for now," Mark said. Brent nodded, eager to hear what Mark had to say.

"She has agreed to marry me." Brent was taken off guard, but the surprise made him happy. "That is just about the best news I've heard in a long time. You two belong together. So when is the big day?" "I don't know we didn't discuss that yet, but as far as I'm concerned the sooner the better." "In more ways than one," Brent muttered quietly.

"What do you mean by that?" Mark asked. "I was just thinking that it would be nice for you two to be married before the baby comes." Mark detected the hesitation and felt that Brent had more to say. "And what?" "Then maybe you'll finally have Sean off your back."

I had thought about the baby, but I hadn't given any thought to Sean. Brent's right, marrying Sabrina would put an end to this damn fiasco with Sean. At least I hope it will.

Chapter 15

Jim made lunch for Sabrina and joined her at the table; noticing that she only picked at her meal, eating hardly anything. Every once in a while he noticed her tense up for a few moments. She was discreet about it, but he could still see it clearly in her face.

"Is anything wrong ma'am?" Jim asked. Sabrina could hear the concern in his voice, and lied to him anyway. "I'm fine; just tired." "Well just so ya know, old Doc Brown lives about a mile away. Just in case you should ever have the need, you don't have to go all the way into Dallas." "Yes, that is good to know," she replied with some pleasantry. "So is there anything that I can do to help with tonight's party?" "No ma'am, everything is well in hand." "Okay then, I think that I'll go upstairs and lie down for a while."

Jim began to clear the table as Sabrina walked slowly away, holding her stomach. The waves of pain had become more frequent, more intense. Walking was difficult. She had to keep stopping, to let the waves pass. The Grandfather clock in the living room chimed one o'clock. She thought of Mark, and wished that he was here with her. She pressed on towards the stairs; only to stop at the bottom, leaning heavily on the railing.

Each step was agonizing. It took her several attempts to reach the last step. Pulling herself with one hand while the other she kept tight against her belly. She was overcome with exhaustion. Her back ached and the muscles in her belly danced with unending spasms. A tear rolled down her cheek. She was scared, and feelings of despair began to consume her. *I don't know what's wrong with me. This is more than a strained muscle, and it's beyond my ability to control. This time I need help.*

She called to Jim; she could hear him in the kitchen, and hoped that he had heard her. After several, long, agonizing moments, he appeared in the living room. "Yes ma'am," he stuttered, as he looked at her leaning on the railing. "That Doctor you mentioned, does he make house calls?" "Yes ma'am, he does. Do you need him?" "Yes, Jim, I think I do." Jim started for the stairs. "Can I help you to your room?" "No, just call the Doctor for me, please."

The unmistakable sound of fear in her voice made him hurry himself back to the kitchen to make the call. Sabrina made her way into the bedroom, using the walls for support. She carefully laid down on the bed, clutching

Mark's pillow to her belly. She wept silently but her mind, her soul, cried out for Mark.

The Dallas arena was alive with activity, the fans restless, anticipating the start of the show; their chants echoed back into the dressing rooms. Sean had arrived unnoticed, and immediately sought the solitude of his dressing room, waiting for his moment. Mark had decided to share the larger dressing room with Brent, Tony and D'arcy; since he wasn't in a match today he was not in need of the privacy to prepare himself.

The guys were all busy getting themselves ready for their matches. Mark paid them little attention. He was lacing up his boots when he abruptly stopped, looked around the room and then went to the door. Opening it, he looked in both directions. Brent noticed the peculiar actions of his friend, and the confused look on his face.

"Hey, Mark, what's up with you?" Brent asked. It took Mark a minute to answer him, and when he did his voice faltered. "I, I thought that I heard Sabrina calling me." "That's impossible." "I know that, but I heard it, as clearly as I hear you." The eerie sensation made Mark shudder. Brent rested his hand on Mark's shoulder. "You know what it is, don't you? This is the first time that you two have been apart; and it's only logical for you to miss her." "Yeah; but Christ it was so real. Maybe I should call her." "Not such a good idea; she's probably resting, and you know that you'd only feel bad if you woke her up." "You're probably right." He returned to lacing up his boots, but her voice haunted his mind.

She had called out to me. No; she had cried out to me. That was the sound that I heard, a bone chilling cry. Maybe it was as Brent had said; our first time apart, and I do miss her.

Jim paced endlessly along the front walk way, waiting for the arrival of Doc Brown; his hands were wet from worry. "Come on Doc," he muttered to himself.

Several years ago Doc Brown had set up his practice from his home. He had wanted to be where he felt he was genuinely needed, and the ranchers around the area were grateful for him being there. Doc, a man in his late fifties, had given up the fast pace of the city, to raise his family in the country. The constant stress of being in the city had turned his dark hair prematurely gray.

At first he commuted into Dallas, but as his patient list grew among the ranchers, he decided to give up his office in Dallas and settled into to the routine of an old fashioned country Doctor. Being available at all hours, and making house calls. For Doc this was the good life, and nothing would make him go back to the city again.

Here he could practice medicine the way it was supposed to be practiced. Treating his patients as people, not worrying whether they had insurance or not. Many times his services had been paid for in sides of beef for his freezer; or stud services for one of his horses. Medicine, for him, was not the practice of getting rich; it was giving the people the best possible care; regardless of their social, or financial status. This new laid back attitude towards life showed in his rotund frame but he was happy. Happier than he had been in many years.

The car appeared in the driveway. Jim breathed a sigh of relief. He waved Doc towards the front door, hurrying him out of the car and up the stairs to the bedroom.

Sabrina was laying on her side; her soft cries made it obvious to both of them that she was in a great deal of pain. Jim brought a chair to the bedside for Doc. "I'm gonna call Mr. Cassidy," he announced. "No! Don't call him, please Jim," she begged. Against his better judgment, he conceded to her request and left the room so Doc could examine her.

"Well, Jim tells me that you're experiencing some pain." "Yes, it's awful." "Can you describe what you're feeling?" Sabrina began to recount the waves of pain that had been afflicting her. After doing a brief exam, Doc sat back, pondering what she had told him.

"Are you pregnant?" Doc asked. She nodded. "How far along are you?" "I don't really know. Is there something wrong with the baby?" "Well from what you have told me, and from what I've seen so far, it appears that you're gonna lose this baby." "No, I can't!" Sabrina began to cry harder. "I'm sorry darlin, but this baby just isn't meant to be. I don't mean to be harsh, but you have to understand what's going on. Your body is doing exactly what comes natural. I am sorry." His words stabbed her in the heart. *I'm going to lose this baby, Mark's baby.* The feeling of loss tore her apart.

"I'll call for an ambulance and get you to the hospital in Dallas." "No! Please, no hospital." Sabrina grabbed at his arm. Doc patted her hand gently. "Okay darlin, don't worry, we can do this here if you like. I'm gonna need a few things though. You rest as best you can, and I'll be right back."

Sabrina clutched the pillow to her, letting it absorb her tears. *Was it the fall from the ring, or the accident here? Which one had caused this to be happening? What's the point of trying to figure it out, I'm losing my baby and I'm probably going to lose Mark too.*

Mark had been incapable of shaking the feeling that Sabrina, somehow, needed him. He had again imagined hearing her voice. It made him very uneasy and with that unease came a nauseating spasm that tormented his stomach. He paced the length of the hallway, unconsciously rubbing his stomach, waiting for his interview to begin.

With each pass, he looked at the pay phone. *Should I? If I did, she'd say that I was being over protective, but if I didn't, and something was wrong, she would be upset, and I would feel like a damn fool. To hell with it.* He picked up the receiver. *Just a quick call, to tell her I love her and miss her, and to see how she's feeling.*

That was the plan, until Nick appeared and disconnected the call. "Come on; I don't have all day," he said pushing Mark away from the phone. *I can call after the promo, no point in arguing and getting Nick pissed off.* Mark followed along, trying to clear his mind, and remember what Nick wanted him to say.

Far off, in a now empty dressing room, a cell phone rang inside a tote bag. "Damn it to hell!" Jim cursed, hanging up the phone. Disobeying Sabrina's plea, he had tried to phone Mark. Jim fetched everything that Doc had asked for. He paced outside the bedroom door, until he could no longer bear to hear her mournful cries. Even downstairs, in the living room, he could still hear her. Mark needed to be here with her. Jim picked up the phone and dialed again. Still no answer. *Calling the arena would be useless, and I don't have anyone else's cell phone numbers. I have to keep trying.*

Sabrina was nearing exhaustion. Her hair was saturated with perspiration and her legs were trembling uncontrollably from being bent for so long. Doc urged her on, telling her she was doing just fine. He had warned her that it wouldn't be an easy process, but she was strong enough to get through this.

"Come on darlin, you can do it," he urged. "I can't! I'm so tired and it hurts so much," she whimpered. "I know darlin, but you have to do this.

Stop fighting it and let it happen. I'll help you." Doc stood up beside her, taking her hand he squeezed it firmly. "Okay on the count of three, we'll give it one big push; one, two, three."

Sabrina pushed as hard as she could. The pain snatched her breath away. "Good girl, it's just about over." Mustering all her remaining strength, she gave one final push and felt her body expel the tiny fetus. She lay back panting, the air burning her already parched throat.

Doc worked quietly on the other side of the sheet. He took the tiny baby, and wrapped it tightly in one of the sheets that Jim had brought in. Sabrina struggled to sit up. "Can I see it?" "No darlin, it's for the best that you don't. Is this your first pregnancy?" "No, I had a miscarriage a few months ago, due to a riding accident." "Have you had any accidents recently?"

"I got knocked out of the ring about two weeks back and then I slipped getting out of the hot tub about a week ago. Why?" "Well, there is some evidence of trauma. When you slipped, did you get a pain something like a pulled groin muscle?" "Yes, I did. Is that what hurt my baby?" "Quite possibly it is, but it would have made no difference even if you had seen a Doctor right away. Nothing would have been able to correct it."

He finished bundling up his package and moved it to one side out of her view. Returning his attentions to Sabrina, he made sure that she was okay. "I'll be back in a few minutes. You rest," he said patting her knees. "You can relax these now too." He picked up his little bundle and left the room.

Sabrina began to cry harder, as she laid her hands on her belly. She whispered Mark's name through her sobs. *How can I tell him? My own stupidity has caused this. He'll never forgive me.* She began to tremble. The shock was taking control. *How can I go on without him?*

The second promo interview was nearly over when Mark again, thought he heard Sabrina's voice. Only this time it was much different; it chilled him even more. He struggled on with the interview, her voice taunting his mind. Out of nowhere, he was attacked, and sent hurtling back into a stack of steel storage crates. With no time to right himself, again his attacker struck, wielding hard blows to his face and his stomach. Marks arms flailed, hitting nothing.

The blows ceased momentarily for him to get a clear view of who was doing this. Scan hovered over him. Mark thrust him backward, enabling himself to get up and launch a counter attack. He tasted blood, his own blood from the cut on his lip. Sean lunged again, striking blow upon blow. Mark retaliated as best he could. He could feel the burning pain of a cracked rib. His knuckles were bruised and bloody from hitting Sean.

Nick stood by watching, making sure the cameras still rolled, capturing every move, so he could use it later as part of the build up to the match they were going to have next month. He still had not been able to find out why these two were so bent on destroying one another, but whatever this personal feud was about it was far better than anything his writers could have come up with.

Relaxing back in the dressing room after their matches, Brent and Tony couldn't hear what was going on, down at the end of the hallway. The cell phone began to chirp again. Tony looked in his bag. "Not me," he said. "Not me either." "Well, D'arcy doesn't carry one, so it must be Mark's."

Brent snatched up Mark's bag, sifting through it until he found the chirping phone. "Hello." "Oh Mr. Cassidy, thank God I got a hold of you; it's Jim." "Jim, this is Brent, Mark's not here right at the moment. Can I help you?" "No! Find Mr. Cassidy for me, and be damn quick about it!" "Jim is there something wrong?" "Damn it man do what I asked, please!" "Okay, hold on; I'll try and find him." Brent covered the phone with his hand and looked at Tony. "We gotta find Mark. Now!"

The two of them headed down the hallway. It wasn't long before they came upon the fight between Sean and Mark. Tony jumped in, pulling Sean away from Mark. He squirmed and struggled, but Tony held tight, dragging him away to the dressing room. Mark's face was covered with blood from the numerous cuts about his head. As he stood up he clutched at his side, the cracked rib made him gasp for breath.

"Why in the hell did you stop it?" Mark yelled. "Look man you've got other things to worry about besides a fight with that asshole," Brent said holding the phone out to Mark. "I don't want to talk to anybody right now!" Mark snarled. "Just take the God damn phone! Don't talk just listen!" Brent again thrust the phone at Mark; this time he took it.

"Hello," Mark said angrily. Brent watched as Mark's face drained of color; he leaned heavily against a cement pillar. The silence was what worried Brent the most; finally Mark spoke. "I'll be there as soon as I can." He closed up the cell phone and sat down with a thump. The nausea that he had been trying to keep at bay now slowly crept up into his throat. The foul taste of bile made him want to vomit.

"Is everything okay?" Brent asked. Mark looked up at him, his face an empty void. "I, I gotta go," he stammered. "Not until you have seen the medics." "I have to go home!" "Not looking like that you don't. You'll scare the hell out of Sabrina if you go home covered in blood."

Brent waived the paramedics over to them. They began to clean up Mark, and assess his injuries. Within minutes they had bandaged his cuts, and taped his ribs. Mark repeatedly insisted that they hurry. At the first sign that they were done, he got up and headed straight to the waiting limo. Brent called to him, but his words only echoed back at him.

Something has to be really wrong for Mark to take off like this. I hope that I'm mistaken, but my gut keeps telling me otherwise.

After he had taken the bundle out to Jim, Doc returned to stay with Sabrina. Jim knew what he had to do. His steps were slow and heavy, as he walked to the barn to get a shovel. Rummaging around in the barn he came across a nice little wooden box, just big enough for the tiny package in his arm. He placed the bundle into the box, nailed the lid shut and carried it slowly up the hill.

Finding a pleasant, peaceful spot, next to a wild rose bush, he set the box down and began digging. When the hole was deep enough, he placed the little box inside. Kneeling beside it he prayed as a tear rolled over his weathered cheek. Losing a child was the worst thing that could ever happen to two people; but Jim knew that the love that Mark and Sabrina shared would get them through this tough time. He finished his task and returned to the house. He had to get a hold of Mark somehow.

Sabrina was in shock; her body shivered uncontrollably. "I think you could do with a shower," Doc said. "No, I just want to stay here; I'm cold." "I know darlin, but you need a shower to get yourself cleaned up and Jim needs to change the sheets on the bed." Doc tried to be comforting, with a soft pat on the hand. "I'll get it ready, and then I'll come back and help you into the bathroom." Without waiting for any rebuttal, Doc picked up the wooden chair and headed off into the bathroom. Sabrina heard the shower start and soon Doc returned for her. "Come on hun," he urged.

It took him a few tugs, but he finally got her out of the bed, onto her feet. It wasn't that she was being uncooperative, she was weak, her legs refused to contribute to the effort. With his arm around her, Doc guided her into the bathroom. He was sturdy enough to support her, but not strong enough to carry her.

"Don't worry about your robe; just take it off once you get in the shower. I'll have Jim bring you a clean one. Take your time it will make you feel a little bit better." Doc held open the shower door, holding Sabrina's hands until she had settled herself onto the chair. "I'll be back in a few minutes to see how you're doing."

Sabrina heard the click of his shoes against the tile floor as he left the room. She slipped off her robe, before it became too heavily soaked with water. Staring at the crimson streaks of blood, that raced across the white tile to the drain; she began to cry again.

Tony continued to struggle with Sean, even after he had him secured in the dressing room. Fed up with Sean's juvenile behavior, Tony struck him, sending him backwards into a table. "What the hell did you do that for?" Sean asked, rubbing at his jaw. "I am sick of this bullshit from you!" Tony began, pacing wildly in front of Sean. "For God's sake man grow up! End this pointless quest!" "Never! I will never give up until she's back with me, and Mark is destroyed!" "You are pathetic, the first time a woman has had the guts to walk away from you and you go off the deep end. Christ we've all been dumped at one time or another. So what, get over it and move on!" "I can't. Ah hell you wouldn't understand anyway." "Try me."

"Sabrina is the most beautiful woman that I have ever met." "There it is! Your attraction to her is purely physical. You're not committed to her the way Mark is; and you never will be," Tony remarked emphatically.

Sean took on a defensive stance. "That's bullshit!" "Oh really; I know you to well Sean. Let's see, when you think of her you think of sex. You look at that body you think of sex. For as long as I've known you, that's how you operate. Every pretty woman that comes along ends up as a notch in your bed post. Yeah, maybe she liked it at first; but brother let me tell you, there is nothing, and I mean nothing, that will change how she feels about Mark. They are so much in love; you must be able to see that. Christ, it even makes me jealous to see how devoted they are to each other. Sometimes it's even down right spooky how they seem to know what each of them is thinking or needing," Tony shuddered as he spoke. "You know I would not be at all surprised if very soon now they announce their wedding plans."

"Screw you! It'll never happen. Mark won't marry her." Sean began pacing the length of the room, mulling over what Tony had said. "Look Sean, I don't know what's gonna happen; but I do know that if you don't change your way of thinking, and soon, you're gonna end up one lonely, pathetic son of a bitch." Tony was tired of lecturing Sean. *If he's going to insist on being so pig headed, then maybe letting Mark beat the hell out of him is the only solution.* He left, to get himself ready for the party tonight, and to let Sean have some time to think.

Sabrina managed to complete her shower; thankful for Doc having brought the chair. Her body hurt, still tormented by intermittent spasms and standing only made her tremble from weakness. Doc had brought her a clean T-shirt of Mark's. She dried herself off in the shower, still using the chair as her support. When she was ready, Doc helped her out, steadying her, as he guided her back to bed.

"This weakness that you're experiencing will pass soon. With a few hours rest you should begin to feel much better." "What about the pain, when will it go away?" Sabrina asked. "Your muscles will be sore for a day or two." "No, I mean the pain in here," she said holding her hand to her heart. Doc patted her free hand gently. "With time and a whole lot of love," he said softly.

How could Mark still love me after this? How could he even tolerate being around me anymore, knowing that I destroyed our child?

"Would you like me to give you something to help you sleep? Nothing too strong that will put you out for hours; but just enough to help you relax," Doc asked. Sabrina nodded, watching as he prepared an injection. The prick of the needle in her hip was barely noticeable. "There, now you try and get some rest. I'll stay around for a little while longer, just to make sure that you're doing okay."

Sabrina didn't need any prompting. Even though she was grievous, sleep was becoming very inviting. The shock had settled in deeply. Doc quietly left the room and went in search of Jim, and a cup of coffee. Jim told him that he had finally got a hold of Mark, and that was another reason why Doc was staying around. He needed to talk to Mark. A conversation that he was dreading.

Death is not an uncommon subject for me; but this, this saddens me deeply. A child is a gift, and I know that this loss is going to leave an empty space in their hearts. It will take time and a strong love to get them through this.

Mark snapped at the driver to hurry up. Jim had been very vague on the phone, telling him only that Sabrina was very ill, and that Doc was with her. His mind was clouded with thoughts, but none of them made any sense. His imagination was exaggerating on the possibilities of what was going on. "Stop it. No point in blowing things out of proportion until I know the facts, but I can't shake this feeling that there's a lot more that Jim didn't tell me."

The car turned into the driveway; Mark was poised to open the door the moment the car came to a stop. He burst into the house like a hurricane. The door flew back hitting the wall, the doorknob leaving a deep imprint from the impact. He hurried to the stairs, but was halted by Jim's voice behind him. "Mr. Cassidy."

Mark turned in the direction of the voice, to see Jim standing in the hallway to the kitchen, Doc Brown at his side. Doc stepped towards Mark. "Good to see you." "Yeah, yeah, whatever. How is Sabrina? What happened?" Mark's questions were quick, and filled with concern. Doc took a breath. "Sit down son we need to have a little chat before you see her." Jim took that as his cue to leave the room. His heart went out to Mark, knowing what he was about to hear.

Mark took a seat on the couch. The tape around his ribs pinched. Doc perched himself on the edge of the coffee table in front of him. "How is she Doc?" "Well, she's doing just fine, considering. Right now she's asleep, and that's good. She's had one hell of a day." Doc's expression turned serious. With pursed lips and a deep inhale that made him sit straight he ran his hands over his knees and made eye contact with Mark.

"How much did Jim tell you on the phone?" Doc asked. "Nothing; only that Sabrina was very ill, and that I should be with her." "There's a lot more to it than that son." Mark waited for Doc to continue, his gut in knots.

Doc sighed heavily, searching for the right words. "God I hate this part. There's no way of making it sound better, or easing into it." "Jesus Doc, tell me what in the hell is going on!" "Mark, I'm truly sorry, but she lost the baby." "No! That can't be! She had an ultrasound; the baby was fine, healthy." "I'm so sorry son, but it is true."

Mark fell back against the couch; his mind couldn't believe what it was hearing. "How could this happen?" "It could have been many things. The accident that she had in the ring, coupled with the other accident that she had." "What accident are you talking about?" "Oh my; she said that she slipped getting out of the hot tub a few days ago." Doc took note of the surprise on Mark's face. "I believe that accident caused a tear in the sack around the baby. Now even if she had sought medical attention right away, it would not have prevented the miscarriage."

Mark rubbed his hands through his hair. He felt cold, chilled to the bone with shock. "Was it; was it a boy or a girl?" Mark asked cautiously. "It was a boy." "Oh God!" His emotions broke loose; he began to weep. Doc touched him on the knee. "She doesn't know that it was a boy. Son, she's gonna need your support and understanding right now. It was an accident, and no one is to blame."

Mark sucked back his tears. "Can I see her?" Mark asked. Doc nodded. "Not for too long, she needs her rest right now, and after two miscarriages her body is gonna need a rest before she tries to get pregnant again."

Mark filed away Doc's advice far in his mind. All he wanted was to see Sabrina, and to hold her. He climbed the stairs slowly. His feet were like lead weights, making him struggle with each step. Pausing outside the bedroom, he rubbed his hands over his face and pulled his hair back. The sharp pain in his ribs made him flinch, but it was inferior compared to the pain in his heart.

Sabrina was asleep. Mark quietly walked to the bed and knelt down on the floor beside her. Her hand lay on top of the sheets; he squeezed it gently. Her eyes fluttered open. Mark stroked her forehead. Sabrina turned; her eyes locked onto his and just as quickly she turned away. Sadness overwhelmed her and she began to cry. Mark brought her into his arms. His own grief surfaced, forcing tears down his cheeks.

"I'm sorry," she whimpered. "There's no reason for you to say that," he said pulling back to look at her. "It was an accident." Through her tears she began to notice the cuts and bruises that colored his face, she touched them lightly. "What happened to you?" she asked. "It doesn't matter." "It matters to me. It was Sean, wasn't it?" "I don't want to talk about that. My only concern is for you." "But Mark." "No buts; my problems don't have any place here right now."

Their silent embrace lasted a long time, until Sabrina moaned softly, tensing her body. "What's wrong? Are you in pain?" Mark asked. "A little," she answered, lying back on the bed. "I'll get Doc." "No need, he said I'd be a little uncomfortable for a while. It'll pass soon. It's a lot better than a couple of hours ago." "Maybe he could give you something for it." "He already has." "God it tears me up to see you hurting like this! Why didn't you call me?" "I couldn't. Maybe I was wrong, but I just couldn't put you through this. I didn't want you to see me that way."

Mark had moved himself up onto the bed with her. "Even during what had to be the worst moment in your life, you were more concerned with sparing my feelings." He closed his eyes, lowering his head to hide his face. Sabrina touched his hand. "I am sorry; but I did what I thought was best." "You don't understand," he began, looking back at her. "I'm not upset I love you too much. I'm relieved that you're okay. I just can't imagine going through this life without you."

"Do you; can you?" Sabrina stumbled with the question that tore at her heart. "Can I what?" "Can you still love me knowing that I have lied to you?" "Yes," Mark answered, looking into her eyes. "Nothing will ever change the way I feel about you Sabrina. I love you; don't ever question that." "I love you too," she managed to say through a yawn. "You need to rest." She began to drift, still feeling the effects of the shot that Doc had given her. A knock came to the door and her eyes snapped open again.

"What!" Mark growled angrily at the noise that had disturbed her slumber. Jim opened the door and peeked in. "I'm sorry Mr. Cassidy, but I need to speak with you." "What is it?" Mark grumbled as he neared the door. "I am very sorry to bother you, but Doc had to leave. He said to call him if she needed him again." "Is that it?" "No sir, the catering staff has arrived, and I wanted to check with you before I dismissed them." "Damn it, I forgot. Yeah, tell them to go, and see if you can catch any of the guys at the arena," he said reaching for the phone list on the desk.

Sabrina had been listening to the conversation. "Mark, don't cancel the party." "I don't feel like having a party tonight, not after all this." She motioned him to her. "Just a minute," he said to Jim. Returning to her side, he sat down to talk to her. "I don't think that this is a good idea," he said. "Well, I do. The guys have been looking forward to this, and we have two reasons to go ahead with it." "What reasons?" "One, we need to grieve for our baby, and this could be a sort of wake, with our friends gathered as support."

"What would the other reason would be?" "This was to be a night to celebrate our love for each other." She was afraid to continue, but she had to know. "Or have you changed your mind about getting married?" "No, I haven't changed my mind. Why would I? More than ever, I want to marry you. You're the best part of me and I want you with me forever." He stopped her from speaking. "Jim, put those caterers to work." "Very good sir," Jim replied as he shut the door.

Now that they were alone, she could speak more freely. "But Mark, I deceived you, I kept things from you and it cost us our child," she said, sniffling back her emotions. He gently wiped away her tears. "You tried to spare me, and that's not deceit. You are one hell of a woman. We'll have the party, but only if you get some sleep; and at the first sign of fatigue it's over and you're back in here." "Okay," she said pulling the sheets up. Mark kissed her on the forehead and quietly left the room. She was asleep before he had shut the door.

The downstairs was bustling with activity; caterers busy with their appointed duties. Mark couldn't tolerate the commotion. Going out to the patio, he stretched out on a lounger, far away from the activity. His ribs were stinging, but his emotional pain still outweighed his physical pain. He had never felt such a pain; not even when he lost his parents so many years ago.

Jim pulled a chair up beside him. "I am so sorry sir. Losing a child is the worst thing that can happen to anyone. I can't even begin to imagine how you're feeling." "No, Jim, you have no idea how I feel. I'm not completely sure myself." "Do you really think that this barbecue is a good idea?" "I don't, but Sabrina thinks that we should share our grief with our friends; and who knows, maybe she's right. There is an upside to all this grief though." "What would that be sir?" "I asked her to marry me this morning, and she said yes." "Well that is something good to hold on to right now sir."

Mark tipped his head back and closed his eyes. Jim returned to his work, allowing Mark to have some much needed time alone. Mark called to him before he had got too far. "Jim, where did Doc take the baby?" "Doc didn't. I took care of the little one; up there on the ridge, near the wild rose. If you like I'll make a nice marker for you to put up there." Mark only nodded; his attention was redirected to the top of the hill.

Jim watched Mark rise and slowly walk across the patio, out onto the lawn. Mark made it as far as the bench under the big oak tree. Unable to go any further; he sat down, his head in his hands. *I will not go up there alone. I will wait until Sabrina is stronger. Then together we will say goodby to our son.* Tears seeped through his fingers. His head throbbed, trying to make some sense of this horrible day; but he had no answers.

I still have her and that's the most important thing. Maybe someday we will have a child together. I know now that it wasn't my imagination that had brought forth the sound of her voice; it was her pain that had cried out to me. Our connection is so strong that even miles apart we can still communicate. I have to marry her. I have to make this up to her, if it takes the rest of my life.

If I hadn't left her behind today, maybe this would never have happened. Wait a minute. She wanted me to leave her home. Did she know? She must have known that something was wrong, that's why she insisted on staying home. Oh God, there were signs, and I ignored them. I let her go through this alone. Grief engulfed him again and shut down his mind.

The arena had quieted down. The show was over. The crew, busy taking apart the ring, hurried with their chores, the sooner they were done, the sooner they could begin their brief vacation. Brent wandered back into the dressing room. "So, what's the deal?" D'arcy asked. "It's still on. So I guess everything's okay at the ranch," Brent answered. "Strange," Tony interjected. "If everything's okay, then why did Mark take off out of here so fast? Didn't change clothes or take his stuff with him." "No point in speculating," Brent responded quickly. "We'll have to wait until we get there to find out."

"Well, I'm ready to go," D'arcy announced, throwing his tote bag over his shoulder. "If you guys don't get a move on you're gonna be walking. I'm going to the car; you guys have got ten minutes." "Yeah, we're right behind you," Tony called, grabbing his bag. "Are you coming Brent?"

Brent was busy stuffing Mark's clothes into his bag, but his mind was back at the ranch; wondering what had made Mark leave so quickly. Even though he had told the others not to make uncertain presumptions, his own mind was stuck on Sabrina, and the secret he had kept for her. *God I hope she's okay.* "Brent, it's now or never," Tony called from the doorway. "I'm coming," he said hoisting the bags onto his shoulder. He slumped slightly, not from the weight of the bags, but from the heaviness that shrouded his heart.

Mark spent the remainder of the afternoon under the oak tree, consumed by his thoughts of Sabrina, of their son. Imagining what the future would have been like, if only their baby had lived. Now and then the sorrow would well up inside him and his eyes would moisten with tears. As the latest rush of emotion began to pass, he rolled his shoulders back to release the tension that had built up.

I have to be strong. I can let my feelings show when I'm with Sabrina, but I don't dare let my guard down around the guys. The sun was skimming over the tree tops. *I need to shower and change before they all arrive. I don't want to disturb her, but I'll have to take the chance.*

Mark was quiet, as he passed by the bed. Sabrina was still asleep. She was so still that it made him stop, watching, waiting for her to breathe. He removed his ring costume, careful not to aggravate his ribs too much. Looking into the mirror; he inspected the tape. It was secure, and waterproof enough to withstand a shower. The water stung as it washed over the cuts on his face. In a way this pain was a relief. It took his mind off of his loss, if only for a moment.

Sabrina was awakened by the sound of the shower. She yawned, and looked at the clock; it was late afternoon and she felt the need to get up. Inching herself over to the edge of the bed, she sat up slowly. The pain was faint, nearly gone, but her head felt light; hung over from the medication. She waited a little longer before trying to stand. Making another attempt to get up, she rose slowly, only to find herself too weak to stand. *Maybe I should rest for a few more minutes.*

"What are you doing?" Mark's voice boomed, startling her. "You should be resting." "I have been, but I also need to be up for a while, or I won't sleep tonight and besides we have guests coming."

She's trying so hard to be strong and spare me her true feelings, but in her eyes I can see the reflections of my own emptiness and pain. Reaching out to her; she melted into his arms. Her heavy sigh heaved her body against his.

"Are you all right?" he asked. "Yes, and no." "Can you tell me what's wrong?" he asked holding her face in his hand. Her lip trembled, fighting back her tears. "Doc never let me see our baby; or even hold it. I never got the chance to say good-by." Her sadness deluged her; Mark held her close, comforting her and himself.

"You still can have your chance to say good-by. We both can." "What do you mean?" she asked rubbing the tears from her eyes. "Doc didn't take the baby away. Jim took care of it; he buried our baby up on the hill." "Take me there; please Mark; take me there!" "When you're stronger, then we'll go together." "No, now! Please I want to go now!" Her voice was filled with urgency; her eyes pleaded with him. It was a difficult decision, but it was something that they both needed to do.

Mark tried to persuade her to put on some comfortable clothes, but she chose to stay in the T-shirt and robe. He pulled on his jeans, and shed his own robe onto the floor. She saw, for the first time, the tape around his ribs. Laying her hand tenderly against it, not asking how it had happened; for she knew that it was courtesy of Sean. "Are you sure that you want to do this now?" "Yes, Mark, I'm very sure." Taking her arms, he lifted her up; she swayed slightly. He secured his hold around her, before attempting a few short steps. He had to slow his stride to match hers, as she moved very cautiously.

The stairs were much easier for her, as she had the support of the railing, as well as Mark. He stopped her at the bottom, allowing her a moment to rest. Sabrina watched the caterers, moving from the kitchen to the patio and back again; she tugged at Mark to move on. Jim stopped himself at the kitchen door as they passed through the dining room; purposely avoiding her, unsure of what he would say. He knew where they were headed and that brought back the heavy feeling to his chest.

Stopping at the edge of the patio, Sabrina picked a single red rose, sampling its sweet perfume before clutching it to her breast. Mark insisted that she rest on the bench under the big oak. She was still drained and willingly took a seat, even though it was uncomfortable. She lay her head against Mark's shoulder.

"Maybe we should wait until tomorrow; when you're feeling better," he said. "I need to do this now." She paused to look up at him. "And so do you." He brushed her cheek with the back of his hand and helped her up. She anticipated a hug, but it didn't come. Only a supportive arm around her shoulders held her.

I want, need him to hold me, but I understand why he doesn't. He's not in control of his feelings. I hope that I have not lost his love.

Forcing herself on up the hill, ignoring the weakness, she stopped only once to catch her breath. As they reached the top of the hill, she spotted the fresh mound of dirt, that was her baby's grave. Letting go of Mark she went to it. Dropping to her knees, her hand resting upon the dirt, tears flooded over her cheeks. Mark stood at her side; unsure of what to do, until she blindly reached for his hand, tugging him down beside her. She locked her fingers into his and squeezed.

The combination of her grief, and weakened condition, made her tremble. He quickly sat down, easing her into his arms before she fell over. Taking a deep, shuddering breath, she released a heavy sigh. "Doc never told me what it was." "It, it was a boy," he said, the words leaving a lump in his throat.

He couldn't see her face, but the frequency, with which her tears dripped onto his arm, told him that it had upset her very much. Laying the rose upon the dirt, she quietly said good-by to her son, and asked for an angel to watch over him. She leaned against Mark, desperately seeking his comfort, and his love. He needed her just as much; holding her tight while she cried.

The limo pulled up in front of the house. D'arcy was the first out, beer in hand. Brent followed, and behind him Tony. Jim met them at the door, showing the rowdy trio through the house to the patio. "Where is everybody?" D'arcy asked, looking about. "You're the first to arrive," Jim answered. "No, I think what D'arcy meant was where is Mark and Sabrina?" Brent added. "They are up on the ridge," Jim said, arching his neck to indicate the direction of the ridge.

"Well, don't they know that there's a party going on down here. I'll have to give them a piece of my mind for being such terrible hosts," Brent responded, as he headed off across the patio. Jim blocked his path. "No, Mr. Shea. Don't go up there. They'll be down soon. When they're ready they'll come back." "Why can't I go up there? What's going on Jim?" "Please, Mr. Shea, no questions. It isn't my place to give you the answers. They'll be down soon."

Brent accepted Jim's explanation with a nod, and returned to join D'arcy and Tony. "Christ Brent, don't look so confused; it doesn't take a rocket scientist to figure out what those two are doing up there," D'arcy remarked, tossing him a beer. "Yeah, there's nothing like a little afternoon lovin to pass the time," Tony added with a wide grin. Brent turned his eyes to the hill. "Maybe you're right. I sure hope you're right."

The haunting sounds of music drifted up the hill, to Mark and Sabrina. They were still entwined in a comforting embrace, sharing their grief. "Sounds like we have company," she said. Mark wasn't ready to let go of her; he kept his arms firmly around her. *I never want to let you go ever. I want to keep you safely in my arms; protecting you from all harm.* "They can wait; you're more important right now," he said. Sabrina rubbed his arm. "I love you so much."

Turning her to face him, he struggled with the questions that still burned in his mind. Sabrina didn't understand the look that was on his face but it scared her anyway. "What's wrong Mark?" "You knew," he said hoarsely, still not in full command of his voice. "Knew what?" "You knew this was going to happen and that's why you sent me away today, isn't it? You've known for a while that something was wrong."

"I didn't know. I thought," she hesitated to sniff back her tears. "I thought it was just a pulled muscle. I had no idea that it would come to this. I've told you that I'm sorry, but I guess it's just not enough, is it?" "You've got this all wrong. I'm not looking for apologies or explanations." "Then what do you want?" she asked, leaning away from him.

"I'm just trying to make some sense out of all of this. Sabrina, I knew, I knew there was something wrong but I ignored the signs." "What do you mean?" "I feel your pain, your physical pain. It started the night you were attacked at the beach house. Everything that your body went through that night somehow manifested itself in me. I felt it all and I've felt everything since then."

"How can that be?" Sabrina asked. "I don't know, but I do know that I am the one who should be apologizing to you. I should have paid more attention to what I was feeling these last few days. If I had, maybe I could have done something." "You couldn't have done anything Mark, and in your heart you know that." "Maybe that's true. Maybe I couldn't have changed the outcome of today but I do know that I can change our future." "How?"

Taking her gently into his embrace, he cradled her in his arms and softly stroked her cheek. "I'm gonna keep you safe and protect you, but most of all I want to marry you." "Are you sure?" "Yes. You are all that matters to me in this world and I promise you, we will never be apart again." Before she had a chance to speak he hushed her with a kiss, that deepened as she responded to his expression of his love for her; it left her breathless.

The sounds of music coming from the house grew louder. Sabrina leaned back slightly so she could look at Mark. "I don't want to leave this place right now but we do have to go back to the house," she whispered, yet her voice had just a hint of a tremor. Mark agreed, only because it was what she wanted. The last thing he wanted right now was to be around people, even if they were his friends.

Before she could even try to get up, Mark had slipped his arms under hers and lifted her straight up. The pain that tore through his ribs snatched his breath away but he kept it hidden from Sabrina. The last thing she needed was to have his problems compounding her own.

His strength still astonishes me, yet he's the gentlest man I've ever known. She rested against him, as she took another look at the little grave. "We can come back as often as you want," he said. With a sigh, she gave in to his silent command to move away. A part of her still wanted to tear apart the earth, to reach in, and if only for a brief moment, touch the tiny life that had once been inside her, to, if nothing else, put this nightmare to rest in her mind.

The party had grown, with the arrival of Sam. The mood was filled with jokes and laughter, as the group exchanged stories, but Brent sat apart from the others, watching the hill, wondering why Mark had left so quickly. Sam dragged a chair over in front of Brent and sat down. "So what's new with you? I haven't seen you for a while, since this damn promo thing kicked in." Sam had been away for over a week, doing an autograph tour, and pushing a new line of merchandise. "Not much; I'm divorced now," Brent answered without even looking at him. "Christ I gotta get back on the circuit. I've been missing all the action." "Hey, it's about damn time you two showed up," D'arcy called.

Brent looked past Sam to see Mark and Sabrina arrive on the patio. As they neared, Brent could see how pallid Sabrina was, yet how vivid her blue eyes were against their red, swollen rims. *She's been crying.* His heart sank.

Mark stopped near the center of the patio. Sabrina couldn't handle the stares, turning her back on the group, hiding her face against Mark's shoulder. He rubbed her back slowly. Mark cleared his throat. "Before you guys start with the questions, I have a few things to say, and I would appreciate it if you would keep quiet until I'm done." Tony and D'arcy each took a seat, quietly waiting for Mark to continue.

Dreading what Mark was about to say Sabrina tightened her hold on him. He responded with a gentle hug. "First of all, I need to apologize for taking off this afternoon; but I think you all understand that Sabrina is my number one priority, and she needed me." He stopped, taking in a deep shuddering breath. "We," he choked up as tears clouded his eyes. "We lost our baby today." "Oh man, you don't need us here. Why didn't you cancel? We would have understood," Tony interrupted.

Sabrina turned back around, rubbing her face. "Mark wanted to, but I asked him not to cancel. You're our friends, and we wanted to share this with you, but this is not going to be a night of sadness. It's not that we don't want you to share in our loss; but we have something else to tell you, the original reason for having you all here." She leaned against Mark, looking at him to continue.

Before he had a chance to make their announcement, he felt her grow weak in his arms. He picked her up, just as her knees buckled. Carrying her to a lounger, he sat her down. "You need to rest," he said. "Yes, I do; but I also need to be with people right now, and more importantly I need to be with you; not locked away in the bedroom alone." Her eyes reached out to him searching for the comfort she so desperately needed at that moment. Mark took her hand, holding it to his heart. "You'll never have to worry about being alone. I'll always be with you, every day and every night; I promise."

He always knows just what to say to make me feel better. It still made her eyes glossy with tears. *Does he really mean it?*

Brent rested his hand firmly on Mark's shoulder. Mark rose; shaking Brent's extended hand. Acknowledging his words of sympathy and kindness. "I need a beer. Would you like anything?" Mark asked Sabrina. "No, thank you, maybe later."

Brent waited until Mark was far enough away before he sat down beside Sabrina. "I'm so sorry," he said, his hand lightly touching hers. "Thank you," she whispered, fighting back her tears. He was about to speak again, when D'arcy, and the others, arrived beside him; Brent relinquished his seat, letting each of them, in turn, offer their condolences to her.

After so many hugs and wishes, Sabrina found it hard to maintain her composure. She broke down into a flood of tears. Sam beckoned to Mark. In seconds he was with her, holding her, soothing her with his voice. The mood of the party had become very somber.

Brent took another beer; his conscience gnawed at him. *I kept her secret, and it cost her, her baby. If only I had spoken up, told Mark, maybe all of this grief could have been avoided.* He lowered his head in shame.

Finally calmed down, Sabrina let go of Mark. *Doc warned me that her mood could change drastically, with virtually no warning, and I have to be prepared. I love her, and I'll do anything for her.*

Sabrina looked over at the long faces of their guests. She motioned for Mark to help her up. Securing herself against him for support, they walked over to the quiet group. She cleared her throat; not to get their attention, but to make sure that she had full command of her voice. "Mark and I, we appreciate your kindness; but we have to move on with our lives. Yes, this tragedy couldn't have happened at a worse time, but it has strengthened our love."

Mark hugged her, pleased with her resiliency; he allowed her to continue. "This gathering originally started out to be the typical end of tour party, but we had our own agenda for this evening. We wanted you all here to share in a very meaningful announcement." Mark couldn't hold back his own excitement she was taking too long to tell them their special news. "We're getting married," he said.

The announcement rippled toward the group like a shock wave. The silence tormented her. The faces before her reflected no emotion. She stared into Mark's eyes, wondering if they had done the right thing. He drew her close to him, his soft embrace taking away her tension.

A strong, firm hand gripped her shoulder; it wasn't Mark's. She looked to see Sam standing near her. His bright, boyish smile warmed her fears away. "You two make a great couple; congratulations," he said. Taking Sabrina from Mark's arms into his; he kissed her cheek, and hugged her gently.

Sam's embrace was uncomfortable, and foreign to her, his strength somehow smothering to her. Wiggling free, she fell back against Mark, back into the loving arms that she so desperately needed. Sam shook Mark's hand. "Man, it's about time you settled down; and I must say that you sure picked a terrific woman." Followed closely behind him, were Tony and

D'arcy, who each stole the opportunity to kiss Sabrina. Something they had both secretly wanted to do.

Brent had opted for another beer, and a seat away from the group. Still tormented by mixed up feelings of guilt, jealousy, and loneliness. *In my own way, I'm happy for them. They belong together; but I hope that their love is strong enough to survive the brutal ups and downs of Mark's career. This business has a way of tearing apart personal lives; my own included.*

Some of the guys, have wives and families, but most opted to stay single, not wanting to subject a wife to the constant stress and worry over injuries, as well as the long road trips. That's what had been the main downfall of my own marriage. Being away so much, we had become strangers. Mark will never let that happen to him and Sabrina. She'll always be with him no matter how crazy the tours get. He would never leave her behind. Someday; I'll find a woman as supportive and loving as Sabrina. He downed the remainder of his beer and opened another. Tonight felt like a good night to get drunk.

An unexpected rustling noise emanated from the dense garden, near the edge of the patio. Brent looked in the direction of the noise, scanning the thick shrubbery for the source of the disturbance. Emerging from under one of the bushes was Patches. Brent disregarded the cat and returned to his beer, that he had been ignoring. Patches stopped for a moment, to look back behind him, before trotting across the patio to his master. To tell her, in his feline ways, of what he had discovered while hunting in the garden.

Sean righted himself after losing his balance. He had been startled by the unexpected appearance of the cat; but more so by what he had overheard from the patio. Fearing discovery from Brent, he had stayed down low, behind the shrubs. He carefully returned to his squatting position, where he could still watch unobserved. As much as he wanted to burst onto the patio, and put an end to their celebration, he couldn't. His despondency forced him to back away from his hiding place. Concealed by the shadows on the far side of the house, he wept quietly.

I still want her, but today isn't going to be the day to get her back. My plan will have to be postponed. A new strategy will be put into place.

Mark settled Sabrina into a lounger, when she began to tremble in his arms. He fetched a blanket, tucking it around her. "I'd prefer it if you would go up to bed; but I know that's an impossible suggestion," he said. "You're right," she said clutching his hand to her breast. "I don't want to be away from you. I've lost so much today and I'm afraid that I'll lose you too." "You never will, I promise; but for now just get some rest," he said quietly. She readily agreed, lying back against the lounger. She welcomed the opportunity to relax. His hand crawled up her neck to her face, stroking her temple, soothing her into a quiet sleep.

I'll stay with you for a little while longer, until I know you're asleep. My heart still aches, but I'm so grateful that you're relatively unharmed. I can bear the thought of never having children, but losing you would destroy me. I wouldn't want to live without you. You will be my wife very soon; very soon.

Chapter 16

Days rolled together undetected. The party was but a memory. The guys had returned to their own homes, to make the most of the free time before the next tour. Brent had stayed on, keeping very much to himself. Having overindulged at the party, he had a hangover that lasted for two days. The solitude of his room, the comfort of his bed was all he needed, or wanted. Embarrassment and guilt compelled him to segregate himself, even for meals. Jim would bring him a tray to his room. Sometimes he returned it to the kitchen partially empty, but most times it was never touched.

Mark and Sabrina maintained a low profile as well, and Jim understood their need for solitude. For a little while each afternoon, he would see them go up the hill, to visit the little grave. Jim spent his free time working on the marker, a genuine craftsman when it came to wood carving; but this project was the most difficult piece he had ever undertaken. Taking his time, making sure that each cut was perfectly shaped and sanded. Periodically a tear would stain the carving, and he would put it away.

Each passing day saw an improvement in Sabrina. Physically, she was mending well; even faster than she imagined, but emotionally, she was strapped to a rocket powered roller coaster, speeding through the highs and lows so fast that even she didn't have any warning. Mark was nearly exhausted from the ordeal. Sabrina didn't sleep for very long, at one time, when she did sleep at all. Sometimes she would wake crying, allowing him to hold her. Most times she would reject him, seeking the solitude of a chair, but she always returned to him, filled with apologies for her behavior.

Out of desperation, Mark finally resorted to calling Doc Brown. She had to have an undisturbed night of sleep, and so did he. He awoke first this morning; Sabrina cradled in his arms, so serene. He was thankful to have had a night of peaceful sleep; not so much for himself, but for her. His hand accidentally slid over her breast, but he kept it there. *I miss making love to her. Holding her fulfills a need for both of us, but I long to really touch her, to show her how much I love her.* Even in sleep, her nipple hardened under his gentle touch; arousing him.

Closing his eyes, he tried to think of something else, to force the feelings from his body. He felt her hand, pushing his harder against her breast. Pulling his hand away, he looked at her. She was watching his face, hoping that he could see the need in her eyes. Replacing his hand, she turned onto her back.

"No, I can't," he said pulling away again. "Yes, you can." "No, Sabrina, it's too soon. Your body." "My body is fine; and it needs you. I need you to fill me with your love, but if you don't want to make love to me I'll understand." She rolled away from him. Deep inside that nagging fear that she had lost his love still gnawed at her soul.

His heart was torn. Raising himself up, he looked down on her beautiful face. "I love you; and I do want you; but it's just too soon. Your body has been through hell and I don't want you to jeopardize your health for anything." "My body has healed Mark, but my heart still aches. I need you so much right now; I need to feel your love to take away my pain." She pulled him to her; he could resist her no longer. He understood her desire to be loved at that moment, not to satisfy the physical urges but the necessity to heal the emotional tear in their bond. They made love slowly, fulfilling their needs to total gratification.

Relaxed, in a lover's embrace, Sabrina nestled close to his side; her hand caressing his chest, listening to the rhythm of his heart. Over the past few days they had barely spoken to each other; Mark felt uncomfortable, but they had to start somewhere. He sighed heavily.

"What's the matter?" she asked. "I was just wondering. When would you like to get married?" "I nearly forgot. Do you still want to?" "Yes," he answered without hesitation. "I want you as my wife, forever." "Well, to answer your question, anytime. My calendar is open. When do you want to do it?" "Anytime you want to get married is fine with me, but you need to make some preparations." "Like what?" "You need invitations, a wedding dress, the date, the place." "Hold on a minute. I have no one to invite. I don't need a special dress, and as for a date and a place, that's something we both have to decide on."

"What do you mean that you have no one to invite? What about your family, don't you want them here?" "I have no family!" "There must be somebody." "I told you Mark there is no one! I have no one, except you. Please don't ask me anymore questions about it because I will not give you any answers. I walked away from all of that and I will not go back, ever." "I'm sorry if I upset you," Mark said calmly as he held her just a little tighter. He understood the pain of the emotional baggage that she was hiding from him, he had carried his own for far too many years.

Someday the pain will be less. It will never completely go away but it will lessen with time. Maybe in the future we will be able to share everything about our lives but not until we're both emotionally ready to travel back down that path.

"So," Mark began with a light sigh. "Getting back to the question at hand I guess as soon as I get the next tour schedule we can take a look at the cities and see if any of them would be appropriate. You know that we're gonna have to do this while on tour, or the guys will be really pissed off for not being invited." "That sounds fine," she said turning onto her side. "But can we discuss it after I've had a rest?" "I told you it was too soon." "No, it isn't," she yawned, pulling his arm around her. "Just hold me."

Brent was feeling considerably better; his hangover had knocked him for a loop. It had been years since he was this sick; even the bout in Vegas wasn't this bad. He continued with his morning swim; the cool water cleared his mind of its haze. Even though his hangover was gone, he still felt the queasy pangs in his stomach; but it was his guilt gnawing at him, not the alcohol. *I still blame myself for Sabrina's miscarriage. I need to talk to her about it, for my own peace of mind. I'll have to wait until she's alone. I don't dare let Mark find out that I have been keeping her secret.*

The beach house was a lonely tomb for Sean; locked away, with only his thoughts for company. He had returned there after sneaking away from Mark's; he couldn't abide being in the state as him. The beach was alive with activity. Part time residents, and tourists, crowded the sandy shores, for days of relaxation, before having to return to their mundane, robotic jobs. He wished that they would all just go away; leaving him alone to wallow in his own pool of self pity.

With so much activity on the beach he had remained inside. Some of the neighbors he knew; but he avoided the tourists. If fans found out where he lived, his private life would cease to exist. Peering out the window now and again, to watch the people, only to turn away when he found himself staring at the amorous antics of lovers.

I still long to be with Sabrina, I remember how she feels; how soft and sexy her body is. I have to get her back; but now, with their wedding announcement, there's more of an urgency. There has to be a way, but not knowing when they'll rejoin the tour frightens me. What if they get married before the tour? I would lose her forever. I have to find out their plans.

Mark and Sabrina spent another afternoon on the hill; each trip, she took with her another rose to lie on the grave. Jim had finished the marker and had secured it into the earth. He had only carved the name Cassidy on it, along with the date. Mark appreciated Jim's gesture but a part of him wished that he hadn't done it. The pain would always be in his heart even without this stark reminder staring him in the face everyday.

I've never asked her if she wanted to name our baby. It doesn't seem right, to name a child that had never really lived. Sabrina never brought up the subject, even after seeing the marker.

Coming back down the hill, Sabrina stopped at the big oak tree, taking a seat on the bench. "Are you tired?" Mark asked, settling in beside her. "Not really, I just don't want to go back yet." "How come?" "When I'm out here, I don't think as much. The change of scenery helps to take my mind off of everything. Not that I'm trying to forget; I just can't let it rule my every thought. Life must go on, and so must we."

Why don't we go somewhere?" Mark suggested. "Where?" "Anywhere you want, maybe Hawaii or Fiji." "I don't know," she answered with a sigh. "Why not? Maybe an exotic, romantic vacation would do us both some good." "Yeah, but those are honeymoon kind of places."

Turning her face to his, Sabrina could see his expression of determination, one that she hadn't seen in a long time. "Then why don't we fly to Vegas, get married, and hop the next flight to some exotic place for our honeymoon," Mark said. "I thought that you wanted to wait until we were back on tour, so the guys wouldn't be ticked off." "Yeah, I did; but I'm marrying you, not them. So what's your answer?"

Still keeping her eyes on Mark, she began to smile, and saw it reflected back to her, through his own expression. "My answer is yes." "So when do you want to leave?" "Anytime; but we should try and find out when the next tour begins, so we will know how long we can be away." "It should have been here by now; but I can make a phone call to find out and then I'll book us on a flight to Vegas."

She pulled back, a look of puzzlement on her face. "What's the matter?" Mark asked. "What do we tell Brent?" "Nothing, except that we are going away for a little while. Come on we have a wedding to get ready for." He helped her up; but instead of starting for the house, she slipped her arms around him, laying her head against his chest. *He fills me with unspeakable joy. The only way I can express it, is to let my body tell him how I feel. I can feel his body responding to mine, growing and pulsating with love.*

Sliding her hand down his body, she stopped just below his belt. "We can't," he said quietly. "Why not?" "We'll be seen from the house." "There must be someplace that we can go." *To take her back to the house would be a dead give away.* Picking her up, he carried her into a densely overgrown area. Obscured from any possible view, he laid her down on the grass. Nothing would abate their ardor this afternoon. Their passion drove them on, reawakening their pleasure, and reaffirming their love.

Jim had the table set for dinner when they returned to the patio. "Dinner's almost ready Mr. Cassidy." "Good, I'm starved," Sabrina announced, taking leave of Mark's arm. Brent was already seated at the table; Sabrina took a seat beside him. "You two have a nice afternoon?" he asked pulling a twig from her hair. "Yes, we did," she smiled and blushed. Mark didn't see the action, or hear the comment, as Jim had taken his attention. He returned to the table carrying an envelope.

"What's that?" Sabrina asked. "Tour schedule," Brent jumped in. "A courier brought it about an hour ago." Mark glanced briefly over the dates. "So, when do you have to go back to work?" Sabrina asked trying to keep her excitement in check. "Not for twelve more days, so you know what that means," he said giving her a sly smile. "Oh yes, I do." Mark smiled at her and picking up her left hand he kissed the back of it. *I can't wait to hear her say those two little words again and when she does it will be to seal our union forever.*

Brent's gaze shifted back and forth between the two of them. *I get the feeling that I'm deliberately being ignored.* "Sounds like you have something planned. What is it?" he asked. Mark cautiously took the lead. "I decided that Sabrina needs to get away from here for a little while. So we're gonna take a little vacation, before going back on tour." "That sounds like a good idea. So where are you going; and when?" "Don't know yet; but soon, very soon."

Brent pondered over what he would do. *I can't stay here, with the two of them away. My only options are to either go back to work early, or to visit my sister.*

"Don't worry man; we're not kicking you out, you can stay here until you have to go back to work." "Thanks anyway, but I think that I'll try and go back to work. Maybe Nick could use me for some promo deal before the tour starts." Sabrina touched his hand lightly. "We really mean it; you're welcome to stay as long as you want." "I appreciate your offer; you have been more than generous, but I need to get back to work."

The smile on her face was cast toward Brent, listening intently to him; but hidden from view, her hand was working its way up Mark's thigh. He abruptly stopped her when Jim brought dinner to the table.

Sabrina devoured her dinner. She didn't understand why she was so ravenous. Passing it off as being that she hadn't had much of an appetite all week, and her body was telling her to catch up. Mark pushed his empty plate away. "I'm gonna make a couple of phone calls," he said. She released a soft sigh, as she watched him walk away. Her heart was filled with love, making her daydream about their wedding.

Brent could see that she was in deep thought. *I have to talk to her before Mark comes back.* "Sabrina," he said gaining her attention. "I'm glad that we have a few moments alone; I really need to talk to you." "About what?" "I feel so terrible about what happened to you." "Brent, you." "Please, just let me say what's on my mind. My conscience has been eating away at me all week, knowing that keeping your secret caused you this grief. I should have told Mark."

"Brent stop, even if you had told him, it wouldn't have stopped this from happening. Doc told me that no amount of medical aid could have changed the outcome. From the moment that I had the accident, the damage was done. It was just a matter of time before I lost the baby." "There must have been something that could have been done to prevent it?" "I'm afraid not. This baby just wasn't meant to be, and I don't want you to beat yourself up over it. There was nothing that you could have done."

Without any warning she began to cry. It still hurt to talk about what happened and all of her emotions were still raw. Brent knelt in front of her, gently taking her into his arms. "I am so sorry," he whispered. She held onto him until her wave of sorrow had settled to a ripple.

Brent had been such a close friend, and when he avoided her, after the miscarriage, she knew that he was bothered by having kept her secret. There was a sense of relief that they had this talk, to clear the air, and restore their friendship. When he tried to release her, she held tighter. "Please, just hold me, for a little while longer."

I can't refuse her request. I need her comfort, as much as she needs mine. His arms tightened around her, one hand stroking her silky blonde hair, the other gently rubbing, caressing her back, her head lovingly against his shoulder. *It gives me a good feeling to know she trusts me enough to let me comfort her, but I dearly treasure the feeling of her shapely body pressed tight against mine. This could very well be the last opportunity I will have, since she is now going to be Mark's wife.*

Mark returned to the patio, smiling to himself, pleased with the outcome of his phone calls. His smile quickly faded when he saw Sabrina in Brent's arms. Brent motioned him over; he felt his heart break. *She's been doing so well, if she has an emotional set back now, it could delay our plans.*

When he reached the chair, Brent released her. Mark took her up; her eyes still showing the evidence of her tears; she willingly went to him. "You should get some rest. Go on up to bed; I'll be up in a minute," he said. She readily obeyed his suggestion. He walked her to the door, waiting, while she climbed the stairs.

Once he was sure that she was safely in their room, he returned to Brent. "So what the hell happened?" Mark asked. Brent was ready for the imminent lecture. "It's my fault." "I figured that. So what in the hell did you do to upset her?" "I never got the chance to tell her how sorry I am; about the baby. You two have been keeping yourselves so isolated, that today was the first chance I had to talk to her."

"Damn it all anyway. I hope this doesn't set her back. She can't get depressed again. She just can't, not now." "Mark I'm sorry; but she's gonna have a few bad days for a while, it's only natural." "I know that; but she's been doing so well. If she has a serious set back now it could ruin everything."

Brent thought about Mark's statement for a moment. "How could that ruin your vacation? Getting away from here could only do her some good." "Yeah, but it could delay a big part of it." *Now I'm even more confused. Delay what?* Like a sudden surge of electricity, the light came on in his mind. "You're going away to get married; aren't you?" Brent asked. Mark glared at him. "What did she tell you?" "Nothing; but that's what you're planning; isn't it?" With reluctance, Mark admitted to Brent's suspicions. "Yeah; but no one is to know! Don't even let on to Sabrina that you know. It has to stay a secret." "Sure, I won't tell anyone, that's a promise."

This cycle of secrets and promises is becoming an annoyance. I don't like being their confidant. Life was much simpler when Mark kept to himself.

Mark excused himself to be with Sabrina. Brent slumped down in the chair, thinking to himself. *When this news gets out God only knows what Sean is gonna do, and not to mention the guys, man are they gonna be pissed off. Wait a minute I'm not even invited, and why should I be? They want to keep this private and that's okay. The less that I know the better, for all concerned.*

He thought back to his own wedding. *I would have preferred the simple way, like Mark and Sabrina, but mine was the typical full blown wedding, with nearly two hundred guests. If I ever get so lucky to do it again, it would be simple and discreet. No family or friends; just me, my bride and a justice of the peace; simple, nothing fancy.* The more he thought, the more it depressed him. Shrugging it off he went to bed.

Sabrina was already in bed when Mark came upstairs; waiting patiently for his body to be beside her. He had barely settled in when she was snuggled up close. "Are you okay?" Mark asked. "I'm fine." "Brent didn't upset you?" "A little, but it's okay. I'd like to say that in time it won't hurt to talk about it, but I can't. It will always make me sad, knowing that I lost a child, your child, but I can't let those feelings drag me down or my life will come to a halt, and I don't want that to happen. I want to move on, with you."

Mark raised himself above her. "I love you," he said softly. She answered him with a kiss. When he deepened his response, she pushed him back. "What?" he asked, confused by her action. "I was just thinking, that maybe we should abstain from sex for a while." "Why? Aren't you feeling good?" "Oh I feel fine." "Then why do you want to stop?" "Maybe we should wait until our wedding night." "Well, that won't be a very long wait," he chuckled.

"What do you mean by that?" "I have us booked on a flight to Vegas tomorrow afternoon, and if you like we can get married tomorrow night."

"Oh yes, yes." "There is a catch; we have to be up early the next morning." "Why?" "We have a honeymoon to go on." "Where?" "I'm not going to tell you." "How will I know what to pack?" "You don't need anything, because I plan on keeping you in bed for at least a week," he answered, a sideways grin giving his face that devilish glow. "I like the sound of that," she said pulling him closer. "I thought you wanted to wait?" "Shut up and kiss me."

The morning came too early. They had stayed up late, not making love, but just enjoying the tenderness of each others touch. Mark tried everything to get Sabrina up; finally when he reminded her of their travel plans, he obtained her full attention. She hurried; getting dressed, grabbing suitcases, tossing clothes wildly about. Mark took hold of her, to slow her down. She trembled in his embrace.

"What's wrong?" he asked. "Nervous, I guess." "About what, or are you having second thoughts?" "No, I have no doubts. It's just that I don't know what to pack." "You worry too much. Just take a few things; anything that's missing we can pick up as needed. Besides we have to stop in Dallas before we go to the airport." "Why do we have to stop in town?" "Every bride needs something special to wear on her wedding day and you are not going to be the exception. I won't have any arguments about it."

She rested against him; he always knew how to calm her. She returned to her packing more in control than before. Mark packed his bag, in the privacy of the closet. When he returned to the bedroom Sabrina was staring at her half empty suitcase. "Are you done?" Mark asked. "I don't know. You're not making this easy for me," she said.

He quickly scanned over the items in the case. "That looks fine, you don't need much anyway; or have you forgotten what I told you last night?" he asked taking her in his arms. "You're not gonna get a chance to wear most of what you've packed, if I have anything to do with it." "I really do like that idea of yours," she answered, reaching up to kiss him. He held her away, before they both became lost in their passion. "We had better get something to eat and say good-by to Brent." "Do we have to leave very soon?" "In about an hour."

Brent was up even before the two of them; he arrived downstairs as Jim was heading out to the barn. Following him, he helped when he could; cautiously quizzing him about Mark's plans, but gained no information. *Either Jim didn't know anything, or he is very adept at keeping secrets.*

When they returned from the barn, Sabrina was seated at the patio table. Jim headed off to the kitchen. Brent made a slow approach, still wary of how he had made her feel last night. As he neared, she rose and greeted him with a warm, unexpected embrace.

"You're feeling much better this morning," he said cautiously. "Yes, I am. I guess the idea of this vacation has helped me more than I imagined. Mark and I both need to get away for a while. We need to put this horrid time behind us and start over." "So where are you going?" "I have no idea. All I know is that we are going to Vegas today, and after that Mark won't tell me." "You're leaving today?" "Yeah, why?" "I just didn't think it would be so soon." "Look, you know you can stay here as long as you want; so please don't feel that we're pushing you out."

Not knowing where to take the conversation at that point; Brent excused himself, returning to his room to phone Nick. *There has to be some work available.*

After a quick breakfast, Mark and Sabrina made a final visit to the hill top. There was no sadness today. Not that they no longer grieved, but they had both come to accept the loss and the pain was not nearly as intense; not like their love for each other. Returning to the house, Jim informed them that the car had arrived, and that their bags were already aboard. Sabrina went back upstairs to pick up a few last minute items; but she really went to say good-by to Brent. She didn't want to leave without saying anything. She stood before him as radiant and beautiful as the first time he had seen her.

"We're leaving now," she said with some hesitation. "Well, I hope that you have a good trip." When the anticipated hug did not spring forth, Sabrina made the move. She embraced him for a few seconds, kissed his cheek and pulled away. "We'll see you when we get back." "When will that be?" Brent asked. "Oh, I'm not sure; but we should be back before the tour starts."

Saying good-by out loud stuck in both their throats; it wasn't an easy thing to say; Sabrina smiled and touched his face. Her hand trailed over his chest, as she turned and walked away. Brent could only watch in silence, as she descended the stairs and out of his sight. *The next time we meet, she will be Mark's wife; completely untouchable and forbidden.* He closed the door on his private fantasy.

While he waited for Sabrina, Mark handed the driver a list of stops that they needed to make in Dallas. He gave Jim a few final instructions along with their travel information, knowing that he could trust him to keep their itinerary to himself no matter what.

Mark relaxed against the luxurious leather seat of the limo; Sabrina solidly by his side. The late night, and early morning had left her drained and drowsy. She drifted in and out of sleep until the forward motion of the limo halted, bringing her to full alertness. Mark slipped away from her, to enter the bank, and returned in minutes.

Their next stop was a bridal shop. Sabrina repeatedly expressed her opinion of not wanting a special dress, but Mark insisted. Escorting her inside, he handed the clerk his credit card and told her to help her find everything that she would need. He wandered down the block and entered a jewelry store. Taking his time, he viewed all of the wedding sets in the showcase. He had to give her ample time to make her selection.

Not knowing where to begin, the clerk tried to offer suggestions, but nothing seemed to ignite Sabrina's passion. She wandered amongst the racks of formal dresses, remembering what her dress looked like when she had married Steve; but this wasn't a formal wedding. *I want something sexy; something that will stop Mark's heart.*

Reversing her tactics, she started with the lingerie first; a long white pair of silk stockings, a corset with garters and a white lace thong. The lingerie began to give her those sexy feelings that she was looking for. She moved back among the dresses, making a couple of selections, before heading to the fitting room.

Mark had made his choice at the jewelry store, including a heavy gold chain for himself. He would need someplace to put his ring when he was on tour, since Nick forbid his wrestlers to wear their wedding rings on their hands when they were exposed to the fans.

While Sabrina waited for the clerk to complete her transaction, she noticed Mark return to the limo. She had found a dress that made her feel sexy, but she couldn't shake the feeling that there was something missing. The driver put her packages into the trunk as she climbed into the back seat. Mark was reclined against the seat with his eyes closed. She carefully stepped over his legs and sat down beside him, staring out the window.

Reaching over he stroked her hair. "Did you get everything?" he asked. "Yeah, I guess so," she sighed, continuing her vigil of staring out the window. The tone of her voice saddened him. He slid closer. "What's wrong Sabrina?" "Nothing." "Then why do you sound so down? Are you sure that you want to go through with this?" "Yes, I'm sure. I want to be your wife." "Then what's the problem?"

"I don't know." She caught that quizzical look of his. "Really, I don't know," she said cuddling closer. "I know that I'm tired, and that's probably all there is to it." Her head came to rest against his shoulder. "I'd like to tell you to sleep, but we're gonna be at the airport soon. You can sleep on the plane. I have something for you," he said as he presented her with a single red rose. "Oh Mark, it's beautiful." She took in a deep breath of the sweet perfume.

Intoxicated by the scent of the rose, and by the feel of his hard, sensuous body beside her, she began to repeatedly kiss him, until she had moved herself to sit astride him. Pressing her body against his, she kissed him passionately. "I thought you said that you were tired?" he asked, holding her back. "I was; but I'm not now." She guided his hand to her breast.

"What are you doing?" "Having a little fun. We can still play and not make love." "You realize that I can't say no to you." With that said she slipped her arms around his neck, resuming her barrage of passionate kisses. She never tired of kissing him; he responded to her so well. It was the easiest way of expressing their love for each other.

The time passed quicker than expected; they were still locked in a loving embrace when the limo stopped at the airport. Mark had the driver pass off their luggage cart to a waiting valet. Taking Sabrina's hand they followed the valet through the terminal; past the ticket counters, and through a set of doors that led out to the tarmac. "Where are we going?" Sabrina asked. "To the plane." "Don't we have to check our luggage?" "Not this time; this is a special flight. We're gonna be the only passengers," he said, directing her attention to the small jet ahead of them.

He had hired the company jet to take them to Vegas; and on their honeymoon. The pilot greeted them just inside the door, showing them into the cabin. The jet was everything she expected, and more. It had every comfort of a well furnished living room, complete with a sofa, chairs, a table and even a bar. Nick had spared no expense.

Once they were in the air, she unbuckled her restraint and stretched out for a nap; Mark covered her with a blanket and took a seat in a chair opposite. He tried not to stare at her, but it was impossible. *She is so beautiful, and in a few hours this beauty will be my wife. You are my eternal mate Sabrina.*

At the other end of the country, in the corporate office in New York, Nick sat at his desk, a pen in his hand, that he tapped rhythmically on a note pad. He had been setting out the match schedules for the upcoming tour, but his mind wasn't into it. The news of Mark and Sabrina's wedding announcement had finally reached him late this morning. He pondered over how he could incorporate it into a show; he kept coming back to one particular idea.

An in ring wedding, the next step in the evolution of the Warlock; it would be a spectacular event, a definite boost for the company, in regard to ratings and profits. When?

He stared at the calendar on the desk. *What would be the perfect day for a Warlock and a Sorceress to get married?* He smiled, drawing a circle around October 31st. "Halloween, brilliant. That will be the day." As he picked up the phone to call Mark, he remembered that Mark had taken the jet. He hadn't told him where they were going, only that they needed to get away for a few days.

Damn. What if they're going away to get married now? So what? The fans don't have to know. The more he thought about the idea, the more he liked it. He picked up the phone, calling to set up an appointment with the company's costume designer. *They will both need a special new outfit for this event.*

Sabrina was awakened by the voice of the pilot, telling her to fasten her seat belt for landing. She stretched and yawned, forcing herself to sit up. "Are you feeling better?" Mark asked, sitting beside her. "Much." She stared out the window at the vast expanse of oasis, called Las Vegas. As the jet taxied in to the terminal, she spotted a black limo. "Is that waiting for us?" she asked. He nodded.

A valet scrambled up the stairs, collected their luggage, and took it to the waiting car. "You go on I need to speak to the pilot for a minute," Mark said showing her to the door. *I want to ask why, but I know what the answer will be.*

When she was near the last step, he took the pilot aside, to go over the details of their next flight, but also to give him a stern warning not to tell Nick where they were going, should he happen to get in touch with the pilot. With his instructions clearly delivered, and received, he left to join Sabrina.

The sidewalks of the Vegas strip were bustling with people; still mainly tourists. *I wonder how many of them have come here to get married?* The thought made her smile; she leaned against Mark, pulling his arms around her. "Happy?" Mark asked. "Oh yes, I'm very happy. So where are we going?" "You'll find out soon enough; just be patient."

She expected that they were going to the same hotel as before; since they were known there; but to her amazement the limo pulled up in front of the largest hotel/casino complex in Vegas. The towering sensation was truly an architectural marvel. Her imagination was flooded with fantasies as they passed through its doors.

She was so very taken with the decor, so much so, that she jumped when Mark put his arms around her. "Sorry," he apologized with a kiss. "Do you like it here?" "Yes, I do; it's so beautiful. "Not as beautiful as you my love." A blush warmed her body. "So what's next on your agenda?" Sabrina asked. "Well, we can't get into our room for about an hour. Why don't we find the chapel, and make sure that everything is in order?"

He had called the chapel from home to make the necessary arrangements, and had faxed them all of the required information to allow them to get married. He slid his arm around her waist as they walked through the hotel. Sabrina stopped just short of the chapel door. "You go on; I don't want to see it yet. Not until it's time," she said. She waited for him by the window, looking out over the sprawling city, taking in the pulsating lights of the other hotels. He was gone for a long time. She was beginning to get restless when he finally returned.

"Everything's ready; we're scheduled for eight o'clock if that's okay?" "Sounds fine," she said checking her watch. "Just over three hours." A cold chill ran through her; she needed Mark. "Hold me," she said almost begging. His massive arms enveloped her, pulling her into him. "You're shaking. What's wrong?" "Nothing, there is just so much to do in such a short time." "There is no reason to rush yourself; we have lots of time. How about dinner first?" "I'm not hungry." "Well then, why don't we find out what kind of room we have, and you can take a nice long shower." "I'll go for that."

While Mark fumbled with the key, Sabrina read the name plate on the door. "The Grand Honeymoon Suite. You booked a suite?" "Yeah, they said it was the best one they had; and you deserve the best." "I already have the best," she said. He smiled and opened the door.

She felt like she had walked into a palace. The suite was as lavish as the rest of the hotel. The decor was done in off white with gold accents and rich walnut furniture, elegant but tastefully simple. "A room fit for a Queen." "Of course; I wouldn't accept anything less," Mark said. She cuddled in close to him. "I love you."

Suddenly she pulled back, looking at him with a serious, yet confused expression. "Don't we need a license?" she asked. "Yeah." "Well, it's after five. Don't the licensing offices close at five?" "Yes, they do; but I already have the license," Mark said with a smile. Her look of confusion intensified. "I got it the last time we were here, just before your accident. That morning that you went shopping and I told you that I was going to the gym."

"So what other surprises do you have in store?" Sabrina asked, trying to contain her excitement. "Only one." "What would that be; or do I have to wait?" "All I will tell you is that you are going to have the most magical wedding you could ever imagine." "What do you mean by that?" "It's not going to be your typical wedding and that's all I'm gonna say; which has been far too much already."

Letting go of him she wandered over to the luggage; picking up the box that contained her dress. *I wonder if I should have picked one more spectacular? By the way he spoke this dress may not suit his plans.* He saw her, stroking the lid of the box, staring into space, lost in her thoughts. "If you're worrying about your dress, don't. What you wear tonight will make no difference, and will in no way effect what I have planned. If it's any consolation, I'm wearing a plain black tux."

Putting the box down, she leaned against him. *His words are of some comfort, but I still wonder what his plans are.* "Why don't you take that shower?" he asked, nuzzling at her ear. "Any chance of persuading you to join me?" Sabrina asked. "As much as I'd like to, I too think we should wait." "I know, but not being able to have you, knowing that I have to wait, makes me want you even more." "I want you too; but just hold onto the thought, that when we do make love, it will be as husband and wife."

The fluttering butterflies in her stomach ceased. She felt warm all over, as her love for him again took control, calming her. After several attempts to release her, Mark finally steered her into the bathroom. He didn't want to let her go either, and it took every ounce of self control within him to keep from taking her to bed. *It will be more meaningful to wait until we're married. Only a couple more hours and she will be mine forever.*

Mark was stretched out on the couch; his eyes closed, resting. From the doorway of the bedroom, Sabrina surveyed her sleeping Prince. *He is my every dream come true. A man who has loved me through all the shadows of time. A love so strong, that it has enabled us to find each other, again in this life, and I know that we will be together in the next. All those years of torment seem so trivial at this moment. I have endured, knowing deep in my heart that I would find the man that had invaded my dreams so many times. I realize now that in a part of my soul I have carried with me, into each life, a portion of his essence. That was how we were able to find each other time after time.*

Quietly she moved over to beside him. Kneeling on the floor, she gazed upon him, watching his chest rise and fall with each breath. His shirt was unbuttoned and she marveled at the strength. *How safe he makes me feel, when I'm pressed close against him, and to be encircled by his massive arms, only makes me more secure. Forever my protector and my savior; he is truly a warrior and a defender just like his name means.*

She could resist no longer; she kissed his chest. He never moved. She kissed him again, her tongue gently teasing at his nipple. She parted his shirt wider, exposing the full width of his torso.

Mark was awake, only pretending to be asleep; fully aware of her presence in the room, the luscious scent of her perfume told him exactly where she was. *I'll wait to see how long it takes her to touch me, and just how far she'll go.* When he felt her hand move over his thighs he stopped her.

"What do you think you're doing?" he asked. She ceased her kisses to look at him. "I was just waking you up." "Oh really!" he remarked, pulling her up onto him. As she settled atop him, her robe parted; her breasts pressed against his chest. *I have to look she's so irresistible. I want her, but I can't.*

"Close your robe," he said as he stared at the ceiling. "Why?" "Just do it, please." She slid off of him, pulling her robe tight while she walked to the window. Hugging herself, not as a comforting gesture because he had pushed her away; but to reaffirm to herself that waiting was the best.

Coming up behind her, he enclosed her in his arms. "I'm sorry." "No apologies needed. You have not upset me." She turned his wrist slightly and looked at his watch. "Besides, we don't have time. We have a wedding to go to in just under ninety minutes." He shifted his arms around her, bringing her closer to him. They stayed quiet, gently swaying, each of them secretly thinking of, and anticipating their future together. The moment was broken by a knock at the door. "Are you expecting someone?" she asked. "As a matter of fact I am," he answered. *He is a puzzlement.*

As he opened the door, she saw a courier; he handed Mark a package and departed. With a broad smile on his face, he returned to her. Breaking open the package he took out a small white box. "This is for you," he said. "What is it?" "Something that means a great deal to me. Open it and I'll explain."

Her hands trembled as she looked at the little white box. Lifting the lid she peeled back the cotton pad to see a large diamond solitaire, fastened to an elegant, antique gold chain. "Oh Mark, it's beautiful." "I knew you'd like it. It's all I have left to remind me of my parents. My father gave it to my mother on their wedding day; and in keeping with tradition, now I give it to you; on our wedding day." *Such a beautiful gesture.* It brought forth her emotions.

"You can't do that," he whispered wiping a tear from her cheek. "Now you have your something old." "Oh shoot; I completely forgot about all that stuff. The dress is my new; but I don't have anything borrowed or blue." "Don't worry; I kind of figured that you weren't paying attention to those traditions, so I took care of it for you."

Mark returned to the package from the courier and pulled out a little velvet box. "Jim said for you to wear these earrings; they belonged to his wife." Sabrina opened the box that held a pair of diamond stud earrings. "Now I have the borrowed, but what about the something blue?" "It'll be here in time don't worry, and speaking of time; we only have about an hour left. I don't want to sound pushy, but you should start getting ready."

She acknowledged his suggestion; collecting her luggage and her parcels, taking them into the bedroom. Mark followed behind; she stopped him at the doorway. "I don't think so. I need to be alone for this. Can you manage out there?" "Yeah, I can," he answered. She gave him a kiss, pushing him backwards. Before she closed the door, she had one last request of him. "Would you do something for me?" "Anything." "Leave your hair loose." She never waited for his answer.

Unzipping his garment bag, he took out the tuxedo. He had it made for him some time ago, to wear to a party that Nick was having; but he never went, so the suit never had been worn. He laid each piece across the back of the couch.

In my wildest dreams, I never imagined that I would be dressing for a wedding, my own wedding. I had resigned myself to the fact that I would spend my life alone; that this recurring vision was merely an illusion, the product of a lonely, desperate imagination.

When his parents had died, he had felt utterly abandoned. Having no other family, he was sent to live in foster homes. His ability to love faded away; as did the memory of his parents. Despite his vigil to maintain their image in his mind, they too, faded away into the shadows. All that remained of them was the necklace, and the story that went with it. That was the only memory his mind had kept intact.

I wish that they could be here today, to see me get married. They would like Sabrina. His mind tried to conjure up an image of them, but it was futile. He could no longer remember what they looked like. *Everything, that was my world, had been taken away from me, but never again. I'll never let Sabrina be taken from me.*

Sabrina had finished with her hair and make up. She opened the packages that contained her trousseau. Slipping on the lace thong, she dropped her robe to the floor. The corset was next. It pushed her breasts up, making them full and rounded over the top. Next the silk stockings, each one she smoothed over her legs very carefully, avoiding any chance of a snag and secured them into the garters. Admiring herself in the mirror, the sexy feelings came over her; it made her smile.

The final piece of the ensemble, the dress, was made entirely of stretch lace. There were no buttons, or zippers to worry about; she stepped into it, wiggling her body as she pulled it up. It was a snug fit that helped to accentuate her figure even more. It fit were it touched, like a second skin. Form fitting almost to her knees, where it began to flair out more and more, laying in a wide sweep against the floor. The front hem was higher, allowing her to walk without fear of stepping on it. She fastened the necklace, put on the earrings, stepped into her shoes, and put on the long lace sleeves that came to just above her elbow; secured to her hand by a single loop attached to her middle finger. A light mist of perfume, she was done. Mark knocked at the door. "It's time to go," he called.

Mark was becoming nervous. He paced about the room, a large box in his hands. The bell boy had delivered it only moments ago. He heard the latch on the bedroom door; he stopped pacing, anticipating the vision of his bride. She stepped into the doorway. Unconsciously Mark gasped at the heavenly sight before him. His pulse quickened with every step she took towards him. "Do you like it?" she asked, her voice so soft. "What?" "I asked if you like my dress." "Uh huh. My God you are beautiful." "Thank you; and I must say that you have never looked sexier."

She admired his black tux; his long dark auburn hair loose about his shoulders, the way she liked it. "What's in the box?" Sabrina asked. "What? Oh, it's for you." He held it for her while she took off the lid, retrieving a bouquet of red roses, nestled in a cloud of white carnations; at the handle was a short blue ribbon amongst the trailing red satin streamers. "Now I have the blue. Thank you so much." She moved to kiss him; he stepped back. "No. Please don't. I'm afraid I won't be able to stop myself." She understood; her own libido was already in overdrive. He took her arm in his. "Shall we go?" he asked. She gazed into his green eyes, smiling. "Marry me."

They never spoke, as they walked through the hotel; around the perimeter of the casino, towards the chapel. She had acquired a permanent blush as she averted stares from the hotel patrons. The women smiled at her, while the men stared, eyes wide, mouth agape. Mark stopped outside the chapel doors. "Are you ready?" he asked. "Yes." "You're sure?" "Mark I'm very sure. I love you and I want to marry you." As he opened the door, she was taken aback.

This isn't a typical wedding chapel. There are no characteristic white bows and bells, no rows of pews, no flower laden archway before an altar. This chapel has none of these things whatsoever.

Inside the door they were greeted by two, very attractive, young women, clothed in fairy tale sprite costumes. The girls ushered them down a path, bordered by an abundance of lush tropical plants; up a set of stone steps onto a platform. There was a waterfall at one end, which emptied into a small pool.

They waited. Sabrina looked about the immense production wondering what was going to happen. A mist began to form around the waterfall, getting thicker until she could no longer see through it. Through the mist a voice was heard. "Who has summoned me?" the mysterious voice asked. One of the young women was quick to respond. "Young lover's sire." "For what purpose?" "They have come seeking your wisdom and blessings;

and they beseech you to join them in marriage," the young woman answered as she stepped away.

As if from nowhere, a figure appeared in the mist. A man dressed in a long purple robe; he introduced himself. "I am the Wizard Merlin," he said stepping forward out of the mist. "You wish that I officiate over your wedding?" "Yes, we do," Mark answered. Mark watched Sabrina's every reaction with great delight. Surprised and captivated, she squeezed his hand.

The Wizard instigated the ceremony. Despite the fairy tale setting, the official part of the ceremony remained very twentieth century. As he concluded the section where they repeated their vows there was an unexpected, startling burst of smoke and flame. A dragon appeared amid the light mist that still swirled behind the Wizard. Sabrina jumped, moving closer to Mark.

The Wizard took up a sword and battled the great beast, lunging toward it, only to be driven back by the flames. The battle continued on for several minutes until the Wizard struck the fatal blow, plunging the sword deep into the heart of the great dragon, slaying him, and saving the wedding.

Adjusting his robe, as he straightened himself, the Wizard then continued on with the ceremony as if nothing had occurred. Sabrina was clutching Mark's hand so tight, that her nails were digging into his skin. He couldn't feel the pain, as he was numb, but he saw the deep indentations.

The Wizard asked Mark for the rings, which he quickly produced from his pocket. Sabrina gave him a curious glance, which he returned with a wink. Their hands both trembled as they each, in turn, placed the rings. Mark removed her eternity ring before placing her wedding band on her finger. The Wizard pronounced them man and wife, commanding them to seal their union with a kiss. As Mark took her in his arms, the mist came again, to reclaim the Wizard. Taking him back into the mystic realm from whence he came.

Engulfed by the swirling mist, Sabrina's lips met Mark's with tenderness. She moved into him, making their kiss deeper. From beyond the veil of mist, the Wizard's voice carried a final message to them.

"Your marriage has been blessed. Your love is strong, strong and pure enough to help me defeat this vile beast. Your love has bound you together for all eternity. It will grow stronger, giving you the power to overcome any obstacle; and with that love nothing will ever be able to defeat you, as long as you cherish and respect each other." The mist disappeared, as did the voice.

Mark released her. "Well, Mrs. Cassidy, shall we celebrate our marriage?" She could only nod, being so overwhelmed with joy, that it left her speechless. One of the young women approached them; she had a camera in her hand. "Would you like me to take more pictures?" she asked. Sabrina hadn't even noticed that she had been taking pictures all through the ceremony. Mark acknowledged her question, pointing to an area away from the stage.

They posed for numerous pictures, standing, sitting, embracing. When the woman announced that she was out of film, Sabrina was relieved. All she wanted was to be alone with Mark; her desires bubbled inside her. She waited patiently, while Mark paid the photographer, and gave her their room number. She overheard the young woman tell him that the pictures could be picked up at the front desk the next morning.

With her departure, Mark turned back to Sabrina. For a second, he thought he detected a glow around her. *She is so beautiful, radiating with love.* He took her in his arms. *The way her eyes sparkle, so soft, yet I can see the longing, the desire in her soul.* He kissed her. "Can we go upstairs?" she asked so delicately that he felt his resistance melt away. He had to stand his ground for a little while longer.

"Why?" "I want to make love to my husband." "Soon, my love." "Why do you make me wait now?" "For one, our room will not be ready for a little while yet." "What do you mean?" "Shhh, just trust me. The other reason is that we have a wedding supper to attend. You didn't think that you were only going to wear that dress for a few minutes, did you? I want the whole world to see how beautiful my wife is." Her body was consumed by a blush, followed closely by a rush of tingles that raced up her spine.

Heads turned, with staring, piercing eyes, as they walked onto the casino floor. Sabrina tightened her hold on Mark. "Do we have to go this way?" Sabrina asked. "No, but I want to go this way. Just pretend that you're going to the ring with me."

They proceeded past the slot machines, that for a brief moment seemed to fall silent. On to the gaming tables; the patrons, seated at the tables, paused their games, turning to view them as they passed by. Occasionally she heard a whistle or two, but never looked in the direction. The entrance to the restaurant was only a few feet away. Her sanctuary was coming closer with each step.

She breathed a sigh of relief when they cleared the casino, only to have it snatched away as a man stepped in front of them, stopping their progression into the restaurant. He wasn't a very tall man; very distinguished with his salt and pepper hair and his black tuxedo. He wore a brass nameplate on his lapel, but she could not make out the writing.

"Excuse me, Mr. and Mrs. Cassidy. I am John Blackthorn, the manager of this hotel. I have been instructed, by the owner, to convey his congratulations to you both." "How did he know?" Mark asked. "You see sir, he is a very big fan of yours, and when he saw your reservation, and wedding arrangements, he felt the need to extend his courtesy to you both. He would like for you to enjoy a fine meal with his compliments, and if you like, a generous amount of gaming tokens is waiting for you at the cashiers cage. We would like your stay with us to be a very memorable one. If you will excuse me, I believe that your table is waiting. Should you require anything, please do not hesitate to call me." He bowed away in silence.

"Well, what do you think of that?" Mark exclaimed. "I would still prefer to go up to our room, and stop being the main attraction." "Hey, we can't disappoint the owner. It's not every day that you get special treatment in any of these hotels. The offer has been made it would look bad to reject it." "As long as you remember that my offer came first," she said slipping her arms around him, pressing herself as close as she could. "Oh I haven't forgotten. Now how about dinner?" He had to tug at her to get her to move. She conceded defeat to her hunger.

The restaurant was grand, a vast open expanse, crowded with patrons; Sabrina saw no chance of privacy here. The waiter guided them through the crowded room to a table in the far back corner. They were barely seated, when a young girl approached the table, begging for Mark's autograph. He was about to cast her aside, when he caught Sabrina's look. He signed the paper and handed it back. The girl bounced back to her family, bubbling with excitement. Sabrina took his hand. "See, now you made someone else very happy today."

In his mind he agreed with her, but his heart didn't want anything to distract his attention away from her. When the waiter returned with a bottle of champagne, Mark whispered something to him and he departed in haste. Pouring out a glass for each of them, he lifted his and toasted his love for his beautiful wife. "What's this?" Sabrina questioned, discreetly pointing to the security guard who now stood near their table. "A little insurance, so we won't have any further interruptions." *I should scold him, but I can't. I too want his undivided attention.*

They never saw a menu; the owner had taken the liberty of ordering for them. Sabrina ate what she could of the delicious meal; but picked at most of it. Her mind, as well as her appetite, was on Mark. They had said very little during the meal. Her desires grew stronger. She stood up. Mark slid his chair out. She motioned him to stay sitting. She was going nowhere, except to his lap, one arm around his neck, the other twirling the strand of hair on his shoulder.

She had forgotten that they were still under close observation from the other patrons; until she heard the familiar clang of cutlery tapping against crystal. They were being prompted to kiss. To appease the onlookers, she took his full lips against hers, taunting his tongue. He intensified his response to her, unaware of the silence that now befell the room; their passion consumed them.

"Take me upstairs," she whispered. Mark summoned the waiter. There was no check to pay, but he left a generous tip anyway. The security guard guided them safely out of the restaurant to the bank of elevators. Mark handed him a thankful gratuity, but the guard refused. It was his job to protect his employer's guests.

Sabrina kept her distance in the elevator. *I have to maintain control of my screaming desires.* Mark unlocked the door to their suite. Stepping inside, she wondered if they had the right room. It had been transformed into the most romantic setting; illuminated by dozens of aromatic candles. A bottle of champagne chilled in a bucket, a tray of fruit on the table, and a small wedding cake beside it. Their luggage was no longer scattered on the floor.

"This can't be the right room," she said. "Yes, it is. It's the same as before, only with a few added details." "I need to freshen up," she said heading for the bedroom. "I'll open the champagne."

The bedroom was also illuminated by candle light, not as bright as the other room, but enough for her to see her way to the bathroom. On her return trip, she paused to look at the bed. It had been sprinkled with red rose petals. On the bedside table, was a basket filled with small bottles of massage oil and bath scents for the Jacuzzi. *He has become a hopeless romantic, one that deserves a night of unending passion.*

Mark was standing by the window, looking out over the city. She snuggled close behind him. He brought her around to face him. "Happy?" he asked. "Oh yes. You have to tell me. When did you do all this?" "Yesterday. It wasn't that hard. The hotel has a florist and I got the rings while you were picking out your dress. Easy when you put your mind to it." "I can't believe this day. You have made this so perfect. I couldn't have imagined anything better." "I love you, Mrs. Cassidy."

Hearing him say it made her warm all over; she smiled. "Make love to me," she said softly, reaching up to him. His hands were gentle against her shoulders, brushing over them, down her arms. She pushed his jacket off, moving quickly to the buttons on his shirt. Her hands trembled, making it nearly impossible for her to loosen them. He took over undoing them, while still kissing her. She frantically pushed, and tugged his shirt off, exposing his chest. Her fingers lightly traced over it. She kissed his neck, moving slowly downward.

He ran his hands down her back searching for a way to free her body. "How do you get this off?" Mark asked. Stepping back, Sabrina took up his hands. "Come with me and I'll show you." She led him into the bedroom. He wanted to take her in his arms but she resisted. "Not yet," she said pointing to the bed. "Just sit there, and don't touch until I say."

He watched her form, in the glow of the candle light. The shadows caressed her jaw line and cheekbones, giving her face a look of mystery, and seduction. His eyes moved across her full breasts, brimming over the top of her dress. *I want her so much.*

Standing just out of his reach, she ran her hands over her body. Pretending that they were his hands, lovingly caressing her body. Locking her eyes onto his, her fingers grasped the top of her dress, and began to pull it down. His eyes grew wide, as she slowly unveiled herself to him. His heart beat faster as more of her body became visible.

The dress fell to the floor. Stepping out of it, she moved closer to him. Raising her foot up, bringing it to rest beside his leg, she unsnapped the garters holding her stockings. With a subtle nod from her, his hands embraced her thigh, gliding the silky stocking down her leg. His heart raced.

She repeated the movement with her other leg. The anticipation was insurmountable. He wiggled out of his trousers, relieving some of the pressure. Kneeling on the bed, astride his legs, she kissed him. "You can do the rest if you like," she whispered, her steamy breath fanning the flame in his body.

Bringing her face to his, he caressed her cheek, kissing her tenderly. Moving his kisses down her neck, to the fullness of her breasts; lingering, while his hands untied the laces of her corset, freeing her body unto him. As he laid her down on the bed, his long hair brushed over her, sending scintillating shivers through her body. His actions were measured and very deliberate, taking her to a new height of erotic pleasure. Making love to him had always been most pleasurable; but tonight she was experiencing an indescribable ecstasy.

Several times she urged him to her, but each time he resisted, covering her with soft, passionate kisses and gentle strokes of his hand. He could have taken her at any moment; but he waited, letting his own ecstasy climb to even a higher place than ever before. She guided him above her, taking him in slowly, with great tenderness; feeling his love strong inside her.

They had consummated their marriage; but it was far more than that. They had united their bodies, but their souls had merged as one. The sanctity of marriage vows had entwined the physical with the ethereal, creating the covenant of eternity that would guide them back to each other in the next life.

Brent rolled over onto his back. He had been tossing and turning for hours. The bed was a mess. The air conditioning was on, yet his body was soaked with sweat. Each time he closed his eyes he could see Sabrina; he envisioned what it would be like to make love to her, but he would never get that chance, she belonged to Mark, heart, soul and body. He looked at the clock.

They're married now, and probably lost in the throngs of passion. I have to stop obsessing about her, or I'll wind up like Sean; the thoughts of which make me sick. I'm grateful that Nick has found a use for me before the tour. I need to be back at work, to take my mind off of Sabrina, and my own loneliness, but if I don't get some sleep I'll be useless at work. He punched his pillow again; forcing his mind to clear itself of all distractions.

Chapter 17

Sabrina was awakened by Mark's subtle touch on her breast; his gentle kisses on her cheek. She willingly surrendered to his amorous advances. There was a new, more intense passion coursing through her veins. Mark could sense her new ardor, but he marveled at his own feelings. A new fire burned in his soul. Flames of passion and hunger fueled his every action; he felt free of any inhibition. He could love her unrestrained, unbound of his private fears. Her soft moans and trembling body thrilled him, as he brought her to complete rapture.

In euphoric exaltation, she rested in his arms; her eyes fluttering, as she fought off the impulse to sleep. "You can go back to sleep if you want. We don't have to leave for several hours," Mark spoke softly. "I thought we had to leave early?" "No, I made a slight change of plans to our honeymoon."

"Where are we going?" Sabrina asked, hoping to learn more. "I'm sorry, but I won't tell you that," he said. She pouted; her lower lip becoming fuller and more sensual but he found the strength to resist. "That won't work this time; you just have to trust me." "Oh I trust you; I love you too much not to." She kissed him, softly at first, but deepening, exploring her lust for him, until he could resist no longer.

It was late morning before they mutually agreed to set aside their desires. Mark had slipped away from her to have a shower; but again succumbed to her advances when she joined him.

She needs to rest and so do I. I've never felt so exhausted, yet so gratified. Once we get to our honeymoon destination we can make love as often as we want. With no deadlines to meet, no place to go; just the two of us, alone, separated from the rest of the world. That's all I've ever wanted; to live life as a normal person away from work and the fans.

Since I've been with Sabrina I've lost that drive that compelled me to go to work just to escape the loneliness of my life, but now, now all I want is to stay home with her. I want to explore all the feelings that she has awakened in me, and for the next week anyway that's just what I plan to do. Alone, together, we can experience the love, the passion and the fantasies.

Mark watched her as she packed her dress back into the box, along with the shoes and the stockings. "Are you going to pack it all away?" he asked, hugging her from behind. "Well, I really don't have any other need for it; unless you have some ideas." "Don't put these too far away," he said, lifting out the corset and the stockings. "Have you forgotten what you told me?" Sabrina asked. His blank expression gave her the answer. "You said that you were going to keep me in bed for at least a week. So why would I need to take this; or any clothes for that matter?" Her hands crawled up around his neck, making him smile. "Humor me," he said.

"What time do we leave?" Sabrina asked. "The plane leaves at three. Why?" "I was just wondering how much time we had left in Vegas." "Was there something that you wanted to do before we leave?" "Well, oh never mind. It's not that important anyway." He grasped her shoulders. "Hey, if there's something that you want to do, just tell me. The plane won't leave without us."

She lowered her head, almost afraid to ask. "Tell me," he coaxed. "I was just hoping, that maybe, if we had time, we could go to that shop were I got this," she said pointing to her tattoo. "You want another tattoo? Why?" "I want to have one to celebrate our marriage." "You got it." "Really! You mean it?" "You bet, as soon as we can get packed up and out of here." She kissed him quick, returning to her packing with speed and recklessness; stuffing everything into her suitcase, folded or not.

Mark called the front desk to have the limo readied, and requested a bell boy for their luggage. Sabrina was ready before he hung up the phone. She paced in front of the window, nibbling on the fruit that they had ignored last night. "Relax," he said taking hold of her. "We have lots of time. The plane will be ready when I say." "I know, but the excitement is almost unbearable." "You're just getting a tattoo." "No, I wasn't referring to that; not that it isn't special as well. I can't wait to get you all alone. I want to make love to you so often that we won't know what day it is, or if it's nighttime or daytime."

Their moment was interrupted by a knock at the door; Mark opened it for the bell boy, giving him brief instructions. Motioning to Sabrina, she was at his side, her arm, lovingly snuggled around him. Checking out of the hotel was even easier. To their surprise the owner had given them the room at no charge. A card of congratulations accompanied the white photo album containing their pictures. Mark penned a quick note of thanks, and they both signed it. Before they left the hotel they stopped at the florist shop to have her bouquet preserved and then shipped home.

Considering the time of day, the tattoo shop had no one in it. Harry was in the back room and didn't hear them come in. Mark had to call to him twice before he got any response. Harry slowly wandered out from his hiding place, muttering to himself at having his lunch disturbed. His face brightened when he saw Mark. "Warlock; well I'll be. Good to see you." "Hey Harry, how ya been?" "Oh can't complain," he said glancing at Sabrina. "I remember you. Now let me think; Sabrina; isn't it?" "Yes, Harry; it's good to see you again."

"So, Warlock; what brings you to Vegas? There's no show scheduled." Harry was always direct and to the point. "Ah, don't tell me, you came here to get married?" "Yes, Harry; we were married last night," Mark proudly announced. "Well, congratulations to both of you. Now what can I do for you?" "I want another tattoo," Sabrina began. "One that will symbolize our marriage." "Do you have anything special in mind?" "I was thinking along the lines of a bracelet, with our two rings joined in the center." "Not a problem; come in and sit down." She settled herself into the chair, putting her left arm upon the table. Mark pulled a stool up on her right side, holding her hand.

Harry used the wedding ring on her finger for his pattern; etching it into her skin at the wrist. He interwove the second ring into the first and joined the two with a Celtic weave bracelet. Before he finished the tattoo Harry scribed the date on the inside of one of the rings. Sabrina admired her new piece of art.

Harry had blended his inks, getting them as close to the gold color as he could. The bracelet he did in black, making the two rings stand out even more. "What about you Warlock, what would you like?" "The same thing for me Harry," Mark said changing seats with Sabrina. While Harry tended to his inks, Sabrina seized the opportunity to steal a kiss from Mark, before leaving him to wander about the shop.

The many designs on the walls intrigued her. She was still drawn to the exotic, and the erotic. Gazing upon them, she imagining what they would look like on her. She was already addicted to the ink. The sound and feel of the needle no longer bothered her; in fact she found it exhilarating.

Harry worked diligently, making little or no conversation. Before he was finished, Mark interrupted him. "Harry, I'd like you to do one more for me." "Sure Warlock; what do you want?" "We lost a child; a son; a little while ago and I," Mark hesitated. "Hey man, I'm sorry. Do you want a headstone or an angel?" "An angel, but of a child." "No problem. How about I put it next to the tat of your wife?" Harry asked. Mark nodded, afraid to speak of it anymore. It still pained him to even think about it; and talking about it was only worse.

Sabrina poked her head back into the room. "Not done?" "No, a little bit longer; I'm having something else done." "Okay; I'm gonna have a look at some of the shops along the block." "Wait a minute," he said excusing himself from Harry. "Take this with you." Mark handed her a credit card. "Just in case." "Always thinking ahead; I won't be long."

The limo driver readied the door for her. She waived him off, walking past him down the sidewalk. There were numerous shops in this block; some empty, their blank facades crying out for a new tenant. A variety, ranging from a liquor store, to a magazine shop, but mostly adult oriented shops; offering a wide range of interesting wares. The one that caught her attention was the one shop that offered a selection of clothing. The windows were darkened, enticing prospective buyers to enter the store. She was intrigued enough to know more.

The shop was dimly lit, adding to the mystery of its goods. More curious than anything, she browsed at the racks containing bondage and fetish gear. Moving on, she went to a rack that was more familiar, but still, in her mind, kinky.

I want to find something for Mark, but nothing in this shop fits his personality, or his physique. Then I'll get something for myself; but in a way it will be for him only I'll be wearing it. She was smiling to herself as she picked out a leather bra, and a pair of short leather shorts, glistening with silver studs.

Everything was safely tucked away in her suit case when Mark came out of Harry's. "You'll need this, I guess," she said returning his credit card. "No. Harry didn't charge me; his version of a wedding present." "So what else did you have done?" Sabrina asked. "Harry did an angel for me." "An angel? What for?" "For our son," Mark said quietly. Sabrina moved into his arms, hugging him. Her silent, loving embrace told him that she was touched with his sentimental gesture. She kept her embrace all the way to the airport.

The plane was already warmed up and ready for take off when they arrived. Impatiently she waited for the seat belt sign to go off. Sliding over to Mark, she stretched out across his lap; the strength of his arms supporting her. "So, will you tell me now where we are going?" Sabrina asked. "No." "There's nothing I can do to persuade you?" She slipped her hand inside his shirt. "You can try," Mark answered with a wide grin.

She lifted herself closer to him, her lips teasing his, kissing him deeply only to back off when he responded. She repeated her question. He stayed fast, revealing nothing. She laid her head on his shoulder. "Don't tell me your giving up?" Mark asked. "Yes, I am. I know when I'm beat; besides I am a bit tired."

Sliding himself to the edge of the seat he stood up, with her secure in his arms. "What are you doing?" she asked. He didn't answer, but carried her to the back of the plane, through a curtain, to a darkened room. There were no windows in this section of the plane, but through the shadows she saw the bed.

"Nick thought of everything; didn't he?" "Sure did," Mark smiled as he placed her on the bed. She kept his hand tight in hers. "Don't leave me here alone; you're gonna need to get some rest too." He had no argument with that statement; he lay down beside her, drawing her close to him.

Brent wandered in to the office building late in the afternoon. Nick had sent a car for him, with explicit instructions that he was to come directly to the office. He wondered why his presence was being requested so formally. It had been a long time since he was last in this building, but it was unchanged; cold and sterile, inside and out, the gray, glass tower, reaching to the sky. He worked his way through the quiet building, on to Nick's office on the top floor. The secretary announced him, and ushered him into the office.

Nick stood up from behind his big mahogany desk. "Brent, good to see you; please have a seat." Brent shook Nick's outstretched hand but wondered about the strange look Nick had on his face. *It's difficult to get a reading on him; he seems almost happy. An emotion that doesn't often surface in this man.*

"Did you have a good flight?" Nick asked. "Yeah, but I'm tired, so enough with the pleasantries. Why am I here?" "I need some information. You've been staying at Mark's; right?" "Yeah, so?" "Well, I heard a rumor yesterday that he's planning to marry Sabrina. Is that correct?" "Yes, it is; but who told you?" "That's not important. What I want to know is when do they plan on getting married?"

"Why is that so important?" Brent asked, annoyed by Nick's interrogation. "Well, I'm hoping that they will hold off for a while because I'd like to have an in ring wedding at the Halloween pay per view." "I don't know Nick; Mark likes to keep his personal life very private." "Well, I'll ask him myself then. Do you know where they are now?" "No. They never told me." *More lies, but I can't tell him that they are already married and off on their honeymoon.*

Brent knows more than he's telling; but to pressure him for information would be useless. "Okay; I guess I'll just have to wait until the tour to talk to them. My secretary has a work schedule for you; see her on the way out."

My dismissal was too abrupt; he's up to something. My gut tells me that he's not about to wait. He'll somehow track Mark down, if only I had some way of warning them.

Nick picked up the phone, but hesitated, struggling with his conscience. The inquisitive side in him won out. He dialed the phone number for his jet. *The pilot will have the information that Brent refused to offer up.*

Picking up his schedule, folding it up; Brent put it in his pocket. *I'll read it later.* The jet lag, coupled with the previous night of restlessness, had finally caught up with him. He leaned against the wall, waiting for the elevator. As the door opened, Brent gasped silently. *Sean! Maybe if I ignore him he'll leave me alone.*

"Hey Brent." "Sean." "What's new?" "Not much." *Just keep the answers short.* "So where is your buddy Mark?" Sean asked. "Not here." "I can see that. So where is he?" "None of your God damn business!" "Christ man, back off; I just asked a simple question." "Sean, your questions are never simple when it comes to Mark. You're fishing for information that's none of your business." "I was just wondering when he was coming back to work."

Brent's anger burst forth, he pushed Sean against the wall his forearm braced under Sean's chin. "I thought I made myself clear; leave Mark and Sabrina alone. They have enough problems without you getting in their face." Sean freed himself, pushing Brent away. "Trouble in paradise, eh. I knew it wouldn't last." "Not likely, in fact their even closer than ever since they lost their son." *Damn it, what did I say that for?*

"What?" "You heard me, now let it be. There is no way that you're gonna get between them; nobody will after today." "What's that supposed to mean?" "None of your business, but if you know what's good for you, you'll give up on this hopeless venture." The elevator doors opened; Brent saw his escape and took it; quickly departing the building.

Sean leaned back against the wall, his mind processing, trying to make sense of what Brent had said. His mind retrieved what he had secretly overheard at Mark's house. *They couldn't, they just announced their plans, they couldn't have gotten married so soon. I have to find out somehow.*

Mark had been awake for sometime. The flight had been plagued with turbulence and that always set him on edge. Fortunately Sabrina was not bothered by it as her sleep was deep. He moved slightly to relieve the pain in his hip but he didn't disturb Sabrina, who was still slumbering in his arms. Her voluptuous body pressed firmly against his; her hand still clutching his arm to her breast. Looking at her sleek body, he realized just how much larger his own frame was. How it cast a shadow over her, making her appear even smaller and more fragile. Yet she eagerly accepted his massive body onto hers, wanting more and more of him.

I wish that I could let her take my full weight just once when we made love, but I couldn't bear to hurt her like that, yet our love always found a way to give us total gratification. Being completely alone for a week will allow us to explore our passions on a new level; nurturing our love slowly.

The pilot's voice on the intercom brought Mark back from his fantasies. *We'll be landing soon, time to wake up my ravishing bride.* He whispered into her ear. She moaned, brushing him away like an annoying bug. He kissed her cheek. When that gesture gained no notice, he nuzzled at her neck, knowing how sensitive that area was. She snickered as his mustache tickled her skin, making her quiver with delight.

"Come on; we have to get strapped in," he said. "Oh?" She turned over reaching out to him. "I didn't know that my husband had a kinky side." "I meant we need to use the seat belts while we land, but if you can keep your yearnings at bay for a little longer, I'll show you a love beyond your wildest dreams." Her heart pounded with desire; her lips found his, sealing his promise.

Darkness enveloped the plane as they departed. Her eyes strained to adjust to the obscurity. The lights of the airport terminal guarded the secret of where they were. She searched through the dark, on into the lights, for some clue as to where he had brought her; not that it really mattered. *As long as I'm with him, our destination is of little concern.*

The windows of the limo were blackened; only the muted glow of a street light penetrated through the glass. To make sure that she could not see anything, Mark had kept the interior light on, devoting his attention to distracting her, and igniting her passion. The limo made abrupt turns. First left, then right, repeatedly causing her to cling to him for stability. She had the impression that they were not traveling along a normal highway.

The anticipation was growing in her; wanting to know where they were, but more, wanting him. "It won't be long now," he said sensing her excitement. The limo continued its series of turns, slowing slightly to maneuver some of them. It slowed again. She braced herself for another turn; but instead the limo came to a stop; the engine went quiet. "We're here!" Mark said with renewed enthusiasm.

When the door opened a delicate breeze entered the car, a warm breeze, filled with the scent of flowers and humidity, a fresh inviting aroma. Stepping out, the amiable breeze embraced her, whispering greetings as it moved through her hair and embraced her body. Closing her eyes and taking a deep breath her mind reveled in the heady scents the wind carried to her. Off in the distance she could hear the sound of waves crashing against rocks, faint but unmistakable.

Opening her eyes slowly she looked about this dark tropical oasis. Before her stretched out a wooden walk way illuminated along its edges by low subdued yellow lamps. Her eyes followed the path as it turned and disappeared into the darkness.

She could see no hotel, nor a house. The limo pulled away, leaving them alone. The strange unrecognizable surroundings gave her a chill, she clung to Mark; looking about for some sign of civilization, but found none. "Come on," he said picking up their bags. "You'll feel better once we get inside." He had sensed her unease. She stayed close to him, keeping in physical contact at all times, grateful for his protection in this strange dark world.

They proceeded along the wooden pathway; the lights only providing enough illumination for them to see where they were going. It offered no clue as to what lay beyond the path. The heavy, earthy tones of their footsteps gave way to a hollow emptiness. Sabrina surmised that they were crossing a bridge. The bubbling sounds of water somewhere below her. Her momentary distraction made her look away from the path. She stumbled, twisting her ankle. Having her arm attached to Mark prevented her from falling.

"Are you okay?" Mark asked. "I'm fine; I wasn't looking were I was going," she said feeling more silly than hurt. "Can you manage, or should I carry you?" "And risk us both falling, I don't think so. Is it much further?" "No, look." Her eyes followed the pathway. Through the foliage, she could see the lights of a building.

"Is that the hotel?" Sabrina asked. "Not exactly." "What does that mean?" "It's not a hotel. It's our house for the next week." "A house? How did you ever find it?" "The travel agent booked it for me. He said it was the most secluded, romantic spot he'd ever seen; I just hope he's right." "Well, we won't know standing out here."

As the foliage opened up, their mysterious trek came to an end; there before them was the house, not overly large but more than adequate for the two of them. The warm glow of the light, through the windows, dissipated her fears. This was no longer a scary, foreboding place, but a place of love and serenity.

Opening the door, with a key he found under the mat; Mark gestured her to stay put while he took the bags inside, quickly returning to carry her into the house. "You can put me down now," she said trying to wiggle free of his hold. "Why?" "Well, I wouldn't mind having a look around," she said. He spun her around quickly. "See, nothing special. Now let me show you the bedroom." "Wait a minute." "I don't want to wait anymore." "Mark, please." With a sigh, he lowered her. Her hand gently stroked his cheek. Her voice was soft and warm. "Have patience my husband. We have a lifetime to love each other." "Yes, but we only have just over a week here, alone."

The want in his eyes. I can't keep denying him this way, but I know that by delaying the inevitable will only make us both more intensely passionate. Moving away from him, she picked up her bag to take to the bedroom. Somewhat disappointed by her actions, he went to the stereo. *Listening to some music might help to take my mind off of her.*

The bedroom was dark. Sabrina groped her hand along the wall searching for the light switch. With a flick of her finger, the room was bathed in a soft pink glow. Her mouth fell open as her eyes took in the sight of the bed; the only piece of furniture in the room. It stood majestically against the wall; a very large, ornately carved, four poster, framed on each corner with veils of fine white netting, that flowed down from the ceiling to the floor.

He has brought me to paradise, to a room that I've only seen in my dreams; now it's my turn to fulfill his fantasies. To make him glad that he's a man, and show him how much I love him.

Taking her bag into the large closet, she found her satin robe, the massage oil, and her new leather outfit. The muffled sounds of music filtered into the bedroom. Her body swayed to the beat, as she stripped off her clothes and wiggled into her outfit. Slipping her robe over top she concealed any evidence of her surprise for him. She placed the bottle of oil beside the bed, and turned down the lights.

Mark was standing at the picture window along the end of the great room. His arms folded across his chest; staring out into the darkness. She quietly moved to him, past the rattan furniture, and the glass tables. Slipping her arms around his waist, she kissed his back. "Miss me?" she asked. "What do you think?" he asked bringing her around to face him. His eyes scanned over the satin robe; the feel of the material excited him.

"I'm sorry that I took so long." "It's okay; you're well worth the wait." The music on the radio changed to a slow love song; she swayed her body to the rhythm, rubbing against him. "Dance with me." "I told you before; I don't dance." "Oh come on; it's easy. Just put your arms around me, hold me tight, and move your body with mine."

Sounded simple enough; he followed her instructions. She rested her head against his shoulder for the duration of the song; fully aware of his body's arousal. As the song faded he started to pull her robe loose, she slipped free of his hold. "Come with me," she beckoned him to follow her. By the time he was able to move, she had disappeared into the bedroom. Her subtle teasing frustrated him, yet excited him. He followed her, turning out lights as he went.

She paced relentlessly. *I need these few minutes alone to affirm my strategy. I can carry out my plan, and not give in to him immediately; no matter how much I want him.* When she turned around he was standing in the doorway, watching her. How the satin flowed over her body, making her more sensual and seductive.

The primal instinct in me wants to go to her, to take her in my arms and release the animal lust that's clawing its way through my soul, but I need to wait, I sense that she's planning something.

She glided across the floor to him; her robe flowing silently against the carpet. She appeared to be floating on air; this goddess of beauty, his wife. She took his hands; her touch sent a rush of electricity surging through him. She drew him closer, their bodies inches apart, he wanted to hold her, but her hands restrained him. She kissed his neck; her breath warm and moist. His body temperature rose, beads of perspiration formed on his forehead. *I must have her.* Taking her in his arms, he kissed her with the passion that he had carried with him for centuries.

Breathless and weak, she found enough strength to free herself. "Not so fast," she panted. "I can't help it; I want you." "Shhh. You need to open your present first." "What?" *I don't understand.* He didn't until she played with the ties on her robe. *She's my present!*

As he moved closer, she instructed him to remove his shirt. His hands trembled when he reached for her, loosening the belt on her robe. She saw the vibration of his heart in his chest; the subtle rhythmic beat of his love. When he touched her neck, her butterflies took flight again.

His hands moved across her shoulders pushing her robe off. "Do you like it?" she asked, her voice quivering with anticipation. Without speaking he guided her hands down his abdomen to the front of his jeans. "I take that as a yes," she said softly. "Most definitely, but you don't have to do things like this to please me." "I know; but I like to do it. I like making you crazy with desire." "You don't need any help in that department; you make me crazy all the time." "In that case, dispatch this outfit and make love to me; like you promised."

Needing no further coaxing, he struggled quietly with the garments, his passion, his lust, building stronger and stronger inside him. *I could easily tear apart the soft leather with my bare hands.* His mind visualized the thought. Seeing the tiny hooks snapping apart, ripping and tearing through the barriers that kept him from having her body. Taking away his hands he stepped away from her. He suddenly felt sick.

In my mind I'm raping her, taking from her, with force, what every woman values the most, respect and dignity. In those few, brief moments, I've come to realize the frenzied lust that drove men to attack women. It scares me to think that I had come so close to doing to her, what I despised other men for doing to innocent women. His stomach churned in disgust.

Stunned by his sudden retreat, Sabrina's mind searched for answers. Her body needed his touch. Mark sat on the edge of the bed, his head in his hands. She went to him, kneeling in front of him, slowly rubbing his legs. "Mark, are you okay?" His silence worried her. She pulled his hands away from his face, making him look at her. His eyes were misty with tears. She moved in closer to comfort him. "What's wrong Mark?" He stayed silent. She kissed his cheek lightly. "Whatever it is you know you can tell me." "No, I can't. Not this time." "Why not?" "Because it's so vile that it makes me sick to think about it."

Her mind was ablaze with thoughts. *What could be upsetting him so bad? Is there some dark sexual fantasy that he wants fulfilled but is afraid to ask?* "Mark, I'm not going to press you for an explanation; but just answer me one thing; and only with a yes or no. Does this have anything to do with sex?" "Yes," he answered lowering his head. Raising it up again, her eyes looked onto his with deep sincerity.

"Mark I love you, unconditionally, totally, with my entire being, as your wife, your soul mate and your lover. I want you to know that if you want to try something new, or different, you should never be afraid or ashamed to ask me, or to initiate anything. I love you and I trust you. Without any hesitation or reservation, I will be a consenting participant to any intimate, erotic act that you desire to explore. I am so devoutly committed to you that I will do anything for you or to you, to fulfill your most secret of fantasies."

Her every word went straight to his heart; he pulled her close. "Sabrina I love you so much, but I can't tell you about this, not now." "It's all right," she whispered as she nuzzled at his ear. "Take off your jeans and lay down." "But." "Shhh; trust me Mark." She backed away, while he slipped off his jeans and stretched out on the bed. Propping himself up on one elbow he watched her as she wiggled free of her leather, reminding himself that tonight this was for the best for both of them.

Crawling onto the bed, she straddled his hips. He reached to pull her to him, but she was already leaning down. Their lips met tenderly, but briefly. "Turn over," she requested. "What?" "Turn onto your stomach and get comfortable." While he turned and settled himself, she reached for the bottle of oil; pouring some into her hand, letting it warm. With a light, sensual touch, she smoothed the oil across his back, working out the tension that he had brought onto himself.

He didn't wait for her to tell him to turn over. She poured more oil in her hand, smoothing it over his chest. The glossy sheen giving more definition to his powerful muscles. All the while she watched his face and his changing expressions. Unconsciously, her body rubbed against him with every stroke of her hands, heightening their arousal. "Do you like it?" she asked leaning in closer to him. "Oh yeah; but you have to experience it too."

Mark took the bottle and raising up his knees for her to recline against he poured the oil onto her throat, watching it run down over her breasts. Leaning back, she closed her eyes, waiting for his touch.

A soft moan, reminiscent of a feline purr, escaped her lips as his hands lovingly smoothed the oil over her body. Her breasts slipped through his hands. He wanted to grasp them more firmly, but held back, keeping his touch light. She leaned into him; she had to have him. Rising up, she found that part of him that her body so desperately desired. Being joined with him was ecstasy beyond extreme; his love filled her soul and made her whole.

Chapter 18

Nick slammed the phone down onto the desk. "Damn it to hell!" he muttered to himself. With his patience wearing thin; the week nearly gone and still he had not located Mark. Pacing in front of the windows, he stared out, but saw nothing. He never heard the door open or the voice call to him.

Getting no response to his greeting, Sean walked over to the desk, knocking loudly on the top. "Hey Nick," he called. Startled by the interruption, Nick spun around. "What do you want?" he asked, annoyed by the intrusion. "Nothing much, I was in the building; thought I'd stop by. So what's got you so pissed off?" "I've been trying to get in touch with Mark, but I'm not having any luck."

The perfect opportunity to worm out information; but I'll have to be subtle about it. "Isn't he at home?" Sean asked. "No, that would be too simple," Nick answered sarcastically. "Well, that's strange. If he's not at home, then where do you think he is?" "That part I already know."

Sean had to push. *I have to know.* "So where is he?" "Somewhere in Hawaii." "What, but how?" "He hired the company jet to take him and Sabrina on a vacation. I've called every hotel that I can think of and they're not registered anywhere. It's as if they dropped off the face of the earth." "Why is it so important that you find him? The tour is gonna start in a couple of days; wait until then." "I guess I'm going to have to," Nick said as he sat down behind his desk, the leather chair squeaking as he pushed himself back in the seat. "If you would excuse me Sean, I have a meeting that I must prepare for."

Sean left the office reluctantly. *My search for answers has only left me with more questions. Nick provided some information, but not what I'd been looking for. Why did Mark go to Hawaii?* His heart ached as he thought about the potential reason behind their disappearance. *It couldn't be. Have I lost her?*

He swallowed, forcing down the lump in his throat. The possibility sickened him, but deep in his soul the flame of desire still burned for her. *I could still get her back. I have to, or lose my sanity trying. I have just over two days to sort out my plan. Since the tour is starting in southern California, I have the advantage. That's my territory, not Mark's.* His eyes gleamed with delight, as his mind pieced together ideas. *I have to get home.*

Calling the airport from his car, he booked himself on the next available flight.

It was still dark outside when Sabrina awoke. *I've lost all track of time since arriving here. Is it morning or still night? I have no idea. Mark kept his promise, finding every excuse to keep me in bed. I don't mind. I never tire of making love to him, or just laying in his arms, talking; this is true happiness.* Her stomach rumbled, begging to be fed. *I can't ignore it any longer; the craving for food is just too strong.*

Careful not to wake him, she slipped out of his arms, pulled on her robe, and quietly crept from the bedroom, as she had done several times before. *I attribute my voracious appetite to all the physical activity that I've been participating in. We did manage to find time for meals, but I seem to be always hungry.* Standing in the light of the refrigerator, she pondered over what would best appease the rumblings in her stomach; settling for an apple and a piece of cheese.

Leaving the fridge door open, for the light, she cut a couple slices of cheese. As she put the knife in the sink, Mark's arms encircled her waist. "Raiding the fridge again," Mark whispered as he nuzzled at her neck. "I was hungry, okay!" "Hey!" He turned her around to face him. "I wasn't being sarcastic. It doesn't matter to me how many times you've done this." "You know?" "Of course I know." "I was so careful not to wake you. How did you know?"

He pulled her close to him. "That my beautiful wife, is just one of the special powers that our love has given me." Reaching up to him, she searched for his sensuous lips. "Come back to bed," he whispered. "I'm not tired." "Good," he answered pressing himself closer to her. "Oh Mark," she sighed pulling away from his embrace. "I thought you liked it." "Oh I do, very much; but we will be leaving soon and we have yet to leave this house," she said as she wandered over to the window. "I want to see the sunrise on this paradise. To know what lies beyond these walls." "If that's what you desire, then that's what we'll do."

She pulled his arms around her. His hands roamed slowly over her stomach. *She feels different somehow, rounder. Probably all the midnight snacks. Keep it to myself, a remark like that would definitely upset her.*

They cuddled together on the sofa, watching the veil of darkness being pushed back by the approaching dawn. Sabrina stared in wonder as this lush paradise was revealed to her. Leaving his arms she went outside to take in the full beauty from the sun deck. The humidity greeted her with a fresh, intoxicating aroma, the mixture of the morning dew and tropical flowers, thrown together with the salty breeze of the ocean energized her. Closing her eyes, she took a deep breath. The scents swirled around in her mind. *This is too good to experience alone.*

She bounded back into the house and straight to Mark, tugging at him to get up. "You have to come and see this; it's so beautiful." "It can't be," he said pulling her against him. "Nothing can be more beautiful than you." "Not this time."

Sabrina wiggled free, continuing to tug him toward the deck. Mark used his weight against her, in a teasing manner; making her struggle harder. Feeling the deliberate resistance, she let go of him, frustrated and angry. "Fine! Stay here then!" she yelled and bolted from the house, down the pathway and out of sight.

He pounded his fist on the door frame. "Damn it!" *I picked the wrong time to tease her, and now I've hurt her. I have to find her, to make it right.*

Running blindly through the vegetation, she took no notice of the direction she had traveled; her tears obscuring the beauty around her. When she could no longer see clearly, she stopped, wiping the tears from her eyes. Looking around only made it worse. The house was no where to be seen and there was no pathway, nothing to guide her back. She dropped to her knees, frightened. *All I wanted to do was to share a special moment with Mark, but my sudden burst of anger made me run away from the man that I love. Why do I do these stupid things?*

Mark called out her name. His heart sank each time his voice was answered by silence. *What if she's hurt? I have to find her.* He followed the pathway until he saw the freshly broken foliage. *She must have gone this way.* Carefully following the newly made path; he called again. Silence. Continuing on, the adrenaline pumped through his veins at a vigorous rate.

Sabrina huddled on the ground, every sound making her jump with fear, bringing her tears rushing harder. Mark cleared the foliage in front of him. To his relief he saw her, her frail form visibly quaking. He was at her side in a heartbeat, kneeling down he spoke softly. "Sabrina," he called as to not startle her. She could not look at him; yet she needed his arms around her. He held her tight, her body shaking uncontrollably. "Baby, I'm sorry. I'm sorry for being such a jack ass."

Her arms tightened around him, acknowledging his apology. She wanted to speak but her sobs had stolen her voice. The sun was climbing toward the tree tops, bathing them in warm golden rays. He stroked her arm. Her skin was cold to his touch and her shaking had slowed some. "I'm taking you back to the house," he said lifting her into his arms. Hugging his neck, she pressed herself close to him for warmth, never had she felt so cold, or so sleepy.

Mark carefully chose his way back to the path. When he stepped into the shadows she shivered. *Her body is experiencing shock. I need to warm her quickly.* His pace hastened along the wooden path to the house. Taking her into the bedroom, he sat her down and proceeded to remove her robe. She pulled it back around her. "Please don't; I, I'm s, so very cold," she stammered. "I know baby; but I have to do this."

The tender, loving look on his face made her more at ease. He stripped her of her robe and helped her to lay down; pulling the full compliment of blankets onto her. Slipping in beside her, he covered as much of her body, with his own, as he could. Her shivering persisted, uncontrollably, until she succumbed to sleep. He stayed awake, aware of every breath that she took, every beat of her heart.

In the dim light of the beach house, Sean reviewed the list, that lay on the coffee table. Each item had a check mark beside it. He smiled, leaning back against the sofa. *The preparations of my plan are complete. Tomorrow I'll put it into play.* He stretched before getting up to wander over to the window. Through the shutters, he caught the fading glimpses of the sunset. *The beach house has been closed up and no one knows that I'm here, not even Charles. This is the perfect place to hide.* "Tomorrow Sabrina. Tomorrow you'll be back where you belong."

Their time in paradise had come quickly to an end. Still consumed with guilt, Mark had done everything he could to make Sabrina happy. She had forgiven him, blaming her untimely outburst on her still mixed up hormones, but his own conscience did not. Putting aside his wants and desires, he listened to his heart, hearing everything that she wasn't saying.

They went for a long walk, amid the tropical foliage, taking the time to fully experience the wonders of the island. He cuddled her while they watched the sunset, and woke her to see the sunrise. His thoughtfulness was recognized by a simple, but subtle, squeeze of the hand; just before she pulled his arms around her.

He sighed, not realizing that he had. She lifted her head from his shoulder. "We have to leave soon; don't we?" she asked. "Yes, but if I had a choice I'd stay here with you forever." "That's a pleasing thought, but we both know that it's impossible, at least not right now. So when do we have to leave?" "We have to be at the airport by nine; that will get us back just in time for tonight's show in Los Angeles." "A show, tonight! We should have gone back yesterday. You're gonna be exhausted." "I'll be fine; I'm used to it. Besides we can catch a nap on the plane." "What about your ring gear, you didn't bring it; did you?" "No, Jim sent it all with the company equipment. Everything will be waiting for us at the arena."

She turned his arm to see his watch. "Three hours, that's not much time." She stood up, pulling him with her. "Come with me." "Yeah, we better get started with the packing." "Packing! I wasn't referring to that," she said pulling him to her. Reading the signals correctly, he carried her back to the bedroom.

The arena was slowly showing signs of life as Brent wandered in. The crew had begun unloading the trailers. Hauling in the components that formed the ring, as well as all the props that made the show more exciting for the fans. He climbed the steps up into the stands, taking a seat where he could watch the activity on the floor. He was tired. The week of doing promotional stops, interviews and autograph sessions had drained him, far more than a two week show schedule. *I'm glad to be back on tour. One more autograph session this afternoon and that will be the end of it.* Reaching into his shirt pocket, he pulled out a copy of tonight's matches.

I'm slated to wrestle D'arcy at the beginning of the second hour, just before Mark. It will be good to see them again, but will they have time for me, or anyone for that matter, now that they're newly weds? I wonder if they will announce their marriage, or keep it a secret a little longer? Considering what Nick is planning, they would do better to tell him and mess up his perfect plan. That thought made him smile.

"Hey man," D'arcy called up to him from the stairs below. "Nick's looking for you, better get a move on before he gets pissed off." With a groan, Brent pushed himself out of the seat. *Just another meeting with the boss and another opportunity for him to grill me about Mark, and another replay of my well-rehearsed lies; or maybe this time it's just business.*

The flight home seemed much shorter to Sabrina. Their honeymoon was over but right now her time with Mark was far more precious than any other. She cuddled up close beside him. "Why so sad?" Mark asked. She shrugged a noncommittal answer. "That's not an answer. No secrets anymore." "I wish we didn't have to go back," she said with a heavy sigh. "You know I have to work." "Yes, I know, but." "But what?" "I just wish that it was any other night than this one." "So what's wrong with tonight?" Mark asked. "I don't know; it doesn't feel right." "What are you feeling?" Mark asked. "Tired. I'm just tired. Forget it, it's probably nothing a nap won't cure," she answered, settling in close to him.

I'm not lying about being tired, but I am hiding what I'm sensing. There's an ominous cloud shrouding tonight's show. Enough that it caused her butterflies to take flight again. She could feel their wings, beating furiously against her belly. She rubbed at it slowly, trying to soothe the trembling turmoil within.

Mark watched her subtle gestures and he slowly rubbed his hand along her arm. *I know she's hiding something, not wanting to worry me; but I have my own misgivings about tonight. I'll need to keep her close to me.*

Sean slipped into the arena unnoticed; his face beamed bright with anticipation. The time was quickly approaching for him to execute his plan. It made him shudder with delight. *There was a revision to tonight's show that offers me the perfect opportunity. Mark is now slated to do a lengthy interview, and that will be my chance to ferret Sabrina away.*

Sitting down, at the table in his dressing room, he went over his list again, double checking every detail for the slightest flaw. Pushing it aside, he drew forth another new sheet of paper, and an envelope. Carefully, and with great thought, he penned a brief note then folded it into the envelope, sealed it and printed Sabrina's name on it. The final piece of the plan was done. Holding the envelope to his chest, he prayed.

A car was waiting, when the plane landed in Los Angeles. The California heat filtered into the car, yet Sabrina shuddered with an icy chill. She hugged herself, not for the needed warmth, but to again calm the tumultuous fluttering in her belly. *Funny, it's almost as if I can actually feel the movement, but that can't be possible. My mind is playing tricks on me, that has to be it. My nerves are on edge about tonight. My imagination is running wild.*

Mark startled her when he opened the door. He was barely seated when she slid herself closer to him, needing the security of his embrace. "It'll be okay. I don't want you to worry about tonight at all, besides if you agree to what I'm about to say, you won't have the time to worry." "What have you got on your mind now?" Sabrina asked.

For a brief moment, he could only gaze into her blue eyes, how they sparkled with love and yet there was something just a bit different, underlying the warm blue of her eyes he could see the hint of fear. "Are you going to tell me?" Sabrina asked. The trance was broken, but his mind was a blank. "What?" Mark asked. "What is on your mind?" "Only this," he said as he kissed her, laying her back on the seat. His kisses long and loving; his hand under her shirt, searching out her breast.

As much as I don't want to, I know that I have to stop this before we both reach the point of no return. "Mark," she panted. His hand pressed more firmly against her. "No, please, we can't," she said squirming free. "Why not?" With all of her strength, she pushed him back enough so she could sit up. "I don't think that this was what you originally had on your mind; now is it?" "Not exactly; but I like this much more." "I can't argue that; but I wish you would tell me." "Okay. How would you feel about telling everybody tonight about our secret?" "If that's what you want, it's fine with me." "You're sure?" Mark asked. Sabrina slid over, straddling his legs. "Yeah; but not before we have a chance to finish what you started." "That's a deal," he said, smiling widely.

Trying to sneak into the arena was next to impossible. Being out of the circuit for as long as they had, was reason enough to get stopped by everyone they encountered. The questions were redundant and annoying to Mark, who muttered and grumbled past each person. With the door of the dressing room locked and their privacy secured, he took his wife in his arms. Her sensual body pressed against his ignited his passion, and hers. They made love until their bodies could sustain no more.

Mark blindly groped through his tote bag. Retrieving his robe, he covered her with it. "One good thing about this show, is that it's not going to be very late," he said. "Why is that good?" "We'll be able to have some time together tonight. Maybe do something special." "You don't have to do anything for me. I'm quite content to just go back to the hotel." "You're my wife now; so get used to being spoiled and treated special." Snuggling closer to his warmth, she hooked her leg over his to secure her position.

If only I could keep him here with me tonight, it would make me feel much better, but he has to work, and I have to be supportive. Time will put an end to this conflict with Sean. I just wish I knew when. Living with this constant worry hasn't been easy for either of us. Mark hides his concerns from me so well, but I don't have that strength. The fear of losing him brings all my feelings to the surface. I may not be capable of making him stay with me, but maybe I can delay his leaving.

In a swift, elegant move she seated herself astride his legs, her lips pressed against his, burning with desire. He held her back. "Hey, what are you doing?" he asked. "What do you think?" "I think we don't have time for this." "Yes, we do," she said rubbing her body slowly against him. "Sabrina, I have a show to get ready for; and so do you. Why now?" "I just want to." Her eyes were pleading, begging him to concede. *I can see way beyond that look, to the true underlying concern.* He pulled her to him, pausing to look at the clock on the wall. *We have over an hour until the match, and if it will settle her nerves.* Lifting her face to his, he tenderly kissed her lips, his love for her taking control of his body.

Their moment of tenderness was shattered by a loud knock at the door. "Warlock, it's Nick. Let me in." Sabrina looked briefly at Mark; her eyes glossed over with a sudden rush of tears. Grabbing his robe, she fled to the seclusion of the bathroom. Nick repeated his command. Mark hesitated, torn between going to the door or going to her. Pulling on his jeans he headed for the door. *The quicker I get rid of Nick, the sooner I can comfort Sabrina.*

As soon as he heard the latch, Nick opened the door, sending Mark backwards, away from the approaching door. "You're not dressed! You've got an interview in twenty minutes," Nick said. "What? I know nothing about an interview." "I sent a memo with all the changes. Oh but you weren't home; were you?" The sarcasm in Nick's voice infuriated Mark. "No I wasn't and as for your interview it will have to wait until after the match." "Fine, but you better get your ass in gear." Nick began scanning the room. "Where is Sabrina?" "She's in the bathroom." "Is everything okay with you two?"

The bait is cast, but I'm not gonna bite. "Yeah, just great." "So where did you go on your trip?" Nick asked. Mark glared at Nick. *As if you didn't know.* "Hawaii." "Very nice, nice and romantic. Anything happen while you were away?" Nick asked. Mark caught the sly glance, as Nick looked at his hands; but Mark had already shoved them into his pockets, purposely hiding his wedding ring. "Not a thing happened, just a much needed rest."

I'm getting nowhere with these questions. I can't just come right out and ask him it wouldn't be proper. As for telling them about the in ring wedding, that can wait for now. "You better get ready for your match; we'll talk later. Say hi to Sabrina for me." "Sure." Mark closed and locked the door. *We need no more unexpected interruptions.*

His robe lay on the bathroom floor. Sabrina was in the shower. Stripping off his jeans, he joined her. She was as still as a statue, the water streaming over her body. He placed his hands on her shoulders; she didn't respond to his touch. Grasping her shoulders more firmly, he turned her around. Her beautiful blue eyes were cushioned amid pillows of red. Even through the water he could see the tears that spilled from her eyes. He drew her close. She resisted, ashamed by her behavior.

He held her firmly, yet gently, calming her tension with his silent reassurance. She looked up at him, attempting to speak; he hushed her with a kiss. "No need to apologize, when this show is over I'm gonna treat you to a very special evening." "But Mark." "No excuses, remember it's my job to take care of you; in every way, but right now we have a show to get ready for, okay?" "Okay."

They had just finished dressing when the knock came to the door, ten minutes until the match. He moved to her, preventing her from putting on her robe. "There is something I have to do first," he said as he began to pull his wedding ring off. "Please don't," she said holding his hand. "I don't want to, but I can't wear it in the ring. It's not permitted. I want you to take care of it for me." "It won't fit on any of my fingers." "That's why I got this."

Showing her the gold chain; he slipped the ring onto it and fastened it around her neck. On her, the chain hung low, hiding the ring between her breasts. "I couldn't think of a more perfect hiding place," he said. "Close to my heart."

The corridor was crowded with wrestlers and crew. Sabrina searched out Mark's hand, entwining her fingers into his. Through the shadow of her hood she searched among the crowd. Some faces she recognized, some she did not. *None of them are Sean, but that doesn't mean he's not here, concealed somewhere, watching us.* Her eyes scanned all potential hiding places.

Their journey ended at the entrance curtain. There was still a match going on in the ring, the fans yelling out the names of their favorite wrestler; individually urging them to win. Sabrina shuddered. *I still get nervous going out there, not at facing all those people, but the potential of an unexpected assault from Sean.*

Lost in her thoughts, she didn't notice that Mark was now standing before her, not until he pushed her hood back. He cupped his hand over her cheek. She nuzzled into it and he kissed her softly. "I love you, and you belong beside me, always," he said. There was no chance for her to answer the music began to play. Mark adjusted her hood. It muffled some of the noise, but not all. She could hear the fans screaming for the Warlock, and for the Sorceress.

The volume increased to a deafening thunder, as they stepped through the curtain. He kept the pace slow, nudging her sideways a little, so that fans could touch her briefly. She felt exhilarated, renewed by the acceptance. By the time they reached the ring she was back into full character, giving the fans the full seductive treatment. As much as Mark enjoyed her seductive performance, he had to end it. *Maybe I should let her rehearse at home, where I could fully enjoy it, and participate. That would make for a few really interesting evenings.*

While Sabrina patiently watched Mark's match, the ring side announcers tried relentlessly to get her to join them for an interview. She politely declined, keeping a vigilant watch for any sign of Sean. The match was over in less than ten minutes. Mark had been victorious, but she already knew that he would be even without the affirmation of a contract.

They both kept in character until they had cleared the curtain. She put her arm around him, stopping him, so she could kiss him. "Now I really have to treat you to a special night," Mark said. He caught sight of Nick coming towards them. "But first, I have an interview to do." He motioned to Nick to wait for him. "I don't know how long it's gonna take." "It's okay; I'm not going anywhere without you." He watched her head off to the dressing room before he followed Nick. Seeing her meet up with Brent made him feel a little better about sending her off alone.

Brent greeted her with a warm smile, and a reserved kiss on the cheek. She responded with a hug that took him off guard. They had no time for conversation as Brent was being summoned to the ring. The last minute changes to the schedule had upset his routine. He ignored it briefly, to take her part way to the dressing room. Her progress was again delayed, as D'arcy took her arm, slowing her pace to a moderate stroll.

Unlike some of the others, D'arcy was always a straight forward, to the point kind of guy. He always said what was on his mind even if he hadn't thought it through first. "So, I hear you two went to Hawaii. I know it wasn't business, so that means it was pleasure," he said with a sideways grin.

Sabrina felt a blush cover her body; she bit her lip and smiled. D'arcy grinned back at her, with his lip curved more to one side. His suspicions were confirmed by her silence. "So, on which island did you spend you honeymoon?" he asked. Her blush deepened. "I'm not really sure. Mark never did tell me." "Well, you must have seen something in town that gave you a clue." "No, we never went out anywhere."

Sabrina continued on to the dressing room, leaving D'arcy to fantasize over her last statement. *It won't take him long to figure it out.* She had just opened the door, when an unfamiliar voice froze her in place. "Excuse me, ma'am," a chauffeur addressed her. "I was instructed to deliver this to you." He handed her a single red rose and a note. Before she could question him, he had retreated back down the corridor, lost amongst the crowd.

Stepping into the room, she took a deep breath, inhaling the sweet perfume of the rose, opened the note and read quietly. "My love, there is a car waiting for you. Join me." A smile warmed her. Mark had begun to fulfill his promise. She left the note on the table and went to find the car. *I'm not going to worry about collecting our stuff; I imagine that he's all ready made arrangements to have it packed up.*

There was no trouble in finding the car, the chauffeur, that had delivered the message, was waiting beside the passenger door of a black car. He opened the door as she approached. She stepped inside, expecting to see Mark, but he was not there. Dozens of roses filled the car, petals strewn across the seat for her to sit on, and bouquets of red, white and pink roses filled every available space. The sight took her breath away. Her heart filled with love. She took her seat to await her husband.

The engine started. *Mark must be coming.* She heard the click, as the door locks were engaged. The forward momentum of the car was evident. She called to the driver to get him to explain what was going on. There was no response. She pushed frantically at the button, that should have opened the partition; it remained in place. Fear overtook her. *Mark would never do anything like this.* The windows were completely blackened and nothing of the outside world was visible to her. Fear instantly turned to panic.

The interview lasted far longer than Mark wanted. Delayed by camera problems that only frustrated him more. *I made a promise to Sabrina, and Nick is keeping me from fulfilling that promise.* As soon as Nick concluded his questioning, Mark left to find her, pushing his way through the crowded corridor to the dressing room.

The door was ajar. He called to her as he entered. Silence was his answer. *She must be with Brent.* He looked back down the hallway. *She'll be okay.* He went inside to change. His attention was diverted to the paper that lay on the table. Picking it up his gut tightened as he read. *Sean!* The dressing room door smashed against the wall, ricocheting back into the frame, as Mark went in search of Sabrina.

Everyone he encountered was asked the same question, had they seen her. His answers were all the same. No one had noticed her. All to consumed with their own petty, trivial duties. Fear crept through him. He pushed it away, letting anger replace it. That unnerved him more, he had not had such intense feelings of rage towards any human being, but knowing that Sean had done this, enraged him to the point that he thought he would explode.

He reached the main area of the backstage, his eyes scanning wildly, hoping, praying, that they were still in the building, that Sean did not have enough time to spirit her away. He tried calmly to gain the attention of those in the area. When his pleas for silence went unnoticed, his rage took over. Blindly, and with little regard for harm to others, he picked up a garbage can, hurling it into the crowd of workers. He followed it with several equipment cases. People scrambled away from the barrage.

Sabrina's fear kept her repeatedly trying the doors and windows to no avail. Her pleas to the driver continued to go unanswered. *In my gut I know that Sean is behind this, but my heart doesn't want to believe that he could do something so foul. Why would he do this? Where is he taking me?* She gasped for breath. *What is he planning to do with me? That question frightens me the most. If he's irrational enough to kidnap me, is he capable of harming me if I resist him?* She wanted to cry but couldn't. Her soul cried out for Mark.

Hearing the commotion, Brent and D'arcy arrived at the scene of Mark's destruction. They approached cautiously, dodging flying debris. D'arcy stepped in front of Mark, stopping him from picking up another case. "Christ Mark, what the hell is wrong with you?" D'arcy asked. "Have you seen Sabrina?" "Yeah, I saw her earlier. Isn't she in the dressing room?" "If she was, do you think I'd be looking for her? That son of a bitch took her!" "What do you mean? Who took her?" D'arcy asked. Mark handed him the note. Brent leaned in to read it while D'arcy held it. "That God damn son of a bitch Sean took her! He took my wife!"

The sudden silence of everyone around and the deep booming voice of Mark's carried his every word to all ears. Nick stepped forward. "If anyone has any information, please come forward and tell me what you know. You," he said motioning to his assistant. "Call the police. Tell them we have a kidnapping situation here." The assistant ran to the office to make the call. Nick turned back to Mark. "We'll find her, don't worry." "Don't tell me not to worry! That bastard took my wife, and God knows what he's planning! If he hurts her in any way, so help me I'll kill him!" "Calm down," D'arcy said, gripping Mark's shoulder. "They couldn't have gotten very far. The cops will find them."

Sabrina cowered in the corner of the back seat. Her body trembled. Her belly rolled over in turmoil, making her nauseous. *The car is traveling faster. I pray that Mark is following us, and soon Sean's plan will be foiled, and I'll be back in the arms of the man I love.* Hugging herself was little consolation. It did nothing to ease her fears or stop her thoughts.

Mark paced relentlessly, while the police took down all information offered by the crew. Listening to the statements, that contained nothing useful, frustrated him more. All they had been able to ascertain was that she got into the back of a black car, with darkened windows. No license plate number, nothing unique about the car that would aid them in finding it.

I feel so helpless; guilty for leaving her unprotected and vulnerable. I have to sort this through and try to come up with some idea as to where he would take her. It would have to be someplace private, someplace where no one would see them. Where?

The police have already checked the hotel where Sean was registered, but he's not there, he had checked out earlier in the afternoon. The search now concentrated on car rental agencies, in hopes of procuring a license plate number, and a better description of the vehicle. All this crap could take hours and Sean could be miles away by then. I can't stand this. I have to do something now before, before. Oh God! He wouldn't? He could! Oh God, Sabrina, please don't let it come to that.

In Mark's mind he conjured a vile vision of the possible outcome of this event. He choked back the vomit that was burning the back of his throat.

"Man, Sean has really done it this time," Brent spoke quietly to D'arcy. "That's for sure. The dumb bastard could go to jail. That is if Mark doesn't get a hold of him first." Brent agreed with D'arcy's statement. *Sean wouldn't stand a chance if Mark found him first.* "Where do you think he'd take her?" Brent asked. "I'm not sure; but he's got over an hour head start. The cops better come up with something soon, for Mark's sake, and Sabrina's."

Mark pushed his way past the detectives, and headed straight to Brent and D'arcy. "Have either of you guys got a car here?" "Yeah," they answered in unison. "Do they know where she is?" Brent asked, handing over the car keys. "No, but I can't sit around here anymore." "I'll go with you," Brent offered. "No! I don't need you with me!" Mark yelled and hurried off to the blue sedan. Brent looked at D'arcy. "Maybe he knows something." "I think you're right. We better follow him," D'arcy answered. Mark's instincts drove him to make this journey; completely unaware of the black truck that followed him.

The car slowed and came to a stop. The engine went quiet. Sabrina heard the driver's door open, then close. Footsteps, slow and measured, paced down the side of the car, around the back, stopping at the passenger side rear door. Her pulse quickened. Fear surged through her veins as the door opened. A hand reached into her. She slid away, striking at the menacing appendage. Sean leaned into the car. "Don't be afraid Sabrina," he said taking her hand. "Come with me." She tried to free herself, but he held fast, pulling her out of the car. Not wanting to anger him, she followed his instructions.

Putting his arm around her, he guided her through the darkness, into a building. Letting go of her only to lock the door behind them. *I want to run, but the darkness is holding me prisoner.* Sean moved past her to light a candle on the table.

Through the dim, golden glow, she scanned the area. Sean lit another candle and more of the room gave up its secrets. *I'm at the beach house!* Sean beckoned her to him. When she didn't move, he came to her. "My beautiful Sabrina, I'm so glad that you're here," he whispered as he kissed her. She lurched away. "Why Sean? Why have you done this?" "Why? You belong here; with me." His arms were around her, guiding her to the sofa. "Come, sit with me," he said calmly.

Sitting in the corner, Sabrina hugged the arm of the sofa. Sean was beside her, turned sideways, so he could look at her. Her eyes had grown accustom to the candlelight. She looked over at the patio door. *Would I be able to get out before he caught me?* She jumped, when Sean put his hand on her thigh.

"Don't bother to look for a way out. All the doors and windows have been shuttered. Only one door opens, and I have the only key." "Why are you keeping me a prisoner here?" "You're here because you belong here, and when you realize your mistakes, then we can get on with our life, together." "You're delusional! I have no life with you!" "You're wrong. Maybe you just need a little reminder," he said leaning over to her.

She tried to pull away, but he pulled her back, sliding her down onto the cushions. His body pressed against her. Struggling was useless as her hands were pinned. Sean leaned in closer; his lips were hot against hers. She resisted. He continued, kissing her harder as his hand moved to her breast. *My worst fears are coming to reality he wants to make love to me. I have to stop him.*

Mark cruised through the city alert to every vehicle that passed, staring at each driver, hoping to catch a glimpse of Sean. He stopped the car in an ocean side parking lot, staring out at the surf. Tears forced him to hide his face against the steering wheel. "Oh Sabrina, where are you?"

D'arcy had pulled his truck into the far end of the lot. Brent was on the cell phone to Nick. "Any news?" D'arcy asked. "No, they haven't located the rental agency yet." "They better do it soon, before Mark has a breakdown." "Nick says that we should stay with him, just in case he comes up with an idea as to where she might be."

Mark's head snapped up. "Sabrina?" he called, looking about the car. *I thought I heard you calling me.* But it was just the wind swirling about the car. "Damn it! Where are you?" He pounded his fist on the dash board. "Where did he take you?" The answer hit him square in the chest. *I've been staring at it all along. The beach house, that has to be it.* The tires squealed, as he sped out of the parking lot, heading to the coast highway.

D'arcy gunned the engine. The truck bumped over curbs as he tried to catch up to Mark. "Where the hell is he going in such a hurry?" D'arcy grumbled, trying to keep control of the truck. "Maybe he got a call that they found her." "I don't think so. He's headed away from the city," D'arcy said.

Brent stared at D'arcy. "What?" D'arcy barked, returning the glance only briefly. "I think I know where he's going," Brent said. "Well, don't keep it a damn secret." "I think he's headed to Sean's beach house." "Oh man, that's a real long shot." "Yeah, maybe it is; but Mark is headed in that direction." "Well, you better call Nick and tell him that we're running on a hunch. See if they can spare a couple of cops to meet us there; just in case your hunch is right."

D'arcy kept his distance behind Mark; only to lose him at a traffic light, but if Mark was headed to the beach house, it wouldn't matter if they were a few minutes behind. Even D'arcy was entertaining the idea of beating some sense into Sean; but if Mark did it first, so much the better.

Sabrina wiggled and squirmed, but could not free herself of Sean's weight. She gasped, desperately needing a full breath of air. Sean backed off, feeling her labored breathing. "I'm sorry I'm not being very considerate am I?" He helped her to sit up. "This isn't a very comfortable spot to get reacquainted; now is it?"

Standing up, he took her hands, urging her to get up. She stayed fast resisting his pull as best she could. "Sean, we need to talk." He pulled harder, jerking her out of her seat, into his arms. "We can talk later," he said, his voice had softened. "You must be tired. Come, I want to show you something."

With his arm cinched around her waist, he dragged her with him, toward the bedroom. Sabrina felt her muscles tighten. Her legs were stiff, as if she had no joints. *I want to cry out, but it would do no good. What is he planning? I don't want to think about the obvious answer.*

Sean opened the bedroom door, and directed her to the closet; he held the candle up. "I kept all your things for you. I knew you'd need them when you came back." All of the clothes, that he had bought, still hung neatly in the closet, just the way that she had left them. She felt sick. "I need to use the bathroom." "Sure, you know where it is," he said handing her a candle.

Mark drove faster, passing cars with every opportunity. He kept seeing Sabrina's face. Only it wasn't the soft beautiful face that he loved, but one of pain and torment. Torment caused by Sean. Rage boiled in his veins. *If Sean has touched her, in any way, I'll make him pay. One way or another, Sean will pay for what he's done.*

Brent closed up the cell phone. "Sean's phone has been disconnected," he said. "Then maybe we're on the wrong track." "Maybe; but it's still worth checking out. The cops haven't come up with any leads, and I don't have any other ideas. Do you?" "Hell no! Man if Sean is fucked up enough to do this, Christ I don't even want to think about the possibilities that he might be capable of. Damn it anyway!" "What?" "I sure hope you remember the way, because I haven't been able to catch up to Mark, and I've only been to Sean's in the daylight."

With the bathroom door locked, Sabrina had the time to clear her head. She went to the window. *It's big enough to crawl through, but the shutters are secured over it.* Her heart pounded. She laid her hand over it, trying to slow it down. Her fingers brushed against the chain on Mark's ring. She held it tight in her hand.

"Sabrina," Sean called. "You can't stay in there forever. Come on out. Don't force me to come and get you." She kissed Mark's ring before tucking it back into its hiding place. She closed her eyes. "Mark, please find me soon," she whispered.

Sean knocked again. "Sabrina, are you okay?" When she opened the door, Sean brought her into his arms. "You must be tired," he said guiding her to the bed. "You'll feel much better after a rest." He lifted her onto the bed, and lie down beside her. *I want to explain to him that this will never work, that I'll never come back to him, but my fear is keeping me silent. I don't want to make him angry.*

Sean's face loomed above her. "I need you, Sabrina. Mark had no right to take you from me. I know that it will take some time for that poison to get out of your system, but you will remember what we had together, and I'll do everything I can to help you remember." He leaned down, kissing her.

She was paralyzed, repulsed by his touch, but helpless to fight him off. His hand found her breast, releasing it from her gown. In her mind, she was screaming, but her voice was silenced by her fear. His kisses moved down her neck to her breast, his tongue teasing at her nipple. She tensed, when his hand came to rest on her leg. His fingers pushing her gown slowly upwards. A tear rolled from her eye. *Can Mark forgive me? Will he still want me?*

I know that I'm getting closer. I don't really recognize the area, but my senses are much stronger. I'm not sure if it's just my hopes, and determination that's keeping me going, or if I'm truly feeling her emotions; her fear and panic. I have to find her before that bastard does anything to her. The thought of Sean, or any man, touching her, making love to her, makes my stomach churn. Our love is strong, but is it strong enough to get us through this? It has to be. I would rather die than to go on with life without her.

Her voice whispered in his head. Mournful, airy cries, filled with despair that stabbed at his heart. Mark pressed his foot harder on the accelerator.

Sean can't see my tears; his body is controlled by his lust. He's lost himself in the pleasures of my body. I can feel his hand creeping slowly up my thigh. How can I stop this? How can I make him understand?

Her fists clutched at the bed sheets. The higher up her thigh his hand roamed, the harder she gripped. She gasped as he forced his hand between her thighs. *I must be dreaming. This has to be a horrible nightmare. At any moment I'll wake up, Mark will be beside me and this will be but a faint memory. Please let me wake up from this.*

The fantasy dissipated instantly, when Sean pulled down her thong and touched her. *His knee is trying to pry my legs apart, but my gown is too tight.* "Take off your dress," he whispered, into her ear. "No, wait a minute. Let me do it. It's been such a long time." Sabrina felt ill. *I don't know what to do.* "No, Sean, I can do it," she said, without thinking. *Maybe it will buy me some time. Mark will find me. He has to. I just have to stall Sean long enough until Mark gets here.*

Sliding herself slowly away from him she sat on the edge of the bed. Sean's T-shirt flew past her shoulder, landing on the floor, next to her feet. "Come on baby; I'm waiting," he said, the eager vibration in his voice more than evident. When she heard the zipper on his jeans, the sound sent ripples of terror up her spine. His hands were on her shoulders and she began to tremble.

"You're cold. I'll have you warmed up really quick, just as soon as you take off your dress," he whispered. Closing her eyes for a moment, she offered a silent plea. *Mark I love you, please forgive me, but if you can't I will understand.* Her dress fell to the floor. Sean's hands roamed over her body, before he pulled her down beside him. *It doesn't seem to bother him that I don't respond to his kiss. His own passions are too strong. I have to try to disconnect myself. Keep my eyes closed and see only Mark's face in my mind. How can I when my heart is breaking?*

Mark stopped the car outside the iron gates of Sean's house. He looked through the bars. *I see no car, no lights, no evidence that anyone is here, but my instincts tell me otherwise. She is here I'm sure of it. This dark, shuttered, bastion is her prison, and I have to set her free; and make Sean regret what he has done.*

He had nearly scaled the gate when headlights blinded him. D'arcy and Brent were at the gate in seconds. "Mark, what in the hell are you doing?" D'arcy called to him. "I'm going to get my wife away from that bastard!" "Wait for the cops," Brent called. "You guys can do that, but I'm not." "Look man, the house is dark and all closed up; they're probably not even here," D'arcy said, trying to reason with him. "She's here! I know she's here!" Mark's large frame landed firmly on the driveway. He glared back at his two friends. "I have to be sure." Mark turned and headed toward the house. D'arcy punched at the air. "Damn it. I'm going with him," he said and began climbing the gate. "God I hope he's wrong."

Sean's body pressed against her, his kisses becoming more intense, as his hand violated her body. *My time is running out. Soon I'll feel the full weight of his body, as he forces his love on to me. Only this isn't love; this is rape. I have to stay subdued and compliant, not because I want this to be happening, but because I'm truly afraid. Afraid of what he might do if I resist, or fight him.* Tears rolled endlessly from her eyes, soaking her hair and the pillow.

His body had pinned one of her arms and it tingled from numbness. With the other, she clenched the sheets, squeezing harder and harder. Sean reached for his jeans; fumbling through the pockets until he found the small plastic package. *I recognize that rustling sound. A condom, thank God.* Her sigh of relief dissipated in a gasp as he eased himself onto her, pushing her legs apart. Her body tensed. She tried to wiggle away, but his weight held her in place.

D'arcy followed Mark, as he vigilantly checked every door and window within reach; only to find every access locked and barred. Completing the perimeter of the house brought them back to the garage door. Mark stopped, looking up at the upstairs window. "What is it?" D'arcy asked. "I've got to get in there now! She needs me." "Man, there is no one here. Can't you see that?" "She's here! I know she is, and if you're not gonna help me find a way in, then just get the hell out of my way!" Mark went on, rechecking doors and windows, hoping to find one that would easily give him access. D'arcy followed; his own conscience hoping that they wouldn't get caught breaking in.

Stumbling in the darkness, D'arcy looked down to see what had tripped him; he grinned. "Hey Mark, come over here." "What is it?" "Do you think this would work?" He pointed to the unshuttered basement window; set deep in a well against the house. "Perfect."

Mark stepped into the well, trying the window before he kicked it in. The glass shattered into a shower of tiny pieces. Mark kicked at all the shards still clinging to the frame. D'arcy took off his jacket. "Here, put this over the sill, so you don't get cut." Taking the jacket, Mark laid it over the broken frame. He lowered himself through the window. D'arcy was close behind him. Just before he dropped to the floor, he saw the police car pull up beside his truck. "Mark, the cops are here." "So what? That bastard's mine first."

Sean hesitated for a second. *I thought I heard something. It's just the wind.* His passion was growing stronger he couldn't stop now even if he wanted to. Sabrina thought she heard a noise, faint and far away. *Please let it be Mark. Let him find me before it's too late, but it is too late, Sean's inside me, his hips heaving slowly, thrusting himself deeper.*

Sabrina tensed with the pain, her body was not ready for him, nor did she want him. *He must know that I don't want him yet still he forces himself into me, his deranged lust compelling him to rape me.*

The pain was indescribably intense and she wished that there was some way that she could disconnect herself from it, but as long as her body was experiencing this anguish her mind would not shut down.

Mark and D'arcy had groped their way up the basement stairs. The lone candle flickering in the living room made D'arcy's stomach turn over. *They are here.* Mark headed for the bedroom and D'arcy grabbed his arm. "Let the cops finish this search." "Screw you!" Mark snapped. D'arcy let him go on. *He's not going to like what he finds, but Sean deserves to have his ass kicked.* Unable to open the front door, D'arcy went out through the garage, and ran to the gate to let in the police.

With each step, Mark's heart vibrated in his ears. Rage, fueled by adrenaline, pumped through his veins. He hesitated outside the bedroom door, praying that his fears were all in vain. Taking in a deep breath he pushed the door open slowly. In the dim light he caught sight of Sean, on the bed, his body moving rapidly. Beneath him lay Sabrina.

Emotions seethed in his gut. He took a run towards the bed; grabbing Sean by the shoulders, he tossed him across the floor like a rag doll. Before Sean had full command of what had happened, Mark was on him, his fists striking wildly at Sean's face and chest. The taste of blood filled his mouth. Sean was defenseless against the attack. Mark had him pinned.

Two police officers burst into the room. Their attempts to pull Mark away were useless; he tossed them aside with little effort. Seeing the situation, D'arcy and Brent took control. Mark's strength was formidable, but between the two of them they managed to pull Mark back; using their combined weight of nearly five hundred pounds to keep him in place.

Mark turned his attention back to the bed, to Sabrina; her nude body huddled into a ball. He struggled to free himself of Brent and D'arcy. They held fast, fearing that he would go after Sean again. "Let me go!" Mark demanded. "Let me go to her!" They backed off. Mark scrambled to his feet, cautiously approaching Sabrina. She cringed and whimpered when he touched her shoulder.

"See!" Sean yelled. "She doesn't want you! She belongs with me!" "Would you get this son of a bitch out of here!" D'arcy commanded the officers. Brent stopped them at the doorway. "You're damn lucky that the cops are taking you away. Personally, I'd just as soon see Mark beat you to death for what you've done." "What I've done," Sean scoffed. "All I did was get back the woman that belongs with me. If anyone has done anything wrong it's Mark, and you two, breaking into my house, assaulting me."

"You still don't get it do you? You're the only one going to jail." "Yeah, for what?" "Oh, let's see; kidnapping, unlawful confinement, rape." "Bull shit!" "What else would you call it; taking another man's wife and then forcing yourself on her? I'm sick of talking to you; take him out of here." Brent turned his back on his once friend. *I can tell by the look on Sean's face, that the poor dumb bastard still hasn't got it through his thick skull.*

D'arcy stepped back to Brent, nodding to him to step into the hallway. "How is she?" Brent asked. "I'm not sure; she's in shock." "Do you think Sean, you know." "I don't want to think about it; but my guess is he did." "Son of a bitch," Brent muttered. Taking a swing at the air, he nearly hit the officer coming down the hallway. "Sorry." "It's okay," the officer said. "This is a volatile situation all around. I have an ambulance on the way for her; but I'm gonna need a statement from her first." "Lots of luck," D'arcy muttered.

Mark had wrapped a blanket around Sabrina, taking her gently into his arms. He rocked her slowly, quietly talking to her. Her senses had temporarily shut down, numbing her to the torment Sean had been putting her through. In her mind, Mark's voice called her name. She thought it only an illusion. The voice grew louder. She opened her eyes slowly, afraid that she would see Sean. A hand lifted her face upwards. Through the blur of her tears she thought she saw Mark. *Is my mind playing a cruel trick?* He spoke again, softly. Her heart broke through the veil of doubt. *It is Mark; he has come for me.*

She threw herself against him; tears poured from her eyes; her body began to shake. "It's okay I got you. It's all over," he spoke softly. The officer approached. "Excuse me, but I have to get a statement." "Not now!" Mark snapped. "My wife is upset enough; your statement can wait." "I'm sorry sir, but it can't wait. I need her to tell me what happened, while it's still fresh; and before the ambulance gets here." "I'm gonna say this one last time your damn statement can wait!" Mark's tone had become stern.

Sabrina loosened her hold on Mark. "It's okay Mark," she struggled with every word. "It has to be done." She never relinquished her hold on Mark, as the officer took her statement of the events. Mark tensed when the officer asked her if intercourse had occurred. His body shuddered when she answered. *Our love is being tested, and I pray that it is solid enough to get us through this.*

The officer closed up his note book. "Now all we need is a Doctor's report to confirm your statement." "Why?" Mark asked. "You can see for yourself her condition, and you have your statement." "Yes sir, but without a Doctor's report, confirming the rape, her statement won't hold up in court." Sabrina tightened her arms around Mark. "Don't leave me," she whimpered. "I won't; ever." The officer motioned to the paramedics, who wheeled a stretcher over to the bed. "Take that away," Mark commanded. He lifted her into his arms, carrying her past the paramedics, out to the waiting ambulance.

Brent and D'arcy followed, questioning the officer, as to where they would be taking her. Brent opted to drive the car to the hospital. They would need a ride back to the hotel. D'arcy got on the phone to Nick; relating the news made him feel sick to his stomach. He kept the story vague. Nick would have to find out the details from someone else.

The paramedics made several attempts to get Mark to put Sabrina on the stretcher; each time their request was met with a stern "Go to hell." He held her, all the way to the hospital. *She needs my comfort as much as I need to hold her.* Carrying her through the emergency room, into an examination room; he kicked a stool over beside her and sat down, holding her hand to his heart and gently stroking her forehead.

"You, out of here," the Doctor announced his entrance. "No way," Mark replied. "I'm sorry, but it's best that you leave." "Please," Sabrina struggled to speak. "I need him here; he's my husband. Please let him stay with me." "Fine; but keep your eyes on her, not on what I'm doing, and do not interrupt me; no matter how uncomfortable she may appear." "Fine. Just get on with it, so I can take her home." Mark locked his eyes onto hers, tears trickled from them and he brushed them away.

The Doctor began his examination, dictating his findings to the nurse, who stood beside him. His descriptions were detailed and graphic. Mark felt sick; but his heart ached every time Sabrina winced from the pain. During the course of his examination the Doctor asked the nurse for an evidence kit.

Through the fog that clouded her mind, Sabrina heard him say that he had found semen. Finding her voice Sabrina stammered over her words. "What you found, that's not, it belongs to my husband." "You had sex prior to your attack?" "Yes." "We'll have to take a blood sample to compare the DNA." "Fine," Mark replied.

Sabrina continued to struggle with her words. She looked up at Mark desperately needing his strength at that moment but she didn't find that in his eyes this time. What she saw made her look away. "Sean, he, he used a condom," she stammered.

The Doctor finished his examination and his verdict was clear; she had been raped. The severe bruises alone, were enough to convince him. Mark found some comfort when the Doctor confirmed that Sean had used a condom. The Doctor motioned to Mark. He wanted to speak to him, away from Sabrina. Mark kissed her hand and laid it down beside her. Pulling the sheet around her, she turned on her side, drawing her knees up, making herself into a small ball. Her eyes were open, but she saw nothing.

Closing up the chart that he had, the Doctor let out a heavy sigh. "You heard my report?" "Yeah." "She's going to be very uncomfortable for a while, but that will heal. What concerns me more is her emotional health." "What do you mean?" Mark asked. "I can't tell you how she's going to cope with this trauma, every woman is different; but I suggest that you encourage her to seek help from a rape councilor. She has to talk about it, and therapy will help her to get through the court ordeal." "Court!" "Yes, she will have to go to court if she wants to see her attacker punished. The only thing that would keep her from that, would be a full confession from the guy who did this."

Mark's mind raced out of control. *If I could have five minutes alone with Sean, I could get the confession. I would do anything to spare her from having to relive this in front of total strangers.*

The Doctor's voice snapped him out of his fantasy. "You can take her home anytime; but you need to be supportive. Don't reject her when she needs you, but don't smother her either. If she wants to be alone, give her that time, but not too much, but most of all try and get her to talk, it will help you both to heal faster." "What about the tests?" "They'll take about a week, but as I said before the evidence speaks for itself."

As the Doctor left the room, Mark caught sight of Brent pacing in the hallway. He slipped out the door. "How is she?" Brent asked. Mark's anger surfaced quickly. "How the hell do you think she is! That son of a bitch!" He choked on his words. "He raped her!" "Christ Mark, I'm so sorry." Mark's anger seethed to the surface. He punched the wall. "When I get my hands on him, I'm gonna put him through the same hell, if I don't kill him first!"

The nurse stepped out of the exam room. "Would you please keep it down," she said quietly, but sternly. "She's been through enough, and hearing things like that, from you, isn't going to help. Now if you have her clothes, I'll get her ready to go while you calm down." "Here," Brent spoke up. "I brought in one of my track suits." He handed it to the nurse who took it back into the room.

Brent put his hand on Mark's shoulder. "I know that you're angry, but you can't show it in front of Sabrina. It's gonna be hard, but for right now, you're gonna have to put Sean out of your mind, and devote your every thought to her." "You're right. It's gonna be real hard, because every time I look at her it's gonna remind me of what that bastard did to her." "You still love her don't you?" "Of course I do! I will always love her!" "Then let that love be stronger than your anger. She needs to know that you still love her." The nurse opened the door. "She's ready to go."

Mark had to take a deep breath, to cleanse himself of the rage within him. Sabrina was still laying on the bed her expression blank and distant. He touched her shoulder lightly. "Come on baby let's go home," he said calmly. She remained motionless. He slipped his hand under her, lifting her up. Her body was limp. It was like lifting a doll. A hint of pain rippled across her face as he sat her up. To relieve her discomfort he quickly lifted her into his arms. Her face calmed and her head tilted against his shoulder.

Brent suppressed a gasp as Mark walked through the doorway. The color had drained from Sabrina's face. Her blue eyes stared right through him. He had to turn away. Sabrina was coherent enough to settle herself into the back seat of the car. Lying down was the easiest, which she did before Mark could get in and claim part of the seat. It bothered him that she didn't want him near her, but he kept it to himself. *She's probably more comfortable this way.*

Brent gripped the steering wheel with force. His knuckles turned white; envisioning his own hands around Sean's throat, squeezing tighter and tighter. *Why would he do that to her? Why?* The drive was long, filled with a tedious silence.

Sean had been taken back to the Los Angeles Police department. Nick was waiting for him. After being finger printed and photographed he was allowed to see Nick. "You've come to get me out of this hell hole?" Sean asked, taking a seat across from Nick. "I can't. The lawyer won't be here until tomorrow morning." "So use your influence." "I can't Sean."

Nick began pacing. "Do you realize just how much trouble you're in?" "Trouble? How can being with the woman I care about be trouble? Let me talk to Sabrina, she'll clear this up; unless Mark has fed her another line of crap." "Sean they have talked to Sabrina." "So everything has been straightened out then?"

"Sean would you just listen for once! This isn't going to go away because you wish it. These charges are serious." "What charges?" Sean asked, still confused by this whole situation. "Christ, you've been charged with rape, as well as kidnapping." "That's bull shit! That's Mark saying that." "No, it isn't. Sabrina has given a statement; and from what I've heard; the Doctor's report confirms her statement."

An officer interrupted their conversation. "Your time is up," he said. Nick stared at Sean. "You had better let this discussion sink in, and figure out what you're going to do, because I don't know if I can get you out of this one. Pray for a miracle, or get used to looking at the world through steel bars."

Mark carried Sabrina up to their hotel room. Brent lead the way, operating the elevator, and opening the doors. He hung around while Mark settled her in the bedroom. Mark laid her on the bed, making sure that she was on her side. Finding one of his T-shirts, he sat beside her. "I'll help you change," he said reaching for the zipper on her top. She pushed his hand away, folding her arms over her chest. "Okay," he said calmly. Not being able to help her or comfort her was tearing him apart. "I'll be in the next room if you need me."

Oh Mark I do need you but I can't. I saw that look in your eyes at the hospital, that look of disgust. I know you're trying to help me but I really don't believe you want to be here, with me. I don't want to be alone.

She tried desperately to wipe away her tears but it was a redundant effort. *I know you're hurting and so am I. We've been through so much but this isn't going to be easy. I need you but if you can't get over this then I'll understand.* Laying back on the bed her mind tried to envision a life without Mark.

"I need a drink," Mark said to Brent, as he closed the bedroom door. "I don't blame you; but the bar is empty. I'll order from room service. What do you want?" "I don't care. Beer, I guess and lots of it. Tell them they have five minutes to get it here." He fell onto the sofa, while Brent made the call; feeling restless, and to some degree helpless.

She had clung to me at first, but now she distanced herself from me, rejecting my comfort, my strength. I want to be with her. I want to take away her pain, to help her through this but if she keeps pushing me away I don't know what I'll do.

Unlacing his boots, he kicked them across the room. It offered little relief for his anger. He paced the length of the room. Brent stayed quiet, watching his friend suffer. *There is little that I can do, other than just be here if Mark wants to talk.* Mark tugged at the neck of his Lycra top. He had worn it many times before, but tonight it strangled him. "I'm gonna check on her, and change my clothes," he said. "Sure; I'll find out what's keeping room service."

Mark was quiet, as he entered the bedroom. The lights were still on. Sabrina was in bed, on her side, facing the wall. Her slow shallow breaths indicated to him that she was asleep. *I want desperately to lie down beside her, to hold her; but I'm still too keyed up to relax enough to sleep, and she needs the rest more than I do.* Stripping off the confining costume, he pulled on a robe. Picking up the track suit that she had discarded, he left the room.

Mark could easily read the question on Brent's face. "She's asleep," he said. "That's good. Isn't it?" "I guess so." "Here," he tossed him a beer. "It may not be the answer, but it'll help you to relax." "Damn it; this wouldn't have happened if I hadn't left her alone." "Mark you are not responsible for this, and you shouldn't even entertain a thought like that." "I promised her that I would always keep her safe." "You have. Look, we all thought that Sean had left. There was no way that you could have predicted his return." "Yeah, but I let my guard down, and she paid the price for it!" He hurled the empty can across the room.

"When I get my hands on him, he's gonna wish that he'd never been born!" "Mark there's nothing more that you can do, it's in the hands of the law, and justice will prevail. You have to believe that." Brent place his hand firmly on Mark's shoulder. "All you need to concern yourself with is Sabrina, being there for her, letting your love help her to recover, and on that note I will leave you. She shouldn't be alone."

"Thanks man, I appreciate everything you've done." "I'll call you in the morning, to see if you're gonna make the flight." "That's all gonna depend on her." "Sure enough, but I don't think Nick would mind if you took some time off, given the circumstances." "We'll see. Knowing Nick, he's probably counting on us to continue the tour." "This is different. Don't let him get to you. If she's not ready, then take the time off and to hell with Nick."

Mark closed the door, leaning against the wall for a moment. He headed for the bedroom, his hand hesitating on the handle. His mind flashed onto the image of Sean on top of Sabrina, forcing himself on her. His stomach turned over. He barely made it to the sink at the bar. Tears clouded his eyes, as his stomach convulsed. The full realization of what had happened was setting in. *I have to push it away, for Sabrina's sake.* The cold water he splashed on his face calmed him but it didn't wash away the vision in his mind.

Sabrina was so still; her body curled up into a ball. *She looks so small and frail, like a child in need of comfort.* Turning out the light, he slipped quietly into bed beside her. His motions were slow; so as to not disturb her. Moving closer to her, the soft fabric of the T-shirt rubbed against him. He positioned one arm above her on the pillow, and with great care he laid his other arm over her, letting it rest on the mattress. Closing his eyes, he prayed for sleep; peaceful dreamless sleep.

Sabrina's level of consciousness began to rise. Her mind becoming aware of the body behind her, and of the arm that held her in place. Her fear surfaced, turning to panic. She now found the courage that had failed her before. She cried out, pushing away her restraints, scrambling out of bed. Her feet became tangled in the sheets and she fell to the floor with a thud. Kicking and struggling, she freed herself, crawling into the corner.

Alarmed by her sudden behavior, Mark slid over to her, kneeling in front of her. Calling to her, he tried to touch her. She fought him, her arms flailing wildly, slapping his hands away. "No! No more, please!" she cried. Mark grabbed her arms, holding them down. "Sabrina! Look at me. It's me, Mark."

Something familiar about the voice registered in her mind. She stopped struggling, staring at the face in the darkness. "Mark?" "Yes, baby, it's me." He released her arms and she fell into him, sending him backwards against the bed. Her cries were heavy, filled with such sadness. He held her tight. "It's okay, I got you; and I'll never let you go." He let her cry. She had to. It was the first step in the healing process. Her tears trickled down his neck to his chest, soaking her T-shirt.

After an hour, she began to tremble, her tears had subsided. Only intermittent gasps still haunted her. He rubbed his hand down her arm. "You're cold. Get into bed and get warm. I'll get you a clean T-shirt." "No!" she yelled, grabbing his arm. "Don't leave me!" "Your shirt is wet." "I don't care. I don't need another." She pulled it off, tossing it across the room. "I just need you. I need to feel you beside me but only if it's what you want." "I'll always be with you; I love you." He let her settle herself, in bed, beside him, before he encircled her with his arms, keeping her safe; protecting her from her dreams.

Mark had slept very little, aware of every twitch of Sabrina's body. Now and then she would whimper. He would tighten his hold until she quieted down. He had begun to doze again when the phone rang. Cursing the interruption, he reached for it, trying not to disturb her. "Hello." "Oh sorry Mark, it's Brent." "This isn't a good time." "Still asleep is she?" "Yeah." "I'll call later, or better yet, you call me when it's more convenient." "Fine; good-by."

As he hung up the phone, Sabrina moved beside him. *Damn, the phone must have woke her.* "I'm sorry the phone woke you." "It didn't. I've been awake for a while; I just didn't want to disturb you." "How do you feel?" "I don't know," she said rolling away from him. "It's not that I don't feel anything I just can't put it into words yet." Covering her face with her hands, she hid the sudden rush of tears. Mark saw the glistening trail that crept out from under them. "What's wrong?" he asked.

"I'm afraid." "You don't need to be; it's over, Sean's in jail." "It's not that. It's," she stumbled over her words. "It's what?" "I'm afraid of what this will do to us." Mark pulled her hands away from her face. "Nothing is going to happen to us. You are my wife and I love you, no matter what."

"How can you say that! I've put you through so much, with the baby, and before. I was raped! I wouldn't blame you one bit if you never wanted to touch me again." Her tears flowed in rivers; forcing her to turn away from him.

Mark pulled her back, leaning in close. "I love you, and I will never abandon you. We will get through this, together, one day at a time, just like before. I know that it will take time for you to recover from this, and until you are ready to accept my expression of physical love, I promise to give you all the emotional love and support that you can handle."

Her lip quivered. "Kiss me," she asked, almost begging. He leaned closer, kissing her cheek. "No. Not like that," she whispered guiding his face in front of hers. Their lips met, tenderly, with warmth and passion. She felt his love wash over her, filling her with strength.

Snuggling against him, holding his arms close to her; she looked at his watch. "What time is the flight?" she asked. "It's not important." "Yes, it is. You have a show tonight." "I'm gonna cancel it, along with a few others." "You can't do that." "Yes, I can. I want to take you home. You shouldn't be around that mess right now." Overcoming her physical discomfort, she sat up. "I don't want to go home Mark. You have to work. You need to work right now, and I need to be with you." "I don't agree; you shouldn't continue this tour."

"I have to Mark. I need to be busy, and so do you. If I'm busy I won't think as much. I just want to forget. So please, don't cancel the tour." "I still don't agree, but if that's what you want. I have a couple of stipulations though. One, there will be no going to the ring. Two, the first sign of stress and the tour is over and we go home." "I can live with that."

She ran her hands through her hair. "I need a shower. I can still." "Still what?" he asked. "Nothing." *I can't tell him that Sean's scent still lingers on my body.* "Will you join me?" she asked almost afraid to hear his answer. "You know I will. Just let me call Brent and tell him that we'll share a ride to the airport."

She inched her way to the edge of the bed. Mark covered her shoulders with a bath robe. "Would you like me to help you to the bathroom?" "No, I can manage." He watched her walk away. Each step that she took was done with deliberate caution. *She's trying to hide her pain from me, but her labored gait cuts through her facade. That bastard really hurt her. God it makes me sick knowing what he did and knowing that I can't help her.*

When Brent didn't answer the phone Mark figured that he must have gone to the gym. He left a message for him to stop by their room, before they had to leave for the airport. He lay back against the bed. *I should have been more firm with her, insisted that we go home, instead of giving in to her, but at least she agreed to end the tour if she couldn't handle it. Enough what ifs.* He headed to the bathroom.

Sabrina was already in the shower. He stepped silently in behind her. She stood under the full rush of water with her arms braced against the wall and her head lowered. *She's crying again.* Reaching out to her, he stopped, calling her name instead. She turned quickly, lunging herself against him. He gently rubbed her back. "Hey, what's wrong?" "I was afraid that you weren't coming; that you didn't want to be with me." "Don't ever think that," he said hugging her.

Her wet body pressed against him. As he held her, it became very evident that his own body showed no signs of desire. *In my heart, I know that I love her, without question, but my body isn't experiencing the usual surges that it did whenever I held her. I just need some time. When she's ready, I will be too.*

"Shall I wash your hair for you?" Mark asked. "That would be nice." She turned around. He poured the shampoo onto her hair, working it through to a thick lather. The soap ran down across her chest. The slippery froth trickled over her breasts.

I so want to touch them, to caress them, to bring back the feeling to my body, but I can't, shouldn't, force myself on her in any manner. I will wait for her to make the first move. I don't care how long it takes I will wait and when we've both healed, our love will again take control.

Sean's patience had begun to wear horribly thin. Spending a sleepless night in a jail cell with a drunken derelict for a companion was the capping of his frustration. *I'm so damn mad at Nick for leaving me in here. He could have hired a local lawyer, instead of waiting for one employed by the company. I still don't fully comprehend why I'm even in here.* His conscience did not bring forth any guilt or remorse.

Maybe it was my altercation that landed me behind bars? Then why wasn't Mark locked up? The guard approached. "Your lawyer is here to see you," he said. "About damn time. I've had enough of this place." "I wouldn't plan on saying good-by just yet," the guard smirked. "What is that supposed to mean?" "Let your lawyer explain it." Despite Sean's nagging questions, the guard remained silent, as he escorted him to an interview room. The silence began to unnerve Sean. *Does the guard know something? Is there more to this than I've realized?* His heart began to beat faster.

When Brent arrived, Sabrina was laying on the sofa. "She's still sleeping?" Brent asked quietly. "No, I'm not," she answered, sliding up against the arm rest. Brent turned back to Mark. "I got your message. So what's up? Are you going home?" "No, we're continuing with the tour," Mark answered. "What?" "Talk to Sabrina. I have to finish packing." Brent was dumb founded. Mark retreated to the bedroom.

Sabrina stretched her hand out to Brent, beckoning him to her. "I don't believe what I just heard," Brent said taking a seat on the edge of the coffee table. "You shouldn't be going on tour. You should distance yourself from that zoo, at least for a little while."

Sabrina took his hand. "I need to be there. Mark needs to work, and I need to be with him. I don't want to be left alone with only my thoughts for company." "Not my place to argue with you; but I can guarantee that you won't be left alone. If Mark can't be with you, then you can count on me to look after you," Brent said.

She smiled, squeezing his hand tenderly. "You're truly a wonderful friend." "Always." Even though he had not completed his sentence, Sabrina knew the thoughts that tormented his mind. She knew about the secret desires that lived in his heart.

Brent withdrew his hand as Mark returned, carrying their suitcases. "Ready when you are," he announced. Sabrina began to slowly sit up. "No, you don't," Mark said, his hand was on her shoulder stopping her.

He quickly scooped her up into his arms. "I can walk you know." "Yes, but not very well, it's enough that you're gonna have to sit for a long time on the plane, and I'm gonna keep you comfortable for as long as possible," he said, giving her that don't argue look. She nuzzled her face into the hollow of his neck. He felt her warm breath against his skin. "I love you," she whispered.

Hot; her breath was hot enough to re-light the fire of desire within him. A feeling of elation washed over him, grateful that their physical bond was still alive. *I'll still have to play it very low key; I will not rush her into anything. Right now she's having a good moment, but that could change, and I will not risk her well being for anything.*

Mark wanted her to have the back seat of the car to herself, but she insistently tugged at him until he joined her. With her legs stretched out, she reclined back into his arms, only because it was more comfortable for her.

The lawyer made several attempts to make Sean understand the seriousness of his charges, but each time Sean cut him off, rambling on about anything but the topic in question. Tired, and annoyed, the lawyer threw his papers into his briefcase, preparing himself to leave. The door opened, and Nick walked into the room.

"How is it going?" Nick asked. "Nowhere! I can't help him when he doesn't want my help." "For Christ's sake!" Nick exploded. "Sean, sit down!" "Why? So I can listen to more lies." "Damn it Sean, sit down and shut the hell up! You're going to listen to everything we have to say, and it damn well better sink in!"

Sean hadn't seen Nick this worked up in a long time. He took a seat at the table. "Okay," Nick began with a sigh. "Now first of all, we need to understand what charges the police have filed." "Charges?" Sean asked. "I told you to keep quiet!" Getting his point across, Nick turned back to the lawyer. "Please continue." "Well, it's a mess to say the least. Mr. Malloy has been charged with kidnapping, unlawful confinement and rape." "Bull shit!" Sean yelled, his fist hitting the table. "For the last time, shut up!" Nick yelled.

The lawyer continued on. "So far the evidence that has been collected is enough to get a conviction. They may never need Mrs. Cassidy to testify." "So what is the worst possible scenario?" "In my opinion, he could get as little as fifteen or the maximum of twenty-five, with maybe the possibility of parole after ten years. This is his first offense."

Nick rubbed the back of his neck, the tension knotting up his muscles. "Is there any other options?" Nick asked. "Maybe. We could always try the psychiatric route and from what I've seen so far it could very well be the only logical answer, but it will all depend on how forgiving the District Attorney is."

"Can I speak now?" Sean interrupted. "Go ahead." "This is nothing but pure bull shit. If I could talk to Sabrina, she'd clear this all up. My fight with Mark was just that, a fight, and who is this Mrs. Cassidy anyway?" "It's Sabrina you fool! You abducted and raped Mark's wife!" "That can't be. She would never marry that overgrown gorilla."

Nick lost his tolerance, striking Sean. "They are married; and if you want us to help you, then you had better come to terms with what you've done!" The guard opened the door. "Your time's up," he said, taking Sean's arm he guided him out the door.

Nick stared at the lawyer. "See what you can do with the psychiatric angle." "I think it's going to be his only defense right now. He's in complete denial of his actions; and I'm sorry to say quite delusional in regard to Mrs. Cassidy." "Do whatever it takes to keep him out of jail; and for God's sake keep it out of the papers."

A story like this, could be damaging to the company, as well as to Sean's career; I don't want to see one of my stars destroyed by an ordeal like this, but mainly I don't want to deal with the press. The company has never experienced a public indiscretion, thanks to me. There have been problems before, but I've always managed to keep it silenced.

If the public knew about the foolish antics of some of the stars, it could very well destroy the organization. Keeping the family problem's quiet was what I paid the lawyers and the PR people for, and the wrestlers know better than to speak about these things outside of the organization. This, this is far more serious than anything I've encountered. It will take a lot to keep this quiet.

As Mark had requested, Sabrina had stayed away from the ring during the first few days of the tour, but she was being deliberately avoided. The guys would see her, but none of them engaged her in a conversation, or even a cordial greeting. *I can sense their awkwardness, even from Brent, even after he made a promise to me. Sean is their friend too; and I understand that; but this has to end.*

While she waited in the dressing room for Mark, she wrote out three notes, one each to Brent, D'arcy and Tony. The message was simple and direct. "Please come to Room #265, at ten, Regards, Sabrina." Positioning herself outside the dressing room door, she delivered each note silently as its recipients walked down the corridor. Brent stopped to read his, he looked up to question her, but she had already retreated into the dressing room.

When Brent entered his dressing room, he caught sight of Tony and D'arcy, each reading a note. "You guys got one too, eh," he remarked, waiving his about. "Yeah," D'arcy answered. "Any idea what's going on?" "Not a clue; but it would be rude not to go; and personally, I'm a little curious."

When Mark returned, Sabrina had already laid out his clothes, and had packed his extra gear into the bag. "Looks like you're in a hurry to leave. How come?" "Please don't be upset with me, but I invited the guys up to our hotel room." "I'm not upset with that, but what's the occasion?" "They have all been avoiding me, us, since, since the incident, and it's time it came to an end." "Are you sure you're ready to face them all at once?" Mark asked. "No, but I'm afraid we might lose our friends if I don't."

He laid his hands upon her shoulders. "I'm pleased that you're moving forward. Making changes like this will only help you to be stronger. Just don't push yourself to hard or to fast." "This is just the first step; there are other things I need to change tonight as well. Now please hurry up and get dressed."

She let him have his privacy while he changed. Over the past few days she had deliberately avoided being in the same room while either of them changed their clothes. *I wonder what else she has on her mind? Her expression offered no clue, and I shouldn't push. When she's ready she will tell me.*

Before Mark's return, Sabrina had called the hotel and requested that a snack tray and beer be sent to their room. Insisting that it be delivered before they returned. Sitting close to Mark, in the limo, she sighed softly.

We haven't been intimate, not even a kiss since that first night. The only physical contact we have had was the odd time, like tonight, when he would touch my shoulder, or like this, when I could sit close to him. I desperately need him; we've been apart for too long. Why hadn't he even tried to initiate anything? Is he repulsed by me, or just being considerate of my physical and emotional feelings? I have to find out. I need to know if we still have a future together.

The hotel room was setup as per her instructions. A tray of cheese and crackers adorned the table, and the fridge chilled the beer. "I'm gonna change," she said, picking up her bag. "Do you think that's a good idea?" "I'm not comfortable in these jeans." "What about our guests?" "This isn't going to be an all night party. What I have to say is going to be short and sweet, and then I'm going to bed." Mark didn't get a chance to analyze her sudden mood change, as the knock on the door changed his mind for him.

The trio arrived together; Mark showed them in. His offer of beer was eagerly accepted by all. "Where is Sabrina?" Brent asked. "Changing her clothes," Mark answered, pointing to the bedroom. "Why are we here?" D'arcy interjected. "I have no idea. All she told me was that she had to talk to you guys." The group talked amongst themselves, discussing their matches from tonight's show, and the remainder of the tour.

Sabrina appeared at the bedroom door. She adjusted her blue satin robe, tightening the belt. Silent stares guided her into the group. "I'm glad you could all make it, if you would please take a seat." She helped herself to a couple of crackers, while the trio followed her instructions. Mark came to her side. "Where do you want me?" Mark asked. "Doesn't matter, this part doesn't concern you," she said turning away from him. He felt rejected, scolded. She had hurt his feelings, whether she realized it or not. He returned to the bar, helping himself to another beer.

Sabrina sat on the coffee table in front of her guests. "Gentlemen, I will keep this brief and direct." She had their attention, but eye contact was being deliberately avoided. "I would appreciate it if you would at least have the courtesy to look at me." She paused for a moment, allowing her less than subtle command to take effect.

"Thank you. As I said before, I will be brief, as it is late. You all have been such very good friends, and in the time that I have known you I have come to appreciate your friendship. Your loyalty and compassion are treasured attributes; but what concerns me right now is what happened to that compassion."

She scanned the group. "Since, the incident, you all have avoided me, like I have the plague, and I don't like it." "Sabrina," Brent tried to speak. "Please, let me have my say. Now, you've probably felt that I needed some space, or that talking to me would be awkward, and I can appreciate all of those feelings, but life goes on and in order for it to go on it needs, rather I need, my friends to help me. So, no more avoiding me, okay?"

"You got it," D'arcy spoke first. "I'm grateful to all of you," she said touching each of them briefly. "Now if you will excuse me, it's late and I have another situation that requires my attention." She bid them goodnight and returned to the bedroom.

"We should go," Brent said, as he stood up. "You don't have to," Mark interjected, hoping to entice them to stay, he yearned for the company. "Yeah, we do," D'arcy began. "She made it quite clear that tonight is not a good night to stay. Besides, now that she's feeling better, we'll have lots of time for parties."

Mark held the door for his friends. *I wish that they would stay, this loneliness is becoming unbearable.* Turning out the lights, he took another beer and dropped onto the sofa, grabbing the remote. *Another night alone, watching TV, since she's gone to bed without me, again.*

With the sound turned down low, he began flipping through channels, his eyes watched, but saw nothing. "Is there anything good on TV?" Sabrina said from behind him. "Not really. I thought you had gone to bed?" "Not yet." "Then why did you dismiss our guests so quickly?" Mark asked. She moved around in front of him. "I sent them away because I want to be with you," she said kneeling beside him. "I miss you." "How can that be? We're together all the time." "I know," she said, slowly running her hand over his arm. "But we haven't shared any intimate time together." She leaned in to him. "You shouldn't," Mark stammered. "Yes, I should; and so should you."

She slid her legs across him, sitting in his lap. "I love you," she whispered as she cradled his face in her hands. The tenderness of her touch made it easy for him to give in to his desires. *She's ready for me. Her body language tells me everything I need to know.*

She leaned back, waiting for him to make the next move. *I have initiated the moment now I have to find out if he is ready to accept me on that level again.* She closed her eyes.

Her head reeled when she felt his touch; but there was something different about it this time, she detected some hesitation from him. "Is something wrong?" she asked fearing the worst. Mark sighed as he removed his hands from her shoulders. He didn't speak, but she had already surmised his answer.

Unable to face him, she ran to the bedroom. Mark followed behind her. She lay on the bed, her back to him. He knelt behind her and touched her shoulder; she jerked it away. "Sabrina, you didn't give me a chance to answer you." "I know the answer; and to make it easier on both of us, I've decided to go home tomorrow." She tried to quiet her sobs. "And if that isn't good enough, then I'll consent to a divorce."

Mark felt like he had been kicked in the gut. "What are you saying?" "I'm releasing you. I understand why you don't want me, and I don't blame you. I'm surprised that you've stayed around this long."

Using his strength he rolled her over. "You're talking nonsense. I don't want a divorce. My God I love you. Our vows said for better or worse, and those vows I take very seriously." "Then why won't you touch me? I need you. You've been here with me but you haven't. You don't touch me or talk to me and you haven't kissed me. Why Mark?"

He lifted her up onto her knees, looking her in the eyes, his hands, firmly grasping her shoulders. "Listen to me, and I mean listen to every word and don't let your thoughts interfere. I love you, and I want to make love to you very much; but I have my concerns. I don't want you to put yourself at risk just to satisfy me. You're entitled to abstain for as long as you need to, and I will not force you into anything that you're not ready for." "Hold me," she begged.

He pulled her close. "I feel like such a fool. I had no right to doubt your love for me." "Hush. Your emotions are on a roller coaster from hell, and you have every right to be confused and to feel like you're alone; but you're not. I'm here, and I will always be here with you, through the good and the bad."

"I'm sorry if what I said hurt you." "It's okay, you're allowed to say whatever you feel; and right now your feelings are being controlled by fear and anger," he said bringing her face around to his. "Am I right?" Unconsciously, she bit at her lip. "Yes you are; but we still need to talk this out. I have to know how this is affecting you." "I'm fine." "I don't think so. What Sean did, it's affected both of us and I want to talk about it." "Maybe you should talk to a councilor?" "No Mark, I want to talk to you. I have to know just how bad he has hurt you."

Releasing his hold on her, Mark sat back and ran his hands through his hair. Sabrina understood the action as he only did it when something was really bothering him. "Please Mark," she urged. "You want to know how I feel?" "Yes." "Anger is what I feel. Every time I close my eyes I can see him hurting you and it makes me so damn angry. I'm angry at him but more so at myself." "Why?" "I let you down Sabrina. I promised to protect you and I failed. I left you alone and vulnerable and it's my fault that this happened to you. I should have kept you with me during the interview. If I had then this nightmare would never have happened."

Sabrina cautiously picked up his hand and gently stroked the back of it with her thumb. "Please don't do this Mark. I can't carry your guilt as well as my own. You are not to blame yourself for this." "And neither are you." "I know, but sometimes I just can't help thinking that I brought this on myself." "Stop it! There is only one person to blame and that's Sean. I can't even begin to imagine what he put you through but it's over." "Is it? Sean raped me but he did more than that and even now I'm still afraid. Sometimes I just want to run away, as far and as fast as I can."

"Maybe we should just go home for a little while?" "No Mark. Running away is not going to make this any easier. What I'm feeling is still hard to put into words right now but I do know that I don't want those feelings anymore. All I want to feel is love, your love, your touch." Her hands slid inside his shirt. "Love me Mark and help me to forget. Even if it's just for this one moment, please help me to forget that night."

Her face was close to his. He could feel her breath on his skin. He moved and their lips met. She still tasted so sweet. He wanted, needed, more of her. With his arms firmly around her, he lowered her onto the bed. "Are you really sure that this is what you want?" Mark asked. "Yes," she answered bringing his hand to her breast. The sensation made her shudder and he removed his hand. "Please don't stop," she said pulling him back to her. "I have to know that we're okay, that you can still love me." "Always baby."

Mark deliberately kept his actions slow and gentle, trying to stay focused on her, watching for any sign that she may be uncomfortable, but all he saw was her hunger. Her unquenchable desire for him, that was equally reflected in himself.

Soaked with sweat, and near exhaustion, their bodies rocked together with orgasmic pleasure, bringing them both to a new level of intensity. With their minds lost in a fog of lust, Mark momentarily forgot himself, letting his full weight come to rest on top of her. Her arms locked around him, holding him in place; until her labored breathing made him aware of what he had done. He moved himself away to her side.

"I'm sorry. Are you all right?" "I'm fine," she smiled. "Are you sure I didn't hurt you?" She slipped her arm around his neck, drawing him to her and kissed him; a long, deep, passionate kiss. "Does that answer your question?"

He smiled, cuddling her close. Still caressing her breast, he couldn't help noticing that there was something different about them. The change was subtle, slightly larger and firmer. He dismissed it as being nothing more than his imagination. She turned on her side, facing him, snuggling into his shoulder. "I want to go back to work, starting tomorrow," she said. "We'll discuss it tomorrow; now go to sleep." "I'm not tired," she said suppressing a yawn. "Then what was that?" "Nothing." "Go to sleep, my love," he said as he pulled the blankets around her.

Relinquishing her position of comfort she kissed him. It seemed like an eternity since she had really kissed him, and what started out to be a simple good night kiss, grew deeper, and more passionate with every breath she took. Mark pulled away.

"You're supposed to be going to sleep," he said. "I know, but I love the way you kiss me. I never want you to stop." She reached for him again. "You know what will happen if we continue with this." "What would be wrong with that?" "Nothing; if you were back to a hundred percent." "Let me be the judge of that. Now, please, stop talking and kiss me."

The request she made was far too irresistible. Their passion guiding them down the same loving path, until they succumbed to the overwhelming exhaustion, falling into a deep sleep, bound together in each other's arms.

Chapter 19

Nick pushed away from his desk. Walking around the office, he ended up at the bar, pouring himself a drink. *It isn't quite noon, but I need something to settle my nerves. Mark and Sabrina will be here soon. I have to remain calm, and not let this meeting get out of hand. Sean's fate rests on the outcome of this meeting, and I hope that we can come to some agreement that will resolve this problem to everyone's satisfaction.*

He poured another drink, savoring the flavor on his tongue. *If only I could talk to Sabrina alone, I know I would be able to persuade her to agree with my proposal, but that isn't going to be easy. Since the incident, she's been closely guarded by Mark, and in his absence, Brent, D'arcy and Tony have watched over her, separating her from the inquisitive stares and questions.* The intercom buzzed, announcing their arrival. Nick finished his drink and went to welcome his guests.

Mark and Sabrina had speculated as to why they had been summoned to the Corporate office, but neither of them dared to tell the other their suspicions. As the door opened, Sabrina reached for Mark's hand. The reassuring squeeze gave her the strength to walk into the office.

Separate chairs distanced them enough that they couldn't touch. With a subtle look from her, Mark moved his chair to her side. She wove her arm around his until she felt the security of her hand in his. Nick took his seat behind the desk. Sabrina noticed the serious look on his face. The deep furrows in his forehead bothered her. *This is not a social visit.* Her stomach began to ripple. She crossed her legs to calm the turmoil.

Nick opened his mouth to speak, but Mark began the conversation. "So why are we here?" Mark asked trying to keep his tension to a minimum. Nick made use of the interruption to take a deep, full breath. "Well firstly, I would like to congratulate you on your marriage. I was a bit disappointed that you didn't tell me right away, but I can understand you wanting to keep your privacy."

Listening to Nick's insignificant ramblings made Mark squirmed in his seat. "Enough with the bull shit! You didn't call us here because you didn't get a wedding invitation. Now cut through the crap and get to the real reason."

Feeling uncomfortable, Nick cleared his throat and pushing himself out of his chair he moved around to the front of the desk. He perched himself on the edge, near Sabrina. Reaching out, he took up her free hand, his eyes, filled with sincerity, looked into hers. "Sabrina, I haven't had the opportunity, until now, to tell you how sorry I am about what happened, what Sean did to you."

Acknowledging him with a nod, she lowered her head to blink away the tears that burned in her eyes. Mark saw her try to hide her sadness and it instantly enraged him. "How dare you bring that up now!" "I'm sorry, but it has to be discussed. The lawyers need to know where you stand." "That's easy. The son of a bitch deserves to go to jail, for as long as possible!"

Trying hard not to let Mark's emotions get to her, Sabrina shifted her gaze back to Nick. "What are the lawyers saying?" she asked. "If he goes to trial, and is convicted, he could get up to twenty-five years in prison." "What are his chances?" "From what I've been told, a conviction is inevitable. Unless." "Unless what?" Sabrina queried.

"No!" Mark interrupted. "There is no alternative. He has to be punished for what he did!" "Mark, please, I need to hear what Nick has to say. Please continue." "Thank you. Now what I have to say is only a suggestion, the ultimate decision is yours Sabrina, and yours alone." "Like hell it is!" Mark was becoming more agitated. "Mark; Sabrina, please just hear me out. I don't expect you to answer me today. I don't want you to. What you don't know is that Sean has been undergoing psychiatric evaluation, and so far it has been determined that he is extremely obsessed with you; to the point of delusional fantasies." "It took a Doctor to figure that out," Mark sneered.

Nick took a moment to survey her reaction, hoping he had tapped in to her compassion. "Now, what I'm proposing is that, if you, Sabrina, agree to it, we could have Sean convicted under the psychiatric evidence. Which would mean that he would receive extensive treatment and still be allowed to return to work, when the Doctor's determine him well enough, but he would be guarded by two officers at all times, at home, and on tour, for a duration set out by the court."

"There would be no prison time?" "No, he wouldn't be behind bars, but his movements would be very restricted." "How long would this be for?" "That I can't say, that would be for the Judge, and the psychiatrist to determine, based on how he responds to treatment."

Unable to listen any longer, Mark pushed himself out of the chair and began to pace. "This is bull shit!" "Sabrina," Nick regained her attention. "All I ask is that you give this great consideration before you give me an answer. I know Sean needs to be punished, but please, weigh the options very carefully before making your decision. Sean's life, his future, rests on you."

"That's it!" Mark yelled, taking Sabrina's hand. "We've heard enough," he said pulling her up beside him. "You've made it quite clear that you don't want anything to happen to your meal ticket! We're leaving!" Sabrina had to run to keep up with Mark's quick, long strides; keeping her close to him, as they left the building.

Nick poured another drink, savoring it with great pleasure. *I'm confident that I've awoken Sabrina's compassion. By the tone of her voice, and the questions that she asked, I'm quite sure that she doesn't want to see Sean sent to jail. If only I had more time with her, I could have convinced her that this solution is the right one.*

The one obstacle that could jeopardize everything is Mark. If he somehow manages to sway her thinking, to get her to agree with his view of punishment, then there will be no hope for Sean. I can't let myself believe that. Sabrina isn't a vindictive person. I have to believe that her gentleness of heart will prevail.

Sabrina stared out the window, as Mark drove back to the hotel. *He is so angry, and initiating a conversation at this point could prove dangerous. I can wait, and hopefully he'll have calmed down enough so we can discuss this rationally.* From the corner of her eye, she could see Mark's hands, tightening on the steering wheel, the back of his hands were red but his knuckles were white from the pressure. *I don't like to see him so tense, especially while driving, it means that he's not fully concentrating on the road.*

Laying her hand on his thigh, she slowly rubbed from his hip to his knee. He covered her hand with his own and gave it a gentle squeeze. "Do you want to go somewhere, other than the hotel?" Mark asked. "No, the only place I want to be is in your arms." She had barely finished her sentence when he pulled the car to the curb.

"What are you doing?" she asked. "Something we both need right now." Unbuckling his seat belt, he leaned across the console, pulling her close. His beard rubbed against her face, reminding her that she was still in command of her senses, not still lost in that void of conversation with Nick. "Take me home," she said softly.

Mark kissed her tenderly. *This is just a quick fix. I need to have her close to me.* He drove on, keeping that thought foremost in his mind; pushing away the conversation with Nick.

Sabrina walked into the hotel room. Stopping near the window, she hugged herself. Mark was behind her. His hands stroked over her shoulders. "You're tense. Why don't you take a long hot bath, and if you like, I'll rub your back." "I'd like that very much," she purred. With a kiss on the cheek, he sent her on her way.

Sabrina poured the bubble bath into the large tub. While the water filled, she stripped of her clothes. Her jeans had become uncomfortably tight lately and it felt good to take them off. Catching a glimpse of her reflection in the mirror, her hands smoothed over her body. *I've gained weight as my no longer flat tummy indicates, too much hotel food and not enough exercise.* Stepping into the tub amid the thick bubbles and the soothing water, she lay back and closed her eyes.

Mark dimmed the lights, before he slipped in beside her, giving her his arm as a neck support. With a push of a button, the water began to boil. The soothing jets of water swirled around them. She snuggled closer to him, turned slightly, so he could fulfill his promise of a back rub. Her skin was soft and slippery, making it easy for his hands to glide over her taught muscles. With each stroke he could feel her relax, settling in closer to him.

"Before you get too comfortable, we should talk about what Nick had to say," he said. Sabrina flipped over onto him; her arms over his shoulders; steadying herself on the edge of the tub. "There will be no talking. Not right now, this is our time, a time for quiet and a time for love."

He didn't wait for her to make the first advance. His arms encircled her, drawing her to him, her lips to his. Sliding her body down over his stomach, she abruptly stopped her kisses and smiled at him. "What?" he asked. "It didn't take you long to get in the mood," she said reaching down to that special part of him. "Baby, all I have to do is look at you and I'm turned on."

With a devilish grin, she resumed her passionate kisses, bringing their bodies together in a fevered release of total ecstasy. Contented and relaxed, she slumped against him, fighting the urge to sleep. Mark nuzzled at her head.

"Why don't we take this to the bedroom, and see what develops?" "We could, or we could stay here and take care of what's already developed," she said acknowledging the firmness that pressed against her thigh. "You're wicked," he said with a wide smile. "I know, but it's because I love you so much. I just can't seem to get enough of you." "I think I can do something about that," he said quietly. She smiled, biting her lip in anticipation. A pleasurable feeling that made her shudder.

Her moment of anticipation became a memory, as an annoying sound drifted into the bathroom. "What was that?" She listened for the sound to return. "There is someone at the door." "Maybe, if we ignore it, it will go away," Sabrina suggested. The knock became louder. "I don't think so," Mark answered, lifting her aside. "I'll go see who it is." He pulled on a bathrobe, closing the bathroom door behind him. With the mood broken, and the bath water getting cold, Sabrina decided to get out. She too was curious as to who had come to visit.

Brent had just about given up, when Mark opened the door. "Damn. I'll come back later." He was embarrassed, knowing by Mark's appearance that he had interrupted an intimate moment. "Don't be like that, come on in." "I just stopped by to see if you and Sabrina would like to join me for dinner." "Nice idea, but I'll have to check with her first. Make yourself comfortable; I'll be right back."

Brent relaxed onto the sofa, while he waited for Mark to return. *Asking them out to dinner is merely a cover. I want to find out what Nick had told them this afternoon. Were they summoned to the office to discuss the wedding or Sean? Sean; no one is talking about him. Either they know nothing, or were sworn to secrecy. Hopefully they would trust me enough to confide in me.*

As Mark opened the bathroom door, his eyes fell wide upon Sabrina. She stood only a few feet from him. Her shapely nude body, barely concealed by the damp towel she held in front of her. "Who was at the door?" she asked.

His eyes followed her hand, as she dried her leg, moving up across her stomach to her breast. He shut the door. "Who cares?" "Mark!" "It's only Brent; he can wait," he said taking her in his arms. "We have left something unfinished." "It's going to have to stay unfinished for a while anyway. We can't ignore our guest."

The disappointment in his eyes was easy for her to read. "I'll make it up to you, I promise," she whispered. The towel fell to the floor, as she reached for her robe. He turned away. The vision of her body made it difficult for him to fasten his jeans.

The unexpected, cold feeling of satin against his back, made him stand straight, as a shiver jolted his spine into place. Sabrina slipped her arms around his chest, running her fingers over the red hair that covered his upper body. "Shall we go and see our guest?" "I guess." He started for the living room, her arms still around him, and she was shadowing each of his steps with one of her own.

Brent stood up when he heard the bedroom door open. "I was about to give up on you," he turned to greet them; a sideways grin crossed his lips. "Hey man, when did you grow the extra set of arms?" "Don't be such a smart ass," Mark sneered at him. Sabrina stepped out from behind him. She went to Brent, giving him a warm hug. He reveled in the brief seconds that her body was close to his.

"I take it that you have declined my offer," he said as he looked at Sabrina. "What offer?" "My fault," Mark interjected. "I forgot to ask her." "Ask me what?" "I came by to see if you wanted to go for dinner." "That's so sweet, but I really don't feel like going out tonight." "I understand, maybe some other time." "Why don't we have dinner here? It's much more relaxed, and I wouldn't have to get dressed." "Are you sure?" "Man, you should know better," Mark said picking up the hotel menu. "When she makes up her mind, there's no changing it." "There, it's settled."

Leading Brent to the sofa, she cuddled up beside him when he sat down. "We haven't spent much time together lately, and I miss it," she said. A strange feeling came over Mark, as he watched Sabrina lean against Brent.

This is a feeling that I don't fully understand, but the more I watch her, the more I don't like what she's doing. With everything that has happened why would she flaunt herself like that? I know that Brent is nothing like Sean but it still isn't right.

Sitting at the far end of the sofa, he observed her behavior. Sabrina's arm was about Brent's shoulders as they perused the menu. She giggled and leaned in closer. Mark's stomach burned. Finished with the menu, she handed it blindly to Mark. When he didn't take it from her hand, she looked at him. The cold, hard stare that met her eyes gave her a chill. *His eyes seem greener than normal, brightened by jealousy. It's been weeks since the incident but it's still very prominent in his mind.*

Turning she knelt beside him. Her mouth silently uttered "I love you." The touch of his hand on her back brought her to him. His kiss was hesitant, until she forced her tongue deep into his mouth. *I feel so foolish, for having those feelings. I have no reason to doubt her she is my wife. It's just so hard to share her with other people but she has a right to have friends.*

He laid her back in his arms, bringing their steamy kiss to an end. Sabrina closed her eyes. As she stretched out, her feet pushed against Brent's thigh. "Oh, I'm sorry," she was startled, pulling herself more upright. "I momentarily forgot that you were here. I just love him so much, that it blinds me to everything around me." "No need to apologize; I understand. You're still newlyweds, and you're in love. You're supposed to be consumed with each other." "Maybe, but it's no excuse for ignoring good friends." "You're allowed to," Brent said patting her ankle. "So have we decided on dinner?" "Yeah," Mark said tossing the menu aside. "I'll have the steak." "Great, I'll call it in."

Sabrina secured her arms around Mark's neck, her face close enough that he could feel her breath. "Any chance of a little dessert before dinner?" he asked. His request made her smile. She eagerly treated him to a sampling of what he could expect later, when they were alone. Instinctively, his hand brushed over her breast. She pressed her body into his touch. Brent cleared his throat, a signal to her to relax back into Mark's arms, and pay attention to their guest.

"Sorry." "Don't be; I remember very well what it's like to be newly married; and frankly, I don't know how you can manage to share your personal time with others." "We'll always have time for you. Mark and I owe you so much." "I'm just glad that I was able to help; but things would have turned out just fine even if I wasn't around." "That may have some truth to it," Mark began. "I know things would have really gotten out of hand if you and D'arcy weren't there to stop me. Christ, I could be sharing a cell with that bastard!"

Sabrina could feel his pulse quicken and she smoothed her hand over his chest. "Well you're not, and I'm so grateful for that." Fearing that she would become upset with the memories Brent quickly changed the subject. "So, I hear that you were summoned to the seat of power, or should I call it the viper's den?" "You got that right. If I wasn't bound by a contract, I'd walk away from Nick, and his damn company, and go to work for somebody else. All he cares about is what's gonna boost the ratings and pad his wallet."

"I know that all too well," Brent sighed. "The only thing that matters, is that he looks good in the eyes of the public." "I take it then that he told you his idea, concerning the both of you?" Brent asked. Sabrina's eyes widened in disbelief. "You know?" "Hell yeah. He wanted my opinion on how I thought you'd react," Brent said. Sabrina shook her head, lowering it until she had concealed her face against Mark's neck.

"Damn him! So much for keeping it confidential; how many others know?" "As far as I know, I'm the only one he's talked to about it." Brent heard Sabrina sniffle. "Hey, it's just a stupid publicity stunt, nothing to get upset about." "How the hell is she supposed to act! A publicity stunt! Christ, Nick is a bigger asshole than I thought. He knows that whatever we decide to do is going to have serious side effects."

Brent was confused by Mark's irrational response. "I don't understand you man. What kind of side effects could a wedding have?"

Sabrina sat back. "What did you say?" "I know Nick has come up with some pretty strange ideas, but I never imagined that having an in ring wedding would upset you so much. I hope you told him to forget it." "Brent, we're not on the same page here." "Hell, we're not even in the same book for that matter," Mark added. "I don't follow you?"

Sabrina looked at Mark. "You explain it to him," she said. "Are you sure?" "Yeah, he's our friend. He should know the whole story." "Christ, where do I start," Mark said running his hand through his hair. "We were with Nick this afternoon, but the only topic of discussion was Sean." Mark proceeded to describe to Brent, the options that Nick had presented to them. Emphasizing the direction that Nick desired Sabrina to go, saving his star performer from a life behind bars.

While Mark recounted the conversation, Sabrina replayed it all in her mind. Blocking out Mark's voice, she rested her head against his shoulder. *Nick has given me so much to think about. He played directly to my emotions, hoping that I would remember that I once had feelings for Sean. Making a decision isn't going to be easy. Sean deserves to be punished, but being in prison would destroy him. On the other hand, he does need psychiatric treatment. It could help him to overcome his obsession.*

Would I be safe? Would I feel safe? Nick said that he would be under guard at all times, but Sean is clever. Clever enough that he could elude his guard. My mind is spinning, which decision would be the right one. I already know which way Mark wants me to go, but would he be understanding, and supportive, if I made the other choice? I want so very much to keep him happy, but the decision is ultimately up to me, whether he agrees or not.

Her thoughts had carried her far away from the conversation between Mark and Brent. It wasn't until Brent got up, that she returned to the present. "Where is he going?" she asked. "Dinner's here. Are you all right?" "Yeah," she answered forcing a smile. "Are you sure?" "No," she sighed. "What can I do to help?" "Hold me." "My pleasure." *Her body trembles so in my arms. I wish that I could erase her memories, of all the bad things that have happened to her over these past few months.*

"Do you two think you can take a break to have dinner?" Brent interrupted, setting plates on the table. Mark let her go. "Feeling better?" Mark asked. "Almost," she answered licking her lips. She kissed him slowly, her tongue tracing over the fullness of his lips. "Now I feel better," she purred.

Wiggling herself off his lap, she stood before him, her back to Brent. Slyly she pulled her belt loose, as it fell away her robe parted, giving Mark a discrete view. He bolted to his feet, pulling her robe closed. "What are you doing?" "Guess?" "Behave yourself," he scolded. "Dinner's getting cold." "Maybe, but dessert is just warming up." "What am I going to do with you?" Mark asked. "I have a few suggestions." "Later." "Promise?" She smiled.

Sabrina took a seat between the two men. The sudden silence that fell over them made her feel very awkward; but that was soon broken, as Brent accidentally dropped his fork to his plate. "I still can't believe it," Brent began. "I knew Nick could be an asshole, but this makes him even worse than that. How he could even think about asking you to make a choice like that is completely tactless?"

Sabrina shoved her plate across the table, glaring at Brent. "I don't want to hear anymore about it! It's my decision to make and I don't want to hear your opinion!" Mark gently squeezed her hand. The look he cast at her made her realize that she was out of line, she turned back to Brent. "I'm sorry; I shouldn't have yelled at you." "It's perfectly okay; you're allowed to. It's only natural to be emotional." "So now that we all know how I feel about that subject, let's just drop it, but what you can tell me, is more about this wedding idea that Nick talked to you about."

Brent leaned back in his chair. "Yes, another one of Nick's fantasies, he has this idea that the Warlock and the Sorceress should stage a wedding at the pay per view on October 31st." "What's his motive?" Sabrina asked. "He thinks that the fans would get a charge out of this unholy union. It would be nothing but a boost to the ratings; and it would take your careers in a whole new direction."

"Why do I sense something more?" she asked taking his hand. "Man, I gotta stop thinking when I'm around you," he chuckled. "There is more. Nick's a little pissed that you eloped. He wanted to be a part of your wedding day; you know, give you a big fancy wedding complete with a full blown reception, but weddings aren't supposed to be dark and sinister, they're supposed to be filled with romance, like I'm sure yours was."

Sabrina looked at Brent and then at Mark, suppressing the urge to laugh. "You haven't seen our wedding pictures, have you?" "No, I haven't. I didn't know you had any." She pushed back from the table. "Don't you tell him anything," she said wagging her finger at Mark, as she headed off to the bedroom to retrieve the album.

Brent cast a long questioning look at Mark, who raised his arms above his head. "You heard her I can't tell you," he said reclining back. "So what direction has Nick planned for my career?" "I'm not completely sure of all the details, but I get the feeling that he wants to turn you into more of a bad guy, Sabrina too." "Me too, what?" "Nothing. Brent and I were just speculating about Nick's plans." "Well, I for one am intrigued with the idea. I think it would be worth finding out more."

Giving Mark a quick kiss, she sat down, laying the photo album in front of Brent. "Our wedding was very romantic, but it was far from traditional. Mark planned everything, and kept it all a secret right to the end." Opening the album, she sat back to watch Brent's expressions. Her hand drifted across the table to meet Mark's.

Brent's eyes widened to match his smile. "I can't believe it," he said staring at the first picture. "What don't you believe?" "That you could be even more beautiful than you already are." Sabrina felt a blush crawl over her. The warmth intensified as Mark's lips kissed her hand. He tugged at her gently until she gave up her chair, for the comfort of his lap. Brent continued to flip through the album. "This is incredible."

"Yes, it is," she answered, her fingers softly caressing Mark's face. "This is without a doubt the most romantic wedding I've ever seen." "Mmmm, incredibly romantic," she purred as she kissed Mark's cheek. "You two were definitely meant to be together." "Forever," she whispered kissing his lips softly. Brent glanced up from the album, staring quietly at the display of affection from the other end of the table. His own loneliness kicked him hard in the gut. *I long to be in love again.*

"Well, I have to get going. Don't get up; I can see myself out. I'll catch up with you sometime tomorrow." He closed the door behind him. Sabrina turned her attentions back to Mark, back to his green eyes. "I think we chased him away," she said stroking his cheek again. "Now where were we?" His lips found the hollow of her throat, making her moan softly, which quickly turned to a gasp, when his hand slipped inside her robe. The sensation of his beard against her skin sent shivers up her spine, as his kisses moved up her neck to her lips. She feverishly engaged him.

He could wait no more. He carried her to the bedroom. She wiggled free, just before he tried to lay her down. Standing close to him, her robe open, her hands gently caressed his chest. "I love you so much," he whispered. He kissed her again, moving her back to the bed. "No, wait. I want to please you." "Baby you do please me." "You don't understand. I want to give you the kind of pleasure that you've only dreamed of."

Loosening his jeans, she pushed them over his hips, to the floor, allowing him to step out of them before she guided him to the bed. Instructing him to lay on his back, she crawled over to his side. "What do you want me to do?" Mark asked. "Shhh," she hushed him with a kiss. "Just let me love you."

With his eyes closed, it permitted his other senses to take over. Her actions were measured. Each time her lips touched his skin the fire of desire raged stronger in him. Her touch was soft, sensual, bringing him to the point of no return, then backing away, denying him the fulfillment of ecstasy.

She repeated her seduction, again and again, still denying him satisfaction. His fists clenched at the bed sheets. His toes curled under from the unending stimulation. His blood was on fire, sweat glistening on his body. Beginning her seduction again, only this time she stopped much sooner than before, she leaned in close to him. "Do you want me?" she asked in a voice so soft.

Mark's eyes snapped open. He rolled her over, gazing into her eyes as she took him in. His senses were so heightened that for the first time he felt all of her as their bodies moved together. It brought him to a climax that seemed endless, the feeling of her body shuddering and tightening around him, prolonged his own rapture.

Perspiration soaked his body, trickling down his forehead, dripping off of his nose, onto her chest. The tiny drops raced across her breast. His body shuddered as another climax ripped through him. His arms trembled from weakness. He wanted to remain in her embrace, but the extreme fatigue forced him to lie at her side. She moved herself close to him. His body was hot, his breath coming in short, rapid pants.

"Are you okay?" she asked, wiping the glistening moisture from his forehead. "Yeah, just give me a minute." Laying her head against his shoulder, her hand on his chest, she felt his breathing slow to a normal rhythm.

Resting her eyes, she had nearly succumbed to sleep when Mark pulled her on top of him. He kissed her, a long, deep, passionate kiss. "I love you so much, Sabrina." "I take it then that you're happy." "There are no words to describe how I feel. I never knew that a man's body could endure such sustained pleasure; but I guess it has a lot to do with having a woman who loves you." "I do love you Mark and I love making you happy." "It's a good thing that I don't have a show tomorrow. I'm gonna need the time to recover my strength, and speaking of time," he glanced at the clock. "You know we've lost nearly two hours." "Maybe we should try for longer?" she asked, laying her head against him. "Not tonight."

In her sigh he detected some disappointment, but then realized what she was doing. She was evading talking about Sean. "I know what you're trying to do," he said staring into her eyes. "You're avoiding a certain discussion, but we don't need to have it; do we? You've already made your decision. You're not gonna let him go to prison." "Are you mad?" "Yes, and no. The decision was yours to make, and you made the choice that was right for you, and I respect that." "I am so blessed to have you." "We're both blessed. We have each other, forever."

The guard escorted Sean to an interview room. A barren gray room, with only a metal table, two chairs, and a telephone. Sean headed straight to the phone. "Nick, are you there?" "Yes, Sean." "Man, I thought you'd forgot about me." "No, I haven't forgot. I've been working on your case, trying to get you out of there." "Well, it's about time; but tell me this, what have all these Doctors got to do with my case?" "A lot, I'm not going to get into it on the phone. The lawyer should be there soon, and he can explain everything to you, and Sean, listen to him, understand what he's going to tell you, and accept it." "You're making it sound pretty bad." "It's not as bad as it could have been, and that's all I'm prepared to say." Sean hung up the phone. He kicked a chair out from under the table, and sat down to wait for his lawyer. A smile lit up his face. *Sabrina must have cleared everything up.* "I knew she would."

Sabrina stood at the window of the hotel room; staring out at the city, seeing and thinking nothing. Her belly rumbled. She smoothed her hands over it, calming the disturbance. Mark put his arms around her. "You did the right thing," he said. "Did I?" "Yes baby, you did." "It's not the choice you would have made." "The decision wasn't mine to make. You have to do what's right for you." "What if?" "No baby. No what ifs, it's over."

Turning herself to face him, she stared deeply into his eyes. "Can you honestly guarantee me that?" she asked. "Honestly, no; but I want you to tell me something. Do you want it to be over or are you willing to live with the fear for the rest of your life?" "I do want it to be over, but I'm not sure if the fear will ever go away. He'll be coming back to work eventually and I don't know how I'm going to deal with that."

"You won't, but we will, together," Mark reassured her. "You're not in this alone Sabrina, you never were and you never will be." He carefully brought her into his embrace, holding her gently. "Why don't we get out of here and do something? Our plane doesn't leave until eight o'clock." "I don't really want to. I'm not a fan of New York."

Mark leaned back to look at her. "Come on; you need to get out of here for a while. I'm sure we could find something to do. Something that doesn't involve a lot of walking." "Why no walking?" she asked. "I'm a bit embarrassed to even talk about it."

She detected the subtle blush on his cheeks. "Embarrassed about what?" "Put it this way, if I didn't have to wear jeans I'd feel much better." "Oh baby," she whispered, running her hands down his jeans. "There's something else," he said lifting her hands up. "What I find even more uncomfortable is the bite mark on my thigh." "I'm so sorry," she said, moving back into his embrace. "I'm not complaining. I don't even remember you doing it." "Neither do I. Sounds like we both could benefit from a long soak in the tub."

He pondered over her remark for a moment, unsure as to her meaning. It didn't take him long to come up with the answer. "I hurt you, didn't I?" "No, my love, I'm just not in a hurry to sit down." "I did hurt you! Damn it!" "Mark no. It's borne of love, and that makes it all right. So then it's settled we're staying here," she said giving him a kiss. "I'd much rather lose myself in your arms, than the city." He held her close for the whole afternoon, ignoring the phone when it rang, and the numerous knocks on the door. Nothing was going to separate them today.

When she walked down the aisle of the plane, toward the rest room, Brent quickly took her seat beside Mark. "Hey man, missed you guys today, I stopped by your room a couple of times, but I guess you were out." "No, we didn't go out today at all." "Then why? Oh, now I understand," Brent smirked. Mark let him have his fantasy. He tugged at the leg of his jeans, looking for some relief, some way of stopping the chaffing on his thigh.

"What the hell is the matter with you? You've been squirming around ever since you got on the plane," Brent remarked. "It's nothing," Mark answered. "Nothing eh; then how come there's blood on your jeans?" "Damn." Mark quickly covered the spot with his hand. "What's going on?" Brent asked again. "Nothing I told you. I had a bit of an accident last night, no big deal." "What kind of accident still weeps blood the next day?" Brent asked.

Mark leaned towards Brent, keeping his voice as low as possible. "She bit me," he whispered. "Bit you!" "Christ, would you shut up!" It was too late; Tony and Sam leaned over the seats in front of them. "Hey Mark," Tony grinned. "I didn't know your wife was a vamp." "Screw off, all of you!"

Sabrina was headed back to her seat, unaware of the loud comment that preceded her. The unusual stares, and quirky smiles from the other wrestlers made her feel very self conscious. Brent returned to his seat, only after he flashed her a devilish grin.

"What's going on?" she asked Mark. "Ignore them. They've all got their minds in the gutter." "Why is that?" she asked. He lifted his hand from his thigh and she saw the dark red stain that had seeped through the denim, she leaned in closer. "You told them; didn't you?" "Are you mad?" "No. Shall I get the first aid kit from the flight attendant and see if I can fix that up?" "No, it can wait until we get to the hotel; and then you can do whatever you want." "Anything?" she asked kissing his full lips. "Anything," he whispered breathlessly. She kissed him harder, beginning the seduction that she would finish later.

Tony leaned back over his seat. "Ah gees, they're at it again." More faces peered at them. "Better be careful Mark, or you'll be too weak to do the show," Tony said with a laugh. Sabrina pressed her lips close to Mark's ear. "I feel like having a little fun, just play along with me," she whispered softly. Mark gave her a nod. *I have no idea what she's planning, but I surmise that Tony is about to be taken down a few pegs, and Sabrina is definitely the one person who can make him lose the smart ass routine.*

Jumping up, she grabbed Tony by the shirt. "It's true he is rather, drained. His body needs to rebuild itself; but I'm hungry now." Her voice was low and sultry. It had captivated him. "Shall you be next?" she asked. He was mesmerized, as her tongue licked sensuously at his neck. "You taste so good. Mind if I have a little bite?" She licked at his neck again.

Mark suppressed a grin as he watched as Tony's dark tanned skin faded to a milky white. Sabrina opened her mouth. Tony felt her teeth dig into his skin. He jerked himself back. "Jesus Christ; you were going to do it!" "I told you I was hungry, but if you're not willing, then maybe you are," she said lunging toward Sam. "No way," he smiled. "I don't think that I'm your type." *I know what she's up to, and Tony deserves what she's dishing out.*

Tony stared at Sabrina, while rubbing at his throat. "Well, I guess I'll have to feed later," she sighed, sitting back down, snuggling close to Mark. Tony peered over the top of his seat before sitting down. He leaned over to Sam. "Did you see that? She really tried to bite me. That is one freaky chick." "Maybe, but you better be careful, no change that, all of us better be careful around her, she may just try it again; and next time she may not ask first." Tony shuddered, as he settled against his seat. *I always thought her to be such a nice girl, but now I'm not sure how I feel about her.*

Sabrina hid her face against Mark's shoulder, as they listened to the conversation unfold. *I've hooked him, and now Sam is playing him like a true sportsman.* "You're full of crap!" Tony snarled at Sam. "No man, think about it. Warlock has always been, well, you know, pale; but lately he's gotten worse and that can only mean that she's the cause of it." "Bull shit!"

"No, just listen. When a body loses blood, it becomes pale, and haven't you noticed her teeth?" "What about them?"

The cue was perfect; Sabrina leaned around Tony's seat. "Changed your mind yet?" "No, I haven't. Now leave me alone," Tony snarled. She returned to her seat and Sam stepped right back in. "Did you see them? I told you man; you better watch yourself." Tony's mind flashed onto her smile, but vividly recalled her fangs; he shuddered. "Leave me the fuck alone!"

Sabrina had very prominent upper canine teeth. They weren't out of place, just a little longer, and sharper than most people, a natural asset for Halloween. "When we land I need to do a little shopping," she whispered into Mark's ear. "What for?" "I'll tell you in the car; but trust me; I want to see this through. He thinks he's the master of practical jokes; well he's met his match." "You're wicked." "I know, but I like it and so do you."

It was late when they landed in Miami. *I'll have to wait until the morning to do my shopping.* On the drive to the hotel, she explained to Mark her plan for Tony. Since he was scheduled to wrestle Mark, it will be the perfect opportunity. The delivery of her plan was perfect, so perfect that it made Mark laugh out loud.

"I love it! You're gonna have him so psyched that he'll jump at his own shadow." "That's the whole idea." "How long do you plan to carry this on?" "Until I tire of the game, or find a new victim." "You know; this could very well be the change that I've been looking for."

He paused their conversation while they checked into the hotel, and went up to their room, mulling over the idea in his mind. "Okay," Sabrina began, kicking the door shut. "Why do you want to change your character?" Mark dropped their bags and took her in his arms. "I'm not ready to tell you just yet. Not until I have it all worked out in my head. Besides," he began kissing her. "You started something on the plane that I intend to finish."

In a swift, effortless move, he hoisted her over his shoulder. It made her squeal and giggle with delight. "What do you think you're doing?" she asked, trying to keep her head up. "I am going to tame this wicked beast that is my wife," he said giving her a playful slap on the ass. A knock at the door halted him. "Go away!" he yelled. "Mark, it's me, Brent." "Oh hell," he muttered, turning toward the door. "You can put me down you know." "And miss out on relieving you of your clothes, no way, besides, I quite like the view," he said caressing her round curves.

"So what's so damn important?" Mark asked, pulling the door open swiftly. Brent's jaw dropped open. "Ah, never mind, I can see that you're busy. I, I'll come back tomorrow. No, wait, you call me when you've got some time to spare." "Fine." Mark began to shut the door. "Good night Brent," Sabrina said curling her body around to see him. Mark never waited for a reply; he shut the door and carried her to the bedroom.

From the hallway, Brent could hear her laughter, as it faded into the distance. *I want to know that kind of love again, unbridled and filled with passion.* He headed for the hotel bar. *I'll settle for one night of lust; and if the bar proved fruitless, then there's always Robbie. She won't deny me.*

Sean took a deep breath. *Los Angeles smog even smells good compared to the cold, damp odor of concrete and dust that made up my cell. I'm free. Free to go back to work, to go on with my life; with the company of my two new shadows. I'm used to having body guards, so this won't be any different; except these guys wouldn't be going home at the end of the day.*

What I still can't figure out is why I have to see all those Doctors? Why all the counseling? If Sabrina had told them how she feels, then I should be free to do whatever I want. The lawyer had explained it as treatment, to get over my obsession; but I'm not obsessed. I care about her. It infuriates me that the lawyer told me that I'm forbidden to talk to Sabrina, or to go anywhere near her. How can we mend our relationship if I can't see her? She must be angry with me, I did deceive her, but I had to. Mark turned her against me. I'll play her little game. I'll prove to her that I'm worthy of her love.

Sabrina stretched, her hand reached out for Mark, but found only the cold emptiness of where he had slept. Pulling the sheet from the bed, she padded out to the other room. Mark was standing at the window. Slipping her arms around him, she kissed his back. "Morning." "Good morning. Did you sleep well?" "Mmmmmm." Ducking under his arm, she cuddled close.

"I wish the window opened," she said. "Why?" "So I could smell the salt air. It's been such a long time. I miss the beach house." "Maybe I can do something about that. How fast can you get dressed?" Mark asked. "Pretty fast, but what's the rush?" "You need to do some shopping, remember, and we don't have a whole lot of time left," he said.

She looked at his watch and was surprised by the time of day. "How could you let me sleep so long?" "You needed it. Now get dressed. I've got a bike waiting downstairs." She was ready in under ten minutes and they were on their way.

The sight of the motorcycle made her tingle. *Having my body pressed tight against Mark; the wind blowing in my face, it's nearly as exhilarating as making love.* She walked around the bike, taking in every exquisite detail. She stopped at the back of the bike. "How come it has Texas plates?" "It's one of mine. I had it shipped out, so we can have it with us on tour." "You are so incredible. Just when I thought I knew all of your special qualities, you surprise me with another one."

"I'm not special. I'm just hopelessly in love with my wife." "Oh Mark, you are special, special to me. You're everything I've dreamed of, hoped for, and I love you." "We had better get going, before we end up back upstairs." "Would that be so bad?" "Hell no; but I'm kind of looking forward to what you've got planned for Tony." "Well then, I guess we had better do some shopping."

She stood to the side while Mark started the bike. The thunderous explosion made her jump. This bike was much louder than any other she had heard before. With a nod of his head, Sabrina climbed on behind him, her arms tight around his chest. Mark cruised through the streets of Miami, giving her a private tour of the city, before he stopped at the theatrical supply store. He waited outside for her. He wanted to go in with her, but he didn't feel good about leaving his bike.

She returned quickly; tucking her parcel into the leather saddle bag. "So where to now?" she asked. "Well, we've got a couple of hours before we have to be at the arena. How about the beach?" "Yes please!" she announced with great enthusiasm.

They cruised along the road that paralleled the beach, passing numerous parking areas, but Mark kept going. *I wish I could ask him why he didn't stop, but he would never hear me over the roar of the bike.* Calming her anticipation, she resigned herself to the fact that this was as close as she was going to get. She laid her head against his shoulder and sighed.

Mark felt her body heave against him. *Only a little further.* Finally catching sight of the landmark that he had been searching for, he slowed the bike and turned off the road, coasting across the hard packed sand, stopping only a few feet from the water. Sabrina gave him a powerful hug before she jumped off the bike. Kicking off her boots, she headed straight to the water. It made him smile, to see her child like behavior. Running into the water, only to be chased back by the surf.

On her second run, she turned too quickly, falling forward into the sand as the surf washed over her. Mark was at her side in a second, helping her to her feet. "Are you okay?" "A little wet is all." "If I'd known you were going for a swim I would have brought a towel." "I don't need one," she said unbuttoning her shirt. "What are you doing?" "Taking these off so they'll dry. I'll hang them on the handlebars of the bike, and let the wind dry them for me." "Sabrina you can't. This is a public beach."

She scanned the beach in both directions. "I don't see any public. Don't tell me you're embarrassed? You shouldn't be; for you see I came prepared." She slipped off her shirt, exposing the top of her bathing suit. "You are such a tease," he scolded.

Wiggling out of her wet shorts, Mark took her clothes and hung them on the bike. Before he returned, he pulled a blanket from the saddle bags. Spreading it out on the sand, he reclined back on his arms, watching her frolic in the surf, wading out into the waves and diving into them. He relaxed when he saw her coming toward him; her golden body glistening with water, barely contained by her bathing suit. She crawled up beside him.

"Thank you," she said. Mark rolled her onto her back. His hand trailed down her body coming to rest on her belly. He leaned back a moment to look at her. "I really like this suit," he said, kissing the top of her breasts, that were being pushed over the top of her suit. "It's a bit too small." "No, it isn't." "It didn't use to be, but I have put on some weight," she said patting his hand. "Maybe; but it all went to the right places." He kissed her breast again.

"I have got to start going to the gym more." "We could work out together," he said. She saw how his eyes sparkled when he said that. "Explain that will you?" "We don't need to go to a gym for a workout; they say that sex burns more calories than any fitness machine." "Well, I'm willing to test your theory; starting tonight," she said with a smile and pulled him closer. As difficult as it was, Mark pulled back from her. "We have to go; but once tonight's show is over I'm gonna make sure that you get your required amount of exercise." "I can't wait." "Come on. We have a plan to execute."

They made a brief stop at the hotel, long enough for Sabrina to change, and help Mark pack their costumes. He wanted to get to the arena early, so that they had enough time to work out all of the details for the show. *I wish that there had been time for the costume designer to create a new outfit for her, but all of this came about so suddenly.*

Traffic was heavier than he anticipated. He had to slow the big bike to a crawl. It gave him a chance to scan the shops along their route. One in particular caught his attention; he pulled the bike to the curb. "Where are we going now?" Sabrina asked. "There," he said pointing to a shop that catered to the gothic trend. "What do you need from there?" "I need nothing; but you need a new costume." Sabrina followed him, as he pawed through the racks of dresses; ignoring the sales clerks offer to help. He pulled a dress from the rack. "This one," he said showing it to Sabrina.

He held up a long black dress, with a quilted bodice that laced up the front, and a full flowing skirt with many layers of sheer black fabric. Attached to the top of the side seams, and to two points on the center back, was a cape of black sheer. Finger loops made it look like wings of a bat. There was a pair of separate pull on sleeves to complete the strapless outfit.

"Sir," the clerk interrupted. "This top is meant to go with that dress." "It needs nothing more!" he snapped, ignoring the item she held up. "Except maybe this." He picked up a black velvet choker, a figure of a bat dangling from it. "We'll take these," he said handing the items to the clerk. "You are going to try it on?" "No, I don't need to. He's never been wrong yet," Sabrina answered, slipping her arms around Mark. "I love you." "I love you too, and I can't wait to see Tony's reaction. Man he's gonna have a heart attack."

The arena was relatively quiet as they drove inside. The fans were beginning to crowd around the entrance gates, waiting, chanting, for the doors to open. The crew was busy checking cables, testing lights and sound equipment. They looked up briefly as the thunderous roar of the motorcycle echoed through the corridors.

Sabrina sought out their dressing room, while Mark went to find the make up artist. While she waited for his return, she laid out their costumes, along with the special effects that she had purchased earlier, a set of reusable fangs, and a package of blood capsules.

"You can get your make up done anytime, the sooner the better though, while it's still quiet. I've told her what look you should have, so don't change it." "Okay." "Damn." "What's wrong?" "Nothing; I have to make a couple of calls. I'll see you back here when Maggies's done with you." Mark started to walk out the door. Sabrina ran after him, grabbing his arm.

"What's with all the orders? Don't I have a say anymore?" she asked. "I'm sorry; of course you have a say. I just got carried away. I have this vision of how you should look tonight. I know I should have consulted you and I am sorry."

"I'm not mad. I just don't understand why we need to make all these changes." "I just want to give the fans something extra special tonight. I want them to leave here with a vision of you etched into their minds forever." "Mark, you're the star, not me. My presence is insignificant." "After tonight, you will be a star; I promise." He kissed her. "Now go on, Maggie's waiting."

It took Maggie, and her assistant, nearly a full hour to create the look that Mark had requested; transforming Sabrina into a Gothic beauty. Maggie had worked for different wrestling companies for nearly twenty years, her talent for make up was exceptional, but Mark's request was proving to be her biggest challenge yet. The coloring had to be just right for Sabrina to be believable. Maggie colored and shaded, and highlighted, while her assistant was employed in the task of turning Sabrina's hair into a thick mass of soft curls.

Maggie took a step back, moving from one side to the other, looking at her creation from all angles. She smiled, pleased with her creation. "You're done," she announced. "Good. Can I see?" "I'm sorry, but I was instructed not to. He wants you to wait until you're in costume before you get your first peak." *That's what he thinks.* Sabrina remembered the big mirror in the dressing room.

Mark was already dressed when she returned. He had his back to her. She went to him, but he turned away quickly. "What's with you?" she asked. "I don't want to see you until you're dressed. I want to see the whole effect all at once, not in bits and pieces." "Well, if you're gonna stay like that and not look at me I might as well get dressed right here, we can at least talk. Can't we?" "Sure; we can go over the plan."

Glancing over to the mirror, Sabrina saw that it was completely covered with newspaper. "Why did you do that?" "Do what?" "Cover the mirror. No, don't bother; I already know the answer." She dropped her blouse on the table, along with her shorts. Loosening the laces on the dress, she stepped into it.

Mark rambled on about what they were going to do. She listened to key points, but her attention was centered on her dress. She tightened the laces, but without a mirror it was hard to know if they were even. She left the space wider across her breasts. Before she pulled on the sleeves, she fixed the velvet choker around her neck. Next were the finger loops on the veil, and her shoes.

"Okay, ready when you are," she announced. Mark spun around; the anticipation was weighing heavy on him. Sabrina had raised her arms up, crossing them in front of her face. Slowly she lowered them away. She watched his eyes as they widened, the lower her arms went.

"Well?" Sabrina asked. Mark stepped closer, walking around her slowly. "It's perfect; absolutely perfect," he said, moving around in front of her. "Can I see now?" she asked. "Oh yeah, sure." He ripped the paper from the mirror; Sabrina walked towards it, staring intently at her image.

"I look ghastly," she remarked on the pale makeup on her face. "It's just part of the effect," he said caressing her shoulders. "Personally, I think you look very sexy. Drop dead gorgeous in fact." "Don't be such a smart ass." He moved his hands around her, settling on her breasts. "What are you doing?" Sabrina asked. "You mean besides having a little fun." "Yeah." "You need to move these up a little higher," he said. Her head tilted back to him. "You lift and I'll tighten." *I want to take her in my arms and kiss her at this very moment, but I can't risk spoiling the makeup.* He settled for kissing her shoulder.

Satisfied with her look, he backed away. "Now for the final touch." He handed her the tooth caps. Sabrina carefully applied the adhesive and placed each cap. "Well?" "Perfect! Baby they're gonna love you." Sabrina lowered her head as she walked away. "Hey now, why so sad?"

"I'm beginning to think that this isn't such a good idea anymore. Those people out there buy tickets to see you, not me." "After tonight they're gonna want to see you. They're gonna make you a star." "I don't want to be a star! I only want to be your wife, your lover, and with a little luck, the mother of your children. What we've been doing is just fine. My presence has had no significant meaning, and that's perfectly fine with me."

Mark put his arms around her. "I think you have a case of stage fright." "I don't think so. I'm just not cut out for all of this; but if it makes you happy." "Wrong answer. I don't want you doing something just because you think it makes me happy. You have to do what feels right to you. Listen; I'll make you a deal. You carry through with tonight, exact revenge on Tony, and if you still feel the same way after, then it's fine with me to keep everything the way it was," he said. She hugged him tight.

"Besides," he continued. "Nick may not like this idea anyway." "You didn't tell him?" "Hell no; and spoil the surprise." "What am I going to do with you?" "Wear that outfit back to the hotel," he whispered, teasing at her ear with his tongue. "Yeah right; like I'm gonna get on that bike dressed like this." "What about undressed?"

She smiled and laughed at his question. "Thank you." "For what?" "For knowing how to make me feel better." "I've just begun." His devilish grin told her more than his words ever could.

The knock at the door was a welcomed relief for Mark. *I was becoming lost in her eyes, and her touch. A few more minutes and I would have given in to the passion.* "Now remember, don't take your robe off until its time," he said fastening it about her. "We don't want to give away our secret too soon." Sabrina had begun to regain her devilish sense of humor, and her love of practical jokes. "By the time I'm through with Tony, he's gonna think twice before he tries messing with anyone's mind." "Come on. Let's give them a show to remember."

Tony was already in the ring, leaning against the turnbuckle. The Warlock's entrance music began; the arena erupted into loud, screaming cheers. Mark checked Sabrina's outfit. He peered in at her face. "Your victim awaits."

They stepped through the curtain together; the volume increased to a deafening roar. Mark deliberately slowed their approach to the ring. Tonight he treated the fans, giving them the opportunity to take more pictures.

Once in the ring, Sabrina began her seductive performance, removing Mark's robe as she rubbed against him. Before she left the ring, she passed by Tony, dragging her finger nails slowly across his chest. His reaction was to side step away from her; but he was curious as to why she still wore her robe. *Every other time she took it off. What's she up to?*

The bell sounded. Mark stalked Tony before engaging him in a hold. Sabrina wandered around the ring. *This won't be a very long match. Mark is supposed to win; but even if he wasn't, his size and strength alone is no match for Tony.*

The two men battled back and forth. Tony struck several blows, but could not get Mark off his feet. Grabbing Tony by the arm, Mark whipped him across the ring. Tony hit the ropes, using them to catapult himself back towards Mark. With his arm outstretched, Mark caught him in a move called a clothesline. Tony hit the mat, stunned, his head pounding from the force.

Mark glanced at Sabrina; her signal. She slipped the blood capsules into her mouth, hiding them under her tongue. Still reeling, Tony was aware that Mark had pulled him up. In seconds he was looking at the audience upside down. Mark had set him up for a pile driver. He felt the downward motion and then nothing. The sudden impact with the mat knocked him out.

Mark parted the ropes for Sabrina. She entered, hovering precariously over Tony. She moved back to Mark as a hush fell over the crowd. They watched in anticipation as Mark gently caressed her shoulders, moving his hands slowly up her neck to remove her hood. Whistles of recognition resounded towards her. Mark pulled her robe off with a swift jerk. The whistles turned to cat calls as she caressed his chest.

He pointed to Tony's body. Spreading her arms to show off the bat like cape, Sabrina moved back to her victim. The crowd was silenced again, as she knelt down, slowly crawling her body up over his. Turning his head, her lips came close to his, but did not touch. He was still out cold. Leaning down to his neck, biting the capsules, she attached her lips to his neck, the blood slowly seeping from her mouth.

Cameras flashed wildly. She closed her eyes to avoid them. Mark touched her shoulder. Lifting her head to look at him, the blood trickled over her lips; there was a gasp from the crowd. Pulling her up, Mark wiped a droplet from her chin, licking it from his finger. "Time to wake him up," he said.

Mark slapped Tony on the face. He flinched; his eyes fluttered open. As he began to focus more clearly, he saw Sabrina; her lips stained red. She smiled at him, showing her teeth. Tony put his hand to his throat. Pulling it away, he saw the blood on his hand. He crawled backwards away from her. Sabrina took a step toward him. "Get away from me! Christ, somebody get her away!" Tony yelled, the fear controlling the vibration in his voice.

I can hear the fear in his voice; but the game is not over yet. Sabrina knelt close to him, reaching her hand to him. He couldn't get away. She ran her fingers along his neck; bringing them back close to her lips, she sensuously licked the red liquid from her fingers. Tony saw her teeth again. He grabbed his neck and rolled out of the ring, setting off at a staggered run back up the ramp.

Mark had taken up a microphone. He called to Tony, still staggering on the ramp. "Your soul belongs to her now, and to me. She has feasted on your essence, your life force. You are the first to be sacrificed to her hunger. All of you are warned. There will be others."

Tony stumbled through the curtain, yelling for a paramedic. The crowd roared; straining to touch Sabrina as she walked past them. She hesitated a moment as fans screamed at her, begging to be her next victim. Mark had to take her arm, to urge her on.

As they passed through the curtain, Sabrina pointed to Tony, running frantically, calling for a paramedic, and recounting his experience to anyone who would listen. Mark tugged Sabrina to the side of the entrance. In the shadows his lust controlled him; he kissed her. The sweet liquid on her lips ignited his hunger for her. He braced her against the wall; his kisses wild.

"Wait," she panted. "Someone might see us." "I don't care." "Well, I do," she said struggling to hold him back. "Take me to the dressing room, where we can have some privacy."

They stole past the small crowd, that had gathered around Tony. He ranted wildly about what she had done to him, while still keeping his hand protectively over his neck. Sabrina giggled to herself. *My revenge has played out perfectly. That will teach him.* Her thoughts quickly changed, as Mark shut the dressing room door.

Lifting her up, she wrapped her legs around his waist. He pinned her against the wall. His kisses were intense. She held him at bay, trying to catch her breath. "If I'd only known that this performance would turn you on so much I would have suggested it sooner." "Stop talking," he said as he kissed her again. "I want you." "Then take me," she whispered.

His beard tingled on her neck. She pressed his head tighter to her, feeling his teeth gently nip at her skin. With her held firmly against the wall by his body, it allowed him the opportunity to loosen the laces of her dress, freeing her breasts for his pleasure.

An unwelcome sound distracted them. "You did lock the door?" she asked. "I'm sure I did." Their answer came as Nick burst into the room. "Who in the hell do," his voice halted, as he looked at them. He turned away quickly. Sabrina slid down over Mark, clinging to him, hiding her nudity, and his arousal.

Mark's anger seethed to the surface. "Man don't you ever knock! What gives you the right to barge in here anyway?" "I'm your boss, or have you forgotten that? And what gives you the right to pull a stunt like that without clearing it with me first!" Sabrina looked up at Mark. "Here it comes," she said quietly.

Mark stared into her eyes. *This view is much more calming than looking into Nick's angry face.* Nick had paused a moment to regain his composure. "Damn it Mark you know better than to try something like this without my approval. Oh what the hell; I loved it!" "You did?" Sabrina asked in surprise. She had expected Nick to hand Mark a suspension. "Hell yeah I did. I'm not forgiving you for excluding me though; but I do understand why you kept it quiet. The element of surprise was definitely the key. Did you see," he began to laugh heartily. "Did you see Tony? He's running around screaming for a paramedic, telling everybody his blood type."

Nick's laugh became infectious, afflicting Sabrina first. Nick loosened his tie as he sat down. "What ever made you think of something like this?" "Let's just say that Tony did something to piss me off," Sabrina answered. "Well, I like how you get revenge." He rubbed at his chin, sorting out the thoughts that suddenly rushed into is mind. Using the silence, Sabrina pulled her dress back together. Mark sighed as he watched her tighten the laces. She touched his chest giving him a pouty I'm sorry look.

Nick summoned them to the table. "You two have come up with a great new angle. You can't use it for every show though. We have to reserve this for pay per views or select televised shows." "I just did it as a practical joke. I didn't plan for it to go any further." "Too late, especially after what Mark said." Sabrina had forgotten; she glared at Mark. "Don't give me that look. I've been in this business long enough to know when the fans are ready for a new twist to the characters," Mark said.

"He's right. It's the only way to keep them coming back. We'll have to see what response we get in the mail; but I think that this idea of yours is going to be a big hit. I should get you thinking about some of the other guys." "In what way?" Sabrina asked. "You might be able to come up with some ideas for their characters."

Rolling her eyes back, Sabrina got up. "Nick, I can't get into this right now; my mind just isn't into it. I'm not turning you down; I just need some time to think about it." She collected her clothes and retreated into the bathroom. Mark saw his opportunity slip away. *She's going in there to change; to take off that dress, and I'm not going to be a part of it.*

He turned a cold hard stare to Nick. "I'm only gonna say this once, and you had better commit it to memory. If she decides to do this stunt again, you are never, for any reason, to come to the dressing room after. Don't even entertain the thought; got it!"

Nick replayed, in his mind, the scene that he had walked in on. "Sure, no problem," he said getting up to leave. "By the way, I would like to talk to you both tomorrow." "About what?" "I've got some ideas for the Halloween pay per view and I need your input." Nick was out the door before Mark could ask any more questions.

With a heavy sigh, Mark locked the door. He pulled off his shirt and sat on the bench, running his hand through his hair. Sabrina peeked around the corner. *It saddens me to see Mark looking so dejected; but I have a plan that will lift his spirits; and maybe something else.*

She crept across the room, coming up behind him, gently laying her hands on his shoulders. "I'll be ready in a few minutes," he said. "There's no need to rush. I'm not in any hurry to leave. Did you lock the door?" "Yeah; but I don't know why; Nick ruined everything." "Oh ye of little faith." She stepped over the bench and stood in front of him. "You're not changed!" "No." She lifted her skirt slightly to sit in his lap and lock her ankles behind his back. "I put it on; but you my love, you have to take it off."

The invitation she's presenting to me is far too tempting to resist. His body readily answered her request.

I like how he responds. It brought a smile to her face; fueling her craving. *The desire I have for him, for his body, has always been strong, but lately it has become even more intense. Wanting, needing, the gratification that he brings to me. I can't get enough of him, or of the feelings that he inspires in my own body. Merely thinking about making love to him brings me to the brink of ecstasy, but why? What is driving my desire; fueling my unquenchable lust? Tonight is no exception. It doesn't matter anymore where or when, just how often, how long and how intense.*

Chapter 20

The flight to San Antonio was long, the plane stuffy. Sabrina slept the entire time, cradled in Mark's arms. *She's exhausted, as am I. I hate tours like this; being bounced from end of the country to the other. I've learned to adjust fairly quickly to the time changes, but Sabrina isn't as resilient. Yet she tries. Pretending that all this traveling is exhilarating, but the truth comes out at times like this. Blaming her naps on the warm conditions on the plane; but I know better. Fortunately, the show, isn't until tomorrow afternoon, giving us time for a much needed rest; but only if she lets me. Between trying to play tourist and being lost in the pleasures of love; a good night's sleep seems like only a memory.*

He stroked her silky hair; she shifted, but stayed asleep. Her hand rubbed gently at her belly. *I've noticed that she's been doing that a lot lately. I can't help wondering about it. She never said that her stomach was bothering her. Maybe she's still tormented by the loss of our child. We haven't really talked about it in a long time, but it must still hurt. I know it hurts me even now. Someday, when her body is healed and the pain is gone from her heart, we'll talk about trying again, but I can be as patient as she needs.*

Having a family is not a top priority, making sure she stays healthy, that is my single priority. Maybe, when we get home to Dallas tomorrow night, I can persuade her to go and see Doc Brown. If nothing else, then maybe Doc can explain to me her increased sexual appetite. Not that I'm complaining, I quite enjoy her amorous advances. Her drive equals my own. Maybe deep down I am making up for all those years of being alone, but what is her excuse? Can it simply be that love drives her, or is there something more, something I don't understand? Doc will have the answers.

The annoying sound of the intercom, accompanied by the scratchy voice of the pilot, brought Sabrina out of her slumber. She stretched and yawned, rubbing the kink out of her neck. "Did you have a good sleep?" Mark asked. "Not long enough." "We'll be at the hotel soon and you can continue your sleep." "That sounds good to me." "Share a ride to the hotel?" Brent asked, as he leaned over the seats. "Sure, why not."

Sabrina stayed quiet, keeping close to Mark, while they collected their luggage. They had barely settled into the limo when she secured herself into his arms, the gentle motion of the car soothing her into sleep again.

"She's really tired," Brent spoke softly. "Yeah." "It has been one hell of a tour, but add in all the extra crap you've had to deal with and I can understand why she's exhausted." "That's for sure. I'll be glad to get her home; she can have a few days to recuperate." "We're going home?" Sabrina asked through a yawn. "Yes, we are." "When?" "Tomorrow, right after the show," Mark answered.

She nuzzled her face into his neck. "Thank you." "You're welcome; now go back to sleep." "I can't." "Why not?" "I'm hungry," she said rubbing at her belly. "You had dinner on the plane." "I know; but I'm still hungry." "When we get to the hotel you can get something from room service." "They won't have what I want." "What would that be?" "Mexican!" she loudly announced.

With a shake of his head, Mark instructed the driver to find a restaurant that would satisfy her strange request. Sabrina rubbed at her belly with anticipation, as the limo pulled to a stop. "Do you know what you want?" Mark asked. "Sure do! Two soft tacos, with lots of hot sauce; the hottest they've got, please." "What about you Brent, what would you like?" "Only a soda for me." "Oh, me too please," Sabrina added. "Thank you." "You're welcome, but I really think that this is a mistake." "Why?" "I'm just afraid that your stomach won't be able to handle it, and you're gonna be up all night regretting this little snack."

Straddling his legs, she looked into his green eyes. "There's only one thing that could keep me awake tonight; and we both know what that is." The impish grin on her face made her irresistible. He pulled her to him. Their lips met tenderly at first, but deepening, as thoughts of making love raced through their minds.

Brent stared at them briefly, before casting his eyes to the floor; but he couldn't escape the sounds. The subtle purring sound that she made every time they kissed; it drove Brent deeper into his own frustration. When the driver returned with their order he was thankful of the interruption.

Sabrina began devouring her taco with great pleasure, savoring every bite. "Is it hot enough for you?" Mark asked. "Not really, here, try it for yourself," she said offering it to Mark. Mark took a bite. Within seconds his mouth felt like it was on fire. His eyes watered profusely as he chewed rapidly, washing it down with half of his soda. He wiped the sweat from his brow.

"Christ, how can you eat that?" "Easy. Do you think that there's something wrong with it?" "Yeah; it's hotter than hell. It feels like my mouth is blistered. Man I've never had anything so hot." "I don't understand; it's not nearly hot enough. Brent, tell me what you think." "No thanks, Sabrina. I'm not partial to Mexican." "Suit yourselves." Perspiration still formed on Mark's forehead, as he watched her consume the last of her snack.

I can't wait to get to the hotel. I've got to get another drink, and to find something to put out the fire that's burning in my stomach. I don't understand her. These snacks have been getting more bizarre over the last few weeks. Her insatiable sex drive and outrageous meal choices are both equally perplexing. Doc will have the answers because I sure can't figure it out.

Brent stayed with Sabrina at the front desk, while Mark stepped into the small gift shop, even though his attention was focused on the bar across the lobby. "Am I keeping you from something?" Sabrina asked. "What?" "If you have plans don't let me keep you, Mark won't be very long." "No, I have nothing special planned for tonight." "Well, the way you keep staring at the bar makes me think that you have a date waiting for you." "I wish! It's been so long I don't remember what that is anymore." "Oh come on; a good looking, sexy man like you should be dripping with women."

"It used to be like that; but since my divorce I can't get much action of any kind. I've almost forgotten what a woman feels like," Brent answered, trying to hide his sigh. The compassionate side of Sabrina surfaced; she stepped close to Brent; her arms outstretched. "Come here," she said softly. He was somewhat reluctant, but he felt the need to be comforted. *She can't give me what I truly need, but just being able to hold her will help to sustain me for the night.*

Slipping into his arms, her body pressed tight against his. Her breasts pushed against his chest as she breathed. With his eyes closed, Brent reveled in the feel of her body. His hands gently caressed her back. Sabrina became very aware of the arousal her gesture was bringing to him; she pressed her lips to his ear.

"I wish I could help you more, but," as she spoke her hand came to rest on the front of his belt. Brent pushed her back. "I'm sorry." His embarrassment made him blush. "Don't be sorry. I've known about your desires for quite some time." "How? Never mind, I know the answer." "I'm very flattered that you find me desirable; but I'm much more impressed by the fact that you haven't let it compromise our friendship." Without hesitation she kissed him full on the lips. "Thank you," he said. "You're welcome. Just promise me that you'll be careful." "I promise; always practice safe sex; no matter what."

The sound of Mark's voice startled them both; Sabrina jumped back. "What's going on?" Mark asked. Sabrina detected not the usual relaxed tone of his voice, but one that was lightly shadowed by anger, and just a hint of jealousy. She went to him; her arms encircled his chest, but his stayed limp at his sides. His eyes were piercing as he glared at her. "Are you going to answer me?" "It was just a little hug between friends, that's all," she said. His expression reflected skepticism.

Seeing, and feeling the tension, Brent excused himself from their presence. *Better to seek the solitude of the bar, than to face an inquisition from Mark. I'm uncomfortable with leaving Sabrina alone like that, but staying would only serve to anger Mark more.*

Mark distanced himself from Sabrina all the way to their room. *For the first time I'm feeling, from him, the rejection that I had experienced with my mother so long ago. It frightens and angers me. We've come so far together, and I'm not about to let a simple hug jeopardize our future.*

Dropping their bags on the floor, Mark headed to the bathroom, Sabrina close behind him. When he closed, and locked the door, she knew she was being punished. *Why? For what reason? It was only a simple hug, or had he seen us exchange a kiss? That shouldn't have upset him. I have to explain, put his fears to rest; if only I could get in there.* The sound of the shower increased her urgency.

Tearing through her cosmetic bag, she found a hair pin small enough to fit into the lock. Working diligently, she freed the barrier that kept her from him. Kicking off her shoes, she carefully stepped into the bathroom. From the shadows on the shower curtain, she knew exactly where Mark was. With great care, she pulled back the curtain enough for her to pass through. Mark did not hear her; his back was to her; his arms braced against the wall.

The water sprayed over his lowered head, soaking her to the skin. She had not bothered to remove her clothes. This discussion was far too important. Sabrina reached out, gently touching his back. Mark straightened up, pulling away from her. "What are you doing in here?" "We need to talk," she said tugging at his arm. "Mark, please look at me." "There's nothing to talk about." "Yes, there is. Something pissed you off and I want to know what it is." "Leave it alone!" "No, I won't. Damn it Mark talk to me."

His silence upset her more than if he had yelled at her. She lashed out, striking him on the back. "Damn you! Why do you have to be so pig headed?" she yelled. He turned around, grabbing her wrists. The look on his face terrified her more than his angry tone.

"How the hell am I supposed to feel! Seeing you kiss him like that; it makes me think that there's something going on between you two." "Don't be ridiculous!" She struggled to free herself. "You're hurting me!" He saw the tears in her eyes, and the bright red marks his fingers made on her wrists. He let her go, pushing himself away from her.

"Damn it Mark; I don't understand you! Why would you doubt my love for you?" "What am I supposed to think? I walk into something like that and you blow me off by lying to me." "Maybe I did, and I'm sorry; but I was only trying to protect Brent from the embarrassment." "Protecting him from me is more like it!" "Would you stop being so damn stubborn and listen to me! Brent is my, our friend, and he was feeling a little sad. I was just trying to cheer him up, to let him know that he doesn't have to feel alone." "If that's your cure for sadness, I hate to think what you'd do if he was really depressed, or have you all ready provided him with that solution?"

Tears burned in her eyes. "I don't believe you! You have the nerve to question my fidelity. You've hurt me Mark, emotionally, and physically." She held out her arms, showing him the deep red marks that he had made in her skin. "I would never break our vows. My life is with you and only you. If you would search your heart you'd know that."

He stared at her in silence; her eyes told him the truth. Focusing on her arms, his anger washed away, as feelings of shame and remorse flooded over him. He pulled her to him. "I'm so sorry that I doubted you. Please forgive me, if you can." Sabrina cradled his face in her hands. "I do forgive you; I love you to much not to; and don't ever doubt that. You are, and will always be, the only man in my life." She kissed him tenderly. "Let me show you how much I love you."

"How can you even think about that now?" "Because I love you and I need you as much as you need me right now." She kissed him again, refusing to back off until he responded to her. His hands struggled to find her body beneath her wet clothes. "Why did you wear your clothes into the shower?" "It's not important; you are important. Now help me get them off." With some reservation, he aided her with her request.

Ever since Sean took her from me I've had this horrid fear that it could happen again. I know in my heart that Brent would never be capable of that but seeing her in the arms of another man brings out feelings that frighten me. No matter how hard I try I can't shake that vision of Sean as he violated her. I can't lock her away from people just because I can't control my fear or my jealousy. She loves me and only me I do know that. I don't deserve her, but her tender touch has broke through my defenses, bringing back the feelings of love that I need at this moment.

Sabrina brought life back to his body. The anticipation pleased her. She urged him to her until he had fulfilled her desire. Mark held her, kissing her ear. "I'm sorry I doubted you." "Hush now," she whispered as her soft kisses came across his cheek to his lips. "Take me to bed, and hold me until the morning." "With pleasure."

Mark was already in bed when she came out of the bathroom. Her hair was still damp and tousled about in disarray. At that moment he thought her to be extraordinarily sexy. He lifted up the sheet for her. She knelt beside him for a brief moment, only to settle astride his hips.

"What are you doing?" he asked. "You said that you believed me, that I would never be unfaithful to you, but we still need to talk this through; so that you completely understand, and are comfortable with what happened." "We don't have to." "Yes, we do. I don't want you to have any doubts about me, or Brent." "I told you I don't."

"Hold onto that thought, and listen to me with your heart." She leaned down giving him a kiss. Mark tried to keep her close to him, but she pulled back. With a slow deep breath, Sabrina entwined her fingers with Mark's, keeping her thumbs free, so she could gently stroke them against his.

"I don't know if you've noticed or not, but Brent is not the same man that I met a few months ago. He's changed, since his divorce," Sabrina began. "I haven't noticed anything different." "The change wasn't dramatic, and it didn't occur over night. Remember back, before his divorce; he was, how can I say this, more energetic, more vibrant; and never lacked for female companionship." "Yeah, I remember. So what's different now?" Mark asked.

"Since his divorce, well, he hasn't really been with a woman for any length of time." "That's crap; Brent always has somebody to keep him warm at night." "Not any more; and it's getting to him. What you saw tonight, was only me offering what little comfort I could. I don't like seeing him so depressed and alone." "Then why did you kiss him like that?" "He needed it. He needed to know that he has friends who care about him." "Wouldn't a simple hug have done that?" "Yes maybe it would, but I kissed him because it had to be done; to put an end to a fantasy." "I don't understand?"

Shifting slightly, she brought his hands around her back. With her own hands free she caressed his chest. "Please do not get upset; but Brent is, well, attracted to me, at least physically." "That son of a." "Mark, please, just calm down. There's nothing to it. I've known about it for quite some time, even though Brent has kept it very well disguised. He knows that it's just a dream, that it would never go anywhere." "How can you be sure?" "I know Brent. He values our friendship too much."

She couldn't avoid the scrutinizing glare from Mark; she lowered herself close to him. "And I know me. I love you and I would never betray that love, ever." The lines in his face began to relax, his eyes lost their intensity; Sabrina smiled. "I'm glad that you understand. Brent is like the brother I never had, and I do care about him; but my heart and soul belong to you, and only you."

Mark quickly flipped her onto back. "I'm sorry that I doubted you; and I'm sorry that I hurt you. My feelings got the better of me when I saw you two together. My imagination took over and that opened the door for jealousy. For an instant it made me remember that night when Sean took you from me. I know the situation isn't exactly the same, but to see another man holding you like that. I'm sorry I let those feelings surface again."

Sabrina stroked his face with the back of her hand. "Shhhh; you shouldn't feel sorry. You're a man. If you didn't have those feelings, then I'd be worried." "That's not an excuse for what I did." He kissed her neck. "And I'm gonna spend the rest of my life making it up to you." He kissed her cheek. "Starting right now." He kissed her lips, as he slowly removed her towel.

Brent rolled onto his side, pushing the sheets down to his waist. His body glistened with sweat. In the darkness of his room, he vividly recalled the sensation of Sabrina's lips on his. *How her touch had set my blood on fire.* He felt movement beside him and a hand slid over his waist. Warm, soft lips kissed his shoulder. *I'm not in the mood for this again.*

"You can go," he said. "I don't want to," replied the sultry feminine voice. "I want to stay here and make love to you." "I said go!" Brent snapped. "Just get your stuff and leave me alone!" "Fucking bastard!" She pushed away from him. He listened, never turning; laying on his back when the door shut.

When he had left Mark and Sabrina, he had gone to the hotel bar. Deliberately avoiding Mark, and the immanent questions. Sitting at the bar, he had consumed half a beer when a young woman sat down beside him. She initiated the conversation; knowing exactly who he was; and his reputation. Brent only had to ask her once if she wanted to go up to his room. *I know I was being ignorant, not even asking her name, but I really didn't care. Sabrina had lit the desire, and I needed it fulfilled.*

Keeping the lights out, he had no need to see her face again, all he needed was her curvaceous body. Weeks of loneliness, and pent up frustration drove him on. Fueling his fantasy, using this body over and over, until exhaustion forced him to back off. *I know I was cold and harsh, dismissing her the way I did, but I had no further need of her. All I can think about is Sabrina. I wonder if Mark accepted her explanation of the situation, or if he's letting his imagination block out the truth?*

The phone was on its fourth ring when Sabrina pawed the annoying device from its cradle. "Hello." "Good morning Sabrina, it's Nick." "Good morning, and what can I do for you?" Sabrina asked. Nick's voice became lost to her as Mark began to nibble at her ear. "I know what I can do to you," he whispered.

Sabrina tried to pull herself away. "I'm sorry Nick. What did you say?" "I said that I'd like to come up and talk to you and Mark, about the Halloween pay per view." In his efforts to distract her Mark found the sensitive spot just above her waist and she flinched. "Don't do that!" she scolded Mark. "Why not?" Nick answered. "Sorry Nick, I wasn't talking to you."

She giggled, as Mark continued to torment her with his scintillating touch. "Sure come on up," she said continuing her conversation with Nick. "I already am," Mark whispered, as he kissed her chest. Sabrina was having difficulty concentrating. "Oh, and Nick, bring something from room service. We can talk over breakfast." "Sure, that sounds good. Anything else?" Nick asked. Mark was on top of her, tugging at the phone. "Yeah Nick, don't rush," she said as Mark gently tugged the phone away from her.

Mark blindly replaced the phone. *I don't want to divert any of my attention from her, or her sweet lips.* She pushed him back enough to look at him. "You're bad," she scolded. "So! I told you last night that I'm gonna make amends for my behavior." "I remember; but you could have waited until I was off the phone." "No, I couldn't. So what does Nick want?" Mark asked. Sabrina began to answer, then hesitated. "I'm not sure. Oh well," she sighed slipping her arms around him. "Now where were we? Oh yes," she smiled guiding his hips. "Right about there." "Now who's being bad?" "Enough talking."

Nick paced the hallway outside their room; he was waiting for room service to arrive. *I wonder if I've given them enough time? I know, by what I heard on the phone, that again I had interrupted them, but time is running out. The pay per view date is just over two weeks away, and I need an answer from them now. There is much preparation to do. New costumes, choreography; it all has to be worked out. The event has to be perfect.*

An evening that the fans will talk about for years, and the after party, their reception, that I so desperately want to give them. Mark deserves it. He's been loyal to me all these years, even when offers from other wrestling organizations tried to lure him away, Mark stayed on. This is going to be the hardest sell of my career. I have to persuade them to go through with it.

The elevator doors opened. A young man pushing a cart stepped out. Nick met him in the hallway. "It's about time!" he snapped. "I'll take it from here." He handed the attendant a generous tip and pushed the cart to the door; straightening his jacket before knocking. Mark opened the door. "Hey Nick, I didn't know that you had another job." "Very funny," he smirked pushing the cart into the room. Sabrina was stretched out on the sofa. "Morning Nick." "Sabrina. Where would you like this?" "Next to the table is fine." "Shall we?" Nick held a chair out for her.

Nick positioned himself opposite Mark and Sabrina; playing the perfect host, serving them before himself. Sabrina cast a discreet look towards Mark, hoping that he would start the conversation. Nick caught the subtle look and took the initiative. "We need to come to a decision about the Halloween pay per view. Have you given it any thought?" "Not really," Sabrina answered. "What exactly did you have in mind?" Mark asked. "Like

I told you before, I think that an in ring wedding would be a tremendous idea. The fans would get a real charge out of something like this. All I need is a yes from you and I can get started on the preparations. We don't have much time left."

Sabrina looked at Mark, searching his eyes for an answer. She could only shrug. "I don't know. The Sorceress, victim thing works; but a wedding, on Halloween; that I'm not sure about," Mark answered. "Sabrina, what do you think?" "I'm not completely sure Nick, but there is one thing I need to ask Mark before I can give you an answer." She rose from her seat wandering around the table before coming to sit in Mark's lap. She ran her fingers through his long auburn hair. "What did you want to ask me?"

She had a far away, dreamy look in her eyes. "I forget. Can you help me to remember?" "I have no idea what was on your mind a few minutes ago." "Try anyway," she whispered leaning in closer, kissing him softly. Suddenly she backed away. "Now I remember," she said stroking his cheek. "Warlock, will you marry me?"

Mark smiled at her. "Yes, I will marry you; again." "Well Nick, I guess you have your answer." "Yes, I most certainly do. This will be a great event." Tearing his eyes away from hers, Mark glanced over at Nick. "You will be taking care of the arrangements?" Mark asked. "Yes, everything." "Good, because we're going home, for a much needed rest." "That will be good, for both of you. If there's anything I need your approval on, I'll call; and as soon as I get the new costume designs, I'll send them over."

Mark had returned his gaze to Sabrina. Nick took his cue to leave. "I'll see you at the arena later," he said. "Sure," Mark muttered, unaware that Nick was now walking to the door. Sabrina casually waved to him as he shut the door behind him. Mark pulled her closer. "We're all alone. Any idea on what we can do?" Mark asked.

Sabrina teased him with short kisses. "I want you, to take me, to see the Alamo." "But I thought." "I know, but we will be home tonight, in our own bed, and." "What?" he asked lifting her face up. "I just don't want to be too tired to go up the hill." "Sabrina, it'll be dark." "I don't care! I have to go. He's been alone for so long." Mark wiped away the tear from her cheek, hugging her tight. "I miss him too baby."

The wind blew briskly off of the ocean, replacing the beads of perspiration on Sean's body with waves of rippling goose bumps. He scanned the horizon. The dark, ominous clouds indicated a storm was approaching, the first of the fall season. *The scavengers will be out tomorrow, combing the beaches for treasures brought in by the wind and the tide. I'll need to stay inside.* When he turned, to continue his jog, he realized that he was standing in front of Sabrina's old house.

It's been so long since I've seen her. It's difficult to remember what she looks like, even though I'm urged to talk about her every day with the Doctors. She still makes my heart warm, when I think about her, but the lust is diminishing. It's taken time, but I've finally come to understand what I did to her and inklings of remorse are beginning to surface.

If only I could talk to Sabrina, but that's still forbidden for now, but soon, the Doctors have been indicating that I may not require therapy for much longer. At least not the intense day to day regime that I've been under going. I'm confident that I can make things right again. All I need to do first is to apologize to her, and hope that her heart is big enough to forgive me.

The Alamo was not as stimulating as Sabrina had hoped. Crowded with tourists, yet she could feel the presence of the others. The ones who had stayed on here, long after their physical bodies had turned to dust. *I can hear them call to me. Please not again, I beg of you. Why do they whisper their torments to me? Why do they want me to feel their pain?*

She stayed close to Mark, keeping her arm around him at all times, deliberately avoiding looking into the shadowy corners. When Mark, sensing her unease, suggested that they leave, Sabrina quickly agreed.

He stopped her from getting on the bike, taking her in his arms. "They bother you; don't they?" Mark asked. "Who?" "The old ones." "No. Senior citizens don't bother me." "Sabrina you know what I mean." "How do you know about them?" "I know; you've talked in your sleep. You're feeling things again; like you did in Salem."

"No, not the same. This is different." "Different how?" Mark asked. "These feelings are; well, they're just different. I know that there are others here, but they just don't want to move on. They need to tell people about this place, about the pain, but they're comfortable here; this was a special place. They gave their lives protecting it, and even in death they continue to guard it."

"Is that what you felt in Salem?" "No!" Her lip quivered, as the tears burned in her eyes. "Tell me Sabrina. I never asked you about it when it happened, but you need to tell me now." "That house, in Salem, it is an evil place, filled with despair. Pain, and suffering, and death permeate its walls." "How do you know that?" "I died there!"

She lost herself in his hold. He stroked her back slowly, waiting for her to calm down. As her breathing slowed, Mark loosened his hold, yet she still trembled. He helped her onto the bike, and seated himself so he was facing her. "Can you tell me all of it now?" Mark asked, not really wanting to know the whole truth. "I'm not sure I know; let alone completely understand." "Please try."

"They were more than just feelings; strong and vivid; but much clearer than anything I've ever felt before. I felt the physical pain that time. My wrists burned from being bound by ropes. My body was covered with wounds, caused by my tormentors. It was so intense, and then nothing. No more pain, just calm, as my soul began its journey to the next life, but so many of them didn't find that peace. I could hear them, crying, begging for mercy."

"Do you know why you were being tortured?" "I had been accused of being a witch but given the times anything that appeared to be not consistent with the church was considered heresy." "I never really understood how people could claim to see the past, or the dead; but being with you has changed my opinion. I've watched you, and what you feel is very real. My own senses have become sharper, but only where you're concerned. I don't have the gift that you have."

"This is not a gift! I wish that I didn't have this. It scares me Mark. I don't understand why they come to me, or what they want from me. Sometimes they try to tell me things, but I can't understand what they want. Are they warning me of my future or helping me to understand my past? There has to be a reason behind it, but I just can't figure it out. Part of me wants to know, wants everything crystal clear, but then again part of me doesn't want to know any of it." "We don't have to talk about this again; unless you need to." "Thank you. I only want to concentrate on the present, and the future. These shadows have always been with me and will continue to be with me, but I'm going to have to learn to ignore them, for the most part anyway."

I wanted to know more, but when she told me that she died in that house, I couldn't bring myself to pursue the issue any further and I pray that she will never feel the need to discuss it ever again. Knowing the intimate details of her death nauseates me. The past is gone; the future is the only thing that matters.

The afternoon could have slipped away completely unnoticed with Sabrina in his arms; their hearts beating as one; but the unexpected interruption from a young fan, made Mark realize that they were close to being late for the show. Taking the extra time to each sign an autograph for the young boy, and to pose for a picture was done in haste. They had to leave before their presence drew any more attention. Mark knew that he was traveling faster than the speed limit, but he had to get to the arena before Nick realized that they were missing.

As they circled around the arena, Mark pointed out that the doors had already been opened, to let the fans in. He didn't have to look at his watch to know that there was less than an hour until the show started. He pulled the bike around back; coasting in to the backstage area.

Nick stood near the doorway; his arms folded across his chest. "Where in the hell have you been?" he snarled, as the bike went silent. "It's my fault Nick. I wanted to see the Alamo; but we're not late." "Well no; but you both know that I like my stars here at least an hour before the show."

Mark had the perfect come back for Nick, but Sabrina had taken his arm, gently tugging him toward the dressing room. "It's not worth it," she whispered. "You're right," he answered. Lifting her up he spun her around quickly. "Mark, stop, please!" He could hear the panic in her voice; he let her down; she ran, staggering, into the dressing room, and into the bathroom. She had barely made it to her knees when her stomach turned over.

When her body stopped its uncontrollable heaving, she pulled herself over to the sink and splashed cold water on her face; her head began to pound. Mark stepped around the corner. "Are you okay?" he asked. When she didn't answer, he proceeded into the room. She was still at the sink, leaning heavily on the edge. He went to her, touching her shoulder. Slowly she straightened up, turning towards him. Her eyes were so vividly blue against her pale complexion.

"What happened?" Mark asked. "I got really dizzy." "That's never happened when I've done that before." "I know, but this time it really got to me." He held her trembling form against him. "When we get home, I want you to make an appointment with Doc Brown." "That's not necessary." "Yes, it is. This is not normal. I won't let you take chances with your health and as for tonight you're not going out there." "This time I will agree with you. I don't feel like doing anything, except sleeping." "Well, there's a sofa out there waiting for you." Guiding her back into the dressing room he helped to lay down, covering her with a robe for warmth.

It seemed that only minutes had passed, when Sabrina was awakened by Mark's touch. "You're not dressed," she said as she turned on her side. "You'll be late for the show." Mark smiled. "I won't be late; the show is over. You've been asleep for nearly two hours." "No. I couldn't have." "You did; but you needed it. So how do you feel now?" "Not bad." "Do you think you can manage the flight home, or would you like to stay over another night?"

Without hesitation, she slid herself closer to him. "I want to go home. The one thing that I might have trouble with is being on the back of that bike." "Not to worry, the bike has all ready been shipped home. There's a car waiting to take us to the airport." "I'm ready if you are."

The rush of take off made Sabrina feel queasy. It began to pass as the plane leveled out. Mark saw how her color had faded out, he put his arm around her. "You feeling okay?" "Not really. Maybe I'm coming down with something." "All the more reason for you to see Doc when we get home." "That's not necessary. It's probably just the flu." "Brought on by these damn tours that you're still not used to. You haven't been getting enough rest." Sabrina leaned into him, as close as the seats would allow. "Maybe, but there's a very pleasurable reason behind that." "I can't argue that. I should ask Nick to reduce my schedule, make it less hectic; it would give us both more time to rest between shows."

"You can if you want, but I will adjust in time; and besides, we both know what free time leads to." "Yes, I do; but that should change the longer we're married." "Don't bet on it," she answered, slipping her fingers in between the buttons of his shirt. "I don't know what I'm going to do with you," he said. "I have a few suggestions," Sabrina answered with a shy grin. "I don't want to hear them; not until Doc says that you're okay. Then we can explore your ideas, as well as some of my own." She looked up at him, her eyes wide with the possibility of hearing more. Mark gently touched her cheek. "I'm not going to tell you, so don't even try. Now fasten your seat belt."

Sabrina forced herself to stay awake during the drive home. Her body begged her to give in, but she persisted, scanning the passing scenery, concentrating on every detail. *I have to show Mark that I'm well enough to go up the hill. If he senses any weakness he will make me wait until tomorrow; but that is not acceptable. I have to go up there tonight. I need to sit with my baby for a little while.*

The feeling of emptiness, of loss, still echoed in her belly. Unconsciously she stroked her hands across it. Mark had been quietly watching her actions. *I too, still feel the pain.* He took her hand into his. "We'll be home very soon, but it will be too dark to go up the hill. We can go in the morning and spend as much time as you want up there." *That's not the answer I want to hear.* Her only response to him was a noncommittal nod.

The house was shrouded in long dark shadows as they pulled up. A gentle fresh breeze greeted them as they walked to the front door. Sabrina casually acknowledged Jim as she walked past him, through the house to the patio door. She searched the darkness for where the top of the hill should be. *I can't wait until tomorrow.*

Glancing over her shoulder, she saw that Mark was occupied with Jim, his back to her. Seizing her opportunity, she removed a candle from the side board and slipped out the door, hurrying across the patio, and on to the bench at the big oak tree. There she paused briefly, allowing her eyes to adjust to the darkness, before setting off on the slow, careful climb up the hill.

Mark called to her; when she did not answer he turned around. She was nowhere to be seen. Thinking that she had gone to the kitchen, he went toward the hallway, the corridor and the kitchen, were in darkness. He called again, still no answer. Turning back, he noticed that the patio door was slightly open. "Damn it," he muttered, looking out into the darkness.

Pulling a blanket from the sofa, and a flashlight from the desk, he headed out across the patio. *Even with a light, I'm having trouble finding my way up the hill. How did she do it without a light?* Every few steps, he paused to shine the light to his left and right, just in case she had become stranded in the darkness. As he flashed the light forward again, he could see the top of the hill only a few steps away. His stride lengthened, until he finally stood atop the hill. Not needing to shine a light toward the grave, he could make out Sabrina's shape next to it. The flickering glow of a candle framed a portion of her form.

Completely lost in her thoughts, Sabrina never heard Mark approach. She jumped when he touched her shoulder. Taking his hand, she urged him to sit beside her. As Mark settled himself, he caught a glimpse of the glistening droplets on her cheek. Sabrina felt the comforting embrace of his arm around her; she leaned into him. Her tears changed from the occasional drop to a seemingly endless stream. Silence became their only companion, with the exception of the gentle whisper of the wind. It wafted through the tree tops, sending light showers of leaves to the ground.

As the wind intensified, Sabrina shuddered from the icy blast that washed over her. Mark wrapped the blanket around her. "We should go back to the house." "Not yet," she said cuddling into him, and the warmth of the blanket. "Wrong answer. You're cold and tired, and if you're coming down with something this won't help." "I guess you're right," she answered with a sigh. Mark helped her up, pulling the blanket tightly around her. He secured it in place with his arm about her shoulders. Sabrina took a moment to look at the little grave. *Someday our love will be complete.*

Mark stayed downstairs, to lock up the house, while Sabrina made her way up to the bedroom. He watched her for a moment. Each step she took was slow and labored; her hand upon the railing, pulling herself up each step. The sight stabbed at his heart. *She needs me tonight.* That thought made him hurry, locking doors and turning out lights.

As he started down the hall to the bedroom, he stopped to pick up the blanket that she once had wrapped around her; but that was only the beginning. At the doorway of the bedroom began the trail of clothes that led across the room ending at the bed. Sabrina was in bed, curled up tight; Patches snuggled up beside her.

Presuming that she was already asleep, Mark turned out the lights and quietly slipped into bed beside her. *I want to hold her. It doesn't feel right to go to sleep without her in my arms; but she does need the rest.* He felt her move, then an icy hand touched his arm, as she slid herself to him. Mark brought her close.

"You're ice cold. I told you not to go up there tonight; now you've got a chill." "I know, but I couldn't wait." She shuddered hard; pressing herself close to Mark's warm body. "Tomorrow I'm making an appointment for you to see Doc." "You don't have to; it's probably just the flu." "Maybe, but I'm sure not going to take any chances." "If it's what you want, then I'll go, but can you do something for me?" "You know the answer to that Sabrina." "Hold me tighter." She shivered harder against his warmth.

Chapter 21

Nick's energy was in high gear. *My plans are coming together better, and faster, than I had expected.* He had on his desk, several designs that the costume department had come up with for Mark and Sabrina. He slipped them into a large courier pouch, along with the matching fabric samples. Accompanying that, he enclosed the notes from the choreographer; all subject to their approval. Sealing the pouch, he called to his secretary, advising her to call the courier service.

The pouch should reach them this afternoon, or early tonight. I'll wait until tomorrow night before contacting them, and hopefully they'll have an answer for me. Putting the pouch aside, Nick pulled a folder from the desk drawer, the catering menu from the hotel in Las Vegas.

Since both of my own children had refused a proper wedding, I'm becoming consumed with all these arrangements, and I actually enjoy it. I've planned dinner parties before, but this is far grander and much more exciting. He sat back, staring blankly at the papers before him. *Am I being too extravagant? Will the others be jealous of my attention to Mark and Sabrina, or will they be supportive, knowing that this is a very special occasion for two special people?*

Nick's fist hit the desk. "Ah, the hell with them! Let them whine and complain. This is important; to me and to the company; and to the fans." "What's so important?" The unexpected voice startled Nick. He looked up towards the door and his mouth fell open. Sean was leaning against the frame. He ambled over to Nick's desk.

"I asked you what was so important?" "Nothing much," Nick answered, still dumbfounded by the unexpected visitor. Sean glanced at the menu on the desk. "Planing a party are you?" "Sort of." "In Vegas eh? Planning my return party perhaps?" "Return party?" "Yeah, I've been given the okay to return to work."

"That's right!" *I have to make it sound like I haven't completely forgotten.* "You know the Vegas pay per view would be perfect for my return, but you've already got that covered, haven't you and a party to boot." "Look Sean; I really don't have the time to get into this right now." "We need to go over the details." "Let me have a couple of days. You are staying in town aren't you?" "Sure, we can talk later in the week." "Sounds good, I'll call you when I've got every thing finished up; but for now, I would appreciate it if you would let me get back to work."

Acknowledging Nick with a quick salute, Sean left the office. Nick slumped back in his chair; his eyes rolled back. "Damn it. Now what am I going to do?" *With my mind solely focused on Mark and Sabrina, I had completely forgotten about Sean's return. It was only a few days ago that Sean was released from medical care. He still has to make regular visits to a psychiatrist, and his two companions are still in place; but the Doctors feel that he's ready to return to work, but is he truly ready to face Sabrina again? Is she ready to face him?* Nick pushed the menu aside, opting for a strong drink to help clear his mind. *I have to stay focused on the wedding. Sean's return will have to take a back seat at this show.*

It was a little past noon when Mark went back upstairs to wake Sabrina. Sitting beside her on the bed, he carefully pulled the hair away from her face. Rolling onto her back, her eyes fluttered against the light. "Morning," she answered as she stretched. "Afternoon." "What!" She became fully awake, looking at the clock. "How could you let me sleep so long?" "You needed to catch up; but now you have to get moving. You have an appointment with Doc in a couple of hours." "You didn't have to; I feel much better today." "Don't make excuses, you promised me that you would go, and I'm gonna make sure you keep that promise." "Okay, okay, I'll go."

She slid closer to him. As her arms encircled his neck, the sheet that covered her slipped down to her waist. Instinctively Mark sought out the soft curves of her breasts. Sabrina leaned into his touch. "Join me for a shower?" she asked.

Her hot breath against his skin was intoxicating; he began to lose himself. Sabrina pulled him down to the bed. She had freed the buttons of his shirt, when Mark forcefully pushed her onto her back. Closing her eyes, she wet her lips in anticipation of his kiss. He fought his desires, her breasts heaved up, beckoning him; his hand trembled above them.

Finding the strength that he needed, he touched her cheek. "Sabrina," he called softly. Her eyes fluttered open. "We really shouldn't." "Why?" "Considering your pending appointment, I just don't think that it's a wise move." With his help she sat up, her arms tight around his neck. "Okay, but you'll have no excuses later on." "I don't know about that; I kind of had something in mind." "Can I ask what?" "No," he answered sternly, wrapping her robe around her. "Now go and have you shower."

He watched her head off into the bathroom. *Her gait has that familiar airy bounce to it. She is feeling better. Was I too hasty in insisting that she see Doc? Better safe than sorry.*

When they arrived at Doc's, Sabrina carefully surveyed the estate. *Doc's house is not as I had imagined it would be. The log home is a far cry from the vision of a stately manor that my mind associated with a Doctor. No rose gardens. No trellis heavy with wisteria. No red brick pathway to guide guests to the house, only gravel surrounded the house. It is an oasis amid the arid sea of stones.*

Clinging tightly to Mark's arm, she carefully picked her path across the stones, feeling them roll and shift beneath her feet. "Nervous?" Mark asked, stopping her at the bottom of the steps. "No," she answered quickly. Mark lifted her face up.

I know that look on his face; he didn't believe my hasty answer. I can never hide my true feelings from him. As he brought her close to him, to the security of his powerful arms, he felt her tension fade away with a soft sigh. "You don't need to be nervous," he said. "I know; but I'm not very fond of Doctors." "That's understandable, given your past history." He felt her press closer to him. "This is much different remember?"

Sabrina lifted her eyes up to meet his. *In the crystal blue depths of her beautiful eyes, I can see clearly what it is she desires the most, what she needs from me at this very moment.* He felt her hands tenderly glide up his back, as his lips met hers. She took from him only enough to renew her strength.

Doc cleared his throat. "Good to see you're still behaving like newlyweds," he said with a slightly chuckle to his voice. Sabrina felt the blush rush over her face. She climbed the two steps up to the porch, her arm still around Mark. Doc held open the door. "Come on in," he said with a smile. Mark stopped just outside the threshold.

"I'll wait for you out here," he said. Her eyes pleaded with him to go with her. "It'll be okay." His reassurance calmed her fears instantly. She followed Doc inside. From the window, Mark watched as Doc led her into his office. When the door shut, he sat down on the log bench, to await her return, and to daydream about his plans for later on.

The office, like the house, is far from what my mind had conjured. This is not a cold sterile office, thick with the smell of antiseptic; but instead it is a cozy den. The appetizing aroma of vanilla calmed her as she relaxed into the rich leather chair. Doc perched himself on the edge of his old chair, the once rich leather, now cracked and faded by age. The brass studs tarnished and dull. Doc opened a folder on the top of the antique oak desk, scribed a quick note before settling his gaze upon Sabrina.

"So, Mark tells me that you've been rather fatigued lately." "A bit, but I told him it was probably just the flu, or if you would like his version, it's all due to the crazy tour schedules." "It could be, but that's what we're going to find out. Have you had a check up since I last saw you?" "No," she answered quietly as she remembered their last encounter.

Doc walked around the desk and opened a door to an examining room. "If you would please come this way, we'll get this over with as quickly as possible. You'll find a clean gown on the table. I'll be back in a few minutes."

The thin cotton gown was cold against Sabrina's skin. An uncontrolled shudder rippled over her body; but was quickly replaced by the warm rush of anxiety as Doc began his examination. He was quick, but thorough. Sabrina had forgotten about how gentle he was, always telling her what he was about to do. As she sat up, she caught sight of Doc preparing a syringe.

"What's that for?" she asked. "Oh this; it's just a vitamin shot. It'll help you to get your energy back." The needle stung as it pierced her hip, and then the burning sensation of the fluid being injected. Sabrina rubbed at it while Doc disposed of the syringe.

Returning his attention to her, Doc pulled a stool up near the table. "Why so serious, is there something wrong?" she asked but afraid to hear his answer. "No, no, nothing's wrong; I think that you're very healthy, and the hectic schedule of Mark's has just got you a little rundown." "That's why the vitamins?" "Yes, but just to make sure that we're both right, I'd like to send you for a couple of tests," he said as he began writing on the pad in his hand. Glancing up he detected the lines of worry on her face.

"Don't worry darlin, they're just standard blood tests, and I'd also like you to have an ultra sound." "Why? Do you suspect something?" "Not at all; I'm just making sure that everything is all right in there. You've had a hard time, what with losing two babies and all and I suspect that you and

Mark have been thinking about a family. This is my way of guaranteeing that you will have your family."

"When do I have to get these tests done?" "Well, you'll have to go into Dallas for them, so I'll have my nurse make an appointment and call you. I'll be away for a couple of weeks; and that should be about the time when the results come back, but trust me, there is nothing to worry about. You get dressed. I'll be outside talking to Mark."

Sabrina sat on the edge of the exam table for a few moments after Doc left, trying to make sense of what he said. Her hands passed lightly over her belly. *Doc must think that there's something wrong, an ultra sound is not part of a standard physical, or maybe it is? Maybe it's what they do in the States.* She let her mind cling to that thought, while she finished dressing.

Mark was on his feet when he heard the latch on the door. "Well Doc, how is she?" "Fine, just fine. She'll be out in a few minutes." Doc rubbed the back of his neck, he was tired and looking forward to his vacation; but he had to talk to Mark. "Sit down son," he said, gesturing to the bench. Mark felt a fist tighten around his heart. He reached for the arm of the bench, steadying himself as he slumped down.

"You found something?" Mark asked, swallowing hard, forcing the vile taste from his mouth. "No, not really. I've ordered some tests." "Tests! What for?" "Calm down Mark; I'm a little concerned about how her body hasn't been functioning the way it should." "I don't understand." "It's hard to explain; but to put it simply, I feel that her body still thinks that she's pregnant. It's not all that uncommon for a woman to experience a false pregnancy, especially after the tragic loss of two babies."

"How can that be?" "It's still a mystery as to how the mind can have such power over the body, but I believe that Sabrina wants so desperately to have your child that somehow her body has refused to accept the miscarriage. So I've ordered a few tests to verify my suspicions." "Does she know?" "About the tests, yes, as to what they're for, no. There's no point in worrying her, once I have all the results, then we can proceed with a treatment." "Should she be taking it easy?" "Not really; so don't change your plans or routines; it could make her suspicious. It'll be a couple of weeks before I get the results." Doc gently grasped Mark's shoulder. "Don't dwell on it son; she'll be fine."

The conversation came to an abrupt end as Sabrina opened the door. "Are you two having a nice chat?" she asked. "Yes, we were," Doc answered. "Just exchanging ideas on vacation spots." Mark had moved over to Sabrina's side. She pulled his arm around her. "We're on vacation too; in the best possible place." "Where would that be?" "Home," she answered with a smile. "And I would very much like to get back there, for you see my husband has something special planned, and my curiosity is getting the better of me." "Well then, get along home, and enjoy what's left of the day." The two men shook hands. Doc giving a stronger, reassuring grip, accompanied by a sly nod. He had retreated to his office before they had reached the car.

The silence between them worried Mark. *Did she overhear me talking to Doc?* Reaching his hand out to her, he moved it lightly over her thigh. "You're awfully quiet; are you feeling okay?" he asked. Sabrina squeezed his hand. "I'm fine; my hip still stings a bit from the shot. It's supposed to help me get some energy back, but right now all I want to do is have a nap." "Well as soon as we get home you can go to bed." "What about your plans for our evening?" "Another night." "No, please don't change anything. I'll be fine." "Let me think about it."

The silence returned for the duration of the drive home. Sabrina kept Mark's hand in hers, gently stroking the palm. *The sensation that her touch is transmitting makes it difficult for me to sort through my thoughts. My first instinct is to forfeit the plan, but I know to well that Sabrina won't let me. Maybe she needs this diversion, and Doc did say not to alter anything. I will tell her when we get home.*

Jim was tending the front gardens when the car came up the drive. He hurried into the house to retrieve the package from the courier. Sabrina was out of the car, and halfway around it by the time Mark had undone his seat belt. "So what's your answer?" she asked as she backed him up until he sat on the hood of the car. "I don't know yet."

Sabrina wiggled her way between his knees, her arms around his neck. "Please say yes. You always know what to do to make me feel better." She pressed herself closer to him. "Please." Mark could feel her breath on his skin, then the sweet taste of her lips. *Her power of persuasion is strong. I've already made up my mind, but I'll let her continue her method of coercion.*

Jim didn't like to interrupt their moment but he couldn't stand there all day; he had chores to do. "Excuse me Mr. Cassidy." "Yes, Jim, what is it?" "This came by courier while you were out." "Where is it from?" "Mr. Manetti." "Put it upstairs; I'll look at it tomorrow. Sabrina and I have plans for tonight, and those plans don't include work." "Very good sir. I've made sure that everything you asked for is in place." "Thank you, Jim." Taking his cue to leave, Jim returned to the inside of the house.

Mark stared at Sabrina, at the woman he loved so much. *Her smile has returned, it makes her glow, and it makes my heart warm.* She pressed herself even closer to him. "Will you tell me?" she asked. "No," he answered with a devilish grin. "I know that it's something you've wanted to do ever since you first came here."

Sabrina took a step back, confused, yet intrigued by his comment. "We had better get going; it's getting late," Mark said. She moved to the car door. "Where are you going?" Mark asked. "To get in the car." "We don't need that tonight. Come with me."

They walked across the front yard to the barn. "What are we doing in here?" Sabrina asked. "I thought we'd take a ride around the property." He spun her into his arms, holding her firmly. "No stunts, just a leisurely walk, got it! I don't want you taking any risks." Sabrina leaned into him. "Okay; I promise, no running the horses."

Mark saddled her horse first, and when he had finished with his own, he took a moment to lean against the beast, to watch her. Quietly talking to the chestnut gelding, she scratched his lip with one hand, while the other she used to slowly stroke the thick muscles of his neck. *Such a gentle person she is; with animals, and with me. As I watch her hand slowly gliding up and down, I can almost perceive her silky touch on my skin.*

Sabrina was aware of his eyes watching her. She glanced over her shoulder. "Did you say something?" she asked. "No, but I was just thinking that I forgot to do something." He moved around the back of the horse, closer to her. "What did you forget?" "I forgot to tell you how much I love you." "Oh Mark, I love you; but you don't have to say it all the time. I feel it, every time you look at me, every time you touch me, and especially when you kiss me."

Her eyes closed. He accepted her tender invitation, only to quickly pull back when he felt the arousal of his own body. Sabrina kept her remarks to herself. *I know that he has our evening all planned out; even though I could easily persuade him to stay in the barn, the perfect place to explore the animal within us both.*

The trail that led from behind the barn was wide enough for them to ride side by side. Mark kept the pace slow by holding Sabrina's hand; not letting her get ahead of him at all. They rode up the hill to the vast field beyond, drifting amongst the trees along the fence line, to keep away from the heat of the afternoon sun.

They were more than halfway across the field when Mark reined them to a stop. "Time to go back?" Sabrina asked. "No, I thought we'd go over to the lake for a little while." "Sure, but not too long, I don't want to be out here after dark." "It'll be okay," he said, squeezing her hand gently for reassurance. "Don't worry."

Even though we're still on the property I still worry, being in the middle of nowhere, after dark, bothers me. I've heard the howl of the coyotes from the safety of the house; but what else lives out here after sunset?

Her preoccupation with watching the sun sink into the horizon made her impervious to the view around her. The horses slowed as Mark eased them to a stop. Sabrina looked away from the sunset; they were beside the lake. Mark had dismounted, and was standing beside her. "Feel like walking for a bit?" he asked. "Yeah, sure."

She slid out of her saddle, into his waiting arms. "You're shaking. Are you cold?" "No, I just need you to hold me," she said. His embrace soothed her nerves, pushing her fears away. *These feelings are absurd. He would not have brought me out here if there was even the remotest possibility of anything happening.*

As his embrace tightened, her feelings changed. The sheer strength of his arms gave her back the security that had momentarily been obscured. "Come with me; there's something I'd like you to see. Something that will make you feel much better." He kept his arm around her as they walked along the edge of the lake; past the thick, tangled masses of wild rose bushes, and old weathered oak trees.

The trail began to widen before them. The dense undergrowth had been cleared away allowing for a thick, lush carpet of grass to take hold. The shadows, cast by the oak trees, crept back as they passed under the last of the branches. Mark stopped Sabrina's progression. She had been walking with her eyes downward, taking care not to become tangled in a shrub.

"What is it?" she asked looking at him. "We're here. What do you think?" She followed his gaze across the clearing to the cottage by the lake shore. "What's this?" "This is our very own sanctuary away from the rest of the world," he said turning her to face him. "This is a place for us, a quiet place to relax and unwind." "And love," she added, taking time to stroke his cheek. "Most definitely, but right now I'd like to show you around." As they walked across the clearing, Sabrina was able to take in the external features of this oasis.

The cottage itself was fashioned similar to the main house, with the exception of a large porch across the front. Complete with a bench swing, and two rocking chairs. Halfway between the cottage and the lake was a fire pit. An old log had been cut into a bench, so one could comfortably sit by the fire.

To the side of the cottage was a corral. Mark led the horses over to it and tied the reins to the top rail. "Why don't you have a look inside while I unsaddle the horses, I'll be in just as soon as I get them bedded down," Mark said. Sabrina bit her lip. *I would sound too eager if I responded to that remark.* She quietly turned away, and climbed the two steps up to the porch. The boards squeaked under her feet. Her hand reached for the door, but her mind was more intent on the swing at the end of the porch.

Sitting down, she tucked her left foot under her, leaving her right dangling, just high enough that she could still give the swing a gentle push. Closing her eyes, her mind drifted, back in time to her family home. The swing wobbled; she came back from her thoughts. Mark was behind her.

"I thought you were going inside," he said. "I started to, but this was much more appealing." "I know what you mean," he answered as he stepped up onto the porch. "This has always been my favorite spot. It's so relaxing to sit here and watch the sunset; even before the cottage was built I used to come here, to this very spot, and dream." "Sit with me for a little while." "Not yet, I'm gonna build a fire, and we should find something for dinner." "Okay, I can take a hint," she sighed as she pulled herself up.

"I take it you've had provisions brought in?" "Oh yeah, you should find something to your liking." Her hand slid across his chest as she walked past him to the door. "I already have; but it's not customary to have dessert before dinner." Mark took a moment to lean against the post. "Oh man, I have got to stay focused." He took a step toward the door. "No damn it. Not yet." He turned away, down the steps to the woodpile.

Sabrina had closed the door, but half expected Mark to follow her inside. *It's fun teasing him. It's guaranteed to ignite his passion, and enflame our night.* A pleasing aroma drifted under her nose, that made her stomach rumble with hunger. Following the scent, she opened the oven door. Jim had left a stew for them. Judging by the temperature dial, she concluded that it was well cooked, and only left in there to keep warm. The table was all ready set; complete with a bouquet of red roses to the side and a bottle of wine chilling in ice.

Nothing for me to do, I might as well look around. The cottage has a very rustic decor to it. It reminds me of a hunter's cabin, with simple white pine furniture, and plush sheep skin covers. Everything is in the one room, kitchen, dining room and living room. Where is the bed? The sofa isn't convertible. She noticed the two doors beyond the sofa. *Must be one of those.*

She opened the first door, a bathroom, nothing special. The second door wasn't as easy. She twisted the knob. *It's locked. Why? Maybe it's not a bedroom; maybe we aren't going to stay here tonight. Enough. It doesn't matter where we are, as long as we're together.*

Mark was sitting on the bench next to the fire. Sabrina laid her hands upon his shoulders. "Looks good," she said. "How is dinner coming?" Mark asked. "Great. It's ready whenever you are." "What? You haven't been in there that long." "Oh come on; don't pretend you don't know." "I have no idea what you're talking about." "Jim made dinner. It's in the oven warming." "That man goes above and beyond. I only asked him to clean up the cabin. I never said anything about making dinner."

"It's nice that he did. It gives us more time for other things." "Well, lead on; all this fresh air has made me hungry." He stepped over the back of the bench and Sabrina placed his arm around her waist. "Make sure you leave room for dessert," she said. "Always."

Mark served up dinner. Sabrina picked up her plate, a glass of wine and headed for the door. "Where are you going?" Mark asked. "To sit by the fire, and watch the last bit of the sunset." She continued on her way out the door. Mark collected his dinner and followed her. She had all ready staked out her claim on the bench when he reached her side. "Now isn't this better than sitting at a candle lit table, all this beauty is too good to waste by staying inside." "You're beautiful in any light." "Eat your dinner and let me watch the sunset."

Stretching back, she watched the last golden fingers of the sun stretch through the trees, searching for something to grab onto, to make these dwindling moments last, but nothing could prevent the cycle from repeating itself day after day.

Darkness quickly followed, leaving only the glow of the fire. Mark had taken the dishes into the cottage. His shadow moved about, stopping briefly to extinguish a light. An unfamiliar sound distracted her; she strained to see through the darkness, listening. The sound came again. *It's only the horses, nothing to be afraid of.*

The weight of a blanket encircled her shoulders. "What's this for?" "I don't want you to catch a chill," Mark said as he stepped back over the bench. "Look what I found," he said, holding a bag of marshmallows in front of her. "Our fire side cook out is now complete."

Sabrina couldn't resist feeding one of the sticky, warm marshmallows to him. Deliberately quivering the stick so that the thick confection stuck to part of his mustache giving her the excuse to kiss away the evidence. Mark drew her close; working his hand under her shirt, moving it slowly up her back.

The sound of brush rustling sent Sabrina's eyes scanning the darkness for the source. "What is it?" Mark asked. "I heard something." "It's only the horses in the corral." "I don't think so. The sound didn't come from there. It could be some other animal." "There's nothing out there." "How can you be so sure that there isn't some wild animal lurking in the darkness, just waiting to make its move?"

Mark lowered his head. "I had hoped that I wouldn't have to tell you." "Tell me what?" Her voice was stressed. "There is one animal you should worry about." "What!" Her eyes were wide with fear. Mark looked into her eyes. "It's me!" He scooped her up into his arms. "Damn you! You know better than to scare me like that!" "I'm sorry. I only meant to tease you," he whispered as he nuzzled at her ear. "Let me make it up to you."

He carried her into the cottage, toward the locked door. "It's locked." "I know, but I have the key." He let her stand while he dug into his pocket, retrieving a shiny silver key. "I've never been in here. I had it decorated, and then locked up; waiting for a special person to share it with. It's been waiting for you." As he unlocked the door she was enthralled in intrigue.

The room was bathed in the soft blue gray rays of the moon, that shone through the large skylight. Sabrina could make out the shapes of the furniture, a chest, a couple of chairs and unmistakably the bed. "Let me turn on the light," he said reaching for the switch.

Sabrina closed her eyes, to shield her from the sudden change, and so she could experience the room fully. Her eyes fluttered open; the moonlight had been traded for a pale pink glow from a lamp beside the bed. The skylight was dark, no longer could she see the stars that twinkled in the night sky.

At her feet lay a large bear skin rug, spreading its limbs out to each corner of the room. "Is this real?" she asked squatting down to touch the head of the beast. "Yeah, they all are," he said directing her attention to the plush, creamy colored sheepskins on the chairs. Straightening herself, Sabrina continued to inventory the room, taking in each object individually and completely. The chest caught her interest, with its ornately carved designs. It was a delight to her eyes, as well as her hands. Her fingers followed the smooth curves of the flowers, admiring the rich grain of the wood. "Jim made that," Mark said.

He had stayed at the doorway, letting her explore on her own. He watched her move to the side of the bed. Her expression changed ever so slightly as her fingers stroked the fur blanket. "What is this? I've never felt anything so soft." "It's llama." "It's wonderful." She continued to run her fingers through the long fur until she reached the border of black satin near the pillows. "Satin sheets?" she queried. "Yes, I only wanted the best of everything for this room, for you." He saw her eyes glisten with a dewy softness just before she turned away from him.

It only took him three steps to reach her; he turned her around. "Why the tears?" he asked as he wiped away the moist streams from her cheeks. "Is there something wrong with the room?" "No, it's perfect. It's just." "What?" "I feel a little sad." "Why?" "It saddens me that no one, except me, gets to see this gentle, loving side of you." "My character doesn't allow it, but I never really knew about this part of me; I never thought that I was capable; until I met you."

"You created this before you met me." "Yes, I did. It came to be shortly after I had my first dream about you, but when nothing came of all those dreams I had this place locked up. I used to come out here sometimes and just sit on the swing, daydreaming, imagining what my life would be like if I knew how to love, but when I met you, you opened the door to my heart, showing me that I could love, and I never want to lose that feeling, or you." "You'll never lose me; I love you too much."

I can see the longing in her eyes. That look of love that makes my heart swell, and ignites my passion. He kissed her, a long, deep kiss, that made her knees buckle with weakness. He laid her down upon the virgin bed. Mark rolled away from her slightly, turning out the lamp. "Why did you do that?" Sabrina asked. "I want to make love to you under the stars, by the light of the moon."

Sabrina looked up at the large skylight above the bed. The dark sky was alive with thousands of twinkling stars. *Just like diamonds on black velvet. They weren't like this back at the main house, only a few of the brightest stars were visible through the skylight in our bedroom. The bright glow of the mercury lamps in the yard obliterated all the other stars.*

The feeling of Mark's beard against her neck sent rushes of electrifying sensations through her body, making her shudder. Mark kissed her ear. "What's your answer?" he whispered. "You should know by now that you don't have to ask. I live for moments like this." With a gentle push, she moved Mark onto his back. As she turned on her side a sharp stinging pain in her hip made her cry out and stand up quickly. "What's the matter?" "My hip hurts, where Doc gave me the shot. I've had shots before but they never hurt like this." "Let me see."

Sabrina stepped out of her jeans and turned her hip towards Mark. "Oh man!" "What?" "You've got one hell of a bruise; and it's warm too," he said as he softly passed his hand over it. Sabrina turned around to face him. "Well you know what this means, don't you?" "Yeah," he sighed. "I get to hold you all night." "No!" She pushed him back onto the bed, straddling his hips. "It means that I get to be on top."

She grabbed his shirt, pulling it apart, the pearl snaps popping open at a furious pace. Mark pulled her T-shirt over her head. He brought her down to him; her breasts pressed against his chest. Their frenzied passion took full control, turning her pain into lustful pleasure.

Nick was pacing around his office. *I promised myself that I wouldn't phone Mark until later, but I have a schedule ticking away.* He picked up the phone and dialed. Jim answered on the second ring, annoyed that he had been awakened so rudely. "Yes," he croaked, clearing his throat. "It's Nick. Could I speak to Mark please?" "No, you can't; he's not here." "Where is he?" "Mr. and Mrs. Cassidy went out for the evening." "When do you expect them back?" "I'm not sure. They could be back for breakfast, or maybe not until supper. I expect them when I see them." "Are you sure that they're not just avoiding me?" "Mr. Manetti, it's not even daylight yet. They'll be back later. I'll tell them you called. Good-bye Mr. Manetti." Nick heard the harsh click of the phone. He looked at his watch; he felt like a fool, not taking into account the time difference. *Jim will pass on the message. I just have to be patient.*

Sabrina shifted slightly in Mark's arms, enough to wake him. He nuzzled at her ear. "It's too early to be awake; go back to sleep," he whispered. "I haven't been to sleep yet," she answered. That brought Mark to full consciousness. "You haven't slept? Are you feeling okay?" "I feel fine, wonderful in fact. I've just been lying here watching the stars. There are so many of them, and so many shooting stars." Mark rolled onto his back and stretched. "Did you make any wishes?" he asked.

The satin sheets suddenly felt cold to Sabrina. She sought out the warmth of his body. "Of course I made wishes." "What did you wish for?" "I can't tell you; it would break the spell." "Then close your eyes and dream about them." "I can't. I'm not at all tired; in fact I have never felt so awake and energized as I am now." She quickly slid atop his body, plying him with soft kisses.

Mark held her back. "You should be totally exhausted." "I'm not." "Sabrina, we made love twice." "No, it was three times." "I must have been asleep for that one," he laughed. She pressed herself closer to him. "Wanna go for four?" "I'm gonna have to start taking those same vitamin shots, if I'm to keep up with you." "The vitamins have nothing to do with it. My love for you is the single driving force. It fills my soul, strengthens my heart and makes me complete. It fills my every thought and with every second that passes, every beat of my heart I love you more than the moment before."

The tenderness of her words, and the soft tone of her voice produced the effect that she had hoped for. Mark's body was aroused beneath her. He brought her to him. His kiss resounded with love. A pure love, a love that brought their bodies together again with renewed energy and endurance.

The heat of the sun, beaming through the skylight, woke Mark. The bed was cold, and empty beside him. *Sabrina is already up; but when? Did I sleep that soundly that I didn't feel her leave my side? She can't be far her clothes are still on the floor.* Pulling on his jeans, he ambled out of the bedroom. He was about to knock on the bathroom door, when he noticed that the front door was open. Stepping onto the porch, he half expected to see her cuddled up on the swing, but it was empty and still. *Where is she?*

Wandering toward the corral, he was stopped by the sound of splashing water. Looking toward the lake, he caught a glimpse of Sabrina before she disappeared under the water. Standing at the lake shore, he watched her dive and swim. When she spotted him, she paddled towards the shore. "Are you just going to stand there, or will you join me for a swim?" she asked. "I'll stay here thank you. How long have you been in there?" "I don't know." "Come on out," he said holding up the towel for her.

The sight of her wet body, glistening in the sunlight, made his heart race. Desire flooded his body and caused him to turn away as she wrapped the towel around her. Coming to his side, she hugged his waist as they walked back to the cottage. "You had better get dressed," he said directing her to the door. "Not yet; sit with me for a little bit." She pulled him towards the swing.

With her feet tucked up, Sabrina cuddled closer to Mark, her head resting upon his shoulder. "Why didn't we come here for our honeymoon? It's so peaceful, and romantic." "I thought about it; but I wanted to get you away from the world." "We are. There's no phone, no television; just us, and that's all that matters." "I can't argue that; but we can't stay here forever. We do have to get back and soon."

Sabrina pushed away from him. "Why do you do this?" she yelled at him and ran into the house. Mark followed her. She was lying on the bed, curled up. "Sabrina, talk to me." He turned her onto her back. "What's the use, you've all ready made up your mind." "About what?" "Why did you even bring me here?" she asked. "I wanted you to see this place that I made for you." "And now you want to take it away!" "No, I don't!" "Then say we can stay. Just for a few days, please Mark. There is nothing at the main house that needs our attention right now. You said that we came home for a rest; well I can't think of a better place to do that than right here."

He had to turn away; his head lowered, his long hair hiding the turmoil on his face. "We don't have any supplies," he said with a sigh. "All you have to do is pull that cell phone out of your saddle bag, call Jim and have him bring a few things." "You've got this all worked out don't you?" "I just don't want to go back yet." "If it makes you happy, then we can stay for a few days." "I'm not asking just for me; you need this too."

Her kiss was soft against his lips, her gentle touch easing him back onto the bed. "Not so fast," he said pulling himself away from her. "I have to call Jim, tell him to bring some groceries, and clean clothes. Anything special you would like?" "Yeah, we need more marshmallows, oh and hot dogs too." "What?" "To cook over the fire, they taste better that way." Mark shook his head all the way out to the kitchen. *She can be a mystery at times; such a marvelous mystery.*

Jim packed the last box out to the jeep. He was glad that Mark and Sabrina were taking a few days for themselves. He took one last look around the house, making sure that he had everything they would need. The ringing phone stopped his exit. He hesitated at answering it, but what if it was Mark.

"Hello," he said with some reservation. "I'd like to speak to Mark please. Tell him it's Nick." "I'm sorry Mr. Manetti, but he's not here." "Well, when do you expect him this time?" "Not for a few days." "Damn it! Where the hell is he? It's very important that I speak to him." "I can pass on the message sir." "Yes, please. Oh Jim, did you receive a package from my office?" "Yes sir." "If there is any way you can get it to Mark, do it. He needs to review the contents and get back to me as soon as possible." "Yes sir; I'll do what I can."

There was no salutation; Jim only heard the echoing click. "Jackass," he muttered, hanging up the phone. Retrieving the package from the desk in the master bedroom irked him. *My employer doesn't need to be bothered with work right now; but if I don't follow Nick's instructions, and it did turn out to be important, there would be hell to pay.* He tossed it in the grocery box and drove off to the cottage.

Sabrina had given in to Mark's request that she take a nap. She was more tired than she realized, and never heard Jim arrive with their supplies, nor did she hear him leave. Mark sat down on the edge of the bed. Sabrina was lying on her side, but more on her stomach. The sheet was down around her waist, leaving her nude torso exposed for him to admire.

How perfect her form is, firm, yet soft and supple. So inviting that I have to touch her. Gently he stroked her back, up to her shoulder and down to the side of her breast. Sabrina took a deep breath and exhaled a sigh; Mark backed off. "Don't stop," she whispered. "How long have you been awake?" "Since you sat down." "Jim has been. Come see what he brought." He left her to get dressed.

Pulling on Mark's shirt, she followed him out. Since there wasn't enough room for both of them in the kitchen area, Sabrina stayed by the table, handing Mark items to put away. She came to the courier pouch. "What's this?" she asked. "I don't know. It's from Nick. Jim showed it to me yesterday. He should have left it at the house." "It might be important," she said.

Mark moved closer to her, taking her in his arms. "I thought you wanted to get away from work?" "I do, but." "If you're that curious, then go ahead and open it." Giving him a kiss, she headed out to the porch swing to examine the contents of the pouch.

Mark had finished putting away the supplies; he had nearly made it to the door when the cell phone rang; his first thought was to just ignore it. *I can't, Jim is the only person who knows this number, and he wouldn't disturb me unless it was important.*

"Yes," he spoke quietly. "Sir, I have a call from Doc Brown's office. Would you like me to put it through?" "Yes, Jim, I'll take it." Mark waited for the click. "Yes, can I help you?" "Is this Mr. Cassidy?" "Yes, it is." "Hi, this is Anne, from Doc Brown's office; I have your wife's appointment date for the tests that Doc ordered." Mark listened quietly as Anne informed him of the date, time and place of Sabrina's appointment. He wrote down all the information, afraid that he may not remember it, since his mind kept wanting to recall his private conversation with Doc.

Closing up the cell phone, he took the note and pinned it to the fridge with a magnetic can opener. *We have the rest of today and tomorrow to be here. Her appointment is for the day after.* Mark made a quick call to Jim, telling him to send a car for them on that morning. *Now to tell Sabrina. I have to keep my emotions in check, and not let on that I talked to Doc, or just how in depth our talk had been.* With his head slightly lowered, he played with his wedding ring. *Someday, when our lives are back to normal then our love will be complete. We will be a family, someday.*

Sabrina heard the squeak of the floor board. "Mark, you have got to see this," she said, without looking up. "Nick is really going over board with this pay per view." Mark took the bundle of papers from her hand. He sat beside her, trying to show some interest in what was in his hand, but it was no use. He tossed the papers onto a table near the swing. Turning to Sabrina, he cupped his hand against her cheek. "Do you know just how much I love you?" Mark asked.

He lifted her onto his lap, making it easier to kiss her. Needing to catch her breath, Sabrina leaned back, her eyes searching deep into his. "Okay, now tell me what's wrong?" "Nothing." "Bull; I know you too well Mark. That phone call did something to change you, and I'd like to know what it is." "No matter how hard I try, you still can see right through me." "That's just part of what makes us so good together. So don't even try to change the subject."

That loving, coaxing look on her face is hard for me to avoid; she has to know. He ran his hands over her shoulders, and down her back. "The call was from Doc's office; they have an appointment for your tests." "Is that all? It's just some routine tests, nothing to worry about. Hey, you told me that Doc was thorough." "You're not worried?" "No. Not at all."

She leaned closer to him. "Now that we have that subject cleared up, where were we?" "We were about to go over Nick's papers." "Not likely! You started something and don't think that you're gonna get out of it now." "With an ultimatum like that I guess I have no choice." "No, you don't!" she answered with a wide grin. Mark lifted her into his arms as he stood up. "Wait a minute. I should take those papers inside. We can go over these later. That is if you're not too tired." "Not a chance," he said with a bright smile.

The chair toppled across the room, as Nick kicked at it with all the force of his growing frustration. *The business day is coming to an end and I still haven't heard from Mark. I'll give them just a little longer. I don't like it when my stars leave me hanging like this. It makes me feel that I'm not in control, and I need to be in control.* He buzzed his secretary, to have her transfer all the business calls to his cell phone before she left for the day.

"Maybe they lost track of time," he thought aloud. "Who's lost track of time?" Sean asked from the doorway. "Nothing you need to worry about. What brings you here at this time of day?" "I thought you might join me for dinner. It's been so long since we've had a real conversation, and with the pay per view just over a week away, I thought we could talk about my return."

"Why not? I have no plans for tonight," Nick sighed heavily. "Great; but can we take your car; it's kind of crowded in mine." "I take it we will have your shadows for company?" Nick asked. "Yeah, but they know to keep their distance. I'll meet you downstairs." Sean disappeared, giving Nick a few moments to straighten his desk. Pausing at the phone, he drummed his fingers on the receiver. "Damn it Mark!"

Sabrina stretched out beside Mark. His breath was quick. His heart beat rapidly. She wiped away the sweat that glistened on his chest. "I think I'm wearing you out," she said. Mark rolled over quickly, pinning her in place. "Not a chance," he said running his hand slowly up her body. "I will never tire of your body, or of your lust for love." "I get carried away sometimes; I don't know why I can't get enough of you. I've never been so completely satisfied. You've brought my senses to new heights, filled me with wondrous pleasures; yet I want more." "You know sometimes you just talk too much. Not that I'm complaining; but I can think of something much better to do with those beautiful lips of yours." He kissed her deeply, making her purr with delight, as his hand tenderly explored her body.

They lay together in silent report. Mark on his back, Sabrina snuggled close at his side. He felt the hollow growl of her stomach. "Hungry?" he asked. "A bit, but I can wait until dinner time." "I think we've kind of gone past that," he said pointing to the darkened skylight. "Oh well." "Not so fast, you need to eat something." "No, what we need to do is go over those papers that Nick sent." "Okay."

With great effort he rolled away from her and sat on the edge of the bed. "You read them to me while I make us some dinner." "I think you have this backwards," she said as she knelt behind him. "I'm supposed to cook while you tend to business." Wrapping a robe around her, he helped her to stand before him; his look was intense as he spoke. "Get that idea out of your head. This marriage, our marriage, is not stuck in stereotypes. We share everything. The word obey was not in our vows, which makes us equal in every way. So if I want to cook," he began to smile. "Then all you have to do is pretend to enjoy it."

By the time she had herself organized and out to the other room, Mark was already busy at the stove. Sabrina sat down at the table, spreading the papers out before her. "So what all did Nick send? New tour dates?" Mark asked without turning around. "No, not schedules, he sent costume designs." "What?" "Yeah, he wants us to choose a new costume for the pay per view; he's even sent fabric samples." "I think he's losin it. We don't need new costumes."

Sabrina was quiet. Mark turned around. "Do we?" he asked. "Well, these designs are pretty nice, and if Nick wants to go to such lengths, I think we should humor him and go along with his wishes." "You're sure that you want to pursue this?" "Yeah, it'll be fun. Besides I have a good feeling about this." "I don't understand." "Neither do I really. It's just that when I think about the show it gives me this warm feeling, like the weight of a burden has been lifted, a new beginning."

"Well, if the show makes you feel like that then go for it, pick out the design that you like and then we can call Nick and tell him our decision." "You should see them too." "Don't need to; I trust your judgment," he said leaning across the table to her. "Just as long as it's very sexy and tastefully revealing." "Yours or mine?" Sabrina asked. "Now who's being a smart ass?" Sabrina blushed and returned her attention to the sketches spread out before her.

Sean avoided the discussion of his return until they had finished dinner. *I can see that Nick is thinking about something else. He's discrete, but he keeps looking at the cell phone on the table.* "So Nick, what has you so preoccupied?" "Nothing really; I've been waiting for a call, but it looks like it's not going to happen; at least not tonight."

Sean was about to speak when the phone began to chirp; Nick seized it quickly. "Yes," Nick answered quickly. Sean listened to the one sided conversation, for any clues as to who was calling.

"It's about damn time you got back to me; I know you received the package. So have you made a decision?" Nick asked pulling a notebook from his jacket pocket. "Just a minute," he said flipping the book open to a blank page. "Okay. Which design sheet? Okay, got it." He scribbled a number down. "Can you send that one back to me? I just want to be sure that we're talking about the same copy." Sean was puzzled by the conversation. *Whom is he talking to?*

"Any other changes to the schedule? Oh really! Good. I'll see you the day before the show to go over the routine." Nick closed up the cell phone and put away his notebook. He stared at Sean. "So let's get down to business. We need to work out your return." Sean could sense the relief in Nick's voice. *Whatever that call was about it definitely changed his attitude.*

Mark put the phone away before he joined Sabrina on the swing. "Did you get a hold of Nick?" "Yeah, he wants me to send the sketch back. I'll do it when we go into Dallas."
There's something different in his touch. He's holding me tighter than ever before. Turning slightly, her hand smoothed the hair on his chest. "What's worrying you?" Sabrina asked. "Nothing. Why do you ask?" "No reason." *I know he's worried about my tests, more than I am; but it's better left alone.*
She continued to stroke his chest slowly. "So what would you like to do between now and the time we have to leave?" she asked. Mark hugged her. "A whole lot of this." He looked at her, lifting her face upwards. "And this." He kissed her. Sabrina weakened, leaning against him. "I like your idea. So when do you plan on executing this idea?" "Now!"

The morning came to soon for Mark. He had been awake for a couple of hours, watching as the sun pushed back the veil of darkness; and watching Sabrina, asleep in his arms. *As much as I wish that I didn't have to, I know that I have to wake her. The car will be coming for us in a couple of hours, and Sabrina doesn't like to be rushed.*
He rubbed her cheek and she stretched. "Good morning," he said softly. "It's too early," she groaned, turning away from him. "Come on," he said rolling her back again. "The car will be here soon, and you need to shower and get dressed." Sabrina stretched again and her arms came to rest around his neck. "Will you join me?" she asked. "I don't know." "Please, I like the way you rub my back." "Okay, as long as you remember that we don't have time for anything else." "I promise."
Mark left her side to prepare the shower, giving her a few more minutes to drift back and forth between sleep and consciousness, before he returned and carried her off to the bathroom.

The car arrived late. Sabrina could see that Mark was trying to hide his frustration. She slipped her arms around him trying to calm his worries. "I don't know why you ordered a car and driver; we could have gone into

Dallas ourselves." "I want to concentrate on you, not the roads. Besides it looks better to arrive at a restaurant in a limo." "Restaurant? What have you got on your mind now?" "I thought we'd go out for dinner after." "Why didn't you say something sooner, I would have dressed accordingly." "Not a problem, we can go shopping first." "I give up!" "Good, now get in the car," he said holding the door for her. "I'm glad to hear that you've finally accepted my promise of spoiling you." "I don't have much choice; but I must admit that I do like it when you're mysterious, just remember one thing, it works both ways."

I like making her happy, and today I'm even more determined, anything to take her mind off of the tests, as well as my own.

Dallas was alive with activity. They had arrived during the noon hour rush. People crowded the sidewalks, busy with their errands. The traffic was heavier than Sabrina remembered, but then again it was Friday, and all these people were probably trying to escape the bustle of the city for an early weekend.

When the limo slowed to a crawl, Mark reached for the intercom button. Sabrina took his hand. "He's doing the best that he can," she said trying to calm his anxiety. "We're gonna be late." "No, we won't. The driver knows his way around; he'll find a way out of this traffic."

Mark settled back beside her. "You're right as always." "I told you that there is nothing to worry about. Surely you've had a physical before." "Yeah, but this is about you, and that gives me every reason to worry. I plan on having you around for a long time." "You're stuck with me; for all eternity." The car came to a stop. "See, I told you we'd get here in plenty of time," she said pointing out the window to the Dallas Medical Center.

For a downtown clinic it was strangely quiet, but they were several hours away from the usual weekend pandemonium of car accidents, overdoses, and street violence, the literal calm before the storm.

Sabrina's blood tests only took a few minutes as there was no one else waiting at the lab. They walked, arm in arm, to the ultra sound unit, again no wait. Mark was asked to wait in the hall. He kissed Sabrina and watched her as she followed the nurse through a set of double doors.
Waiting is not my strong suit. I have to do something.

The nurse came back out to her station and Mark approached her. "Excuse me, but how long will this test take?" "About thirty minutes," the nurse answered. *That's plenty of time for me to run a little errand. Sabrina won't even know that I've gone.* He headed off toward the lobby.

Sabrina sat quietly in a small changing room. She had disrobed and put on the silly hospital gown as the nurse had instructed. A voice from the other side of the curtain called to her. "Mrs. Cassidy, we're ready for you." Sabrina pulled the curtain back; there was a nurse standing there, dressed in a rose colored uniform. She proceeded down the hallway and Sabrina followed.

Passing through a doorway, they entered a darkened room where Sabrina was instructed to get on the stretcher at the far side. When she was settled, the nurse covered her with a sheet and pulled her gown up, exposing her belly up to her chest. The technician, who was fiddling with the equipment, turned to her. "Relax Mrs. Cassidy, this is a painless test." "I know, but the jelly is still cold." She tensed as he squeezed the gel onto her stomach.

He began to carefully pass the wide wand over her belly. Sabrina tried to get a look at the monitor, but it was turned away from her. Only the technician could see it clearly. Continuing his pattern of passes he stopped briefly to freeze the image and take a picture. Putting away the wand, he turned back to Sabrina. "Lay back and relax. I'll be back in a few minutes."

She saw his form disappear at the foot of her stretcher. A door opened, briefly filtering in more light and then was gone. She closed her eyes; but her rest was all too brief, as the technician returned with the nurse. "All done, you can get dressed. We'll forward the results to Dr. Brown in a few days."

The nurse cleaned the gel from Sabrina's belly and helped her to sit up. Sabrina politely thanked them and padded off to her cubicle to change, the sooner she was rid of this drafty gown the better.

Mark had returned to the waiting area, but found it difficult to sit. He paced the length of the hall. The nurse couldn't help noticing him as he passed her station. His thick soled boots fell heavy on the tile floor and echoed off of the concrete walls. An annoying echo that prevented her from completing her duties.

The double doors opened; Mark pivoted around; Sabrina was walking towards him. He met her halfway. She touched his cheek and smoothed away the worry lines in his forehead. "I'm okay; really." "I love you," he whispered. From behind his back, he produced a large bouquet of red roses, presenting them to her. "Oh Mark they're beautiful; but you didn't have to." "Yes, I do. You're my wife."

The nurse, who had been pretending to work, kept stealing brief looks at them. Admiring their devotion to one another; and wishing that her own husband was that attentive. As Mark and Sabrina strolled away down the corridor, the nurse who had been with Sabrina appeared at the nursing station. She frantically patted her coworker on the shoulder.

"What is it?" "Do you know who that is? It didn't hit me until I saw him." "It's Mr. and Mrs. Cassidy, so what?" "You obviously don't watch wrestling." "Yeah I do; but only because my husband does." "Then you must recognize them?" A blank stare and a shrug came her way. "That's the Warlock and the Sorceress. My God, wait until I tell my boy friend. He's gonna freak." "That's against hospital policy you know." "Screw policy. This is the best thing to happen in a long time. It's sure gonna make working tonight a whole lot better."

Sabrina was quick to take her place close to Mark's side. Close enough that she could kiss him with little effort. "What's this all about?" he asked. "No special reason. So what's on your agenda for the rest of the day?" she asked. "Feel like shopping?" "I guess; but we should find a courier for this," she said waiving the envelope. "And maybe a brief tour of the city." "Sure."

Mark passed on the instructions to the driver and settled back with Sabrina. Putting his arms around her, he spoke softly. "Now, where were we?" "Would you like a reminder?" Sabrina asked in her soft sultry voice. "Sure!" Sabrina shifted, sitting across his lap. She pushed the hair away from his face.

"I know I've said this before, but it's worth repeating. I never tire of kissing you. It serves as a reminder of just how gentle, and loving you are; and of how much I love you." "I love you too," he answered. But between the tone of his voice, and the heavy sigh, Sabrina felt that there was more that he wasn't saying.

"Why do I get the feeling that there should be a but after that remark?" "No!" he answered avoiding her piercing eyes. "No more secrets, remember?" "There are times that I wish that our love was complete, that we were," Mark said with some hesitation. Sabrina hushed him. Her eyes glistened. "I know. I still miss him too, but we will have a child someday; when the time is right."

The limo stopped abruptly. Sabrina was lurched forward onto the floor. "Are you okay?" Mark asked frantically. "Yes, the only thing wounded is my pride." "That stupid ass! How could he do something so ridiculous?" Mark reached for the intercom. "No, Mark, I'm okay. There's no need to be angry with him. Just let him send that package off to Nick and then we can go home." "I thought you wanted to go shopping and out for dinner?" "I did." She pulled his arm around her. "But right now I just want to go home." "I've upset you." "Mark we only have a week left before work takes control again. I would like us to spend that time alone together, at the cottage."

Holding her close, her tears began to soak through his shirt, yet he kept his silence. *I know that she's hiding her pain from me. A pain that I've caused. If only I had kept my feelings silent, we could be enjoying the enchantments of Dallas instead of going home.*

He slowly stroked her arm. His hand come to rest on the side of her belly. A feeling of a knife in his chest made him choke back his own tears. *I have to protect her. If she is to learn of Doc's suspicions it would devastate her. To want a child so badly that her body is mimicking being pregnant; it would crush her. I have to keep her safe; but most importantly I have to get her mind off of the sadness that she now feels.*

"We're home," Mark whispered. Sabrina scrambled past him and into the cottage. By the time he got inside she was nowhere in sight. The bathroom door was open, but the bedroom door was shut. He laid the flowers on the table as he headed toward the door. Hesitant, his hand trembled against the knob. *Maybe I should give her some space. No damn it, the last thing she needs is to be alone.*

Opening the door, he looked toward the bed. She wasn't there. He scanned the room. She was sitting in a chair with her arms wrapped tight around her. Mark knelt in front of her. "I want to be alone!" she lashed out angrily. "No way, I've upset you and I'm sorry. Please let me make it right."

After what seemed to be an endless silence, Sabrina lifted her eyes to meet his. Her bright blue eyes were edged in red. Mark swallowed his heart. "I'm so sorry for saying what I did. I didn't think of how it would affect you.

Please forgive me." He waited for her to respond. *I've tried to say that I'm sorry. I never meant to break her heart, but is my apology enough.*

From the corner of his eye he saw her hand move. He closed his eyes, bracing himself for the cold, sharp sting of her palm against cheek. To his surprise, her touch was gentle, moving the hair away from his face, her thumb slowly stroking the contour of his cheek. Mark looked at her, the moist trail of her tears so vivid against her skin.

"Oh Mark, there are so many feelings I want to tell you about, but I don't know where to start." "You don't have to give me any explanations. I'm sorry that I hurt you; but you can still believe in me, and believe in my love for you." "I do believe in you, and every time I look at you, and hold you, it eases my pain. It makes everything right again. You mean everything to me."

Mark brought her close. "I'm gonna take the time to show you just how much you mean to me. You are everything I will ever need, or want in this life; and I will never again cause you any sadness." Sabrina held him tighter, nuzzling her face into the hollow of his neck. "Come on. You need a change of scenery," he said. "I only need you." "Well, I was planning on going with you." He secured her close to him. Picking up a folded blanket they walked out of the bedroom. "What's that for?" she asked. "In case you get cold."

He guided her outside, past the fire pit to a path that led to the lake. They walked along the shore line without engaging in conversation; until Sabrina stopped. They were in a grassy area, surrounded by low growth brush, a large oak tree partially shading the area. "Can we stop for a little while? I'm a bit tired." "Sure. This is the end of our journey anyway." Sabrina wandered closer to the lake. It was so still and clear, inviting her in, but she didn't feel like swimming.

Mark came up behind her, folding his arms across her chest. "What are you thinking about?" Mark asked. "About how peaceful it is here, it's like being in another world." "That's why I had the cottage built out here. I've spent a lot of time in this spot, and I always dreamed of sharing it with someone I love. Thank you for making my dream come true." "You're very welcome." "Come. Sit and rest for a while."

He had spread the blanket out upon the shaded grass. He helped her down and then stretched out beside her. The thick grass cushioned them from the hard earth below. Laying on his back, he waited for her to join him; but she sat there, staring out at the lake. Mark sat up.

"Are you all right?" he asked. He was still concerned that she was thinking too much. "Yeah. I was just remembering a special day." "Which one? Because since I met you every day has been special." "I was thinking about when you took me riding; the day you opened your heart to me, and gave me this." She held up her right hand with the silver ring. "I remember; it was the first time that I felt alive."

He leaned in, kissing her, while he eased her down upon the blanket. Sabrina held him back. "I wish that you had let me love you that day." "Oh baby, I wanted you to; but I was concerned for your health, and I had to be sure that you were the one that I had been waiting for." "I can appreciate that; but you have no idea just how much I wanted you that day." "Yes, I do. That overwhelming feeling of desire, that burning lust, it's exactly what I'm feeling right now." "Then let me quench that thirst. Let me love you now, like I wanted too then."

Their love brought them together with a new tenderness. A new found sense of discovery. All inhibitions, all doubts and fears had been swept away. At that moment their love was renewed. They had put behind them all of the times of sorrow and pain, freeing their hearts to explore their love to its fullest. It was a new beginning, the opportunity to solidify their deep commitment to each other. To become consumed by the emotional and physical power of pure love. This rededication of devotion sustained them for the entire week; oblivious to the outside world. All that mattered was that they were together.

They spent the week taking walks, or sitting by the fire, but always in physical contact. The need to be touched and held was strong in both of them. Here they could express their love openly, away from the scrutinizing eyes of the public, and their coworkers. Privacy had always been important to Mark, but since being with Sabrina, he had opened up more, becoming more comfortable with expressing his feelings. She had found the tender, gentle side of him that had been lost for so many years. The part of him that he never imagined being capable of showing. As the week progressed, Mark became even more confident. At the pay per view the whole world would see how much he loved her.

Chapter 22

For the first time during the week, Mark awoke with his arms empty. He reached for his jeans, but the unexpected bite of the crisp fall morning made him take his robe as well. Sabrina was right where he knew she would be, on the porch swing; with only his shirt on, she huddled in the corner. Her legs were tucked up under the shirt seeking all possible warmth.

"What are you doing out here so early?" he asked. "I wanted to see the sunrise." "You should have woken me." "No, sorry, this one was for me only." "I don't understand?" "You are not supposed to," she answered. Mark took her hand. "You're freezing; come back inside. Maybe when you've warmed up you can explain this better." He helped her back into the cottage and back into the warmth of their bed, holding her tight, warming her trembling body with his own.

Not until her shivering subsided did he speak. "Can you tell me now what compelled you to sit out there in the cold?" "I'm not sure, when I woke up I felt different somehow. I can't find the right words to describe it. I just have this feeling that today is the first day of many special things." "I don't follow." "I'm sorry; I'm talking nonsense. Something wonderful is going to happen Mark, and I needed to complete the feeling by watching the sun come up. It sounds strange I know, but it's an old habit of mine. In simpler terms, it's like receiving a blessing."

It was a blessing that I was seeking, but one I can't share with Mark. I have been up long before sunrise, standing in the moonlight, reciting my prayers. Reconnecting with who I really am; and whom I need to be again. I wish that I could tell you all of my secrets Mark but I can't. In time, maybe, when I'm sure you're receptive. This wedding is going to bring up questions from you but I can't give you all the answers just yet. I can't let you in to that part of my life yet.

Mark kissed her forehead bringing her back to the moment. "Something special is going to happen. We're getting married, again, but this time the whole world will share in our love." "It's more than that, not that marrying you again isn't special; it's. Damn it; I wish I could get a better feeling on it." "Hush now. If something is meant to happen it will happen just don't dwell on it. You know we don't have to leave until after lunch," he said freeing the buttons on her shirt. "Maybe we can make this a special morning for both of us?" "I like how you think," she answered with a smile.

He pulled her on top of him; their kisses soft, filled with love. Sabrina sat back, finishing the few remaining buttons on the shirt. Mark watched the cotton fabric rub against her breasts; her nipples were hard, taunting him. He parted the shirt, pressing his hands against her breasts; how firm and full. This time he realized that they were larger.

My own hands are large, but her breasts now overflow the confinement of my palms. He forced the thoughts of how and why out of his mind. *All I need to concentrate on is giving her the pleasure she deserves, and anticipating the pleasure she will give to me.*

Their love making had always been slow, but over the past few days it had become even slower, allowing more time for them to explore their fantasies with great care. Even though their love was lingering, and completely fulfilling, it was also exhausting for both of them. Leaving them sleepily enveloped in each other's arms; adrift in an endless ocean of love and contentment.

Mark let Sabrina sleep longer than he should have, and now he felt guilty for rushing her to get ready to go. Sensing his anxiety, she slipped her arms around him. "We won't miss the plane; so stop worrying." "I know, but I feel like I'm rushing you." "No, you're not. I'm ready, and if I know you, you've had Jim pack everything we need before he sent the car for us." "Well, it looks like I'm gonna have a hard time hiding anything from you." "That's right. I know your heart and your soul," she said taking a step back. "And I also know that it's time we left."

As the car pulled away from the cottage, Sabrina turned herself to look out the back window. Watching the cottage grow smaller and smaller until it disappeared from view. She sighed. Mark rubbed his hand over her thigh. "We will come back Sabrina; I promise." "I hope so."

Sliding back around, she moved close to him. "It's a special place for us, a place to relax after a tour. Don't get me wrong, I still love the main house; but I like the privacy out here, to be able to live our lives as a real couple, with no servants catering to our needs, just us." "I like it too, especially the freedom to love you."

At that moment Sabrina was lost for words. She laid her head against his shoulder. They were made for each other in every aspect. He kissed her head. "What was that for?" she asked. "Do I need a reason?" "Never! You can kiss me anytime you want to." "Well then." He lifted her face up. "I think that I'll take advantage of that open invitation."

His kiss was soft, sensual; Sabrina shuddered. "Are you cold?" Mark asked. "Not in the least." "Then why do you shiver every time I touch you." "Oh my love, it's because you electrify me. With every kiss, every touch of your hand, I feel this surge of raw power run through me. I felt it the very first time I met you, and I've felt it every day since then. It's the most wondrous feeling; powerful and magical."

Mark leaned back; he ran his hands through his hair. "What is it?" Sabrina asked. "I don't know what to say." "You don't need to say anything when actions speak louder than words." Their lips had barely touched, when the car came to a stop.

The valet had their luggage stacked onto a cart when they exited the car. The airport was crowded with people. Sabrina anticipated problems, but they slipped through without being noticed.

Checking in was just as quick and simple; the tickets were waiting for them as usual. Mark opened the ticket folder. "I'll be damned," he muttered. "What?" "Look; first class," he said handing her the tickets. "So what's so unusual about that? You always travel first class." "Yeah, but only when the other guys are on the same flight, during the same tour. Nick never books first class for flights prior to a tour. I wonder what he's up to?" "I guess we'll have to wait and see." "It's probably nothing. So what would you like to do tonight in Vegas?" he asked.

Sabrina hooked her arm around his. "I can think of lots of things; but I think that we should wait until we get there before making any plans, just in case Nick already has our evening planned." "He can plan all he wants, but we will have some time for ourselves tonight, no matter what." She snuggled herself closer to him. She found his masculine assertiveness so sexy, and secure.

Nick had done far more than just book them first class seats; he had booked the entire first class cabin for them, complete with champagne. Sabrina kept her thoughts to herself. *I know that we aren't going to have the evening to ourselves. This is Nick's way of preparing us for the events to come.*

Mark fidgeted in his seat. His mind was running thought's one after the other, trying to figure out what Nick had up his sleeve. *It angers me to think that I won't be able to have time alone with Sabrina. I had our day all planned out. Check into the hotel then visit Harry for another tattoo, a romantic dinner, a show. Maybe even some gambling, and then back to the hotel for a night of love.* His hand clenched the armrest.

Sabrina watched his knuckles turn from red too white, as he squeezed harder and harder. Deep lines appeared across his forehead and Sabrina stroked his cheek. "Don't think about it. Nick can't occupy all of our time. We'll make sure of that." She laid her head against him; watching his tension ease, as his fingers slowly let go of the armrest.

The stretched limo was waiting at the curb for them. Mark expected to see Nick step out, but when the driver opened the door and nothing, or no one sprang forth, Mark relaxed just a little. The not knowing was gnawing away at him.

They checked into the hotel easily and quickly. Too quickly, Mark thought. Nick had booked them into the bridal suite. Mark cautiously opened the door, unsure of what to expect. Other than a few flowers, the suite had no surprises. Sabrina took her bag into the bedroom and returned quickly, not wanting to waste any time hanging around the hotel.

Mark was standing near the window, rubbing his shoulder. Sabrina stood behind him and ran her hands up his back. "You're tense. Why?" "I can't stand this not knowing; waiting for the other shoe to drop, waiting for Nick to make his move. Damn it! I really hate this," he said, the agitation in his voice taking full control, causing more tension to creep up his neck.

Sabrina moved around in front of him. "You need to get rid of this tension, and I have the perfect solution. Come with me," she said taking his hands. She led him into the bedroom. "I don't think I can; at least not right now," he said looking at the bed. "Did I say anything about making love? We have a Jacuzzi, and you need a long soak to get rid of this tension that you're creating." "How is it you always know what I need?" "Being your wife, makes it my job to know what you need. Now get yourself into that tub." "Yes ma'am. Will you be joining me?" "Of course, but I need a minute first." She left the bedroom while Mark undressed and got into the tub.

In the privacy of the outer room, Sabrina called the front desk, instructing the operator to not let any calls through for at least an hour. Hanging up the phone, she began to strip away her clothes, leaving a neat trail into the bedroom. Mark reached for her as she stepped into the tub.

"No, you don't," she scolded. "Now turn around." She picked up the thick sponge. "You need to relax; remember?"

Soaking the sponge in the water, she squeezed it out over his back. When his back was completely wet, she began to smooth her hands across his shoulders and down his spine, pushing away the tension, freeing his mind of all the nagging thoughts.

When he began to slump, she stopped her gentle massage. "Feel better?" "Like a new man; you have the magic touch, but how are you feeling?" "Great; but if I stay in here much longer I'm gonna need a nap. I forgot how warm these things are." "There's nothing wrong with that; if you're tired you should rest." "Later. We should sneak out of here before Nick comes looking for us." "I'll second that," he said rubbing her shoulder.

"Feel like going to see Harry?" "Yeah; it's about time I got a new piece of art." "After that, maybe we can take in a show, if you're up to it." "That would be nice; but I won't get my hopes up, at least not until we've made our escape from the hotel." "Well, how fast can you get dressed?" Mark asked. Sabrina didn't answer, she was out of the tub and in the bedroom before he could blink. Mark wrapped a towel around himself. Sabrina's massage had left him so relaxed, he knew he should be hurrying, but he just didn't have the energy.

Sabrina was pawing through her suitcase. Mark watched her from the doorway. Her sexy body scantily covered by the bath towel. *I need to hold her, to have that body against mine.* He took her by the shoulders, turning her around. Pulling her close, he kissed her passionately. Sabrina felt her towel loosen. She grabbed at it, backing away from him.

"No way, you said we were going out," she scolded. "Yeah, but we have plenty of time." "Oh no you don't! You're gonna have to put those thoughts out of your mind until tomorrow night." "What?" "You heard me, no sex until after the wedding tomorrow night." "We're already married; why wait?" "Humor me Mark; please." "Okay, we'll wait," he said, stroking her shoulders. "But can we at least share the same bed?" "Of course, and you can still hold me." "I'll be happy with that; at least until tomorrow."

The unexpected knock at the door startled them both; Sabrina reached for her robe. "Ignore it," Mark said. "We both know who it is; maybe he'll give up and go away." "Not fair; it's better to face the music now, than the wrath later." "Fine; I'll let him in." "Better let me," she said tying her robe. "You need to put some pants on." She pulled off his towel as she walked away. Mark grabbed it back, giving her a quick flick on the ass with the damp towel.

Sabrina reached the door as the third barrage of loud knocks echoed into the room. "Come in Nick," she announced, opening the door. "How did you, never mind," Nick muttered, stepping past her. "Where is Mark?" "Getting dressed; he'll be out in a minute. So what can I do for you?" "Well, to start with, you both need costume fittings. Then we need to go over the ceremony with the choreographer; some preliminary photos."

"Not tonight," Mark interrupted. "It has to be done tonight! Christ, the show is tomorrow afternoon." "I said not tonight," Mark answered, moving closer to Nick. "We already have plans, and you're not gonna make me break a promise to my wife." "These things have to be done." "Not tonight! Got it!" "Fine," Nick scowled. "But nine o'clock tomorrow morning, you both had better be downstairs, and no excuses for being late." Nick headed for the door. "Remember, nine o'clock, not a second later!" The door slammed behind him.

Sabrina bounded over to Mark; she hugged him tight. "What's this about?" he asked caught off guard by her actions. "I am so happy, and so proud of you, for standing up to Nick like that." "I'm just tired of having him control our lives. I promised you a night on the town; and that means you and me, not you, me and half the company." She stretched herself up to kiss him. "I love you," she whispered as she stretched herself higher. "Maybe I shouldn't make you wait until tomorrow night."

He was about to answer when he saw on her face the expression of pain. She pulled away from him grabbing at her side. "What's wrong?" "I'm fine; it's just a muscle spasm," she answered, rubbing at the annoyance. "You're sure?" "Yes, I'm sure; I over extended myself, that's all."

With his piercing green eyes he scrutinized her expression. Sabrina knew that look all too well. She turned away and headed to the bedroom. "While you're trying to decide if you believe me or not, I'm going to get dressed. You're not going to get out of taking me out tonight." Mark sank down onto the sofa.

Why do I worry so much? If she said she was fine then I should believe her. There should be no doubts. She's young and healthy, no need to worry, but I love her too much to ignore what she calls her little aches and pains. What if, what if Doc suspects more than he let on? Enough; I'm making something out of nothing. We are going out tonight, and all that matters is that she has a good time.

The phone rang six times before the switchboard cut in. "Would you like to leave a message?" "No, thank you. I'll try again tomorrow." Doc hung up the phone and picked up the file in front of him. Being away for two weeks had left him with a great deal to catch up on. His patients were all very important to him, but this one took priority over all. *How could I have been so negligent? I should have recognized it for what it really was.*
Doc laid Sabrina's file down. "I'm so sorry darlin. I've been a stupid old fool," he said quietly as he patted the folder. "But I'm gonna make it up to you. You're gonna get the best care possible, I promise." *I'll call them again tomorrow; Sabrina has to know. They both have to know, and it has to be soon. I will not give up; time is important. I have to reach them before they became locked into the tour, and too far away from home.*

The plan for the evening hit a snag. Mark was dumb founded as he stood before the door to Harry's shop, reading the closed sign. In all the years that he had been coming here, never had Harry been closed. "I hope he's okay," he said to Sabrina. "I'm sure he's fine. Maybe he took a vacation." "Maybe." "Why don't we try someone else?" "No! I trust Harry; especially when it comes to you." "Okay then. So what was next on your agenda?" "It was a show; but it's way too early. What would you like to do?" Sabrina thought about it while she settled herself in the car.
Mark started the engine. The interior was flooded with the cool breeze of the air conditioner. "Well?" "I really don't know. It's too early for dinner, or a show. Too late for shopping, and I'm not overly excited about sitting in a casino. So what's left?" "Well, if you're not into gambling then why don't we tour some of the hotels?" "I don't understand?" "We could go and watch a jousting match, or we could take a ride down the Nile River, and then visit." "That one," she interrupted. "That sounds romantic." "Okay, that one it is then."
The immense hotel was a magical wonder. The glass pyramid towered high, reaching to the sun. They had only traveled a few blocks, but seeing this giant monolith made Sabrina feel like they had actually traveled to ancient Egypt. The authentic costumes, and lavish decor enhanced the magic, and mystery of this strange land. Mark arranged for a private barge

to take them along the man made river. He held her close as they drifted through the past.

From the barge, they took a leisurely stroll through a recreated tomb. Mark stopped when he felt Sabrina leaning heavily against him. "What's the matter?" Mark asked. "It's just so warm in here; it tires me." "We'll leave then. How does an air conditioned restaurant sound?" "Fine." Her usual enthusiasm wasn't there. Mark lifted her face up to his. "Maybe not; you're really tired; aren't you?" "I'll be fine once I've cooled down." "We'll see."

Mark steadied her as she got into the car. He started the engine and directed the air vents towards her. Sabrina leaned back, closing her eyes, as the cool breeze engulfed her. With Mark's soothing touch on her temple, she was lulled into a brief slumber, only to be startled awake as her body involuntarily jumped from the speedy relaxation. He squeezed her hand. "I have my answer. We're going back to the hotel and you're gonna get a good night's sleep." "But our night out."

"Not now, this tour is gonna be a long one, and I don't want you exhausted before it even starts. We can have dinner in the suite, and then you can go to bed. You know I'm not at all surprised that you're so tired. I think that the longest you've slept, at one time, this week has been about only four hours." "Yeah; but we just have too much fun when we're awake," she said as she slowly rubbed at his thigh. "Not tonight, you made that promise yourself; tonight you rest." "And prepare for tomorrow."

"Are you worried about tomorrow?" Mark asked. "A little I guess; but I know I shouldn't be. It's just another show." "Yeah; but it's what Nick's cooking up for after the show is what bothers me," Mark answered. "It's just a party." "Is it? I'd prefer to be alone with you, than stuck at some party being the center of attention."

The party I can deal with; but if Mark were to find out the true significance of the ceremony. I don't know how he would react. During our time at the cottage, I had penned the ceremony for Nick; unnoticed by Mark. I know it off by heart, so scribing down the script was easy. Then hiding it in the courier pouch that went back to Nick; along with a note with suggestions for costumes and decor.

This couldn't have come at a better time; being Halloween and all, it's perfect. I have to renew myself; become strong again. It's wrong not to tell Mark about it. He wouldn't understand, but by bringing him into my world, I will be able to protect him better. With any luck, he will think that this is just another story cooked up by Nick and the writing staff.

When they returned to the hotel Sabrina was out of the car quickly, waiting for Mark. She snuggled into him when he neared her. "Maybe we can sneak out of the party," she said. "Not likely, if I know Nick, he'll either have us separated, or he'll be stuck between us the entire evening." "Don't dwell on it. Just hold onto the thought that we will be leaving together, and we will be spending the night together."

"Don't get me thinking about that now." "Why?" "Because I have to help you keep a promise tonight." "Maybe, maybe not." Her hand slid slowly down over the buckle on his jeans. Mark was quick to lift her hand back up. "Please don't. It's difficult enough just being back here with you." "I know. I can still remember every wonderful moment."

"Excuse me, Mr. and Mrs. Cassidy." The unexpected voice startled them both. Sabrina turned. "I remember you. You're the manager; Mr. Blackthorn." "Yes ma'am; and may I say it is a pleasure to have you both back here with us." "Thank you," Mark answered. "But you know this is more business than anything." "Yes sir I do. I have been overseeing tomorrow night's festivities; and before you ask, I have been instructed not to discuss it with you. However, I have been informed by my employer to extend to you the hospitality of this hotel." "Come again?" "My employer would be pleased if you would accept his offer of a fine dinner, and special seats at the evening show."

"I don't know. We were planning on ordering from room service. My wife is a bit tired." "Hey!" Sabrina interrupted. "I'm feeling better now." "You're sure?" "Yes, very sure; besides you promised me a night out, remember?" "Okay." Mark turned back to the manager. "We accept." "Wonderful." "Do you think there would be any room at the dinner show, instead of the late show?" "Of course, I will make the arrangements myself. You should be at the theater in about forty-five minutes. I will meet you there." He quietly bowed away from them.

Sabrina smiled at Mark. "What?" he quizzed. "I told you that something special would happen this weekend." "Yes, you did," he said, turning her toward the elevator. "Now use your intuition to figure out what you're going to wear to dinner."

Mark had begun to pace as he waited for Sabrina. She had banished him from the bedroom while she changed her clothes. He knocked on the door. "We have ten minutes to get downstairs," he called. Getting no response, he wandered over to the window. *There is no need to make her rush; the table is guaranteed.*

Sabrina quietly opened the door. She stuck only her head out to see where Mark was, then leaned back against the frame. "I'm ready if you are," she called. Mark started to turn. "It's about." His words froze in his throat. He gasped for breath, as his brain demanded him to breathe. His eyes followed the contour of her ankle up to the shapely curve of her thigh, the full expanse of her tanned leg, exposed by the wide slit in her dress.

Continuing his visual examination upward, over the pink fabric that wrapped her body, up to her bare shoulders, to the blonde hair that was pulled up, except for a few wisps that swirled down around her neck. Sabrina moved toward him. Her slow, sultry gait made his heart pound, his breath keeping time with the sway of her hips.

She touched him, gently wiping away the beads of perspiration on his forehead. "Do you have nothing to say?" "I, I'd like to," he stammered. "But my mind just can't find anything appropriate to describe how beautiful you are." "You don't need words, actions speak far louder, and clearer," she invited.

Stepping blindly into his arms, she tasted the gentle warmth of his lips on hers. The taste of love that she hungered for. She teased at his tongue until it plunged deep into her mouth, bringing her closer to him. Mark pulled back suddenly. "Why do you torment me like this? We made a promise." "I know; but I do know what I'm doing. By teasing you now, guarantees me that when we make love tomorrow, it will be a night far more intense than any other."

Mark ran his hand lightly across her cheek. "It's our second wedding night. It should be a night of tenderness and lasting pleasures." "No, my love, tomorrow is a fantasy; and that's how we should think of it. A chance for us to fulfill all the desires that we've kept secret."

"What would your fantasy be?" Mark asked. "I won't tell you that now; but I will let you know part of it. I crave to have your body pressed against mine, to feel your weight, as you fill me with ecstasy." "You can't handle it. I'll hurt you." "Oh my sweet love," she whispered, kissing him softly. "You can never hurt me. We were meant to be together; in body and soul, completely, joined together for all eternity."

Mark stepped back, holding her at arm's length. "We need to end this conversation; for more than one reason," he said sternly. "Okay, but please think about what I've said. I want to fulfill your fantasies, and I will do anything to give you the pleasure that you deserve." "Sabrina you are my fantasy come true; in every way; and as much as I would like to continue this, we are going to be late for dinner." He wove her arm around his and guided her to the door.

The manager was quick to whisk them away from the stares, from the other patrons, lined up for the show. They were directed to a row of private booths near the stage. The high backs secluding them from the view of the theater behind them. Sabrina glanced down the row of booths. The sight of a familiar face made her smile. "I'll be right back," she said to Mark.

He hadn't seen the person sitting six tables down. He presumed that she was off to the ladies room, so he sat down to peruse the menu. Her approach had gone unnoticed; she stopped at the edge of the booth. "Hey good lookin," she spoke in a subdued voice.

Brent looked up. The sight of Sabrina made him stand up in haste. The table rocked, toppling glasses. "Easy," she said, taking another step closer. "You'd think you hadn't had any human company for a while." "Not as pretty as you." Brent took a long look at her. "My Lord, you are hot! You could stop traffic dressed like that." "Thank you. So, are you here alone, or are you expecting someone?" "No, just me, I got tired of staring at the walls in my room. Where is Mark?" "Down there," she answered tilting her head to the side. "Why don't you join us?" "I don't want to intrude." "Since when is friends having dinner together an intrusion? Come on." She took his hand firmly into hers.

Brent was glad of the company; being alone so much was beginning to take its toll, slipping into moments of depression, after days of sleepless nights filled with frustration. Just being able to be near her made him feel much better.

Coming up behind Mark, Sabrina announced herself. "Look who I found," she said, tugging Brent to the front of the table. "Hey Brent. Good to see you man." Mark stood up extending his hand to receive the firm grip of Brent's handshake. "Yeah, same here." "I asked Brent to join us." "Great idea." "You're sure? I don't want to intrude on your evening." "It's not an intrusion; make yourself comfortable," Mark said. Brent slid in on the opposite side of Sabrina. Mark welcomed the company. *At least it might help to take my mind off of her incredible invitation for tomorrow night.*

"I really didn't expect to see you two until tomorrow night. I figured that Nick would have you locked up, going over the details," Brent said. "He wanted to," Sabrina answered. "But Mark took care of him." "Good for you, Nick gets carried away sometimes. He forgets that we have personal lives, away from the ring."

Sabrina wiggled a little closer to Brent. "Speaking of; anything new I should know about?" she asked. "With me? Nothing new," Brent answered. She squeezed his hand gently. "Don't worry. You will find someone; and it will be worth the wait." "That's right man. I went through years of hell, until God sent me this angel, the most beautiful, loving, sensitive and sexy woman to ever walk this earth." Sabrina blushed as her eyes glistened with moisture. *How dare I make him wait?*

The conversation during dinner was light, focusing on anything but the tour. Brent leaned back, setting down his cup of coffee. "You two ready for tomorrow night?" Brent asked. "According to Nick we're not," Sabrina answered. "He wants us at the ring at nine o'clock, for costume fittings, and a rehearsal with the choreographer." "That sucks. He never knows when to quit, but what I was really referring to was if you were prepared for Nick's other plan." "What other plan?" Mark asked. "Oh shit! He didn't tell you did he? That sneaky son of a bitch!" "Brent please." Sabrina began to worry. "What has Nick neglected to tell us?"

Brent stared into her blue eyes, wide with anticipation, and just a hint of fear. "Sabrina, I'm sorry that you have to find out this way," he paused to take a deep breath. "Sean is coming back tomorrow." "What!" Mark exclaimed. "Yeah. He's been cleared to return to work. Sabrina I'm so sorry. Nick should have told you a week ago."

Sabrina hugged herself as she began to shake uncontrollably. "Are you okay?" Mark asked. "I, I'm cold," she stammered. "So very cold." Mark had no jacket to give her, and neither did Brent. He pulled her close, holding her tight against him. Her quaking slowed, and then stopped abruptly. "You better get her upstairs," Brent said. "She'll be fine." "No man, she's in shock."

You need to get her upstairs, now." "Sabrina," Mark called to her, trying to bring her back from her thoughts. "Come on baby."

She inhaled deeply, and began to shiver again, only harder. "I'm so cold." She snuggled into Mark. He slid off the bench, taking her with him. "We're going upstairs." She didn't have the energy to argue with him, but did find the strength to reach out to Brent; who, reluctantly, tagged along behind. *I may be intruding, but maybe I can give them the answers that Nick had kept from them.*

The elevator stopped on their floor. Blocking the door with his foot, Mark shifted Sabrina into Brent's arms. "Take her to the suite," he said handing Brent the card key. "Wrap her in a blanket." "Where are you going?" Brent asked, even though he knew the answer. "I've got something to take care of; and it won't take very long." Mark moved his foot and the door shut. Pressing the floor button, the elevator began to move down, stopping three floors below.

In Sabrina's current state, she didn't even notice Mark's absence. Brent settled her onto the sofa, tucking a blanket around her. Sitting at her side, he intended to put his arm around her, but Sabrina laid her head on his lap, curling up into a little bundle beside him. He made sure that the blanket covered her trembling body. With some hesitation, he rested his hand upon her shoulder. He rubbed at it gently, as he thought about what Mark was about to do. The repercussions could damage them both.

Mark forced the elevator door open. Pushing past a room service clerk he went down the hall, stopping at the last door. He pounded on the door relentlessly, until he heard the click of the lock. The door swung in, out of Nick's hand, hitting the wall with a vibrating thud. Mark's fist found it's target. Nick staggered backward to the floor.

Towering above him, Mark began to yell. "You son of a bitch! How could you not tell me?" "Tell you what?" Nick asked, rubbing at his jaw. "You should have told me that your star asshole was coming back to work tomorrow. How could you do this to Sabrina? You knew that she'd need time to prepare herself, but no, you decide to keep this a secret! As far as I'm concerned the show is off!"

Nick pulled himself up, making sure that he was out of Mark's reach. "The show will not be canceled! It will go ahead as scheduled. Sean knows that he's not allowed anywhere near Sabrina. Besides she's strong enough to." "Strong enough! Bull shit! Then why is she upstairs shaking with fear; thanks to you!" "I'm sorry Mark. I didn't think that." "That's right; you didn't think, and as far as your damn show, that will depend on her condition tomorrow! If she's not up to it, it's off, simple as that! Got it!" "Fine; but she's going to have to face him sooner or later." "My preference is later; very much later." Mark stormed down the hall. Nick closed the door; a smile crept across his face. *It is going to be a great show.*

Standing before the door to his suite, Mark took a deep breath. *I have to be calm. Sabrina doesn't need to see the anger. I have to support her.* Shrugging off the tension in his neck, he opened the door. Brent motioned to him to be quiet. "How is she?" Mark asked. "Sleeping, I think. How did it go with Nick?" "Fine. I introduced him to my fist." "Do you think that was a wise move?"

"I don't care anymore," Mark said quietly as he brushed the hair from Sabrina's face. "Let the son of a bitch fire me if he wants. She's the only thing that matters anymore. I'm tired of the lies and the bull shit. The things he does just to sell tickets, and get ratings; it's not right. He has no right to hurt people like this; especially her." "Maybe; but he does sign your paycheck."

"I'll quit before I let him destroy her with his mind games. She doesn't deserve it." "It's a mess that's for sure. Look, you should get her to bed, and I should get out of here." Brent slipped out from under her. "Thanks man." Mark patted Brent on the back. "Hey no problem." Brent paused at the door. "I'll stay close by tomorrow; just in case."

Sabrina moaned and stretched. "How are you feeling?" Mark asked, as he perched himself on the edge of the coffee table. "Tired and cold." "You should be in bed." He lifted her up. She staggered at first. Mark held her tight, supporting her against him. He helped her to put on one of his T-shirts and tucked her into bed. Dropping his clothes on the floor, he slipped in beside her, bringing her close to him. Within minutes she was asleep again; Mark stayed awake. Periodically she would shudder; but her mournful whimpers fueled his anger.

She's remembering, in her dreams, what that bastard, has done to her. I feel so helpless, if only I could free her mind of this damn torment. Maybe I should quit. Other organizations had offered a substantial amount if I would work for them; but it still wouldn't be a better life for Sabrina. We would still be on the road, maybe more than now. Tomorrow will be the deciding factor. If being around Sean is too much for her, then I will quit, and take her far away from this man made hell.

The night was too short. Mark awoke alone, Sabrina no longer in his arms. He found her huddled on the sofa. "You're up early," he said taking a seat beside her. "I needed to think." "About what?" "The past." "Baby don't torment yourself." "I'm not. I need to get over it; but to do that I have to face him; and that means going through with today's show." "Don't push yourself into something that's going to upset you." "I can't let it upset me anymore. I won't let it. As long as you are with me, I can be strong." "I won't leave you alone for a minute; I promise. We will face him together, but with any luck it won't come to that."

Straightening herself, she saw the bruise on his knuckles. "Where did you disappear to last night?" she asked. "I had something to take care of." "That would be what?" "Let's just say that I might be tempted to pay more attention to those other job offers." "Oh Mark you didn't?" "Yeah; but I was just so angry at Nick. I didn't think clearly." "Is he hurt?" "He was still talking when I left, so it couldn't be too bad."

"I admire how you defend my honor; but you can't let that side of you get control. You have to let your head control your heart." "You're right; but it makes me crazy to see you hurt." Shifting herself slightly, she looked at him. It was a look that he didn't understand. "What?" he asked. "You definitely live up to your name." "I don't understand what you mean."

"Your name means a warrior and defender, and that's exactly what you are. You have fought for me and protected me, all true admirable qualities and," she hesitated while she shifted herself onto her knees. "And I love you," she whispered as she kissed him, her hands softly caressing his face. "How do you know so much about names?" he asked. "Let's just say that it's an old habit of mine and leave it at that."

Still holding his face gently in her hands, she softly nuzzled her face against his. "Mark, will you marry me today?" she asked in a soft, breathy voice. "Yes! I will marry you again, without hesitation." "Then shall we see what kind of screw ups Nick has made to our wedding plans, and, to see if I can affect some sort of damage control."

There was a light knock at the door. "That will be Brent," Mark said. "We should go as soon as you're dressed." He waited until Sabrina had shut the bedroom door before he let Brent in. "I didn't wake you, did I?" Brent asked. "No, Sabrina's getting dressed." "How is she feeling this morning?" "Amazingly well. I don't know whether to feel relieved, or worried." "What makes you say that?" "She wants to face him; to see Sean face to face." "Not alone I hope." "No way! I will not allow this confrontation that much latitude." "You can count on me to be close by." "Thanks man."

"Thanks for what?" Sabrina asked. "Oh, I was just thanking Brent for helping me out last night." "Yes, Brent, thank you. You are such a good friend; to both of us." "That friendship could be in jeopardy if Nick's in a bad mood," Mark interjected. "Let me handle Nick," Sabrina said, taking Mark's arm. "Now shall we see to this wedding?"

The costume designer, Gene, was the first to snare them as they arrived. He had fitted Mark many times, but never having designed for Sabrina before, he wanted to spend as much time as he could with her. His instructions were to make her outfit perfect, or find a new employer. Nick had never been so fanatical about a costume before. Per Nick's instructions, Mark was not allowed in during Sabrina's fitting. He pulled up a chair outside the door and waited. More like a guard, than an impatient husband, he methodically checked the hallways for intruders.

Brent had wandered off, but soon returned with a tray of coffee. He handed one to Mark before sitting down on the floor across from the doorway. "Sabrina's still in there I take it?" Brent asked. Mark only nodded, as he sipped his coffee. "Have you seen Nick yet?" "Nope; and I'm not looking." "How long are you two tied up here?" "Probably right up to show time; and beyond."

"I didn't see a breakfast tray in your room; so I'm guessing that you haven't eaten yet." "That's right," Mark answered. "Well, Nick can't hold you here without food. When Sabrina's done we should sneak out for an early lunch." "Nick will have a fit if we leave." "Screw him, or do you think he'd be pleased to see her faint from hunger? We don't even have to leave the hotel." "You're on. I've got to keep her healthy."

As the trio headed back into the hotel, Matt, the security chief called to them. "Hey Mark; you got a phone call." "Tell who ever it is that you can't find us and take a message." Matt related the information to the caller, but received no message. "Damn it to hell!" Doc cursed as he dropped the phone into its cradle. He looked at his watch.

Maybe I should fly up to Vegas, since trying to reach them by phone is proving to be fruitless. Picking up the phone again, he called the airlines. With each call, he became more frustrated. Each airline he called had the same answers. No more flights today, or all booked up. Tapping the phone index on his desk gave him an idea. *One of the ranchers near by has his own plane. It's a long shot, but one I know I have to take.*

Lunch was abruptly cut short with the arrival of Nick. "I thought I told you that we had plans for today," Nick lashed out angrily. "Oh come on Nick," Brent took up the conversation. "They've been in costume all morning. Do you really want Sabrina to be ill because you've kept her from revitalizing herself with a meal?" "Well, no." Nick's stern voice had softened. "Just don't take too long. The choreographer will be waiting for you." Nick turned and wove his way back out of the restaurant.

Sabrina leaned over to Brent and kissed his cheek. "What's that for?" he asked. "For standing up to Nick. It's not all that hard to do, and he does respect you for it." "Sure it's easy, when it's on your behalf. If I was making my own stand, he'd walk all over me." "Only if you let him Brent, only if you let him."

Leaning back in his chair, Brent's expression took on a more quizzical look. "Enough about that ass. So what's your costume like?" he asked. Sabrina looked at Mark and back at Brent and her grin widened. "You'll both have to wait until show time," she said with a smile and turned back to Mark. "But it will be well worth the wait. It might even help you to come up with an answer to my proposal." "I gave you my answer," Mark replied, not wanting to get into this conversation in a restaurant. "No, you gave me a very nice comment, but you did not give me an answer."

Seeing the all absorbed look on Brent's face, Mark put an end to the discussion. "We can talk about this later," Mark said. "Don't stop on my account; you have me intrigued. Just carry on like I wasn't even here," Brent said with a smile. "Not likely!" Mark pushed his chair back. "I'm sorry, but this is personal, between Sabrina and myself." "Oh now you've really piqued my curiosity; but I'll leave it alone. My imagination can fill in the blanks quite nicely thank you."

"Oh for Christ sake!" Mark grumbled as he stood up. "I'm leaving. Are you coming Sabrina?" "Yeah, I'll be right there." Mark wandered over to the cashier. "I'm sorry. I embarrassed him; didn't I?" Brent asked. "A bit, but don't worry about it. Mark's more confused by me, and what I have asked of him." "I wouldn't know about that; but I think he's also on edge about today." "You're probably right. I'm not going to think about it anymore. We better get going, before Nick comes back."

Mark was waiting by the door. Sabrina slipped her arms around him. Knowing that he should disappear at that moment, Brent kept on walking. "I'm going on. I'll tell the choreographer that you're on your way."

Sabrina moved her hands up Mark's back, bringing herself closer to him. "I'm sorry for upsetting you," she said softly. Mark sighed, but did not answer her. "Please forgive me," she pouted. "I love you; and I know you are a private person when it comes to sharing our love in public; but I just want the whole world to know, and to see, how much I love you." "They will," Mark answered, stroking her hair. "In a few hours our love will be on display for all to see, but our real love will still be our own private secret and tonight I will tell you my fantasy." Sabrina could only respond with a soft moan, as Mark's kiss had taken her voice.

The choreographer, Erik, was relentless. Even though he had a slight feminine air about him, he was still a boisterous and arrogant little man bordering on obsessive compulsive. Over and over he made them rehearse the routine without a break. Down the ramp to the ring, through the entire ceremony less the written portion of the script.

The arena area was being kept off limits to all. Even Brent was barred. The show was going to be a surprise for the fans, as well as the crew. All the others involved with the ceremony had been given their scripts, showing only their parts. Nothing of the other roles was being revealed to anyone, and talking about it was forbidden.

Sabrina had lost track of how many times they had walked through the routine. She knew it off by heart. Her feet ached. She sat down on the edge of the ring, much to the disgust of the choreographer. "We must continue; it's not perfect yet," Erik said, a hint of sarcasm in his voice. Sabrina stopped rubbing her foot; she glared at this tiny man. Her patience was long past worn out and all of her nerves and emotions were raw.

"Fuck you!" she yelled at Erik. "Sabrina!" "I'm sorry Mark, but I've had enough of this bull shit. We've been over and over this, more than I can count. I'm tired, my feet hurt, my back aches; and his highness here still thinks it's not right." "Well, I never!" Erik exclaimed. "Yeah, you probably never; and it might change your attitude if you did!" "Sabrina stop it!" Mark stood in front of her. "What is the matter with you?"

He saw her eyes well up. He quickly glanced over his shoulder to Erik. "Rehearsal's over; leave us!" Mark commanded. Turning back to Sabrina, her tears had already spilled down her cheeks. He brought her into his arms. After a long silence, Sabrina pulled back. Mark wiped away the lingering moisture from her cheeks.

"Feel better?" "Yeah. Mark I'm sorry." "Don't be. I don't blame you for getting pissed off. He did go a little overboard." "It doesn't excuse what I said." "It doesn't matter. In a few short hours this will be nothing but a memory, but right now I'm going to take you back to the dressing room and get you into a nice hot shower; and hold you in my arms until its time to get ready."

Sabrina slid from her perch. "I love it when you know what I need, when I need it." "It's my job," he said as he caressed her cheek. "Now let's sneak out of here before Nick catches us, and our brief interlude is snatched away."

He sent her on to the shower. When she was out of sight, he locked the dressing room door, and as an added safeguard, braced a chair against the knob. He wandered back to the shower. Sabrina's clothes were strewn on the floor. "How are you feeling?" he asked. "Lonely. I'm waiting for you. You did promise to hold me." "I meant; ah, hell."

He stripped off his clothes and joined her. Sabrina backed up to him; pulling his arms around her. She handed him the soap. "I don't think so," he said setting the soap aside. "We made a promise," he reminded her. Sabrina repositioned his hands, one on her breast, one on her thigh. "I know we promised; but I need you, want you, now. I need to feel your strength." She felt his lips on her neck, his hand slowly sliding between her thighs.

"You make me so crazy," he whispered. Sabrina turned around to kiss him. "That's good," she whispered. Mark lifted her up. She locked her arms around his neck, her legs around his waist. "This is not what I hand in mind," Mark said, bracing her against the shower wall. "No excuses; just make love to me. It won't change the passion that I have planned for tonight."

She kissed him, preventing him from answering, but letting him know just how much she wanted him. Mark was more than pleased with her spontaneity. It was quietly driving him crazy having to wait. Their love, their lust, rewarded them with the pleasures they both longed for.

Nick kicked over a garbage can, as his anger boiled to the surface. "Where the hell are they?" he yelled to anyone who would listen. Brent came around the corner. "Who are you looking for?" "You damn well know; Mark and Sabrina. They're not where they're supposed to be. Have you got any ideas?" "I don't know," Brent shrugged. "Did you try the dressing room?" "What the hell are they doing in there?" "Taking a break from your minute by minute controlling agenda of their lives." "Knock it off! Another wise ass remark like that and you'll find yourself on suspension!"

Nick turned away toward the dressing rooms; Brent sneered at him, and followed along. Without knocking, Nick grabbed the doorknob; expecting it to open, his body ran into it when it didn't. "Damn it," he muttered, twisting at the knob. Nick began to thump on the door with his fist. "God damn it Mark; open the door!"

"It was nice while it lasted," Sabrina sighed, dragging herself away from Marks arms. "Yeah, but it will be better later, and that's a promise." Nick's persistent thuds were becoming annoying. Mark kicked the chair aside and opened the door. Nick burst into the room. "Why aren't you at rehearsal?" "We were! Sabrina was tired, so I ended it." "You have to rehearse, or it won't be right."

"Look! She's not like the rest of us. You can't push her hour after hour. She does need to rest now and then, or would you like to see her worn out and making mistakes?" "No, of course not, I just have to be sure that this show goes smoothly. Can you guarantee me that?" "Yes, Nick," Sabrina said as she ambled over to him. "I can. I know that routine inside and out. I wrote it; remember?"

Mark's headed snapped around to look at her. That look of bewilderment on his face, she knew she would be in for a very long interrogation. She avoided his stare and looked straight at Nick. "You just better make sure that the rest of them know the script. I don't want any screw ups either."

"Good," Nick answered, taking a deep breath. "Sabrina I need you to come with me." "Why?" "There's only ninety minutes until show time, and I need you in makeup, and then into costume." "Fine," she said, taking up Mark's hand. "Lead on." "No. Mark can't go." "Why not?" "I would prefer it if you two didn't see each other until the ceremony." "I guess it's okay." "Well, I don't like it," Mark said, glaring at Nick. "Can we have a few minutes?" *I need answers, now.* "Sure, but not too long." Nick stepped into the hallway to wait.

"I'll be fine," she said, taking Mark's face in her hands. "My guardian angel won't be very far away." Seeing the look of puzzlement on his face, she glanced toward Brent. "Oh yeah, I guess I won't have to worry as much." "No, you won't. In fact you can use this time to work out your fantasy for tonight." "You're completely wicked." "Maybe; but I know you love it."

"I know I love you; and the rest is just a wonderful bonus. Baby I have to know. What did you mean, you wrote this script?" "Please don't question me now. Let's just get through this and then, maybe, I'll explain everything." They shared one last kiss. A long, passionate kiss, to sustain them until they were together again.

"Okay, okay," Nick interrupted. "We have to go." Mark walked Sabrina to the door. She held his hand tight, even though she had wove her other arm around Brent's. As she began to walk away, her arm stretched back, her hand slowly slipping loose from his. Her fingers glided over his palm to the tips and then her touch was gone. Mark felt his heart sink; his stomach knot up. *She'll be fine, but with Sean on the loose somewhere in the building, makes me uneasy.* Sabrina glanced back at him. She smiled, a forced smile. *I want to go to her, to tell Nick to go to Hell. Screw his plans. No, Brent will stay close to her.*

Before being barred from Sabrina's private dressing room, Brent checked it out thoroughly. Only one door, no windows, no closets to hide in; she would be fine. Brent placed his hands lightly upon her shoulders. "It'll be okay. I'll be right outside the door, should you need me to get Mark," he said with a reassuring smile.

Sabrina shrugged off his hands and hugged him. "I know; and thank you." "For what?" "For showing me what a real friend is. I never understood what true friendship was until I met you. You have stood by Mark and I through the best, and the worst; and I am so very grateful of that." "I'll always be here for you, and for Mark. You two are like my family."

"I am sorry that we didn't include you in our real wedding." Her face suddenly lit up. "I have an idea! Nick, I have something to add to the ceremony." "What would that be exactly?" Nick asked. "I want Brent to escort me to the ring." "No way. Not possible. I don't like last minute changes, especially with a production this big." "Yes, it is possible. Just give him a robe, like the others, and a copy of the script. It won't alter the routine at all. Please don't ask me to explain, but it would give me peace of mind."

Nick thought about it for a moment. *I know her reasons, and I really don't blame her. I can't even guarantee that I'll be able to maintain control of Sean.* "Fine, not a bad idea at all." "Thank you, Nick." "Whatever. Now can we get this show on the road? Brent you can't stay here." "I know I was just leaving." Brent picked up a chair and placed it outside the door. Nick followed him out, shutting the door behind him. "Well, since you're going to be waiting out here then make sure that the only people to go in or out of that room are those from makeup and costume, understand?"

"Yes boss," Brent said sarcastically saluting Nick's back. D'arcy passed Nick at the corner and then he spotted Brent. "Hey man, what's with the chair? Did you piss off the boss?" "No, Sabrina's in there, I said that I'd watch the door." "Where is Mark?" "Down the hall. Maybe you should keep him company." "I get it. This is part of Nick's big plan for tonight's show." "Yeah, and I can tell you that separating these two is the worst thing that Nick's ever done. Neither of them are handling it very well." "I guess not. Where did you say Mark was?" "Down the hall, turn left, name's on the door." "See you later."

Doc paced the tiny airport lounge, checking his watch repeatedly. The rancher had agreed to fly Doc up to Vegas, but Doc grew impatient as the plane was readied for take off. He tried the number of the hotel again, muttering to himself as the phone rang endlessly. Looking at his watch again, he realized that they were probably at the show by now; the next dilemma. *How will I get back stage to see them? Damn it I'm their physician. I shouldn't be denied.* The rancher tapped on the window. He beckoned to Doc; it was time to leave. Collecting his briefcase Doc wished silently that they would be there in time. They just had to.

Chapter 23

Sabrina felt edgy. Her hair and makeup were complete. The costume designer, Gene, had been in to help her into her outfit; but now she was completely alone, isolated from everyone. The show had started. She heard the arena fill with screaming fans, the sound of entrance music for the matches. Leaning against the door she imagined the events in the ring; a poor substitute. The loneliness of this empty cell had become unbearable; she had lost count as to how many times she had paced the perimeter like that of a caged and frustrated animal. Going to the door, she opened it just a crack.

"Brent?" she called. "Yeah right here." "Oh good." "Are you okay?" "Lonely is all." "Open the door and I'll keep you company." "I wish that I could, but I can't. Nick told me I had to wait in here alone. Any idea how much longer I'll be in exile?"

"Let me see," he said pulling the schedule from his pocket. "Tony's in the ring now, then there's five more matches until the main event; which is you and Mark." "Why did I ever agree to this nonsense?" Sabrina asked but expected no answer as the question was solely meant for her own conscience. "I can't answer that. Hey, why don't you pull up a chair next to the door. We can at least talk for a while," Brent suggested. "I'd like that. I'll go crazy in here alone." With the door just barely open, they passed the time talking about anything and everything.

D'arcy left Mark and headed towards the ring, stopping briefly at Sabrina's door. "How is Mark holding up?" Sabrina asked. "Driving me nuts! All he's doing is talking about you. Which isn't a bad thing, but it's the damn pacing that got to me. He hasn't sat down once since I got there." D'arcy's entrance music began. "I'd love to stay, but duty calls. I'll stop on my way back if I can."

Sabrina heard the fans chanting D'arcy's name and it made her smile. The thrill of the crowd was still in her. The music faded away. As it came on again, her smile was washed away by the cold spear that shot up her spine. It was music that she hadn't heard in a long time; Sean's music.

Brent knew by the sudden silence that she was upset, and the position of her chair prohibited him from opening the door. He squeezed his fingers through the opening and found the round curve of her shoulder. He pawed at her gently, calling to her. The volume of his voice went up when she didn't respond to him. "Sabrina!" he yelled through the small opening. "I'm gonna get Mark."

"No! Don't. Don't go. Mark doesn't need to know." "You're obviously upset; he should be with you." "I'll be fine. I was just taken by surprise that's all." "I don't know." She opened the door, enough that she could take Brent's hand. She clutched it tight. "I'm fine," she said.

He felt her warm, moist lips against his palm. The sensation electrified him. For a brief moment he allowed himself to feel the lust that he had for her. *A dream, a fantasy that I will live with for the rest of my life. A moment that I can draw on when I'm alone and lonely.*

Brent quickly pulled his hand away when he heard Nick approaching. "What is it?" Sabrina asked. "Nick's coming; better shut the door," Brent said quietly. Nick stopped in front of Brent. "No one has been in there?" Nick asked. "Not a soul, but tell me, why does she have to be locked away like this?" "The element of surprise; if everyone saw her before the ceremony it would take away from the mystery; no mystery, no ticket sales, and speaking of sales, this place is completely sold out, and the pay per view connections are tripled." Brent shook his head as he listened to Nick. *Asshole, always concerned with the bottom line, never about the people who make you the money.*

Nick rapped on the door and waited for Sabrina to answer. When the door opened, he entered. "Trick or treat," Sabrina said. "Definitely a treat," Nick replied with a grin. "You look so beautiful," he said lifting up her hands to give himself a better view of her costume. "I'm so glad that you've allowed me to do this for you and Mark. You two are a very special couple, and you deserve the best." "Nick please. We know you're doing this more for the ratings than anything."

"Sabrina, listen to me," he said guiding her to a chair. "I admit that profits mean a lot to me; but I do have a human side. When you eloped with Mark I was hurt, like a parent would be, but then I decided that I was going to do something very special for you two. Yeah, the wedding is for the fans; but the reception is for you."

Sabrina blinked rapidly. She wanted to cry. "Nick I had no idea that you had such a," she hesitated searching for just the right words. "Kind heart?" "That wasn't the words I was looking for, but yes." "I'm not normally such a hard ass; it kind of developed over the years. Dealing with some of these guys isn't easy; but you two are different. I admire the way

Mark stands up to me, where you're concerned, and the way he loves you is remarkable. It's so pure that it makes me jealous." "Oh Nick." Sabrina patted the corners of her eyes. "If you don't stop it I'm gonna cry."

He leaned down and kissed her head. "Try and hold off until later, okay?" "Okay; but how much longer?" "Thirty minutes or so. I'd better get Gene in here for the last minute touch ups." "They better not decide to make any more changes to this outfit. It's so tight now that it's hard to breathe." "Try to hold on for just a little longer. I'll be back in a few minutes."

Looking into the mirror, Sabrina checked her makeup. She had visions of her black eyeliner being rubbed away. Her blue eyes stood out so vividly against their black frames, and pale canvas. *The entire look is most pleasing, a perfect compliment to the ceremony. If they only knew just how important this night is to me, and now my worst fears, I have to tell Mark about this. I'm not ready and neither is he. I'll have to find some way of distracting his mind and hopefully he'll just let it pass.*

There was a light rap on the door. "Who is it?" she asked. "It's Brent; open the door. There's someone who wants to talk to you." "I can't. I'm not allowed to, and you know that." "Sabrina please." It was Mark. She opened the door a crack, keeping herself clear of the opening. Her fingers reached through, searching for him. Feeling his touch, she grasped his hand tightly.

"Let me in." "Oh Mark, you know I can't. I want to, but Nick will have my head." "Screw him; I need to see you. I need to hold you." "Soon my love, very soon." "This is insane. We're already married." Sabrina pulled his hand through the opening, pressing her lips against his palm. The sensation flooded through his body.

"Sabrina stop." "Why? Don't you like it?" "That's the problem; I do like it, very much; and if you don't stop, now, I'm coming in there." "Okay," she sighed releasing his hand. "Just make sure that you keep those thoughts close by, for later." "I don't know how I'm supposed to think of anything else," Mark replied with a subtle hint of a sigh.

"Get away from that door!" Nick yelled. Mark backed away. "I was just talking to her," he said. "Are you sure you didn't see her?" "I'm sure damn it!" "Fine. Get yourself to the staging area; the show starts in about ten minutes."

Nick slipped into the dressing room behind Gene. Mark laid his head against the closed door and sighed heavily. Brent placed his hand on Mark's shoulder. "Come on man; it's almost over." Mark made a move down the hallway. "Aren't you coming?" "Not yet," Brent answered holding up a robe. "I have been selected as the bride's escort; so I'll see you in the ring."

Mark continued on; his steps slow and heavy, like a man shackled to a chain gang. *This waiting is the hardest thing I've ever had to do; but in thirty minutes it will all be over. She will be in my arms, her lips, her body, pressed close to mine, wanting me to love her, begging for my tender passion to fill her soul, to take our love to a new level.* He leaned against the wall. Walking had become difficult; he needed to relax.

Gene placed the black robe around Sabrina. Nick motioned him to wait before placing her hood. Nick stood before her with his hands gentle on her shoulders. "You are so beautiful," he whispered, leaning in to kiss her cheek. "I feel so very proud at this moment. I think of you as a daughter Sabrina, and my heart is filled with happiness. Thank you for allowing me to do this for you."

Sabrina brushed the corner of her eye, but there was no time for tears. Nick checked his watch. "It's time to go," he said. Her hood was placed carefully as to not disturb her hair. The shiny satin band along the edge of the hood reflected a small fragment of light, but not enough to see her face completely.

Nick guided her out the door, placing her hand on Brent's arm. "Take it slow her vision is limited," Nick said. Brent deliberately walked slow. Unaccustomed to wearing a robe himself; he found it tedious to maneuver. Sabrina was relieved with the slower pace; her nerves were on edge. She slowed her breathing to match her steps. They stopped near the heavy black curtain, that separated the wrestlers from the fans.

It's eerily quiet. "What's going on? Why is it so quiet?" Sabrina asked. "Well, from what I can see on the monitors, they're still setting up props in the ring," Brent answered. "Where is Mark?" "I'm not sure. He's not in the ring." "Why aren't the fans yelling?" "I don't know. I think they're mesmerized by what they're seeing. You know that none of this was leaked to the press. Nick promoted it only as the main event that would never be forgotten. No details about who was in the main event, nothing." "Now I'm really nervous, but it's too late to back out now."

As she spoke the last word, music began to play. Not the normal tune that had been associated with the Warlock, but a new one, a slower, deeper, more ominous melody. Sabrina shuddered. "This sounds more like a funeral than a wedding," she said. *But it fits with the scene perfectly.*

A dozen robed figures walked past them and vanished through the curtain. Brent watched the monitor as the figures spaced themselves evenly along both sides of the ramp that led to the ring, each of them holding a lighted candle. Behind them were four more robed figures who descended the ramp and entered the ring. From the shadows at the far side of the curtain, Mark made his appearance. He did not look at Sabrina, but parted the curtain and stepped through. "Are you ready?" Nick asked her. "I don't know," she answered nervously. "You'll be fine. Just follow the routine that you rehearsed, and try not to let anything throw you off."

Before she could speak, Nick gently pushed her toward the curtain. "It's show time," he said, unable to hide his enthusiasm. Sabrina gripped Brent's hand hard. "Give me a second," she said, needing to take a deep breath.

This is only a show to Nick and the others but for me it has a much more significant meaning. I'm about to resurrect my beliefs in front of thousands of people and no one, not even Mark will be aware of the full meaning. I can't let him find out yet. Not until I'm ready.

Brent kissed the back of her hand. "You'll be fine. Come on beautiful, your husband, and your fans await." He gave her a little tug. "Now give these people a show to remember." The curtain parted and they stepped through onto the platform. The arena was hushed with profound anticipation. Thousands of people inside this building and the only thing that Sabrina could hear was the sound of her heart pounding in her chest.

Afraid to look at the crowd Sabrina chose to only look forward, to the ring, to Mark. Her eyes fixated on his large frame. It grew closer and closer with each step that she took. The majority of the arena was in darkness, but the ring itself was illuminated by blood red spot lights that shone down from a frame high above the ring.

With every beat of my heart, I'm closer to the arms of the man I love, but we are forbidden to touch during the ceremony. Just being near him will have to sustain me.

A special set of stairs had been set up between the ring posts, wide enough for two people to walk up. As Brent and Sabrina neared the steps, two of the robed attendants climbed the stairs, and entered the ring. The ring ropes had been removed from the side before them; they walked up into the ring. Brent led her to where Mark was standing, and kept his place at her side. The two attendants had taken up a position behind Mark and Sabrina in the ring.

The anxiety is insurmountable, only inches away from Mark, yet I can't touch him, or look at him, but his scent is so sweet, it fills my mind with pleasant memories. He has only worn that cologne a few times before, and I remember each one vividly; with all the magic and passion of those special days. Her body shuddered. *I have to stay focused.*

Pushing the feelings aside temporarily, she visually took in the scene before her. There was a man standing before them, robed as they were, yet his identity was concealed by a mask in the likeness of a wolf. Behind him was an altar; adorned with many black candles, a skull, burning incense, and statues. All the items were readily associated with the practice of the black arts. He picked up a large book from the altar. Opening it, he began to read in Latin. A microphone, discretely attached to his robe, carried his voice through the arena.

Raising a sword from the altar, he lightly touched the point of it to Sabrina's chest, and then to Mark's. "Whence come you?" he asked in a deep voice. In unison they replied to his question. "From the North, the place of great darkness." "Whither goest thou?" "To the East, in search of light." "What passwords dost thou bring?" "Perfect love and perfect trust." "I, the Guardian of the watchtower of the North, forbid thee entrance. Thou canst not enter this place from the North; save thou first be purified and consecrated. Who vouches for you?"

"I, Guide of Souls, so do," Brent replied, suppressing his urge to laugh at this situation that he found to be so theatrically amusing. "Children of Darkness," the priest continued. "Approach thou the watchtower of the North and receive of me the bonds of death and blessings of earth."

The attendant, behind Mark, stepped forward and removed Mark's robe. A gasp echoed through the audience. The arena was quickly silenced again as the fans looked at their idol. His costume, made entirely of black leather, consisted of a vest, held together in font by a single lace. The wide opening allowed the fans a first time look at his powerful chest. The back of the vest bore his trademark design. The leather pants left nothing to the imagination; the power of his muscular form stretched the lacings that spanned the full length of his legs. Because he had taken a step forward, Sabrina could see how good he looked. It made her body tingle.

Sabrina's attendant removed her robe. The echoed gasp returned, but was quickly followed by cheers and whistles. Her hair had been transformed into a mass of long spiraling curls that shrouded her bare shoulders. Like Mark's, her costume was also all black leather. The tight bodice, with it's under wire supports, pushed her breasts up full and round, the lacing down the front, cinched her waist in. From the bottom of the vest, to the floor, ran lengths of leather ribbons, barely concealing the leather thong beneath.

Mark felt his heart skip a beat as it kicked into overdrive. *Never have I wanted her so much as I do at this moment.* Fortunately the tight leather pants concealed and restricted his physical feelings.

The attendants were again behind Mark and Sabrina ready to proceed with the next step of the ceremony. Taking Mark's and Sabrina's hands and pulling them behind their backs the attendants carefully tied them together with a red cord, that was then drawn up, and loosely fitted around their necks, leaving a length hanging in front. Another red cord was tied around their ankles; long enough for them to walk freely.

The priest at the altar sprinkled a few grains of salt on their foreheads and placed a coin between their lips. Picking up the cord, the attendants led Mark and Sabrina slowly in a clockwise direction around the ring, stopping before another robed figure.

Removing the coins, this priest issued the same challenge as before. Mark and Sabrina again replied in unison. "From the North, the gate of death." The figure, who indicated that he was the guardian of the West, offered them a drink from a chalice, and then purified them by sprinkling a few drops on their foreheads.

Continuing in the clockwise pattern, they were led to the guardian of the South. Again they were challenged, now by the figure representing fire. Taking a sword and laying it on their right shoulders, he sprinkled them three times with incense and spoke. "I bestow upon you the sword of power and the consecration of fire."

They were next led to the figure that represented the East, who, by breathing upon their heads three times, bestowed them with the breath of life and the gift of light. Finally returning to face the priest at the altar, their bindings were removed, and they knelt before him. The priest extended the sword and Mark and Sabrina placed their right hands upon the blade. "Having been purified and consecrated by the four elements of the wise; are you now prepared to take the oath?" "Yes, we are," answered Sabrina and Mark.

For the first time during the ceremony Mark and Sabrina were allowed to look at each other. Starting their recitation separately, they completed their lines together. "I Warlock." "And I the Sorceress." "In the presence of all here assembled, man or god, living or dead, do of my own free will, most solemnly swear, that I shall ever keep secret, those things entrusted to my ears alone, by thee; and that I shall never deny thee what is thine or mine. All this I swear upon my life, now and hereafter, and may those powers I possess, now and hereafter, turn against me should I break this most solemn oath. So mote it be."

Still kneeling before the priest at the altar, he opened his book and Mark and Sabrina each signed their character names and the date. He then laid his hands on their heads and recited a blessing in Latin. When completed he made them rise. Opening the book again, Mark saw their wedding rings. He picked up Sabrina's rings and placed them back on her finger. Raising her hand to his lips, he kissed her ring. Sabrina picked up Mark's ring; her hand trembled as she pushed it onto his finger.

The crowd erupted with deafening cheers and thunderous applause but they didn't hear it. Mark had taken her into his arms. She felt weak. Their lips met and as the passion deepened, the arena was rocked by a thunderous explosion of red flame from pyro set up across the entrance stage.

The distraction brought them back to the reality of the moment but could not silence their own private thoughts. The fans cheered and yelled as they moved to each side of the ring, sharing this special moment with everyone in the arena. Cameras flashed rapidly. Sabrina tried to blink away the sea of bright light.

Exiting the ring, Mark escorted Sabrina around the ring, allowing the fans to reach out and briefly touch them. Sabrina looked at all the faces. All of them beamed with smiles, some wiping away tears. She was glad to return to the ramp. She wanted Mark alone; but before they passed through the curtain Mark stopped, turning her around for one final look. She began to back up. With Mark's hand firmly in hers, she gently tugged him to follow her.

The fans remained standing; cheering and applauding. Sabrina managed to tune all of it out; she had but one objective. In the shadows behind the curtain, she melted into his arms; needing to continue the kiss that had been taken from her in the ring. Their kiss was long, passionate. Sabrina making up for their hours apart, and Mark responding to the erotic way his wife was dressed.

Nick had stood back, giving them their special moment, but when there seemed to be no end, he stepped in. "Okay you two," he said maneuvering his way in between them. "Great show, just great. Listen to them out there; you've excited them so much; they don't want to leave. Give them another look at the most beautiful, in love couple on the planet."

With reluctance, Sabrina followed Mark back through the curtain. The eruption of cheers overwhelmed them both. Mark kissed her, and the volume increased ten fold as he gently cradled her back in his arms.

Still waiting on the other side of the curtain, Nick put his arms around them both when they returned. "See, you've made all those people very happy; not to mention me. Now we have a reception to go to." "Give me a minute," Sabrina replied. "I'd like to get out of this outfit." "No way! You can't change. It's not customary to change before the reception. Besides, if I let you two disappear, we may not see you again until the next show." Sabrina blushed at his remark. *Nick knows us too well.* "I've had your dressing rooms packed up and sent back to your suite; so there is no reason for you to go anywhere else."

Keeping his arms around them, Nick guided them through the backstage area. Except for some of the ring crew and a few technical staff, Sabrina didn't see any of the other wrestlers. "Where is everybody?" Sabrina asked. "They've already left for the reception, and we better get a move on as well."

Sabrina wiggled free of Nick's hold. "No offense but I didn't go through all this to end up holding your hand," she said, stepping into Mark's embrace. "None taken," Nick smiled. "Follow me and don't get lost."

Mark secured her at his side; Sabrina slipped her arm around his waist, occasionally letting it slide down over his hip, only to have him return it to its original, higher position. Nick guided them through a series of corridors to a service elevator, where Sabrina took the opportunity to steal a kiss from Mark. From the elevator, Nick led them through another series of hallways, stopping near a set of double doors. "Wait right here," he said, opening the door. "I mean it. Don't go anywhere."

With no one to see them Mark spun Sabrina around in front of him and lifted her high against him. She locked her arms around his neck and kissed him. Being unprepared for her hunger, Mark had to break away to catch a breath. "You look so incredible," he whispered. "You like my selection then?" "Definitely. Can we keep it for a while?" "Forever sound good." "Oh yeah; but you can send mine back anytime." "No way! I like how you look in leather; and I definitely like how it fits you." "You have the most wicked thoughts." "No, I just happen to be very much in love with the sexiest man alive."

Mark ran his fingers over the top of her breast. "We've given the fans a show to remember; and when I get you upstairs, I'm gonna give you a night to remember." "Not until you let me," she was cut off by Nick's return. "Sorry, I didn't mean to be gone so long." "We hadn't noticed," Mark said still staring into Sabrina's eyes. Even though she had not been able to finish her sentence, Mark knew exactly what she was going to say. His vivid imagination was filling in all the erotic blanks.

"Well, don't just stand there; this party is for you two," Nick reminded them. Mark wove Sabrina's arm around his. "Let's get this over with," he said. Nick opened the door for them and they entered the small ballroom to a volley of applause. The room was filled to capacity with people. Most of them Sabrina recognized, others she didn't, wrestlers and the crew, in the company of their wives or girlfriends. As they wove their way through the tables, Mark recognized faces that he hadn't seen in many years. Nick had invited wrestlers that no longer worked for the company, but they were people that Mark had worked with in the early part of his career.

Brent beckoned to them. He was standing behind what Sabrina knew to be the head table. They took their place beside him, behind the long table with its bright white table cloth and glistening crystal. No sooner had they sat down, when the familiar clang of cutlery against crystal rang out.

"We'll be lucky to finish our dinner," Sabrina said to Mark as she leaned over to kiss him. "What do you mean by that?" "They're gonna keep us busy doing this. Do you think you can handle it?" "Sure, all I have to do is to look at you and they all disappear, but I'm still holding onto the thought that soon we will be able to disappear ourselves." "I can't wait." She kissed him again to appease the insistent clanging.

The evening progressed as Sabrina had predicted. Their dinner had gone cold, due to the constant interruptions, but one thing remained constant. Mark's hand never left her leg, gently massaging the inside of her thigh, keeping her libido running wild.

Nick made the customary speech as the surrogate father; but when Brent offered a toast to Sabrina, the speech he gave made her cry. His words touched her heart so deeply that when he sat down she kissed him.

Nick asked Mark and Sabrina to join him at the end of the table. "What now?" Mark asked her. "I don't know." Their questions were soon answered when the caterer wheeled out a large wedding cake; all decorated with red and black roses. People, with cameras in hand, flocked around them. The photographer, that Nick had hired, posed them for the traditional cutting of the cake.

Sabrina carefully fed a piece to Mark. He followed her lead, but when he saw the faint traces of icing on her lips he could not resist the urge to kiss it away; much to the delight of all the onlookers. For just a brief moment the annoying flash of the cameras was halted and a hush befell the room as Mark cradled Sabrina back in his arms; losing himself in the sweet taste of her lips. When he released her from his gentle embrace it was to a loud applause. Sabrina turned away to hide her blush.

Nick had the microphone again. "In keeping with tradition, the first dance shall be solely for the Bride and Groom," he announced. Mark stared at Sabrina. "It'll be okay," she said touching his cheek. "All you need to do is hold me, and let the music take control."

I feel so awkward, never dreaming that I would have to reveal my flaw in front of all these people. Sabrina took his hand. "Hold me close," she whispered. The music began. Nobody watching, realized that there was any inadequacy; their bodies swayed together slowly in time to the music; tender kisses took them far away from the staring eyes. When the song ended, Mark hugged her to him. "Can we leave now?" Mark asked. "No, now we have to mingle. Just relax; it won't take long." "I hope not."

Doc took the first cab waiting at the curb. He told the driver where to take him and told him to hurry. He checked his watch. *I hope it's not too late.* Given the time of day, he was surprised by the amount of traffic on the streets; but the cab made good time getting to the hotel. Doc rewarded the driver handsomely for his efforts. He went straight to the front desk.

"Are Mr. and Mrs. Cassidy still guests here?" Doc asked. "Yes, they are," replied the clerk, after checking the computer for their registration.

"Could you please ring their room for me?" The clerk obliged. "I'm sorry sir but they are not in." "Damn!" He thought for a moment.

"They're with the wrestling show. Is it still going on?" "No sir, that ended a couple of hours ago. They may still be in the ballroom though. The company is hosting a private party in there." "Fine; can someone take me there?" "I'm sorry sir, but as I said it is a private party." Doc's patience was worn out. "I'd like to speak to your manager!" The clerk, not wanting to get into a verbal altercation, called his manager without question.

Mark and Sabrina made the rounds together, but like any wedding, they became separated by people each wanting their attention. Sabrina had reached D'arcy's table. She sat down to wait for Mark to catch up. He had become engaged in a deep conversation with a wrestler he hadn't seen in ten years. One of the catering staff approached her. "Excuse me, but your presence has been requested on the patio." Sabrina thanked him. She looked around for Mark. Not seeing him, she surmised that he was the one summoning her. Excusing herself from D'arcy, she wandered out to the patio.

It was dark. No outside lights had been turned on. Her eyes strained through the darkness. "Mark," she called. "No, it's not Mark," a voice answered. *I know that voice.* It made her blood run cold. "Sean, is that you?" "Yes, Sabrina." He moved out of the shadows. "I'm sorry for deceiving you; but I had to talk to you alone." "You could get yourself into serious trouble for this." "I know, and I don't care. I had to see you, to apologize." Sean gestured to Sabrina to take a seat on a bench. "I have to tell you how sorry I am. I never meant to hurt you." "You did hurt me Sean." "I know; and every day I have regretted that mistake."

She had heard enough. He still made her nervous. She went to get up; Sean held her down. "Please Sabrina; hear me out." The icy chills raced up her spine. "All right, but please don't touch me," she answered, even though her first instinct was telling her to run. Sean backed off.

"Fine, I understand. You know that I've been going to therapy; but you have no idea how grateful I am to you, for not sending me to jail. During my therapy I came to realize that my feelings for you were not those of love, but of possession. I didn't want to see that you loved someone else. I wanted you for myself, and the thought of another man winning your affection infuriated me. Saying that I'm sorry may not seem like much to you, but understand that I am truly repentant."

"So what do you want from me; forgiveness?" Sabrina asked, still wary of him. "No, I wouldn't dream of asking you to forgive me. What I did, what I put you through, was the most vile thing imaginable, all I ask is that you hear my apology and take it to be sincere. I am happy that you and Mark have found such a special love, and I wish you all the best." He stood up, backing away into the shadows. "I will never contact you again. Be happy Sabrina." "Wait, please come back; please don't leave yet. There is more I need to know." Her plea went unanswered.

"Who are you talking to?" Brent asked from behind her. Startled, Sabrina turned around quickly. She stared at Brent. "How long have you been standing there?" she asked. "Not very long. Who where you talking to?" "I was," she hesitated, glancing over her shoulder into the shadows. "Sean was here."

"What! That son of a bitch, he knows he's forbidden to have any contact with you. Are you okay?" "A little shook up, but otherwise fine," she answered, more in control of her feelings. Brent put his arm around her. "Come inside, before Mark comes looking for you."

She stopped at the doorway. "He came to apologize." "Yeah right." "No, Brent, he was sincere. He truly is sorry for all the trouble he caused." "Sean doesn't know the meaning of the word." "You're wrong; he came to me only to tell me how sorry he was. He didn't ask me to forgive him. In fact he was glad that Mark and I are so much in love. The last thing he said was that I should be happy." "Either his therapy has done some good, or he's up to something." "I'd like to think he has recovered." "Only time will tell. Come on. You owe me a dance."

She took a last look back; she thought she detected some movement, but dismissed it as the wind. Sean watched her from his hiding place. *I know I'm risking my freedom by talking to her; but I had to see her one last time. To talk to her; to try and atone for my cruelty was all I wanted. There is always going to be a secret place in my heart for her. For as long as I walk this earth I will carry her memory. She really loves Mark, I know that now; but it doesn't make me bitter, I'm happy for her. Someday.* He watched her dancing with Brent. *Someday I'll find that kind of love.*

Mark's mind slowly tuned out Tony's voice, as he watched his wife on the dance floor. *Her moves are so graceful, so sexy. The sway of her hips makes me think about making love to her.* Tony gave him a light tap on the shoulder. "Hey man; get your mind out of the gutter," he chuckled. "What?" Mark stared at him. "I said to quit thinking those nasty thoughts. You'll be alone with her soon enough. Christ, it's all you think about, isn't it?" "Most of the time; but man, being married to a woman like her; I just can't help it." "I'd say give me specific details, but I don't want to spend the rest of the night looking for my teeth." "You got that right. So now you know the rules about discussing my wife in my presence." Mark moved on to another table. Sabrina was now dancing with D'arcy.

Doc was prepared for the hotel manager when he arrived, not even giving the man a chance to speak. "Look, I'm normally a patient man, but I can tell you that my patience is shot to hell!" "Sir, if you would please explain the situation to me, I may have an answer." "I have been on a plane, from Texas, specifically to see Mr. and Mrs. Cassidy. I am Dr. Brown, their personal physician." He opened his identification and pulled Mark's and Sabrina's medical files from his bag. "It is of great importance that I get in touch with them tonight." "I'm sorry sir, but they are part of a private party this evening and cannot be disturbed. If you would like to leave a message at the desk, I will personally see that it is delivered."

Doc lost his cool. "Look you pompous ass! I didn't fly up here to leave a message! They have to be informed of Mrs. Cassidy's test results; and it has to be now! She needs to be in a hospital, as soon as possible, but if you are prepared to risk this woman's life, then go right ahead and keep being a jackass!"

Mr. Blackthorn straightened himself. *If I stand my ground and the owner finds out the circumstances, my job will be gone.* "Very well sir, please follow me and please accept my apology." "Fine, just take me to them." The manager walked quickly; Doc kept up as best he could. When they reached the ballroom, the manager stopped at the door. "If you would like some privacy, there is a small room attached to the ballroom that you can use." "Good, take me there and bring Mr. and Mrs. Cassidy to me, but I warn you, do not alarm them or tell them who has requested the meeting. I can not afford to have her upset." "Very good sir."

The manager led Doc along the perimeter of the ballroom, to the room at the far side. Doc dragged an extra chair in and set his bag on the small table. The manager worked his way through the room, searching for

Mark and Sabrina. Doc rolled his head. His neck cracked from the tension. *This isn't going to be easy. If Mark is so inclined, I could lose my license; but more importantly I could lose their trust, and Sabrina doesn't need to be looking for another Doctor at this point.*

Feeling a little claustrophobic, Mark was not one for parties at the best of times, but this was far too big for his liking. *Sabrina's still dancing with D'arcy; she won't miss me for a few minutes.* He headed out to the patio for some fresh air. Seeing where his friend was going, Brent worked his way to him. "Mind if I join you?" Brent asked. "Not at all."

Brent scanned the patio. Knowing that Sean had been out here earlier, he wasn't taking any chances now. *Telling Mark would be a mistake; he would go crazy. If he's meant to know, then Sabrina will have to tell him.*

"Nick sure knows how to throw a party," Brent began the conversation. "Yeah, but it's a bit extravagant." "Hey, you two deserve it. With everything that you've been through together, it's only right that something good happens now and again." "Maybe, but this is still too much. That's why we got married privately, to avoid this." "Oh come on, admit it, you're having as much fun as she is." "To tell you the truth, I'd rather be having fun with her, alone, but I know she likes to dance." "Hey man, you've done your required time here; if you want to leave, then leave. This is the beginning of your second honeymoon."

Mark smiled. "That's right; but actually we're still on our first one." "So why are you sitting around here when you could be, well you know." "That does it. Soon as I find her, we're out of here," Mark announced. They stopped at the patio doors, each scanning the room for Sabrina. "Do you see her?" Mark asked. "No, but she has to be here. She was dancing with D'arcy; maybe he knows where she is."

D'arcy was back at his table, finishing a beer when Mark approached. "Hey man, that wife of yours is something else on the dance floor," D'arcy remarked. "Where is she?" Mark asked. "I don't know; some guy in a monkey suit interrupted our dance, said that there was somebody here to see her and she left." "Where did they go?" "Sorry, I wasn't watching."

D'arcy left their company and headed back to the bar. "Oh shit!" Brent gasped. "What is it?" "Sean was here earlier. He talked to Sabrina out on the patio. I should have known that he was up to something." "Damn it

Brent! Why the hell didn't you tell me?" "I'm sorry man; I didn't think." "That's right; you didn't think. Now help me find her."

Sabrina followed the manager to the side room. Her jaw dropped open when she saw Doc. "Doc; this is such a nice surprise. Why aren't you enjoying the party?" "Sabrina, you look wonderful. Here, please have a seat." He pushed the chair toward her. "I'm here on business." Turning to the manager, Doc glared at him. "Would you please find Mr. Cassidy and bring him here at once." "Yes sir."

"So Doc, what kind of business brings you to Vegas?" Sabrina asked. "Please don't think anything wrong, but I'd like to wait until Mark is here." "Is something wrong with Mark?" She jumped to her feet, panic surging through her body. Doc took her by the shoulders. "Sabrina please sit down; Mark is fine." She slumped into the chair. "If Mark's okay, then it must be me. All those tests; you found something!" Her panic grew, making her tremble. "Sabrina, let's just wait until Mark is here."

"No, I have to know. You have to tell me first. It must be something pretty bad for you to fly up here." Doc pulled a chair up in front of her; he tried to brush away the tear that rolled down her cheek. "Darlin, I must apologize for being such a stupid old fool. For not recognizing the symptoms, and for not doing a proper examination after you had your miscarriage."

Sabrina began to rock in her chair. "Oh God," she whimpered. "Sabrina hush now. Your imagination is just making it worse." "It is worse; you're just trying to ease me into it." "I'm trying to explain; and in doing so I could be opening myself up to a lawsuit." "I don't care about that, I just want to know what the tests found." "Are you sure you don't want to wait for Mark?" "I'm sure. It concerns me; my body, and I'll decide when and if Mark should know."

Doc picked up her hands and squeezed them gently. "If I had examined you properly after the miscarriage, I would have found out then, but when you lost the baby, the thought never occurred to me that this was even a possibility. It wasn't until Mark called me about his concerns that I started thinking; but still I didn't even entertain the possibility. When I sent you for the tests, it was a complete surprise to me to get the results that I did."

"Doc you're really scaring me. Are you trying to tell me that I may not be able to have any more children?" "No, that's not it." "Then cut through the bull shit and just tell me." "Sabrina I need you to be strong. You're gonna have to spend a little time in the hospital, and you will be the subject of many examinations."

He gripped her hands tightly, as the trembling increased. "Sabrina, what we both didn't know, when you miscarried, was that you were carrying twins. Now I've only read about this happening on extremely rare occurrences; but when you miscarried, you only lost one baby. The other one was completely unharmed by the ordeal." Sabrina stopped shaking. Her face went blank as she stared into Doc's eyes.

"When I got your test results back I couldn't believe it myself, so I sent for your medical file, when you had the ultrasound just before your accident. Whoever did your scan wasn't paying much attention to what he was looking at, both babies were visible but to somebody in a hurry it could have been passed off as a shadow." "What are you saying Doc?" Sabrina asked utterly confused by what she was hearing.

"The ultrasound that you just had confirmed it all. The other twin is alive and healthy, and from the size of it, well, I can't really tell you how far along you are, or the baby is just taking after its father, but we can try and determine that once we get you in the hospital."

Sabrina rubbed at her belly. "I'm pregnant?" she asked, still in complete disbelief. "Yes darlin, very much so. You're both a medical miracle. I am sorry for not catching it sooner, but to be perfectly honest, I was convinced that you were so desperate to have a baby that your body was going through a false pregnancy."

Tears flooded down her cheeks. "I'm really pregnant?" "Yes, Sabrina you are. There's no mistake. The tests, and the ultrasound confirmed it, but like I said, you need to get into the hospital for a few days. We're gonna make sure that this baby is strong and healthy." Without warning she flung herself into his arms, her body racked with sobs of joy.

The manager located Mark, who was near panic, unable to find anyone who had seen Sabrina leave. "Excuse me, Mr. Cassidy." "Yeah, what do you want?" "Your wife has sent me to find you." "You know where she is?" "Yes sir, she is in the side room with a Dr. Brown." "Doc? What's he doing here?" Mark looked at Brent as if he would have an answer. "At least she's not with Sean," Brent answered.

"Why would Doc be here? Unless," Mark's voice faltered and stopped. Brent watched his friends face turn cold with shock. "Unless what?" Brent asked. "I can't explain now!" Mark snapped. Looking back at the manager, Mark commanded him to take him to Sabrina. Brent stayed behind; he had no place with them right now.

D'arcy wandered back from the bar. "Where is he going in such a hurry?" "To be with Sabrina." "Hey, that's the guy who broke up our dance. So do you know who stopped in for a visit?" "Yeah, unfortunately I do," Brent sighed. "Well, don't keep me in suspense. Who is it?" "Their Doctor from Texas." "That's strange; don't you think?" "Yeah it's strange all right. For him to fly up here and want to speak to them privately; that tells me that he wasn't invited to the party. Damn it. There is no point in speculating. I'm just glad that it isn't one of Sean's sick tricks."

"Sean? What would make you think he was part of this? The bastard knows he's forbidden from seeing her." "Yeah, he knows, but it still didn't stop him from luring her out to the patio earlier." "Tonight? That dumb son of a bitch! Did you tell Nick?" "No, not yet; and I don't think I will." "Why not? He's broken his probation; he deserves to go back to jail for that." "Maybe; but Sabrina wouldn't like it. She told me that he came here to apologize, not to scare her. She really believes that he's repented. He even wished her and Mark a good life together." "I don't believe it; that bastard is too sneaky. You should still tell Nick, and let him decide Sean's fate." "Maybe," Brent muttered. His mind was still fixated on the possibilities as to why Doc was here.

Mark's gut was in knots, that grew tighter the closer he got to the door of the side room. Thoughts raced through his mind. All questions; that led him to one recurring answer. *What would bring Doc to Vegas? It must be serious. Why didn't he just phone? Sabrina; that's why he's here. All those tests. It must be worse than he originally let on. Oh God, I can't live without her.*

He hesitated outside the door, swallowing hard, pushing his heart back into his chest. Sabrina was in Doc's arms. By the way he patted her back, and the way her body heaved, he knew she was crying. *No matter how much it hurts, I have to try and stay calm.* "What's going on?" Mark asked.

Doc released Sabrina and stood up. "Mark, good to see you." Sabrina wiped the tears from her face before going to Mark. She tried to hide her face from him, but he lifted it up, staring into her blue eyes. "Are either of you going to tell me what's going on?" "I will," Sabrina answered. "But not here, not now."

"Sabrina, I think you should, now. I'm here to make it all clear." "Doc, please. It's something that I need to do, not you." "Damn it!" Mark bellowed. Sabrina jumped, scared by his sudden, angry outburst. "Don't talk like I'm not even here." " I'm sorry Mark. Sabrina has made her choice, and as her Doctor I have to respect her request." "I don't like this!" Mark snapped at them; his anger growing stronger from being ignored.

Sabrina clung to him. "Take me out of here please Mark." He could sense her need for privacy. "Okay," he answered, somewhat calmer. Sabrina looked back at Doc. "I won't forget anything that you've told me. Just leave a message at the front desk about where and when." "Okay darlin, but remember that you can't put this off for too long."

Stopping at the mirror, she wiped away the traces of makeup that had been loosened by her tears. *I can't go back into the ballroom looking like this.* "We have to tell them that we're leaving," she said to Mark. "I don't care! You're keeping something from me and I don't like it; not one bit!" "Mark just bear with me, please. Get me out of here, to where it's quiet, and it's just us."

Reaching up to him, she kissed his cheek. Mark pulled away from her. She wanted to cry again, but she understood how he was feeling. *I hate doing this to him, but he deserves to hear it from me not Doc.* Rather than make a spectacle of themselves, Mark left her by the door while he told Nick of their intentions.

Seeing her leaning against the wall, Brent went to her. "Hey beautiful." He saw the redness in her eyes. "Why so sad?" "Not now Brent; I'm not in the mood for conversation." "Okay." "Don't give me that tone! Just because I want to be alone with Mark doesn't give you the right to jump to conclusions." "Sorry, I didn't mean to upset you." Realizing what she had done, she hugged him. "Forgive me. I'm just tired and I've got a lot on my mind." Brent softly kissed her ear. "You're forgiven. I'm just concerned about you; it's something that just happens between friends."

With Mark's return, he took her hand and dragged her from the ballroom. The journey back to their suite was quiet and tedious, the tension between them thick, the silence smothering like a heavy blanket of fog. Sabrina had to speed up as Mark pulled her along the hallway. She sensed an anger in him that she had never felt before, and it scared her. *Maybe I should have let Doc tell him? No, I have to do this; it'll be better this way.*

They had come to a stop outside the suite, Mark searched his costume, but there were no pockets. "Damn it!" "What is it?" Sabrina asked. "I don't have the God damn key!" He raised his foot, about to kick the door in. "Don't!" Sabrina cried. "Well, I don't see any other option; do you?" "You could use the house phone by the elevator to have a bell hop bring up a replacement," she answered, trying to remain calm. "Fine, I'll make the call; and you stay here," he said, a strong commanding tone in his voice. Sabrina grabbed at his arm. "Please remember to come back," she said softly. She still fought the urge to cry. Mark grumbled something she couldn't understand and walked off down the hall.

Leaning back against the door, she slowly slid down to sit on the floor. Her belly rumbled; she smoothed the turmoil with her hands, quietly talking to herself. "All this time I thought it was just a bad case of nerves; but it wasn't. You were just trying to get my attention, to let me know that you were here. I know I've been sad for a long time, but no more. I still miss your brother, but I still have you and I do love you and when your Daddy finds out about you, he's gonna love you just as much as I do. Don't be afraid little one, your Daddy may sound angry, but he's not like that. He will love you as much as he loves me. I can't wait to hold you; and if Doc is right, it won't be much longer." The turmoil in her belly calmed and disappeared. "That's right; you sleep now and grow stronger."

"Have you always talked to yourself, or is this something new?" Brent asked as he approached her. "What?" "You were talking to yourself Sabrina. Are you all right?" "Fine," she replied, pushing herself back up the door. "Where is Mark?" Brent asked. She heard that unmistakable tone of concern in his voice. "He forgot the room key. He should be back soon."

Brent positioned himself directly in front of her; he kept his eyes focused on hers. "Is there anything wrong between you two?" "Nothing. Why would you ask such a thing?" "Maybe because both of you are acting really strange. Mark got all fired up when I told him that Sean paid you a visit; but he really fell apart when he heard that Doc was here. So what's up?" "Brent I can't tell you. I'm sorry, but I just can't."

Her eyes suddenly became glossy. Brent held her by the shoulders. "You know I won't pry; but I'm here if you need someone to lean on. I'll always be here for you, and for Mark." "Thank you. I do appreciate your support. Once I talk to Mark, clear everything up; he'll come around to his old self again."

"You two having a good chat?" Mark sarcastically interjected as he neared them. "Man this is really cozy, isn't it? You must have one hell of a sense of radar." "Mark what are you talking about?" Sabrina asked. "Oh come on. Every time I leave you alone he shows up; rather convenient." "You're way off base. I was going to my room, which happens to be on this floor, I saw Sabrina, so I stopped to talk. Would you prefer I ignore her?"

"Why should you?" Mark glared at Sabrina. "Is this why you dragged me up here; to tell me about your involvement?" Sabrina snatched the key from him. "Why are you being so cruel?" she asked opening the door. "How could you even think such a thing?" Her tears forced her to retreat into the suite.

"You're a God damn son of a bitch!" Brent snarled. "You have become so single minded and possessive that you can't stand her to have any friends!" "You're not denying anything; so my suspicions are true," Mark sneered. Brent shoved Mark against the wall. "You bastard! That woman loves you, and only you, and if you value your marriage I suggest you find out what is upsetting her; and why Doc showed up here tonight!"

Mark slumped forward slightly. "Doc. Brent; man I'm sorry. I let my imagination create a scenario to avoid the truth. I know why Doc is here and," his voice began to crack. "And I don't want to face it. Somehow the idea of losing her to another man instantly became easier to deal with than the reality of the situation." "You're talking in riddles. What is going on?" "A couple of weeks ago Doc did some tests on Sabrina. It can't be good, for him to fly up here like this. I can't imagine my life without her. Man I've never been so scared as I am right now."

"Christ Mark, no wonder you've been actin so crazy. You have to talk to her." "I know, but I'm afraid to hear what she's got to say." "Look man; whatever it is; she's gonna need you; your strength and more importantly your love. Talk to her Mark, and love her. With all your heart love her."

With a gentle nudge, Brent pushed Mark through the open door. He closed it behind him and leaned against the wall. Tears burned in his eyes, closing them only forced the droplets to spill out. He prayed quietly for a moment, and then sought the solitude of his room, and the comfort of the liquor in the bar.

Sabrina wasn't in the living room. The bedroom door was closed. Mark could not bring himself to open the door. He stood outside and called to her. "Sabrina, I'm sorry. If you can find it in your heart to talk to me, I'll be waiting for you out here." He wasn't at all surprised by her silence he expected it. *I hope that it won't last too long. Our marriage means everything to me and I promise I'll do anything to save it.* Taking a beer from the fridge, he sat on the sofa, in the dark and so very much alone.

Hearing Mark's voice at the door, made Sabrina cry even harder; tears dripped from her jaw like rain. She had heard his apology. *That's the man I know. The man in the hallway was lashing out in fear. We have to talk; once he knows, it will be okay. I need to feel his love again. We have a wonderful reason for celebration.* She went into the bathroom, washing away the traces of her tears and her makeup.

There was the sound of the latch on the bedroom door; Mark stood up quickly, awaiting her entrance. She slipped into the room without a sound. Mark could not move, frozen in time by her beauty, and by the fear that she would reject him. She moved toward him, gliding silently through the dimness, until she was now just inches away from him. "Sabrina I'm so sorry." "Shhh, I know; but I don't need your apologies. I need you, and only you. I need you to hold me."

He welcomed her into his arms and kissed her forehead. "I was such a damn fool. I love you Sabrina, with all my heart I love you." She kissed his chest, moving slowly up his neck, seeking out his warm lips. Cradling his face in her hands, she spoke softly. "Make love to me." "You know I want to, but we need to talk. You have to tell me why Doc is here." "Not now; we can talk later." "Baby I can't. I need to know; it's tearing me apart. Please tell me why Doc made a special trip up here." "Okay, but you had better sit down, and so should I."

Mark dropped to the sofa; Sabrina sat across his lap, leaning against the arm rest. She ran her fingers over her face and through her hair. "Where do I begin; and how?" Mark wanted so desperately to know, but pushing her into it may not be the best way; best to start with something else first.

"Did seeing Sean upset you?" Mark asked. "You know?" "Brent told me, but don't be mad at him." "I can't; he's just looking out for me; and seeing Sean didn't upset me. It was a shock at first, but after talking to him for a little while, the fear went away." "Why would he risk going back to jail just to see you?" "To apologize; that's all he came for. He didn't ask me to forgive him his sins; only to say he was sorry, and to wish us a good life together." "Do you think he meant it?" "Yes, I do. I feel that he has come to terms with what he did, and he is repentant. He even promised to never contact me again." "I'm still not sure about that; but he'll never get the opportunity as long as I'm around."

They both went silent, neither of them knowing how to continue. Mark played with the curls that rested on her shoulders. Sabrina unconsciously ran her fingers along the edge of his vest. Taking a deep breath, Mark took the next step.

"Can you tell me now why Doc is here?" "I'll try. What I'm going to say may sound unbelievable, and somewhat confusing, but I'll try my best." "That's all I ask," he said as he began to rub her shoulders. "It has something to do with all those tests; right?" "Yes, but it goes much further back." "What were the results?" "Well, the just of it is Doc wants me to spend a few days in the hospital."

Mark felt the color drain from his face. "It's that serious?" "Yes, and no," she answered. Now he was even more confused and at a loss for words. Sabrina felt her belly turn over. She picked up Mark's hand and laid it across her belly. "Can you feel that?" "Feel what?" "Our baby."

Mark's eyes snapped wide open. "That can't be!" "Yes, it can. That's what all those tests found. Oh Mark it's so incredible. A miracle is what Doc called it. When I had the miscarriage, I was pregnant with twins; but I only lost one baby. By some miracle the other baby survived, unharmed."

He stared at her belly, moving his hand slowly across, searching for that sensation again. "Doc's absolutely sure; there's no mistake?" "No mistake." She lifted his face to meet hers. "Forgive me, for not letting Doc tell you." "I'm the one who needs your forgiveness. For the way I yelled at you, for the horrible things I accused you of. I was so overwhelmed with fear. Fear that you would be taken from me."

"Mark stop; I understand how you felt, and I'm not angry at you. I forgive you; I love you too much not to. Deceiving you was wrong, but I didn't want you to find out down there. This is our moment, not theirs."

The gentle touch of his hand wiped all the tears from her face. "You said that something special was going to happen, and you were right," he said softly. She brought him close to her. "This has been a magical day, but the day is far from over and we promised each other a night of love, of passion and of fantasies fulfilled."

He pulled back, gazing into her eyes. He wanted to tell her no, but he remembered what Brent had told him. Bringing her to him, he held her tight; his mind and body in turmoil.

Feeling her breath on his neck, her breasts pushing against his chest made his decision easier. Picking her up, he whisked her off to the bedroom. They had every reason to celebrate their love. Sabrina slid out of his arms, loosening his vest. "Now my love, tell me about your fantasy." "There will be no fantasies tonight Sabrina. I won't risk it." "Okay, maybe mine will have to wait a few months, but yours doesn't." "You are my fantasy," he said loosening the leather laces on her dress. "Your body next to mine, your perfect love, that's all I'll ever need."

The costume fell to the floor. Mark laid her back onto the bed; he lay down beside her, propped up on one elbow. "I love you Sabrina; and I owe you so much that its gonna take me the next three life times to make it up to you." He placed a finger over her lips, a signal for her to stay quiet.

"Before I met you, I was a lonely, empty man. Convinced that my life was worthless, convinced that love was for other people, not me; but then you came into my life. You melted the ice that contained my heart, and you showed me that there was a life outside the ring; a life worth fighting for. You have shown me that perfect love can overcome anything, and it can create the most magical thing of all, a new life." He gently stroked her belly.

The tenderness of his voice, and the gentleness of her touch, guided their love and their passion through a night of ecstasy never before obtained. With the sun, now awakening a new day, Sabrina became lost in the need to sleep. Mark cradled her close, closing his eyes, he dreamed. Dreams of their new life, dreams filled with the sounds of children playing, of ponies and puppies, and sleigh rides in the snow. Of growing old with Sabrina, spending his days and nights loving her, thanking her for making him whole, for showing him just how wonderful life could be outside the ring.

Chapter 24

Doc had kept a close watch on Sabrina. After spending a week in the hospital, and undergoing countless examinations, the exact stage of her pregnancy could not be determined. It would be a waiting game for all of them, but that was all right, this was how it should be, not knowing when the baby would be born, it put the mystery back into the pregnancy.

Sabrina continued to work with Mark, until it became too difficult to hide her condition under costumes. Her height and body type had concealed her pregnancy much longer than other women. It was as if her body was deliberately concealing her pregnancy until the moment they found out. She still traveled with Mark on the tours, much to Doc's disagreement. The baby grew quickly, and Sabrina's belly blossomed at an amazing rate, making it hard for her to walk or keep her balance.

Being on tour was made as comfortable as possible for her. Nick had a special seat for her near the backstage monitors. She could watch Mark, and Nick could keep an eye on her. Not having any grandchildren of his own gave Nick the opportunity to take part every chance he could. Spoiling her and making sure she wanted for nothing.

The guys had become much more involved, always asking how she was or if she needed anything, but what struck her as quite cute, was that as each of them passed by on their way to a match, they would stop for a moment to rub her belly, and talk to the baby.

They're all so attentive; D'arcy, Sam and Tony, but especially Brent. They all act as if this is their baby. It pleases me to see that our friendship has grown into such a close family.

When it became too difficult for Sabrina to maneuver without help, Doc ordered her to stay home. It was an ultimatum really. Stay home, or go to the hospital, no more touring. Mark had two weeks left on his tour before he would have time off. She went with him to the airport, staying close to him for as long as possible and trying very hard to keep her emotions well hidden from him.

When Mark had to finally leave her, Jim consoled her as best he could. He wanted to take her home but she insisted on staying until the plane left. Sitting beside her near the window that faced the runway, Jim made sure her supply of tissues never ran out. For nearly an hour she wept quietly.

When the plane finally left, it took Jim several attempts to get Sabrina up out of the chair. They walked slowly to the car. Jim knew how deep her pain was but it was beyond his ability to ease it for her.

Being apart was a strain on both Mark and Sabrina, even though they never said it aloud, it was very clear every time they spoke on the phone. Mark could hear her sniffle back her tears. Sabrina could hear his muffled sigh, but somehow one of them would turn the conversation around, and soon they would be laughing. This pattern repeated itself with every phone call.

On several occasions, Mark would deliberately phone late at night, knowing that she would be in bed. In the darkness of the bedroom, with a pillow against her back, and the phone close to her ear, she pretended that Mark was holding her; the sound of his voice lulling her to sleep. In those special moments, the hundreds of miles between them disappeared; and in their dreams they were together.

Jim had moved upstairs, to the guest room, that was slowly being converted into a nursery. He set up an intercom system between the two rooms; in case Sabrina needed him, he could be there a lot sooner. Sabrina thought him to be a bit overprotective, but when she found it next to impossible to get out of bed by herself, she was glad he had made the suggestion.

The baby was so big now, that sleeping through the night was not to be. Two or three times a night she would call Jim to help her to the bathroom. She felt bad at disturbing his night. He had a ranch to run all day; but he never complained. He fixed a chair in the shower so she could bathe, and always brought her breakfast in bed. While she ate, he would run out and do his chores and then return to help her down the stairs.

Every day he would recount a story to her about when his wife was expecting, always finding something humorous to lift her spirits. He knew how lonely she felt, having to be away from Mark right now and he made sure that she had very little time to herself. Sabrina would have preferred to stay in bed, as it took the pressure off of her back and her ankles; but Jim insisted that she come down stairs. He told her that fresh air and sunshine was better for her and the baby.

The days dragged on slowly. The early morning air had an unusually crisp bite to it. Sabrina could only spend a few minutes outside before she began to shiver. In those moments she would hug herself tight, imagining Mark's strong arms around her, keeping her warm. Her vivid imagination helped her to sleep better. She found that by putting some of Mark's cologne on the pillow and then holding it tight helped to ease her loneliness, but the only thing that would dissipate it completely would be to have Mark home with her.

The calendar on the desk, in the bedroom, counted off the days until Mark would be home; and Christmas was fast approaching. *It's my second one away from home, and our first one together. The last one had slipped by completely unnoticed, but no more. This is going to be the best Christmas ever. There is so much to do.*

Sabrina kept a list beside the bed, checking it every night, and making changes as things were completed, or if she thought of something else to make this holiday more memorable for them. She had made sure that Brent and D'arcy would be spending the holidays with them, after all, they were like family now; and neither of them seemed to be too interested in spending time with their own families.

It took a lot of convincing to get Jim to take her with him while he picked out a tree. The house had to be perfect for Mark's return, their first Christmas together, their baby and their friends. Jim had to rearrange the furniture to accommodate the large fir tree. For as long as he had been with Mark, there had been no celebrating of any holiday.

There were no special decorations, no fancy dinner, not even a conversation. Mark always isolated himself on holidays. Jim wasn't sure how Mark would react to a Christmas tree; but since it was her wish, then maybe he would be tolerant. Insisting that she give him the decorating instructions from the sofa, Sabrina sat back and watched Jim, a pitcher of his special eggnog at her side.

I love the smell of a fresh evergreen tree, especially a fir tree. After my father died we never had a fresh tree at Christmas. Mother always complained about the mess they made. I hated that little plastic thing that she had bought with its tacky little ornaments and virtually no lights. Christmas never meant anything to her, and surprises, well, forget that. I always knew what I was getting, whether she told me about it or whether I was with her when she bought it. Sometimes it was things that I wanted but most times it was just more useless crap to put in my closet.

As for dinner, that was even a bigger joke. We never had anybody over for dinner and even though we had invitations to go out for dinner, mother always declined. She would spend hours cooking like we were having company but it was always just the two of us, with enough leftovers to last more than a week.

Things will be a lot different now. I have Mark and a baby due any day; I have the family that I've dreamed about for so long. Everything has to be just perfect, not just for Christmas but for every holiday now. I can't wait to celebrate every one of them with him and our child.

Putting down her glass of eggnog she picked up two special ornaments from the box beside her. One for their first Christmas together and one for their baby. They would be the last decorations to go on the tree, but not until Mark was home.

The last square on the calendar was finally marked off. *Today, he will be home today. I want to look good for him, but trying to look sexy, when my belly has expanded so far that any resemblance to my shapely figure is now but a memory. The baby has grown so much that even maternity clothes are uncomfortable. Even Mark's largest T-shirts are stretched to the maximum. If I'm this big on the outside, then just how big is the baby inside me? Is this baby going to take after Mark right from the get go? Can I deliver this baby, or will there be problems? No more. Mark will be home soon and that's all I have to worry about. I miss him so much.*

She waited by the front window, standing like a statue, watching the driveway for any sign of a car. Finally Jim had to take her by the arm, and make her sit down. The fire crackled and popped in the fireplace. Jim covered her with a blanket and soon she had given in to the warmth of sleep. Everything tired her, standing, walking, sitting. It was all such a strain, and she found herself napping more and more.

Something was rubbing against her hand. She flicked it away, but it returned to torment her and disturb her nap. Forcing herself awake she opened her eyes. She saw Mark, perched on the coffee table in front of her. He laughed, as she wiggled and struggled to sit up, only to sink lower onto the sofa.

Seeing the glistening desperation in her eyes, he carefully lifted her up, holding her gently. She pushed herself close to him. *I've missed him, needed him. Two weeks without making love to him has made me hungry. With Brent and D'arcy not expected until at least supper time, maybe I can persuade him to go upstairs. He should rest after his long flight; but I have my own agenda.*

Mark carried her upstairs to their bedroom. Her kisses made him forget all about resting. They hadn't abstained, they couldn't, but Mark had slowed his actions to keep her, and the baby safe, but being apart for so long made them both forget. As their bodies came together, Mark felt the intensity of her body around him.

Being pregnant had increased all of her senses. Just a simple touch from him brought her to the brink of orgasmic pleasure, but making love now always disturbed the baby, causing it to kick and roll inside her belly and bringing their moment of passion to an untimely end. It had become a ritual, after they made love, Mark pulled her into his arms, and together they slowly rubbed her belly, watching it shift and move.

I can tell that she's become a lot bigger, but I don't dare say anything about it, she's self conscious as it is. Every day of her pregnancy has filled me with wonder, to see her body growing with my child. A child created from a perfect, timeless love, but can her body stand the strain? Doc could only guess at her due date, because the size of the baby made it difficult to determine the age.

The baby is taking after me all ready; and I hope, pray, that her body can deliver this baby without any problems. Only time will tell, but I'll be with her, no matter what. The company has suspended tours for the holidays, but I've already told Nick that I wouldn't be back until some time after the baby is born. It doesn't feel right to leave her alone too soon; and I want to spend as much time as I can with both of them.

With Mark now home, the time seemed to speed by. Brent and D'arcy had stayed on as promised, always keeping her company when Mark made little trips into town. They came and went as they pleased, like they were at home, and that made Sabrina very happy, knowing that they were that comfortable here. It put a strain on Jim, having so many people around all the time, but he liked it, even though he didn't show it very often.

Sabrina was awakened suddenly one morning, by the thundering knocks on the bedroom door; it was Brent and D'arcy. "Come on sleepy heads," they called. "It's Christmas and Santa Claus has been." Mark chased them off with his gruff morning voice. He rolled Sabrina over to him and kissed her. "Merry Christmas my love," mark whispered softly as he kissed her cheek and caressed her belly. "Merry Christmas Mark." "Shall we see what Santa left or shall we stay here and spend the whole day in bed together?" "We can't disappoint the guys, or my curiosity," Sabrina smiled, and stretched her arms out to him, to help her up.

She stood beside the bed rubbing her back. It wasn't the usual ache that she had become accustom to over the past few weeks but dismissed it anyway. "Are you feeling all right?" Mark asked. "Oh yeah, my back hurts a little. I must have slept twisted; or." "Or what?" Mark asked. "Maybe it was just too much activity last night." "I'm sorry." "I'm not complaining," she said moving closer to him. He pulled her robe around her, the edges didn't meet anymore and the tie was barely long enough but she still looked good in it. "Shall we join the boys?" Sabrina asked.

Much to her dismay, Mark carried her down the stairs to the living room. Brent and D'arcy stood shoulder to shoulder near the tree, each of them grinning devilishly. "Merry Christmas Sabrina," they said. Promptly stepping aside, they revealed a large rocking chair. "It's from both of us," D'arcy said. "For you and the baby," Brent added. "You guys."

She waddled over to them, giving them each a kiss on the cheek. "It's so beautiful." Running her hands across the glossy finish, she stopped at the carving on the backrest. "What's this?" "We had it personalized," Brent began. "So you can pass it down through your family." Her gaze turned to Mark. "Don't look at me," he said. "I had no idea what so ever. These guys don't tell me everything you know." Mark helped her into her new chair and she began to rock slowly, as she rubbed her belly.

D'arcy sat himself down on the floor next to the tree, his excitement getting the better of him. "Let's see what else Santa brought," he said. "Wait," Sabrina said looking at Mark. "Where is Jim? We can't start without him." "I'll get him," Brent answered. "Just hold off until I get back."

Once Jim was with them, the exchange of gifts began. So many of the presents were for the baby; from the other wrestlers and their families. Sabrina was overwhelmed. She slid to the edge of her seat. Her back ache was much worse. She managed to stand up and stretch to relieve the tension.

Pawing through the branches of the tree, she retrieved a gift that she had hidden away. "This one is for you, Mark." As she handed it to him a strange sensation washed over her, she steadied herself against the rocking chair. As the feeling diminished, the sudden realization hit her. She smiled to herself. "Mark wait; don't open it yet; I have one more very special gift for you."

He stared at her in wonder. *Her face is different, softer and more radiant than I can ever remember.* As he waited for her to continue, he watched her face change. It lost the glow and now reflected pain. She grabbed her belly and leaned forward. "What is it?" Mark asked; panic very evident in his voice. Sabrina gripped his arm. "It would seem that our baby wants to play with his new toys." "What?" he responded, completely missing her meaning. "I'm in labor," she panted as another contraction seized her body.

"I'll call the ambulance," Jim said. "No, Jim, I'm afraid that will take too long. Call Doc, and tell him to hurry." "Why didn't you say something sooner?" "I wasn't sure. I thought it was just a back ache."

Brent scrambled to her side. "Let's get her into the downstairs bedroom." "No way!" Sabrina pulled herself free of his arm. "If our baby is going to be born here, then it's going to be in our bed." "Okay." Mark hugged her as she doubled over. "We need to get you there quick."

Jim had returned from making the phone call. "Doc is on his way." "Good," Sabrina answered. "This baby isn't wasting any time." She looked down at the warm puddle around her feet. "My water just broke." Mark's heart began to race.

The event that I've dreamed of is finally here; but instead of joy, all I feel is uncontrollable panic. I am no longer the master of this situation. Someone much smaller is directing this scene. I have no idea what to do.

"Can you manage or do you want some help?" Brent asked. "What?" Mark stared at him blankly. "Getting her upstairs; do you want some help?" "No, I can manage; I think." He waited until Sabrina's contraction had stopped before he picked her up in his arms. Jim had gone up ahead to prepare the bed. Stripping away the designer sheets, he covered the mattress with plastic and then two layers of soft flannelette. He had just finished when Mark walked in. He left them to wait downstairs for Doc.

Sabrina paced herself as she pulled off her robe. She left her T-shirt on, and Mark helped her into bed. Getting her as close to the middle of the bed as he could, he propped her up against a thick bank of pillows.

The contractions are becoming more intense. I feel so helpless. She's in pain and I can do nothing to ease it for her. All he could think of was sitting beside her, stroking her hair and gently massaging her belly, but even that had no effect for her, as she would push him away when another contraction came.

Doc finally arrived, and immediately dismissed Mark from the room while he examined Sabrina. "This baby is in one hell of a hurry," he said. He was trying to take her mind off of what he was doing. "Must have heard about Jim's famous turkey dinner," Doc chuckled. He finished his exam as another contraction ripped through her body. "Well?" she panted. "Well, you're not gonna miss dinner; in fact, you'll be having company for lunch," he said patting her belly. "I'm gonna get Mark. You just hang in there and remember to breathe properly."

Mark paced frantically in the hallway. Brent and D'arcy stayed near the stairs, well out of his way. Doc came out of the bedroom, greeting Mark with a wide smile. "Well son, are you ready?" "Oh hell Doc, I don't know." "If you don't feel up to it, I can get Jim to help me." "No," Mark said, taking a deep breath. "Sabrina and I are in this together." "Okay then, let's go and meet your baby."

When the bedroom door closed behind them, Brent, D'arcy and Jim sat down on the steps to wait. "Maybe we should call Nick," D'arcy said. "You don't call anyone," Jim scolded. "It's not your place. Mr. Cassidy will make the calls when the baby is born." Brent jumped to his feet, slipping off of the step. "What the hell was that?" Sabrina's cry had caught him off guard, and it chilled him to the bone.

Doc encouraged her to yell. It would help her to focus on delivering the baby, not the pain. "You're doin just great darlin; it won't be long now," Doc encouraged her. Mark wiped the perspiration from her forehead with a cool cloth. When her contractions ended, he would kiss her, and tell her how much he loved her.

Doc draped a sheet across her. He didn't think that Mark was ready to see everything, maybe the next time. He checked her progress and looked over the sheet with a smile. "Are you ready to have a baby?" Doc asked.

Sabrina nodded; Mark squeezed her hand. "Okay then, you follow my instructions exactly and we'll get through this just fine. Now give me a big push when you're ready." The next contraction gave her the urge; relaxing back, exhausted when it had passed.

The pattern continued until Doc told her to stop. He talked to her the entire time, telling her what he was doing and why. "Okay hun, one more time, and give it all you got." Sabrina pushed, the pain was blindingly intense, she cried out, and then suddenly the pain stopped. She lay back, panting hard. Her heart pounded in her ears. Through the hum she heard the cry of a baby. Doc looked over the sheet. "Would you like to meet your son?" he asked.

He placed the baby on her stomach while he cut the cord. Sabrina reached out, touching her son. His cries stopped. "He knows his mother," Mark said. Through the tears, she looked up at Mark. His own eyes were wide and misty; he leaned down and kissed her deeply. "I love you," he whispered.

Doc lifted the baby up and wrapped him in a blanket. "Hey you two," he said with a wide smile. "In case you have forgotten, that behavior is exactly what got you into this in the first place." "I haven't forgotten," she said smiling at Mark. "And I'd do it all over again, just for this one precious moment." Mark kissed her again. "You just rest easy for a few minutes," Doc said. "This little guy needs to have his first bath."

Sabrina laid in Mark's arms, tired and exhausted. Doc was only gone a few minutes it seemed, when he returned with the baby all clean and bundled up. He handed the baby to Mark. "No, I can't," Mark said backing away. "I might break it." "Nonsense! Now hold your son while I get your wife cleaned up."

Doc positioned Mark's arms and laid the baby into them. Frozen with fear, Mark stared at the little face of his son. Sabrina touched him. "Breathe," she said quietly. "What?" Mark exhaled. "That's better. He won't break you know. You can touch him."

She laid back and watched Mark discover his son. His confidence came back slowly. He began to find that he could easily hold the baby with his left arm alone. He parted the blanket and found the tiny hands, so small against his own fingers. His heart was full; their love had created this wonderful miracle.

The baby began to squirm; Mark felt his confidence disappear. "What do I do?" Mark asked a slight hint of panic in his voice. "Hold him close to you and let him feel your heart beating," Doc answered. "I'm just about done and then I'll take him." Doc had moved over to the desk, where he set up a scale and opened a file.

Looking up from the desk, something caught his eye out the window. "Well, I'll be damned," Doc muttered. "What did you say Doc?" "Look at this," he said pulling the curtain aside. "It's snowing. It never snows here." Mark looked down at Sabrina. "Two miracles in one day," he whispered to her. "Come on young man," Doc said, taking the baby from Mark. "You and I have some business to do." He took the baby over to the desk. He had to be weighed, measured and foot printed.

Sabrina wiggled beside Mark. "How are you feeling?" Mark asked. "Good. Could you help me sit up a bit?" she asked. He put his arms under her and carefully lifted her up. "Did we do good?" she asked. "Baby you did fantastic. He's beautiful; just like his mother." He couldn't resist the urge to kiss her again. He had so much love for her that words alone were not enough. "What are we going to name him?" Mark asked. "Well, since it is Christmas, what do you think about Christian Mark Cassidy?" "I like it. Did you get that Doc?" "Sure did," he answered, bringing the baby back to Sabrina. "Well, Doc, what are the stats?" Sabrina asked.

"Well, he's the biggest one I've ever delivered. Eleven pounds, two ounces, and twenty-three and a half inches long." "Ouch," Sabrina winced. "Yes, but you made it look easy darlin. Anyway, I'm all done here. You'll have a few minor contractions for a while, but that's normal. Just take it easy." "How long should she stay in bed Doc?" "Oh she can get up anytime she's ready. Just don't let her take the stairs alone."

Doc picked up his bags and headed for the door. "Merry Christmas all." He opened the door, and saw the three anxious faces in the hallway. "Ready for visitors?" "Sure," Sabrina answered. "Just give us a few minutes; but don't tell them anything." "Okay, I'll stop by in a couple of days. Congratulations you two." Doc closed the door. "Well?" Brent was the first to speak. "They're all fine. Mark will come and get you in a few minutes." "No, what is it?" Brent pressured him. "A baby," Doc said with a smile and walked down the stairs.

Sabrina held the baby up to Mark. "Could you put him in the cradle, and give me your arm?" "Why?" "I'd like to get up." "You shouldn't." "I don't want them to see all this," she said, looking at the blood stained sheets. Mark looked at the squirming bundle in her arms, unsure of what to do.

"Keep one hand under his head and you'll do just fine," she encouraged him. After a couple of attempts, Mark finally picked up the baby. Holding him close, he carried him to the cradle. "See it's not that hard," she smiled at him. "My turn now." She reached out to him.

"You need something else to wear. I'll get you a clean T-shirt." "No, I need something with buttons. Your son is going to get hungry, and I won't be able to feed him if I'm wearing a T-shirt." Mark searched through the closet and brought out one of his old shirts, one that was softened from age and many washings. "Is this okay?" "Perfect. Now could you help me up?"

He stood before her; with his arms around her he lifted her up. She swayed a little and he held her close. "I don't think that this is a good idea." "I'm just a little weak, but it will pass." Mark helped her into the bathroom. He put the chair next to the vanity and eased her down. When she had assured him that she would be all right, he went back to the bedroom and stripped the sheets from the bed. Finding a clean set in the closet, he quickly made up the bed as best he could. Sabrina was standing in the doorway when he turned around.

"What are you doing?" he asked. "Waiting for you." Her legs trembled and Mark caught her as her knees buckled. "I told you," he said picking her up. "You're not going to get out of bed for a while." He set her down upon the bed. "You need to get some sleep." "Yes, but there's two god fathers and a grandpa waiting patiently to see our son." "Fine, but they're not staying very long."

Sabrina settled herself against the pillows as Mark opened the door, inviting the three men in. He stopped them beside the cradle. "Gentlemen, I'd like you to meet our son, Christian Mark Cassidy." "A boy! Congratulations," Brent said, leaning over the cradle. "A fine looking boy Mr. Cassidy," Jim added. "He's gonna be a giant like you man; but at least he's got his mother's good looks," D'arcy added with a smile.

Brent sat down beside Sabrina. "How are you feeling?" "Exhausted, elated." Her tears ran freely. "And very emotional." "Hey now, you're allowed to be. You did good Sabrina. You have a beautiful new son, born on Christmas Day; can't get any better than that."

The baby began to fuss and squeak. Jim picked him up immediately. "Okay you two, time to leave," he said, bringing the baby to Sabrina. "Come on, let her get some rest." Brent leaned over her and kissed her cheek. "Merry Christmas beautiful."

Jim hustled them out of the room, taking the dirty linen with him. Mark took his place on the bed again. "Why is he crying?" Mark asked. "Birth is traumatic, but too he's probably hungry." "Oh! Ah, what do you need?" "Only a pillow."

She laid the baby upon the pillow on her lap, talking softly to him as she opened her shirt. Mark watched in total amazement as she put the baby to her breast, and with little coaxing he began to nurse. Sabrina loosened the blanket, freeing his tiny hands and feet. "Won't he get cold?" "A little, but if he's too warm and cozy he'll go to sleep and not get enough to eat. He's not going to get much for a day or so anyway, until I have enough milk to feed him."

"Amazing. For nine months your body has provided a warm, safe place for him to grow, and now that he's born it provides him with the nourishment he needs." "Come here," she said holding out her hand. Mark eased himself closer to her. He put his arm around her shoulders.

"Does it hurt?" he asked. "A little, but it feels really good. You can be a part of this to you know." "Excuse me!" "Don't look so shocked; all I'm asking is for you to massage my breast; to help bring the milk in." His hand trembled. "It's not like you haven't touched them before. Here like this." She guided his hand; his touch was gentle. "See, you're doing this for your son."

With the baby fed and asleep in his cradle, Sabrina slid down under the blankets. "Stay with me," she said reaching out to Mark. "You need to rest." "I need you to hold me." Mark knew that look all to well. He lay down beside her, bringing her carefully into his arms. "I love you Sabrina. Of all the gifts you could have given me today, this is by far the best of all. We have a son." He kissed her softly. "Thank you."

Sabrina suddenly sat up and with eyes wide with the look of discovery she stared at Mark and smiled. "I think I can give you one more gift," she said. "What?" Mark asked completely confused. "Bring me the calendar from the desk please." Mark did as she asked. She flipped back through the pages stopping at March.

"Oh my God," she gasped. "What is it?" "I think I know when I got pregnant," she said looking up at him with a wide smile. "It was that first night we were together." "Are you sure?" "I think so. It's exactly the right amount of weeks, right to the day." "That was my birthday," Mark said. "I didn't know that then. You never let me know until much later." "Well," he said helping her to lay down. "That is one hell of a gift." "Happy belated birthday." "Thank you, again." "For what?" "For loving me, and for giving me a son, two of the most precious of gifts I could ever receive. My life began the day I met you and now it's complete."

He looked down at her. She was sound asleep, a smile still on her lips. He held her tight for most of the morning and on into the afternoon, until Christian again announced his needs.

After his feeding, and peacefully asleep in the cradle, Mark took Sabrina down stairs. He loudly objected, but she insisted that they all be together for dinner. Jim brought Christian down, along with his cradle, putting him within reach of Sabrina.

Seated at the table, Mark looked around at the bounty before him. *I've been given a gift that has long been only a fantasy. Years of wandering aimlessly through life were gone. I have a future, a direction, a purpose for being here, on this earth, in this time. I have wonderful, caring friends. A house that is now a home, a loving wife and a new baby son at my side, a family.*

No more is this a dream that haunted me night after night. This is real; I can touch it and feel it. Life couldn't be any better than this. I feel stronger than ever before. This is how it is meant to be; a future filled with endless possibilities, and love. Pain and loneliness will never again find their way into this home of perfect love.

About the Author

G I Thompson has many achievements to her credit. With a solid background in business management she is a multitalented woman who rarely backs away from any challenge.

Of all of her accomplishments her first love is still that of writing. For her, writing is a very useful diversion from the stressors of being a single parent of a special needs child.

Her many interests include being a family historian, a small business owner and a motorcycle enthusiast. She is currently working on her second novel, a sequel to *Outside The Ring*.

Printed in the United States
20865LVS00003B/301-306